3D Imaging in Medicine

SECOND EDITION

Edited by

Jayaram K. Udupa, Ph.D.

University of Pennsylvania
Philadelphia, PA

Gabor T. Herman, Ph.D.

University of Pennsylvania
Philadelphia, PA

CRC

CRC Press

Boca Raton London New York Washington, D.C.

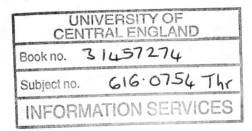

Library of Congress Cataloging-in-Publication Data

Catalog record is available from the Library of Congress.

International Standard Book Number 0-8493-3179-X
Printed in the United States of America 1 2 3 4 5 6 7 8 9 0
Printed on acid-free paper

Preface

Research in three-dimensional (3D) imaging in medicine started in the 1970s. The activity in the field became very brisk in the 1980s. During this period, the technical developments — design of algorithms, software, and machines — have galloped ahead, accompanied by a considerable increase in clinical applications, but clinical validation and the study of clinical usefulness have generally lagged behind. Yet it is the latter aspects that will decide whether or not 3D imaging for medicine will survive and prosper. It is mainly for this reason of fostering acceptance in clinical practice that we organized a meeting entitled Three-Dimensional Imaging in Medicine in December 1987 in Philadelphia. Since prior meetings on medically oriented three-dimensional imaging, such as those sponsored by the Society of Photo-Optical Instrumentation Engineers and by the National Computer Graphics Association, catered mainly to the technical aspects, our second prime reason for the 1987 Philadelphia meeting was to provide a forum for dialogue between the technical developers and the clinical end users. Encouraged by the very positive response to that meeting, we decided to organize further meetings of the same type. We also thought that a compendium of articles from leading clinically oriented researchers on their own areas of expertise, supplemented by a technical tutorial article tailored to non-specialists, would form a useful reference book on 3D imaging for medical researchers and for practicing clinicians, as well as for technical developers. The previous edition of this book was a collection of such articles from the invited speakers of the second meeting on Three-Dimensional Imaging in Medicine held in Coronado, California, November 16 to 19, 1989.

Although the applications that were pursued for 3D imaging in the early 1980s were for imaging the bone via CT, with the advent of MRI in the mid-1980s, soft-tissue 3D imaging became a hot topic. This also initiated research in the better utilization of functional imaging modalities such as PET in conjunction with CT and MRI for a variety of applications. The 1990s saw the re-emergence of CT with the advent of spiral technology, and the rapid acquisition of 3D volume data made possible new 3D imaging applications for CT. The 1990s also witnessed rapid advances in the use of 3D imaging for interventional and surgery procedures. The difficult problem of acquiring image data and processing and analyzing them for studying dynamic organs also continued to be pursued with steady progress.

Keeping in mind the developments that took place during the years since the first edition of the book was prepared, we have rewritten this book entirely. The chapter by Udupa (Chapter 1) gives a comprehensive tutorial overview of the 3D imaging principles and algorithms with numerous practical medical examples. Chapter 2 (Zonneveld) gives a comprehensive review of the use of 3D imaging operations in a variety of areas of clinical research and practice with ample examples. Chapter 3 (Herman) reviews efforts in quantification of object information contained in medical images with several detailed examples taken from particular applications. Chapter 4 (Vannier) gives an overview of the methods required for evaluating the usefulness of 3D imaging with illustrative examples. Chapter 5 (Lavallée et al.) describes the various strategies and approaches currently taken in utilizing 3D and other imagery in assisting surgery and therapy. Chapter 6 (Kalender and Prokop) reviews the progress made in spiral CT technology and its ramifications for 3D imaging. Chapter 7 (Pelizzari and Chen) describes the use, requirements, and shortcomings of 3D imaging for radiation treatment planning. In Chapter 8, Fishman and Kuszyk describe several orthopedic applications that utilize their volume rendering technique. The last chapter, by Hirsch et al., describes how 3D imaging can be utilized for the kinematic analysis of joints, concentrating on the tarsal joints of the foot.

As with any new discipline, 3D imaging is not without its controversies. The views expressed in this book by the individual chapter authors are their own; they do not necessarily agree with those of the editors. While we provided all contributors with our editorial comments, we felt that we should leave them to the final decision of what to include in their chapters. Thus we present the state of the art: diverse and vibrant.

Finally, we would like to express our sincere gratitude to all chapter authors for their contributions and to the staff of CRC Press for their cooperation.

J.K. Udupa
G.T. Herman

Editors

Jayaram K. Udupa received a B.Eng. degree in Electronics and Communication from Mysore University, Malnad College of Engineering at Hassan, India, in 1972 and a Ph.D. in Computer Science from the Indian Institute of Science, Bangalore, in 1976. After working briefly at this institute, he joined the Medical Image Processing Group at the State University of New York, Buffalo, as a postdoctoral fellow. He subsequently moved to the University of Pennsylvania with this group in 1981 and became the director of the group in 1982. Since 1991, Dr. Udupa has been the Chief of the Medical Imaging Section in the Department of Radiology, where he has been a Professor of Radiology since 1994.

Dr. Udupa has made numerous seminal contributions in 3D imaging, image processing, graphics, visualization, and their medical applications. Many of these have initiated new areas of research and applications and have been widely used. He spearheaded the early transfer of 3D imaging algorithms into the medical imaging industry via software development and dissemination. He continued recently the public dissemination of his methods and algorithms through an extensive software system called 3DVIEWNIX, which was designed by him, developed by his team, and widely distributed worldwide. This was named one of the top 10 visualization software systems of 1993 by the journal *IEEE Computer Graphics and Applications*. He is on the editorial board of *IEEE Transactions on Biomedical Engineering* and *Computerized Medical Imaging and Graphics*.

Gabor T. Herman received the M.Sc. degree in Mathematics from the University of London, England in 1964, the M.S. degree in Engineering Science from the University of California, Berkeley, in 1966, and the Ph.D. degree in mathematics from the University of London, England, in 1968. From 1969 to 1981 he was with the Department of Computer Science, State University of New York at Buffalo, where in 1976 he became the Director of the Medical Image Processing Group. Since 1981 Dr. Herman has been a Professor in the Medical Imaging Section of the Department of Radiology at the University of Pennsylvania. He is involved editorially with a number of journals; in particular, he was for a while the Editor-in-Chief of the *IEEE Transactions on Medical Imaging*. He is the author or editor of numerous books on medical imaging and related topics, including *Image Reconstruction from Projections: The Fundamentals of Computerized Tomography,* published by Academic Press in 1980, and *Geometry of Digital Spaces,* published by Birkhauser in 1998.

Dr. Herman has been an influential pioneer in 3D imaging in medicine; each of the following papers of his have been cited in the research literature over a hundred times: Three-dimensional display of human organs from computed tomograms. *Computer Graphics and Image Processing,* 1979; The theory, design, implementation and evaluation of a three-dimensional surface detection algorithm. *Computer Graphics and Image Processing,* 1981; Three-dimensional reconstruction of craniofacial deformity using computed tomography. *Neurosurgery,* 1983; Analysis of brain and cerebrospinal fluid volumes with MR imaging. Part 1: Methods reliability, and validation. *Radiology,* 1991. He is the recipient of many honors; in particular, he was made an honorary member of the American Society of Neuroimaging and received honorary doctorates from the University of Linkoping, Sweden, and the University of Szeged, Hungary.

Contributors

Eric Bainville
TIMC Laboratory
Grenoble University Hospital
La Tronche, France

Ivan Bricault
TIMC Laboratory
Grenoble University Hospital
La Tronche, France

George T.Y. Chen
Department of Radiation and Cellular Oncology
The University of Chicago
Chicago, Illinois

Elliot K. Fishman
Department of Radiology
Johns Hopkins University Hospital
Baltimore, Maryland

Bruce Elliot Hirsch
Department of Anatomy and Cell Biology
Temple University School of Medicine
Philadelphia, Pennsylvania

Willi A. Kalender
Institute for Medical Physics
Friedrich Alexander University
Erlangen, Germany

Brian Kuszyk
Department of Radiology
Johns Hopkins University Hospital
Baltimore, Maryland

Stéphane Lavallée
TIMC Laboratory
Grenoble University Hospital
La Tronche, France

Charles A. Pelizzari
Department of Radiation and Cellular Oncology
The University of Chicago
Chicago, Illinois

Mathias Prokop
Institute for Medical Physics
Friedrich Alexander University
Erlangen, Germany

Eric Stindel
Service d'Orthopédie et Traumatologie
Laboratoire d'Anatomie
Hospital de la Cavale Blanche
Brest, France

Michael W. Vannier
Department of Radiology
University of Iowa College of Medicine
Iowa City, Iowa

Frans W. Zonneveld
Department of Radiology
Utrecht University Hospital
Utrecht, The Netherlands

Contents

1 3D Imaging: Principles and Approaches

Jayaram K. Udupa

CONTENTS

0-8493-3179-X/00/$0.00+$.50

1.1 INTRODUCTION

1.1.1 Scope

The main purpose of this chapter is to give an overview of the current status of the science of 3D imaging. Loosely, *3D imaging* here refers to all processing operations that are applied to acquired multidimensional image data to facilitate visualization, manipulation, and analysis of the information captured in the image data. The chapter will also identify the major challenges currently faced and point out the opportunities available for advancing the science of 3D imaging.

This chapter covers all commonly used 3D imaging operations. It will delineate the main concepts and algorithms without detailing the underlying theory. Although most of the techniques described here are applicable in areas other than medicine, such as microscopy,[1] industrial inspection,[2] geoscience,[3] meteorology,[4] and fluid mechanics,[5] all examples are drawn from medical applications, particularly from those in which we are currently engaged. The description will also attempt to clarify some common misconceptions.

The target audience is developers of 3D imaging methods and systems, developers of 3D imaging applications, and clinicians using 3D imaging methods and systems. The description will assume some familiarity with medical imaging modalities and some knowledge of rudimentary concepts related to digital images.

1.1.2 Background

The purpose of 3D imaging is:

> *given* a set of multidimensional images pertaining to an object/object system,
> *to output* qualitative/quantitative information about the object/object system under study.

1.1.2.1 Sources of Images

There are several sources of digital multidimensional images, in medical imaging, as indicated below:

> *2D:* A digital radiograph, a tomographic slice from a data set from computerized tomography (CT), magnetic resonance imaging (MRI), positron emission tomography (PET), single-photon emission computed tomography (SPECT), ultrasound (US), functional MRI (fMRI), magnetic source imaging, and surface light scanning.
>
> *3D:* A time sequence of radiographic images or tomographic slice images of a dynamic object, a volume of tomographic slice images of a static object.
>
> *4D:* A time sequence of tomographic volume images of a dynamic object.
>
> *5D:* A time sequence of tomographic volume images of a dynamic object for each of a range of values of an imaging parameter (e.g., MR spectroscopic images of a heart).

It is not feasible at present to acquire 4D images to truly capture dynamics. Hence, various approximations are made to capture "stop-action" or "gated" images. 5D images cannot be acquired in a routine fashion with adequate resolution, and hence are not practically feasible at present. Higher dimensional images can also be generated computationally, as we will indicate at appropriate points in the description of the various processing operations.

Among tomographic modalities, CT, MRI, and US provide structural/anatomical information. They do so by measuring within each elemental volume, tissue-differentiating properties, such as X-ray attenuation (in CT), various relaxation times upon magnetically exciting the tissues (in MRI), and acoustic impedance (in US). Other modalities, namely PET, SPECT, and fMRI, as well as doppler US provide information about function (rather than structure) of objects including fluid flow, perfusion, and diffusion. See Ref. 6 for a description of some of the common medical imaging modalities.

Given a set of multidimensional images, possibly acquired from different modalities, but pertaining to a given object system, the aim of 3D imaging is to extract certain qualitative and/or quantitative information relating to the object system.

1.1.2.2 Objects of Study

Here, an *object* refers to any physical object such as an anatomical organ or a prosthetic device, or a pathological entity such as a tumor, or a conceptual entity such as an isodose surface in a radiation treatment plan, or an activity region in a functional image provided by a modality such as PET, SPECT, and fMRI. An *object system* refers to simply a collection of physical or conceptual objects. The objects encountered may be rigid (e.g., bones), deformable (e.g., soft-tissue structures), static (e.g., skull), or dynamic (e.g., heart, joints). In most applications, the object system of study consists of a few static objects. For example, an MRI 3D study of a patient's head may focus on three 3D objects: the white matter, the gray matter, and the cerebrospinal fluid.

The qualitative information that is sought via 3D imaging is usually visual in nature. Hence, for this purpose, how to extract and display such information for human visualization become the predominant issues. The quantitative information that is sought via 3D imaging usually pertains to the morphology of the object/object system or its function. Toward this goal, therefore, the extraction of such information from images is the main issue to be tackled.

1.1.2.3 References

Most background material on 3D imaging is scattered in archival journals and conference proceedings. Several edited books, particularly for medical applications, have been published.[7–9] Books on specialized applications[10] and on scientific visualization[11,12] also cover some material relevant to medical 3D imaging and applications. The proceedings of the following conferences also contain useful related information: Visualization in Biomedical Computing,[13–16] the annual Image Display and Image Processing conferences sponsored by the Society of Photo-Optical Instrumentation Engineers, Bellingham, Washington (proceedings also published by the sponsor), and MRCAS: Medical Robotics and Computer Assisted Surgery. Perhaps the best opportunity to gather information about available 3D imaging products is at the annual convention of the Radiological Society of North America, usually held in Chicago, Illinois.

1.1.3 Classification

1.1.3.1 Operations

3D imaging operations may be broadly classified into the following four groups:

Preprocessing: The operations under this group are aimed at defining the object system. The input is a set of multidimensional images, and the output is a set of multidimensional images or a computer representation of an object system.

Visualization: The emphasis of these operations is on viewing and comprehending the structure and dynamics of the object system. The input is a set of multidimensional images and/or a computer representation of an object system, and the output is a set of pictures depicting the multidimensional structure and function of the object system.

Manipulation: These operations are for virtually altering the individual objects or the relationship among objects in the object system, as in a virtual surgery operation. The input is a computer representation of an object system and the outcome is a computer representation of the virtually altered object system.

Analysis: The aim of these operations is to quantify morphological/functional information about the object system. The input is a set of multidimensional images and the output is a set of quantitative measures.

The four groups of operations are highly interdependent. For instance, some form of visualization is essential to facilitate most operations in the other three groups. Similarly, object definition through an appropriate set of preprocessing operations is vital to the effective visualization, manipulation, and analysis of the object system.

1.1.3.2 Viewing Medium

Since visualization is an integral component of 3D imaging, a viewing medium is essential for any system that supports 3D imaging operations. Three types of media are currently being used and investigated: computer monitor, holography, and head-mounted display.

The video display unit of computer workstations is the most commonly used viewing medium. Unlike the 2D nature of this device, holography offers a 3D medium.[17] However, the long processing

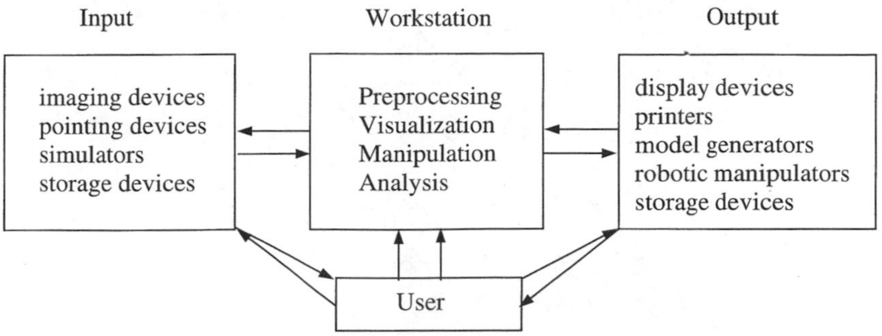

FIGURE 1.1 A schematic representation of 3D imaging systems.

time and the cost associated with creating holograms and the lack of human intractability with image data are the major hurdles for the effective use of this medium. Head-mounted displays[18,19] consist basically of two tiny monitors presented in front of the two eyes through a helmet-like device that is worn over the head. The display offers the sensation of being free from our natural surrounding and immersed in an artificial environment provided by the data being displayed. Through appropriately creating renditions of the object system and displaying them on the two monitors, it is possible to create a visual sensation of being inside the object system. By far, however, the video computer monitor is the most desirable medium at present because of its flexibility, low cost, speed of interaction, and resolution over other media. Stereoscopic viewing on these monitors is possible through appropriate hardware and software enhancements. However, this facility is not utilized commonly in actual applications.

1.1.3.3 Systems

A generic representation of 3D imaging systems is shown in Figure 1.1. A workstation with appropriate software implementing the four groups of 3D imaging operations forms the core of the system. Human interaction is an essential component of the system. Depending on the application, a wide variety of input/output devices are utilized.

Common input devices include storage and graphic pointing devices. In intra-operative situations, imaging devices may directly and continuously provide input data during the operation in real time.[20] More sophisticated pointing and navigational devices are often used whose position relative to the object system of interest is continuously tracked using optical/magnetic position sensing devices. These are often used in interventional/intra-operative situations.[21] Common output devices include hard-copy printers, high-resolution/stereoscopic/special-purpose monitors, and storage devices. More sophisticated and specialized devices include model generators and robotic manipulators. The former are used in creating physical models of objects from their computer representations. The latter are used in assisting surgeons and interventionalists in invasive treatment procedures. (See Chapter 5 for details.) Considering the core of the system (independent of input/output), the following categorization of 3D imaging systems can be made:

- Physician display consoles provided by imaging device (scanner) vendors.
- Image processing/visualization workstations supplied by workstation vendors.
- 3D imaging software supplied by software vendors independent of workstations.
- University-based 3D imaging software often freely available via the Internet.

Systems provided by scanner manufacturers and workstation vendors usually have a strong application focus and may cost \$50,000 to \$150,000. These systems often depend on specialized hardware engines to achieve interactive speed for 3D imaging operations. On the other extreme,

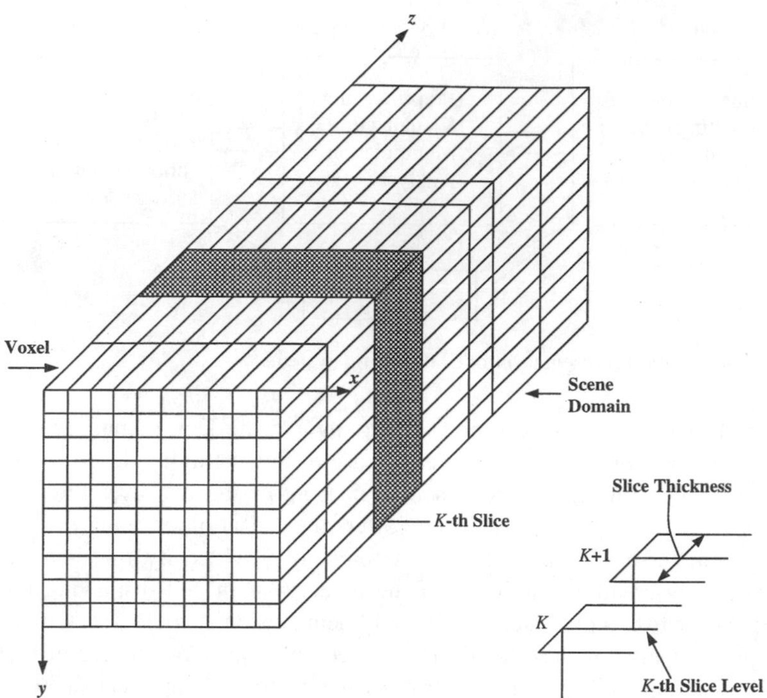

FIGURE 1.2 Illustration used for the definition of basic terms. The slice location and thickness for the K-th and (K+1)th slice here are so chosen that they do not overlap, or abut. As we increase the thickness for both slices, they first abut and then overlap.

general-purpose, platform-independent software systems are available that do not have application-specific focus but that provide the same speed as or better than that of specialized hardware devices when configured even on PCs such as a 300-MHz Pentium.[22] Since such software systems are available either freely or for a nominal fee, if the user has the know-how to install and configure such software on an appropriate platform (such as a Pentium), a system comparable in performance to that of the costly devices mentioned above can be set up for under $5000. In between these two extremes, commercial software packages with application focus are also available for various platforms. Their cost falls in between the extremes indicated above. The speed of processing varies considerably.

All examples of processing operations illustrated in this chapter are produced using a software system called 3DVIEWNIX.[23] The executable binary codes for this software system for several platforms are freely available via the Internet at http://www.mipg.upenn.edu. The reader is encouraged to use the system to gain practical processing experience while learning the concepts presented in this chapter. We will point to particular 3DVIEWNIX commands to help the reader in experimenting with various processing operations as the operations are described in various sections.

1.1.4 Basics and Terminology

For brevity and later reference, some terms that are used throughout this chapter are defined in this section. (See Figures 1.2 and 1.3.) Although many of the (especially preprocessing) operations are applicable to image data of dimensionality greater than three, our description will focus in detail only on the 3D case but will indicate briefly the higher dimensional generalizations where appropriate.

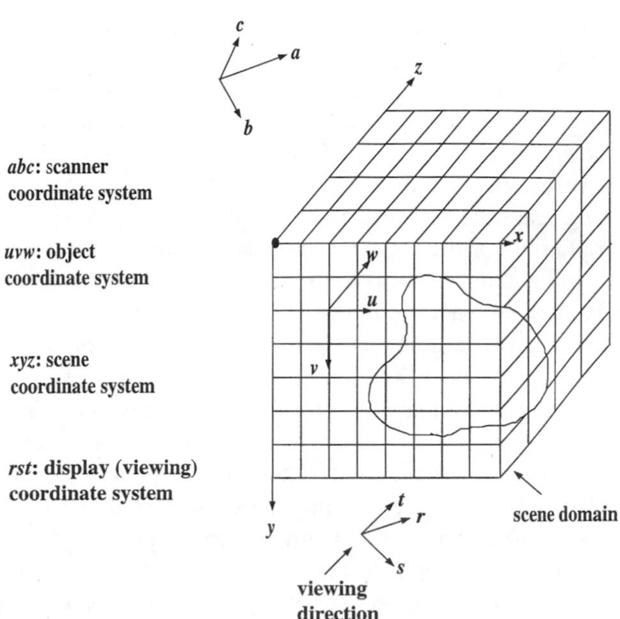

FIGURE 1.3 Definition of the coordinate systems associated with the imaging device, scene, structure, and display (viewing).

Object: The original physical object of study. This may be a particular organ within a live/dead human body, a human-made physical object (a prosthetic device or a phantom created for carrying out scientific experiments), a purely mathematically described geometric object such as a mathematical phantom, regions within a live human organ that are "activated" by some physiological or other processes, or pathological entities such as a lesion or a tumor within a human body.

Object system: Simply a collection of objects. In a brain study of a patient, for example, the object system may consist of three objects — the white matter, gray matter, and the cerebrospinal fluid (CSF). The objects in the system may be of mixed types; for example, the collection consisting of a dynamic organ, a mathematical phantom simulating a static organ, and a prosthetic device. For fulfilling most 3D imaging objectives, it is necessary that the objects in the object system have the proper (spatial) relationship.

Body region: A finite region of the 3D space within which the object system of study is embedded. For anatomical entities, the meaning of this term is obvious. For other objects, body region represents the mathematical or physical space within which the objects are embedded.

Imaging device: Any device or computational/simulation process that produces a digital image of the body region with its object contents. Tomographic scanners and software systems[24] that enable simulating objects and their tomographic reconstructions are examples of imaging devices.

Pixel, voxel: For a variety of reasons and to facilitate processing by a digital computer, images of the body region must be acquired in a digital form. This means that the body region is virtually partitioned into small abutting cuboidal volume elements and the imaging device estimates an aggregate of property of the material within each such element. The volume elements are usually abbreviated as voxels. The 2D analog of a voxel is a pixel (abbreviation for picture element). For higher dimensional spaces, we retain the term voxel to denote a higher dimensional volume element.

Scene, scene domain, intensity, binary scene: Scene is a short name for a digital image. A 3D scene of a body region is a 3D rectangular array of voxels together with a value assigned to each voxel in the array. The rectangular array represents a digitization of the body region in terms of voxels. Since the body region may not be of cuboidal shape, extra voxels are added to yield a rectangular array. We represent any scene $\mathcal{V}$ by a pair (V,g), where V is a rectangular array of voxels and is referred to as the domain of $\mathcal{V}$, and for any voxel v in V, $g(v)$ represents the aggregate value, called the intensity of v in $\mathcal{V}$, estimated by the imaging device for the material in v. For the same reasons that the body region is virtually digitized, the intensity values estimated for the voxels are also discretized into (positive) integer numbers. The voxels used for padding are usually assigned the value 0. A scene in which any voxel has the intensity value either 0 or 1 is called a binary scene.

K-th slice, pixel size, slice thickness, slice location, slice spacing: Typically, imaging devices acquire data in such a fashion that two fixed sides of all voxels have identical length and the remaining side is several times larger than the other two. Usually the third direction in the array is considered to be the direction of largest voxel side. In an $L \times M \times N$ scene $\mathcal{V}$ (meaning a scene with $L \times M \times N$ scene domain), the subscene defined by the set of all voxels with indices (i,j,K) in the array for all i and j from 1 to L and 1 to M, respectively, and for a fixed K between 1 and N, together with the voxel intensities in $\mathcal{V}$ is called the K-th slice of $\mathcal{V}$. Note that the lengths of the largest side of voxels may not be equal in different slices (see Figure 1.2). The length of the equal sides is called the pixel size of $\mathcal{V}$. When acquisitions are isotropic (i.e., all sides of all voxels are of identical length), the directions and hence the meaning of a slice are determined by the imaging device operator.

In slice-by-slice data acquisition, imaging devices collect data from a "slab" within the body region to determine the K-th slice of $\mathcal{V}$. The thickness of this slab is called K-th slice thickness, and the location of a plane passing through the center of the slab is referred to as K-th slice location (see Figure 1.2). The spacing between any two slices is simply the difference in their locations. The slice thickness within a scene is usually fixed; however, the spacing between successive slices (which actually determines the length of the voxels in the third direction) may not be fixed in a scene. Slice thickness is usually ignored by most 3D imaging operations.

Structure, structure system: A computer representation of an object/object system. For real physical objects/object systems, this representation is arrived at from a scene of the body region containing the object/object system. Because of the finiteness of precision of the various computational processes of the imaging device and of the 3D imaging system, and because of heterogeneity of object material properties and their variation from subject (patient) to subject, the process of arriving at this representation with high (acceptable) reproducibility, accuracy, and efficiency remains the greatest challenge in 3D imaging.

Rendition of a scene/structure/structure system: A 2D rectangular array of pixels, together with a gray/color value assigned to every pixel, that portrays some aspect of the object information captured in the scene/structure/structure system. Usually, in a gray rendition, every pixel in the rendition has a single (positive) integer gray value associated with it, and in a color rendition, three (positive) integer values are associated with it representing the red, green, and blue components of color.

Imaging device coordinate system: An origin together with an orthogonal axes system affixed to the imaging device.

Scene coordinate system: An origin plus an orthogonal axes system affixed to the scene (see Figure 1.3). The origin is assumed to be at a corner of the first voxel in the scene and the axes are assumed to be parallel to the edges of the voxels. Knowing the location and orientation of the scene coordinate system with respect to the imaging device coordinate system is helpful in some 3D imaging operations; because of this, many imaging devices automatically store this information in the file containing the scene.

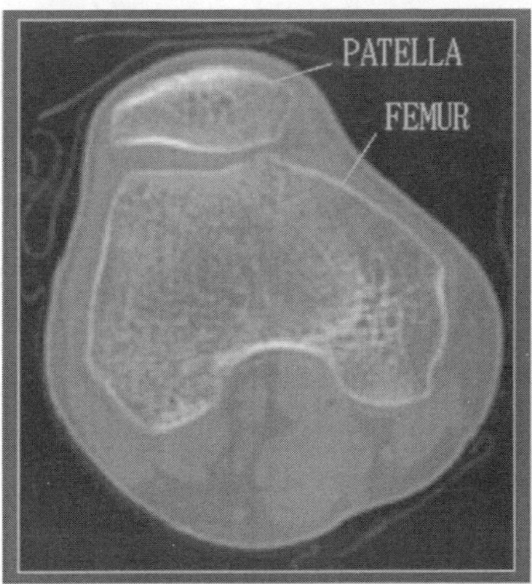

FIGURE 1.4 Illustration of graded composition and hanging-togetherness of voxels in scenes. Voxels constituting the femur have a gradation of density values. In spite of this, they hang together to form the femur.

Structure coordinate system: An origin plus an orthogonal axes system affixed to the structure/structure system. Knowledge of the location and orientation of this coordinate system with respect to the imaging device coordinate system is useful in some 3D imaging operations; thus, some 3D imaging systems keep track of this information in the file storing the structure/structure system.

Display (viewing) coordinate system: An origin plus an orthogonal axes system affixed to the viewing plane. A knowledge of the location and orientation of this coordinate system with respect to the imaging device is useful in some 3D imaging operations; as such, some 3D imaging systems keep a record of this information in the file storing the renditions.

1.1.5 Object Characteristics in Images

Any scene of any body region displays two important characteristics of the objects contained in the body region. Appropriate handling of these characteristics is vital to the effectiveness of all 3D imaging operations. These are described below with an example — a slice of a CT scene of a human knee. The objects of interest in the body region (knee) are the two bones that appear in the slice — the femur and the patella, displayed in Figure 1.4.

1.1.5.1 Graded Composition

Objects in any body region have a heterogeneous material composition. In the example under consideration, both objects are composed of hard (cortical), soft (cancellous), and intermediate type bone tissue. In addition to this, imaging devices blur object information captured in scenes due to various approximations. Thus, even if an object is composed of perfectly homogeneous material (such physical objects may be very difficult to create, but they can be created mathematically), the scene of its body region will invariably display a heterogeneous intensity. We refer to this property as graded composition of object information in scenes.

1.1.5.2 Hanging-Togetherness (Gestalt)

In spite of the graded composition, human viewers usually perceive objects as distinct in a display of the scene such as that shown in Figure 1.4. The fact that there are voxels in the femur and the patella that have identical intensity values which are similar to the intensity values of some of the voxels in other objects in the body region such as muscles, does not interfere with the viewers' ability to form a mental grouping of the voxels into objects — a phenomenon referred to as "Gestalt" in psychopictorics.[25] Devising precise, accurate, and efficient computational methods that can identify these groupings in scenes is essential for fulfilling most 3D imaging goals. We refer to this grouping property as hanging-togetherness. Note that voxels in the cancellous part of the femur should hang together more strongly with voxels in the cortical part than with voxels in the cancellous part of the patella. Although for ease of illustration we have given a 2D example in Figure 1.3, hanging-togetherness is a property that is applicable in the 3D space to 3D objects (and in higher/lower dimensional spaces for higher/lower dimensional objects).

In the remaining sections of this chapter, we will describe preprocessing and visualization operations in considerable detail, followed by a brief outline of manipulation and analysis operations. In the final section, we will identify some of the main existing challenges faced in 3D imaging.

1.2 PREPROCESSING

1.2.1 Overview

The purpose of preprocessing operations is, given a set of scenes of a body region, to output a structure/structure system corresponding to the objects in the body region or another set of scenes which facilitate structure definition.

The commonly used preprocessing operations may be classified under the following five groups:

Volume of interest: Converts a given scene to another scene by reducing the size of the scene domain and/or the intensity range for the purpose of minimizing the storage space requirement.

Filtering: Converts a given scene to another scene by suppressing unwanted information and/or enhancing wanted information.

Interpolation: Converts a given scene to another scene of a specified level of discretization.

Registration: Converts a given scene/structure to another scene/structure by matching it with another given scene/structure. The aim here is to combine information about the same body region from multiple sources.

Segmentation: Converts a given set of scenes to a structure/structure system.

1.2.2 Volume of Interest (VOI)

Often the object of study occupies only a small portion of the scene domain. The volume of interest operation allows us to create another scene whose domain is again a cuboid which encloses information about all aspects of interest of the object of study but as little as possible of irrelevant objects (Figure 1.5). The main purpose of the VOI operation is to minimize the computer storage space required for further processing of the scene. As an example, a $512 \times 512 \times 64$ scene contains more than 16.5 million voxels. If the region occupied by the object of interest is $200 \times 200 \times 64$, then the number of voxels — about 2.5 million — is nearly seven times less than that for the whole body region. Another reason for the VOI operation may be to exclude a part of an organ and to image the remainder so as to reveal its interior. For example, if we wish to create a 3D display of a part of the spinal column of a subject revealing the spinal canal, then we specify a rectangle of fixed size and location on all slices of the scene such that only half of the spinal vertebra falls inside the rectangle. By specifying a fixed rectangle in this fashion and a subset of slices in the given scene, we have essentially indicated the scene domain for the output scene. Creation of the output scene consists of just collecting all voxels (along with their intensity) that fall inside the rectangle in each slice of the set. For higher dimensional scenes, the extent of the output scene domain in each direction should be specified.

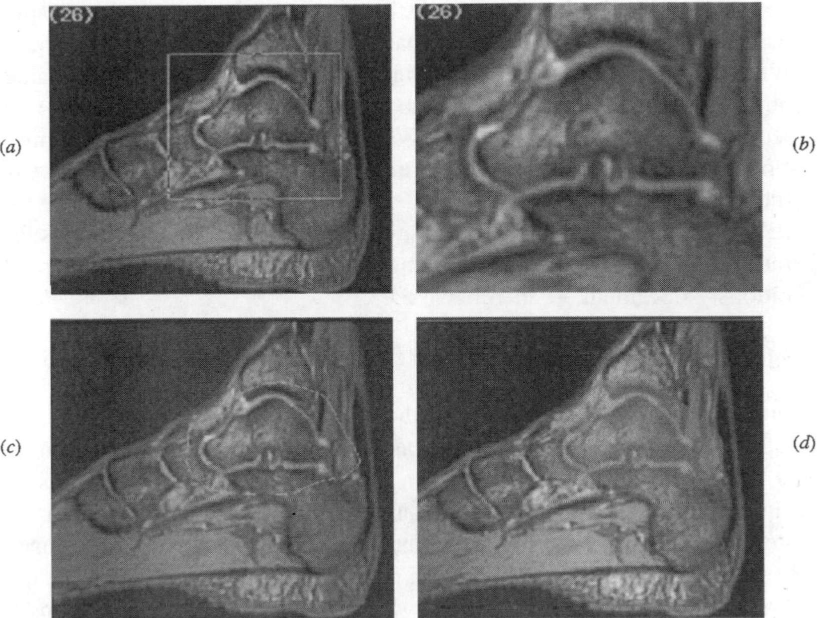

FIGURE 1.5 A region of interest specified by a rectangular box in the scene (a). The output scene is shown in (b). Regions of arbitrary shape are indicated by drawing (c) and painting (d).

A somewhat more sophisticated VOI operation[26] is to specify a polyhedron instead of a cuboid (of course, the scene domain of the output scene should still be a cuboid). A simple way of doing this is to specify two rectangles, one on the first of a set of slices and the other on the last slice. The polyhedron is defined by joining the corresponding vertices of the two rectangles, which of course may have different locations and sizes. This operation gives the effect of cutting by oblique planes (planes not orthogonal to the *xy* plane of the scene coordinate system), which is often useful in the spinal canal example given above. To compute the output scene, we simply have to collect all voxels that fall inside the polyhedron and then appropriately pad the exterior region with just enough voxels to create a cuboid scene domain.

A still more sophisticated VOI operation is to specify regions of arbitrary shape. One approach to this[27] is to indicate on each slice displayed on the screen a region by drawing closed curves or by "painting" using "brushes" of various size and shape (see Figure 1.5). In the output scene, the voxels belonging to such regions are assigned their respective intensities in the input scene, and voxels lying outside this region but inside a cuboid scene domain are assigned a fixed intensity value, usually 0. Such operations become indispensable in many situations, not for storage reasons, but because structure extraction from scenes would otherwise be impossible. An example is the visualization of the articular surfaces of a joint for which scene data are acquired via MRI. It is very difficult to identify the individual bony components by automatic methods because bony components and other structures such as tendons and ligaments that generate feable MR signals are very close together. Instead of indicating a structure by precise drawing/painting of its boundary/region, it is often possible to specify a VOI more loosely. By indicating a region that contains information about the object of interest but that excludes information about other objects of similar image property, it is often possible to subsequently extract structures within the VOI automatically. For example, in an MR scene of the head of a patient, automatic extraction of the brain and its component tissues (gray and white matter) is often greatly facilitated if the scalp and other regions outside the brain are excluded from the VOI.

VOI may appear to be a trivial operation. In large applications requiring the routine processing of a large number of scenes, devising an effective VOI (even of the rectangular box type) can save considerable storage space and human operator time by making subsequent operations faster and more effective. This underscores the need for making this operation automatic especially in large applications. While this is feasible if we are dealing with scenes pertaining to the same body region in different subjects, it is clear that an ability to define structures (even roughly) will be useful, and perhaps necessary, to completely automate VOI. We will see a similar dilemma in all preprocessing operations; namely, the need for structure definition (segmentation) to make the operations optimally effective.

The 3DVIEWNIX command that supports the rectangular box VOI operation is PREPROCESS → SceneOperations → VOI. The manual drawing and painting is provided under PREPROCESS → SceneOperations → Segment → Interactive2D.

1.2.3 Filtering

These operations convert a given scene into another scene. Their aim is to enhance wanted (object) information and to suppress unwanted (noise, background) information in the output scene. The output scene $\mathcal{V}_o = (V_o, g_o)$ created by filtering an input scene $\mathcal{V}_i = (V_i, g_i)$has the same domain as that of the input scene (i.e., $V_o = V_i$), but their intensities may be different. The main idea behind most scene filtering operations is to assign an intensity value to a voxel v in V_o usually based on the intensities of voxels in a small neighborhood of v in V_i. Depending on how the intensity values are used and how the neighborhood is defined, we get different filtering operations.

Filtering operations may be classified into two groups: enhancing, wherein wanted information is enhanced hopefully without affecting unwanted information, and suppressing, wherein unwanted information is suppressed hopefully without affecting wanted information.

1.2.3.1 Enhancing

In enhancement (also known as high-pass filtering), the idea is to emphasize edges in the scene. Clearly, since edges appear where there are significant differences in intensity, to enhance edges we simply have to compute differences of intensities of neighboring voxels. We can get different types of effects depending on how the differences and the neighborhood are defined. Figure 1.6 illustrates some commonly used neighborhoods. (Neighborhood definitions are also needed in other 3D imaging operations, as we will see at various points in our discussion.) We give two examples of this type of filter:

(i) Using the neighborhood of Figure 1.6a:

$$g_o(v_0) = \left| \frac{w_2 g_i(v_2) + w_1 g_i(v_1) + w_8 g_i(v_8)}{w_2 + w_1 + w_8} - \frac{w_4 g_i(v_4) + w_5 g_i(v_5) + w_6 g_i(v_6)}{w_4 + w_5 + w_6} \right| + \left| \frac{w_6 g_i(v_6) + w_7 g_i(v_7) + w_8 g_i(v_8)}{w_6 + w_7 + w_8} - \frac{w_2 g_i(v_2) + w_3 g_i(v_3) + w_4 g_i(v_4)}{w_2 + w_3 + w_4} \right|. \tag{1.1}$$

(ii) Using the neighborhood of Figure 1.6b:

$$g_o(v_0) = \frac{w_1 |g_i(v_1) - g_i(v_3)| + w_2 |g_i(v_4) - g_i(v_2)| + w_3 |g_i(v_6) - g_i(v_5)|}{w_1 + w_2 + w_3}. \tag{1.2}$$

In these equations, $|x|$ represents the absolute value of x, and the weights are positive numbers. Figure 1.7 illustrates the enhancing filter of Equation (1.1) with $w_1 = w_3 = w_5 = w_7 = 2$ and $w_2 =$

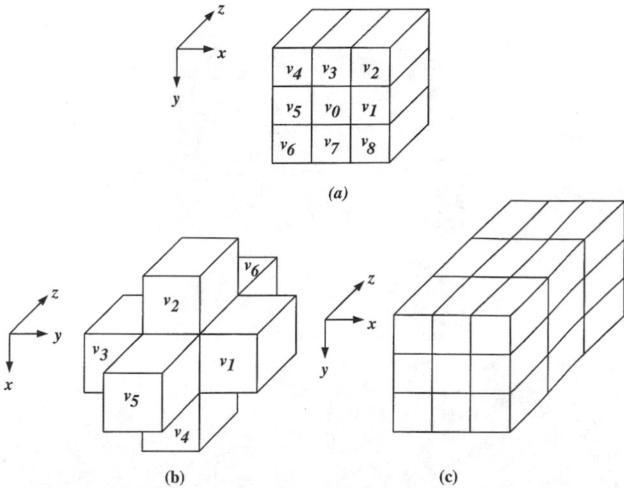

FIGURE 1.6 Neighborhood definition for the filtering operation. (a) Neighboring voxels are defined in the same slice. (b) Neighboring voxels (total of six) share a face with the voxel v_0, which is in the center. (c) The total number of neighboring voxels is 26, and v_0 is in the center.

$w_4 = w_6 = w_8 = 1$, which is known as the Sobel operator, applied to a slice of an MR scene of a patient's head. It also shows the 3D version of this filter applied to the same slice. Note that the 3D filter in this instance enhances the edges more strongly than the 2D version. It is readily seen that the voxel intensity $g_o(v)$ in the output scene is simply the sum of the differences of input intensities in the vicinity of v along the principal directions. It represents an estimate of the spatial rate of change of voxel intensity at v_0; in other words, the magnitude of the mathematical gradient of g_i at v_0, denoted $|\nabla g_i(v_0)|$. How to devise effective digital approximations of the gradient operator is an intensely researched topic in image processing.[28] The gradient is a vector whose direction indicates the direction in which scene intensity increases most rapidly at v. Using the neighborhood of Figure 1.6b, one commonly used approximation for this vector is

$$\nabla g_i(v_0) = \left(g_i(v_1) - g_i(v_3), g_i(v_4) - g_i(v_2), g_i(v_6) - g_i(v_5)\right). \tag{1.3}$$

Gradient operators are used in locating object boundaries (discussed later) as well as in finding ridges and crest lines in object surfaces.[29]

1.2.3.2 Suppressing

If we assign to v a weighted (with positive weights) average of the intensities of the voxels in the neighborhood of v, then the local variations are averaged or smoothed. Hence, after the whole scene is filtered this way, if we display the same slice from the input and the output scene side by side, the latter appears smoother than the former. Thus, in this filtering operation (commonly known as low-pass filtering), the intensity $g_o(v_0)$ assigned to a voxel v_0 in the output scene is given by

$$g_o(v_0) = \frac{\sum_{j=0}^{n} w_j g_i(v_j)}{\sum_{j=0}^{n} w_j} \tag{1.4}$$

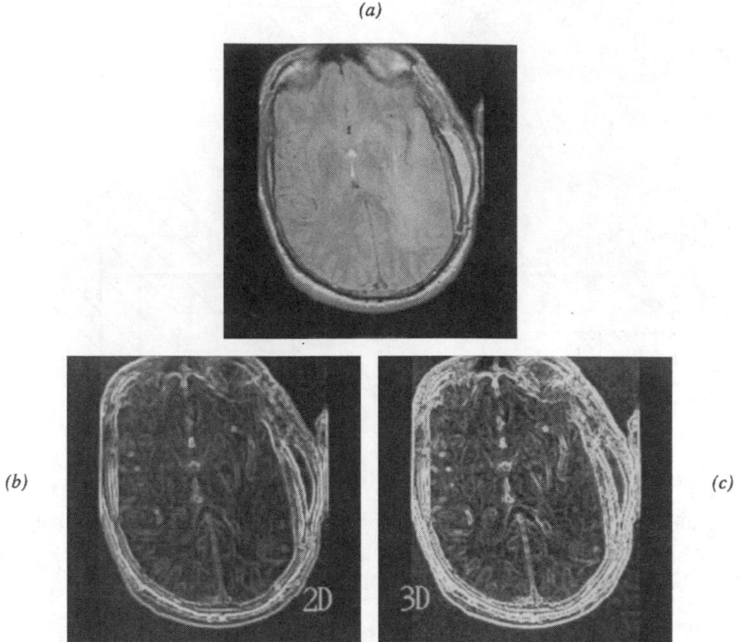

FIGURE 1.7 A slice of a 3D MR scene of a patient's head (a) and its edge-enhancing filtered output with a 2D (b) and a 3D neighborhood (c).

where $g_i(v_j)$ is the intensity of voxel v_j in the input scene, w_j is the weight (a positive number) associated with v_j, and $v_1, v_2, \ldots, v_n$ are the neighbors of v_0. Note that the neighborhood defined by Figure 1.6a is within the same slice and hence filtering in a slice is not affected by its adjoining slices. The other two definitions in Figure 1.6 allow 3D operations. The weights are usually chosen such that the voxels closer to v_o are given more weight than those that are farther away. Note that the range of intensities in the output scene remains roughly the same as that in the input scene. The weights w_j are often chosen as the values at the level of w_j of a Gaussian function of two or three spatial variables with the maximum of the function occurring at the center of v_0. If the weights are selected in this fashion, we refer to the resulting filter as a Gaussian filter.

Another type of smoothing that is often used is called median filtering. In this operation, $g_o(v_0)$ is taken to be the median value of the intensities $g_i(v_0), g_i(v_1), \ldots, g_i(v_n)$. For example, suppose we use the neighborhood of Figure 1.6b and the neighbor intensities around v_0 (including that of v_0) are 130, 100, 120, 110, 200, 90, 80. To find the median value, we arrange these intensities in ascending order (80, 90, 100, 110, 120, 130, 200) and then take the middle value (110) and assign it to $g_o(v_0)$. Figure 1.8 illustrates the smoothing operation using 2D and 3D Gaussian filters and a 3D median filter on the slice in Figure 1.8a of a CT scene of a human knee.

The use of low-pass filtering in 3D imaging is mainly to suppress noise. One undesirable aspect of this operation is that along with noise, the real sharp intensity variations due to the presence of tissue boundaries (wanted information) are also smoothed out. It is possible to detect such discontinuities through high-pass filtering and to do low-pass filtering selectively. See Ref. 30 for a survey of such techniques. A method designed along these principles that is often used in 3D imaging is called anisotropic diffusion.[31] See Ref. 32 for an example of how this method is utilized in smoothing MR images of the brain. Here, smoothing is formulated as a process of diffusion. Intensity gradients in a given scene $\mathcal{V}_i = (V_i, g_i(v))$ are considered to cause a "flow" within the scene whose functional dependence on gradient is controlled through a parameter κ. The given scene $\mathcal{V}_i$ is influenced by

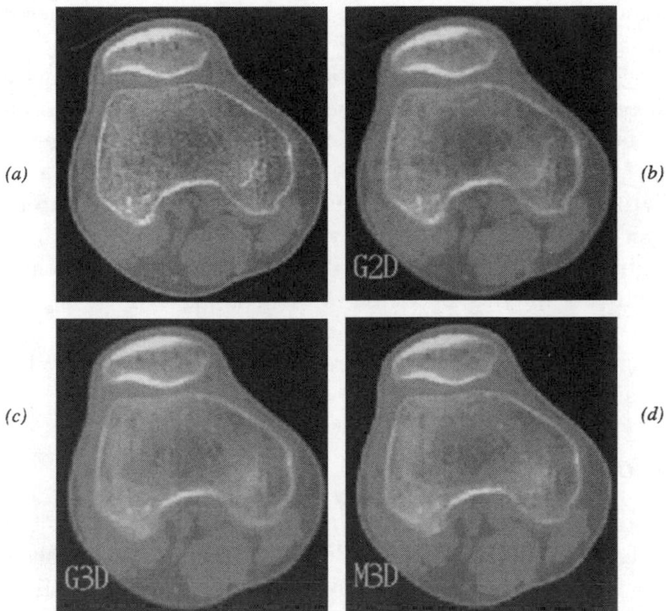

FIGURE 1.8 Illustration of a smoothing 2D Gaussian filter (b), a 3D Gaussian filter (c), and a median filter (d) for the scene in (a).

flow and results in a time-dependent scene (V_i, $g(v,t)$) which initially is $\mathcal{V}_i$. The diffusion process is governed by

$$\frac{\partial}{\partial t} g(v,t) = \mathrm{div}\big(c(v,t)\nabla g(v,t)\big) \tag{1.5}$$

where

$$c(v,t) = \exp\left(-\frac{|\nabla g(v,t)|^2}{\kappa}\right) \tag{1.6}$$

and div is the mathematical divergence operator. The flow $\phi(v,t)$ at a voxel v is given by

$$\phi(v,t) = c(v,t)\nabla g(v,t). \tag{1.7}$$

A solution to the diffusion process[31] leads to an iterative method for estimating the time-dependent scene as follows for the 2D case:

$$g(v,t+\Delta t) = g(v,t) + \Delta t\big(\phi_{\mathrm{right}} - \phi_{\mathrm{left}} + \phi_{\mathrm{bottom}} - \phi_{\mathrm{top}}\big) \tag{1.8}$$

where ϕ_{right}, ϕ_{left}, ϕ_{bottom}, and ϕ_{top} represent flow from v in the different directions, computed from Equation 1.7. κ is chosen according to noise level and edge strength. The method blurs discontinuities dependent on κ. Since the flow phenomenon is defined based mainly on gradient magnitude, information about subtle objects (such as small lesions of the brain in multiple sclerosis [MS]) may be lost in this (and other) methods of filtering if object intensity characteristics have significant overlap with that of the noise that we are trying to suppress.

Low-pass filtering is useful in several operations including surface rendering, surface filtering, and surface normal estimation,[33] as we will study later. The median filter, on the other hand, is often quite effective in suppressing noise and at the same time in preserving the sharpness of real boundaries.

Ideally, any filtering operation should not suppress wanted (object) information and enhance unwanted (non-object) information. This ideal is difficult to achieve, which implies that structure definition (even roughly) is perhaps necessary to meet the above requirement. How to incorporate object knowledge into the filtering operation without doing explicit segmentation is an open problem.

Several enhancing and suppressing filters are incorporated in 3DVIEWNIX under PREPROCESS → SceneOperations → Filter.

1.2.4 Interpolation

Medical imaging systems collect data typically in a slice-by-slice fashion. Usually, the pixel size p of the scene (see Figure 1.2) within a slice is different from the spacing between adjacent slices. In addition, often the spacing between slices may not be the same for all slices. For visualization, manipulation, and analysis of such anisotropic data, they often need to be converted into data of isotropic discretization or of desired level of discretization in any of the three (or higher) dimensions. Often the resolution of the acquired data may be too high to be handled comfortably in an interactive situation; for example, to visualize the surfaces of an object of interest that is captured in the data via surface or volume rendering. A possible solution is to keep a low-resolution iconic representation of the object for interactive use and the full-resolution representation for detailed non-interactive study. If data are acquired for the same object of study, say a patient's brain, from two modalities such as MR and PET, upon registering the two data sets, one of them needs to be redigitized. In addition, the data sets may differ in their resolution, whence the level of discretization of one of them needs to be converted to that of the other, so that they can be analyzed together. A similar situation arises in longitudinal acquisitions using the same modality for the same body region. For example, we may wish to study how the lesions in an MS patient's brain change over time in the natural course of the disease or in response to a therapy. Upon registering the scenes with respect to a common coordinate system, the slices representing exactly the same location (plane) in the patient's head need to be computed to facilitate this comparative study. Finally, often the slices of a scene are not or cannot be acquired along desired orientations. In such situations, the scene needs to be "resliced" so that the desired aspects of the objects can be visualized in the new slices. Interpolation is an operation that can be used to help in all these situations. It converts a given scene $\mathcal{V}_i = (V_i, g_i)$ to another scene $\mathcal{V}_o = (V_o, g_o)$ of a specified level of discretization. So, usually $V_o \neq V_i$, although the two scenes cover roughly the same body region.

Broadly, interpolation techniques can be divided into two categories: scene based and object based. In scene-based methods, interpolated scene intensity values are determined directly from the intensity values of the given scene. In object-based methods, some object information extracted from the given scene is used in guiding the interpolation process.

1.2.4.1 Scene-Based Interpolation Methods

Suppose that the pixel size p and p' of the input and output scene are identical. Our aim is to create an output scene of cubic voxels of side p' $(= p)$. The interpolation operation can be described by concentrating on one column of voxels in the input scene in the z direction with coordinates (I,J,k) for some fixed I and J and for $1 \leq k \leq N$, since the same operation is repeated for all columns. The simplest way of determining the intensity to be assigned to the voxels of the output scene in this column is by using the "nearest neighbor rule":[34] assign to an output voxel v' the intensity of the input voxel v that is nearest to v'. One possible definition of nearness is using the distance between the center of v' and that of v. Nearest neighbor interpolation is equivalent to duplicating thinner slices.

A better approach in this case of $p' = p$, called linear interpolation,[34] assigns different values, that vary in a linear fashion, to the voxels falling within the same voxel of the input scene. One commonly used model of this form of variation assumes that the intensity varies linearly along z from one voxel center to the next. To compute the intensity of any voxel v' in the output scene, we simply have to determine the voxels v_n and v_{n+1} of the input scene whose centers C_n and C_{n+1} are closest to the center C' of v' in the $-z$ and $+z$ directions and then compute the distances d_n and d_{n+1} of C' from C_n and C_{n+1}. The intensity of v' is then given by

$$g_o(v') = g_i(v_n) + \left[\frac{g_i(v_{n+1}) - g_i(v_n)}{d_n + d_{n+1}}\right] d_n \tag{1.9}$$

Note that we cannot estimate interpolated intensity at voxel centers which fall outside the line segment connecting the centers of v_1 and v_N, the voxels in the first and the last slice of the input scene in the column under consideration.

A more sophisticated method is the so-called trilinear interpolation method. As the name implies, instead of interpolating in only one (z) direction, as in the previous method, this allows (linear) interpolation in all three directions. It is not necessary to assume $p = p'$ as in the previous method. This implies that we can create a scene that is more finely or more coarsely discretized than the input scene. Imagine that we build the new voxels of side p' starting from one corner of the scene domain. Our problem is to determine the intensity $g_o(v')$ at the center of each new voxel v'. The principle is similar to that of linear interpolation except that the step indicated by Equation 1.9 is applied a few times to compute $g_o(v')$. The steps involved are illustrated in Figure 1.9. We make a slight change to the assumed model of variation of intensity across the old voxels. In this model, we assume that the intensity $g_i(v)$ of the old voxel varies linearly from the center of its front end (face) to the centers of the front ends of its six neighbors in the principal directions, where the neighbors of v are defined as in Figure 1.6b. Given this model, to determine the intensity at any point C' (which represents the center of a new voxel v'), we find eight old voxels $v_1, v_2, \ldots, v_8$ such that their centers $C_1, C_2, \ldots, C_8$ are closest to C' as illustrated in Figure 1.9. The trilinear problem then is to determine the intensity at C' knowing the intensities $g_i(v_1), \ldots, g_i(v_8)$ at the centers $C_1, \ldots, C_8$. Note that, since we know the coordinates of C' as well as the distance between these centers, we can calculate the distances marked d_1', d_2', and d_3' of C' with respect to the centers $C_1, \ldots, C_8$. The actual computation of the intensity at C' now consists of seven calculations similar to that in Equation 1.9: first we compute the intensity at P_1 knowing the intensity at C_1 and C_2, then at P_2 knowing the intensity at C_5 and C_6, and then at P_3 knowing the intensity at P_1 and P_2. Similarly, we compute the intensity at P_4 using three calculations. Finally, $g_o(v')$ is computed knowing the intensity at P_3 and P_4. Clearly, if C' falls on a face of the cuboid $C_1, \ldots, C_8$ we need only three calculations (in this case, interpolation is called bilinear since it takes place in a plane), and only one (linear) if C' is on an edge of the cuboid.

Higher order polynomials may also be used as gray-level interpolation functions instead of the linear function used above. Their waveforms are often chosen to be approximately Gaussian in shape. One notable member of this class is the cubic B-spline.[35] When higher order polynomials are used, more neighboring voxels will need to be considered for estimating output voxel intensity. For example, compared to the situation for linear, the intensity of 4 voxels will participate in the calculation of an output voxel intensity by the cubic B-spline method, two on each side of the voxel center C' under consideration. For the more general situation depicted in Figure 1.9, intensity of 64 voxels will participate in the computation.

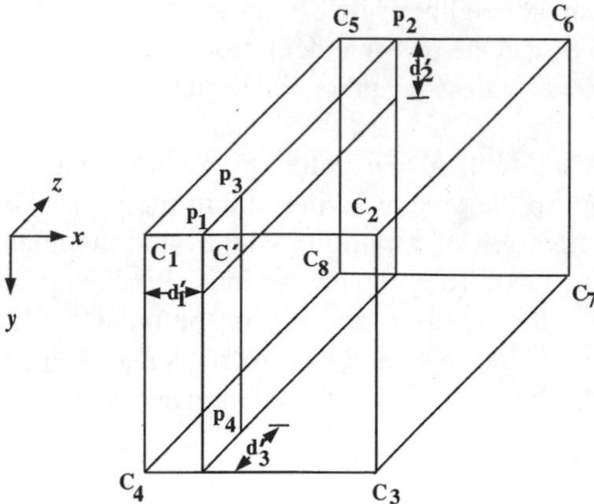

FIGURE 1.9 Trilinear interpolation. C_1, C_2, …, C_8 are the centers of eight voxels that are closest to C', the center of v', whose intensity we want to estimate. Note that the cuboid C_1, C_2, …, C_8 does not itself correspond to any voxels, new or old.

A statistical process, called kriging,[36] is also used for interpolating gray values based on their statistical variations, rather than on the gray values themselves. In this method, interpolation is cast as a statistical estimation process. For any voxel v' in V_o it defines $g_o(v')$ to be the estimate

$$g_o(v') = \sum_{\ell=1}^{m} w_\ell g_i(v_\ell) \tag{1.10}$$

where m, a parameter in the method, is the number of neighboring voxels v_ℓ in V in the vicinity of v' used in calculating the estimate. Further, g_o becomes the best linear, unbiased estimator when $E(g_o - g_i)=0$ and $E(g_o - g_i)^2$ is minimum, where E denotes expected value.

1.2.4.2 Object-Based Interpolation Methods

The first object-based method appearing in the literature seems to be what is known as shape-based interpolation, originally developed for binary input scenes.[37] The main idea in this technique is to first convert the given scene into a binary scene (we will discuss such scene transformations later) such that the voxels with intensity 1 in this scene represent the structure of interest and those with intensity 0 represent non-structure regions. Shape-based interpolation uses this binary scene as input and creates another binary scene for the specified level of discretization. The method consists of first converting the input binary scene $\mathcal{V}_b$ into a scene $\mathcal{V}_g$, both with the same scene domain, by assigning to each voxel v in $\mathcal{V}_g$ a number that represents the shortest distance between v and the (2D) boundary in $\mathcal{V}_b$ between the 1-voxel and 0-voxel regions within the slice that contains v. The number is positive if v has an intensity 1 in $\mathcal{V}_b$; otherwise the number is negative. Now we interpolate $\mathcal{V}_g$ using linear, trilinear, or other interpolation rules to create another scene $\mathcal{V}'_g$. Remembering that the numbers associated with voxels in $\mathcal{V}'_g$ represent distances from boundary, we create the final interpolated binary scene $\mathcal{V}'_b$ by assigning to a voxel in $\mathcal{V}'_b$ the intensity 1 if the corresponding voxel in $\mathcal{V}'_g$ has positive value. All other voxels are assigned the intensity 0. Several extensions of this method have been developed.[38–40] For example, Ref. 38 extends this method to images containing tree-like objects to improve the performance of interpolation of these structures. These publications have shown that, in certain aspects of structure measures, shape-based interpolation produces more accurate results than the scene-based interpolation (linear, cubic B-spline) followed by an application of the same segmentation method that was used for creating the input binary scene for the shape-based method. Whether or not this improvement helps in a specific medical task is unknown at present.

If a slice-by-slice VOI (see Section 1.2.2) or segmentation (see Section 1.2.6) operation is indispensable in an application, we strongly recommend the use of shape-based interpolation. The reason is that if a scene interpolation scheme is used instead, user interaction will be required on a much larger number of slices. As an example, suppose we wish to segment a 4D scene representing time-varying cardiac MR images consisting of 10 slices for each of 8 time instances, with (cuboid) voxels of uniform size $.7 \times .7 \times 5$ mm. Assuming we create an interpolated scene with cubic voxels of size $.7 \times .7 \times .7$ mm, the interpolated scene will have close to 560 slices. If we wish to create more, say 16, time instances, also through interpolation (often desirable for providing a smooth depiction of dynamics), the resulting 4D scene will have more than 1100 slices! Any slice-based user-assisted operation quickly becomes impractical. If we use shape-based interpolation, the operation is required on only the 80 (original) slices (often less, since the operation can be duplicated by the computer for a set of contiguous slices), irrespective of how much interpolation is needed or desired.

The shape-based method extends easily to higher dimensional scenes. For example, in 4D, to interpolate along z and t (representing, say, time in the fourth dimension), we generally need to carry out bilinear (in z and t) interpolation in order to generate more slices and time instances. To determine the intensity of a voxel v' in the output scene, the four voxels v_1, v_2, v_3, v_4 whose centers are closest to the center of v' are determined and then a bilinear interpolation (involving three computations of the form expressed in Equation 1.9) is carried out. Note that these four voxels have the same x, y coordinates.

Recently, the shape-based method has been generalized to gray-level scenes.[41] The basic idea in this generalization is to first "lift" the given 3D scene into a 4D binary scene by having the fourth dimension represent scene intensity. For every voxel in the 3D scene, a column of 4D voxels with intensity value 1 is added in the fourth direction whose length equals the voxel intensity in the input scene. All other 4D voxels that make up a 4D array are assigned the value 0. Binary shape-based interpolation is then applied to this 4D binary scene and the resulting 4D binary scene is "collapsed" (inverse of "lifting") to get the final 3D gray scene. Other examples of attempts to generalize shape-based interpolation to gray scenes are provided in Refs. 42 and 43.

The object-based method presented in Ref. 44 casts the problem as interpolating to increase the number of slices in the z direction. The method uses information only from pairs of neighboring slices during interpolation. One slice of the pair is referred to as the reference image; the other slice is referred to as the target image. The voxels with high gradient magnitude values (i.e., above some threshold value) are referred to as feature points. A matching process determines the correspondence between the feature points in the reference slice to those in the target. Correspondences such as one feature point in the reference slice to one feature point in the target, one feature point in the reference slice to many in the target, and one feature point in the reference to no feature points in the target are allowed. To interpolate points on the intervening slices, a line is drawn between each pair of matching points on the reference and the target slice. One then linearly interpolates the values along the lines that intersect the intervening slices. For points with low gradient magnitude, conventional linear interpolation between slices is carried out.

The method described in Ref. 45 involves the use of cores[46] as the transform domain of the images. Cores are based on the medial axes of structures in the image which are produced at multiple scales. To form the core of a 3D scene, one first produces a 4D scene by smoothing the original 3D scene by (typically Gaussian) filters of various standard deviations (scales). This fourth dimension indicates the scale, the idea being that a greater degree of blurring is needed to smooth out larger aspects of the objects. The next step is to assign a fuzzy measure of boundariness to each voxel v in the 4D scale space and to determine the orientation of the boundary at v. In the next step, a degree of medialness is assigned to each voxel via the Hough-like-Medial Axis

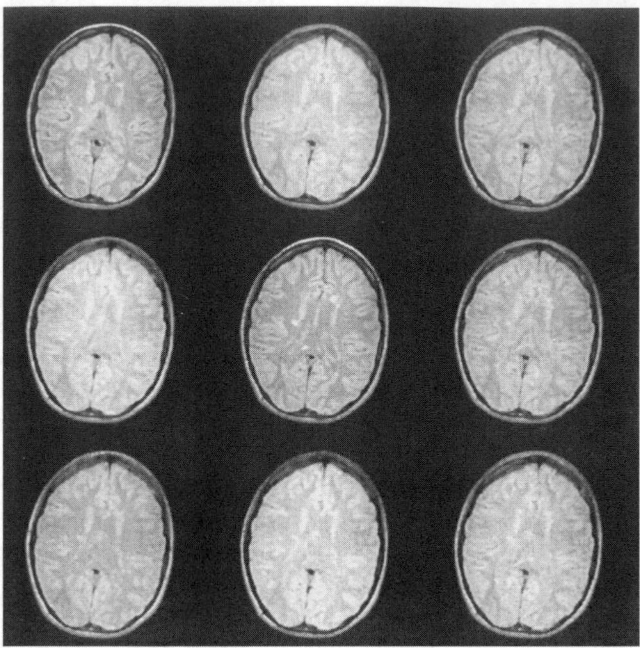

FIGURE 1.10 A display of the same slice estimated by different interpolation methods from the adjoining slices of an MR brain image data set. From left to right, row 1: nearest neighbor, linear, cubic spline; row 2: shape-based 1, original slice, modified cubic spline; row 3: shape-based 2, shape-based 3, and the method of Goshtasby et al.[44] Shape-based 1, 2, and 3 represent different versions of the shape-based method, 1 being the best as per the evaluation studies.

Transform. Ridges in this medialness image form the cores. Cores can be used in interpolation as follows. Say our input scene consists of two slices and we wish to interpolate an intervening slice exactly in the middle. First apply the core method independently to each of the two given slices. If the slices contain more than one structure, then a matching process must be used to pair the structures' cores. Additional problems may occur when objects are present in one slice but not in the other. Given two matched cores, the rotation, translation, and scaling to transform one core into the other is estimated. Then half of this transformation is applied to the first slice and half to the second. The two transformed slices are then interpolated (typically linearly) to determine the intervening slice. The core is used, in effect, to determine the transformation (rotation, translation, and scaling) of the first slice into the second, in a manner somewhat analogous to how the feature points are used in Ref. 44.

The performance of three methods in the shape-based (gray-level) family[41] has been compared objectively[47] with that of several scene-based and object-based methods, including nearest neighbor, gray-level linear, two methods in the spline family,[35,48] and the method of Goshtasby et al.[44] Twenty 3D scenes of different body regions of different subjects from different modalities have been used for this purpose. Each slice in each scene has been estimated by each method from the adjoining slices and compared to the original slice using several measures. The results[47] indicate strong evidence of the superior performance of shape-based methods over other methods compared. Figure 1.10 shows one slice of one of the 20 scenes that is estimated by each of the methods. The original slice is also shown for reference.

Figure 1.11 shows an example of a 3D rendition of a child's skull at a coarse and a fine level of discretization obtained from a CT scene. Gray-level trilinear interpolation was used in both cases.

The motivations for the development of object-based methods and the associated results indicate that for optimal (ideal) results, full structure information (segmentation) becomes necessary. The

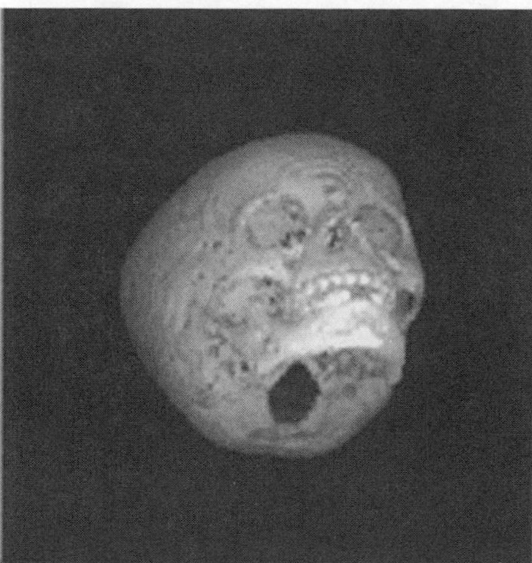
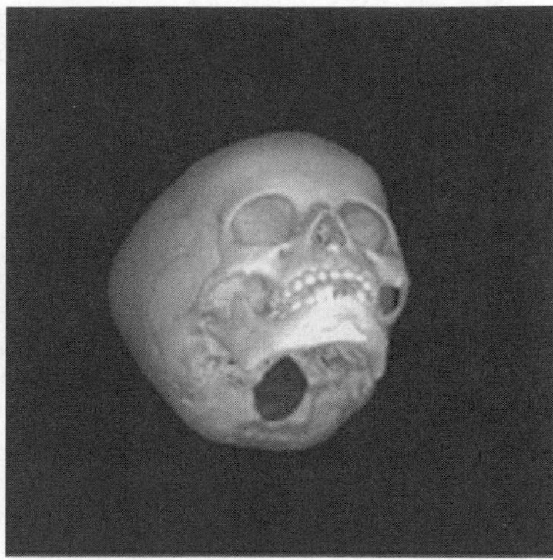

FIGURE 1.11 Illustrations of renditions derived from a CT scene of a child's skull at a coarse (left) and a fine (right) level of discretization. The two scenes are obtained from the original scene by trilinear interpolation.

challenge in interpolation then is how to approach the ideal results without doing explicit and complete segmentation. Further work is needed in understanding how the various methods fare in specific medical applications. The study of how the methods influence the quality and accuracy of 3D renditions is also an open area.

Several scene-based and object-based interpolation methods are available in 3DVIEWNIX for scenes up to 4D under PREPROCESS → SceneOperations → Interpolate.

1.2.5 Registration

The purpose of these operations is to represent information pertaining to the same object system of study in a common coordinate system. Broadly, registration methods may be divided into two groups: scene based and object based. In scene-based methods, the transformation needed to convert a given scene to match spatially with another given scene is estimated by matching the intensity pattern in the two scenes. In object-based methods, structure information derived from the two scenes are matched for this estimation.

Registration becomes necessary primarily in the following situations: (1) Scenes are acquired for the same body region from different modalities — for example, CT, MRI, fMRI, and PET for a patient's head. The need for registration comes from the fact that fMRI and PET provide mainly functional information and lack anatomic details, and vice versa for CT and MRI. Registration helps associate the functional activity information with specific anatomic regions. A similar situation arises when using different protocols within the same modality for the same body region — for example, T1-weighted images of the brain before and after administration of Gd DTPA contrast agent. Here registration helps to identify the regions that enhance and thereby to study certain disease processes. (2) Scenes are acquired for the same body region using the same modality for different time instances. The time instances may be close to each other for studying the motion or displacement of an object in the body region, or they may be far apart for studying longitudinally the growth or change in an object. (3) In certain interventional procedures, information derived from acquired scenes is utilized to provide navigational aids for the devices used in the procedure. In these situations, it becomes necessary to register the device, the body region, and the scene. (4) Scenes acquired for a given body region are to be matched to a computerized atlas for the same body region. This is often helpful in studying statistically the variations in certain object measures over a subject population as well as in scene segmentation.

No registration is needed between two scenes if both the following conditions are satisfied: (1) The same objects of study are observable in both scenes and they do not change shape. (2) The relationship among them and to the scene coordinate system does not change. For any objects, even static, in any body region, these conditions are difficult to meet, and therefore, registration becomes necessary in the situations described earlier.

1.2.5.1 Scene-Based Registration Methods

In these methods, input is a pair of scenes $\mathcal{V}_{i1} = (V_{i1}, g_{i1})$ and $\mathcal{V}_{i2} = (V_{i2}, g_{i2})$ of the same body region and the output is a pair of scenes $\mathcal{V}_{o1} = (V_{o1}, g_{o1})$ and $\mathcal{V}_{o2} = (V_{o2}, g_{o2})$. Assuming that $\mathcal{V}_{i2}$ is to be matched with $\mathcal{V}_{i1}$, the output scenes are such that

$$\mathcal{V}_{o1} = \mathcal{V}_{i1}$$

and

$$\mathcal{V}_{o2} = T(\mathcal{V}_{i2}) = (V_{i1}, g_{o2}) \tag{1.11}$$

where T consists of a geometric transformation T_G to register $\mathcal{V}_{i2}$ with $\mathcal{V}_{i1}$ and an interpolation operation T_I to estimate scene intensities at the new locations for each voxel v in $\mathcal{V}_{i2}$. That is, the registered scene T_G ($\mathcal{V}_{i2}$) needs to be redigitized. An appropriate scene-based or object-based interpolation method described in the previous section is utilized for this purpose. The registration transformation itself may be rigid or elastic. In the rigid case, the mismatch is assumed to be due to a global translation and rotation of one of the scenes. Scaling, if required, is usually handled easily by an interpolation of one of the scenes prior to registration to make its voxels equal in size to that of the other. In the elastic case, it is assumed that local deformations are needed, in addition to a global translation and rotation, to achieve a match.

1.2.5.1.1 Rigid

A majority of the existing scene-based methods[49–56] are of the rigid type. They can all be characterized, more or less, by the following process, along the lines suggested in Refs. 49 and 50:

1. Interpolate $\mathcal{V}_{i1}$ and $\mathcal{V}_{i2}$ to make voxels cubic and equal in size in both scenes.
2. Choose a criterion function $G_{2,1}$ for determining the degree of match/mismatch of (the transformed) $\mathcal{V}_{i2}$ with $\mathcal{V}_{i1}$ and a stopping criterion S.
3. Do an initial translation and rotation of $\mathcal{V}_{i2}$ to roughly align with $\mathcal{V}_{i1}$.
4. Compute $G_{2,1}(P)$ for the current pose (location and orientation) P of $\mathcal{V}_{i2}$. Compute $G_{1,2}(P)$ reversing the roles of $\mathcal{V}_{i1}$ and $\mathcal{V}_{i2}$ and the average $G(P)$ of $G_{2,1}(P)$ and $G_{1,2}(P)$.
5. If $S(P)$ is satisfied, stop; else go to Step 6.
6. Modify P incrementally (e.g., by one voxel translation and/or 1° rotation) using partial derivatives of $G(P)$ to decide in which direction to move, and go to Step 4.

The essential differences in the different methods are in Steps 2, 3, and 6. Here is an example of $G_{2,1}(P)$ and $S(P)$:[49]

$$G_{2,1}(P) = \sigma_r / r_{\text{mean}} \tag{1.12}$$

where r_{mean} and σ_r are the mean and standard deviation, respectively, of $g_{o2}(v)/g_{i1}(v)$ over all v in the domain of $\mathcal{V}_{i1}$ such that both intensities are non-zero, and $S(P)$ is a threshold criterion

$G(P) \leq$ a threshold. Examples of other criterion functions used include correlation coefficients of intensities or of intensity features,[51–54] and similarity measures such as the sum of the absolute values of differences.[55,56] Other strategies used for seeking optimum solutions (Step 6) include random search and simple methods.

When $\mathcal{V}_{i1}$ and $\mathcal{V}_{i2}$ are from the same modality (and protocol), excellent results are obtained by these methods. When the meaning of similarly ranked intensities is different in the two scenes, either due to different modalities or due to protocols (such as Tl- and T2-weighted MRI protocols), these methods tend to go astray. Although several solutions have been suggested, this remains as the main challenge in scene-based methods. Figure 1.12 shows an example of scene-based within-modality (and protocol) registration. Figure 1.12a shows an MRI slice approximately at the same location of an MS patient's head taken at eight longitudinal time instances. Since the scenes are not registered, the progression of the MS disease, which is manifest as hyper-intense lesions in these protein density (PD)-weighted scenes, cannot be properly discovered. Figure 1.12b shows the slices estimated at the same location upon registering in 3D each of the first to the seventh scene to the eighth. The progression of the lesions at this planar location in the patient's brain is now clearly demonstrated.

1.2.5.1.2 Deformable

These methods are far fewer than the rigid scene-based approaches. The method suggested in Ref. 57 consists of an initial global translation and rotation of V_{i2} to roughly align the two scenes. This is followed by a local deformation at the level of voxels. This deformation (local translation and rotation) is estimated based on a measure of correlation of the intensity and gradient magnitude at voxels in a neighborhood of each voxel.

A more basic approach is taken in Refs. 58 and 59, which, as presented, is applicable only to scenes depicting normal (or close to normal) anatomy. The basic idea is to match (and transform) all scenes to a standard atlas or textbook. Formally, a textbook is a triple $(\Omega, F, \mathcal{F})$. Here Ω is a subset of R^3 and constitutes a body region. F is a function that assigns to a point in Ω a vector from $\mathcal{F}$. The components of the vectors in $\mathcal{F}$ constitute features of the tissues in the body region. These may include image intensities for various modalities and protocols as well as tissue labels. A set $\mathcal{E}$ of elastic transformations E: $\Omega \rightarrow \Omega$ consisting of local dilation and contraction is constructed. The maps of these transformations form a set of normal anatomies $\{F \circ E | E \in \mathcal{E}\}$, where $\circ$ stands for composition, generated from the textbook. Given a patient study consisting of a set of scenes, the textbook is brought into the coordinates of the patient's study by finding the transformation $E' \in \mathcal{E}$ that corresponds to the mean of the posterior distribution induced by the elastic energy. To establish a correspondence between $\mathcal{V}_{i2}$ and $\mathcal{V}_{i1}$, the textbook is transformed in this fashion to match with each scene.

1.2.5.2 Object-Based Registration Methods

In these methods, input is a pair of structures ST_1 and ST_2 representing some same object information from a given body region, and the output is a geometric transformation T_G to be applied to ST_2 to match ST_2 with ST_1. This transformation may be rigid or elastic. In the rigid case, the mismatch is assumed to be due to a global translation and rotation of one of the structures. If the structures are derived from acquired scenes, their scale differences are handled easily by appropriately interpolating the scenes prior to the extraction of structures from them. Otherwise, scale differences should be handled in the transformation. In the elastic case, it is assumed that local deformations are needed, in addition to a global translation and rotation, to achieve a match. Unlike in scene-based methods, explicit interpolation of ST_2 is usually not necessary, and T_G can be stored conveniently along with ST_2 for whatever purpose ST_2 is used subsequently. However, if the aim of object-based registration is indeed to match the scenes from which the structures are derived, then interpolation of one of the scenes becomes necessary.

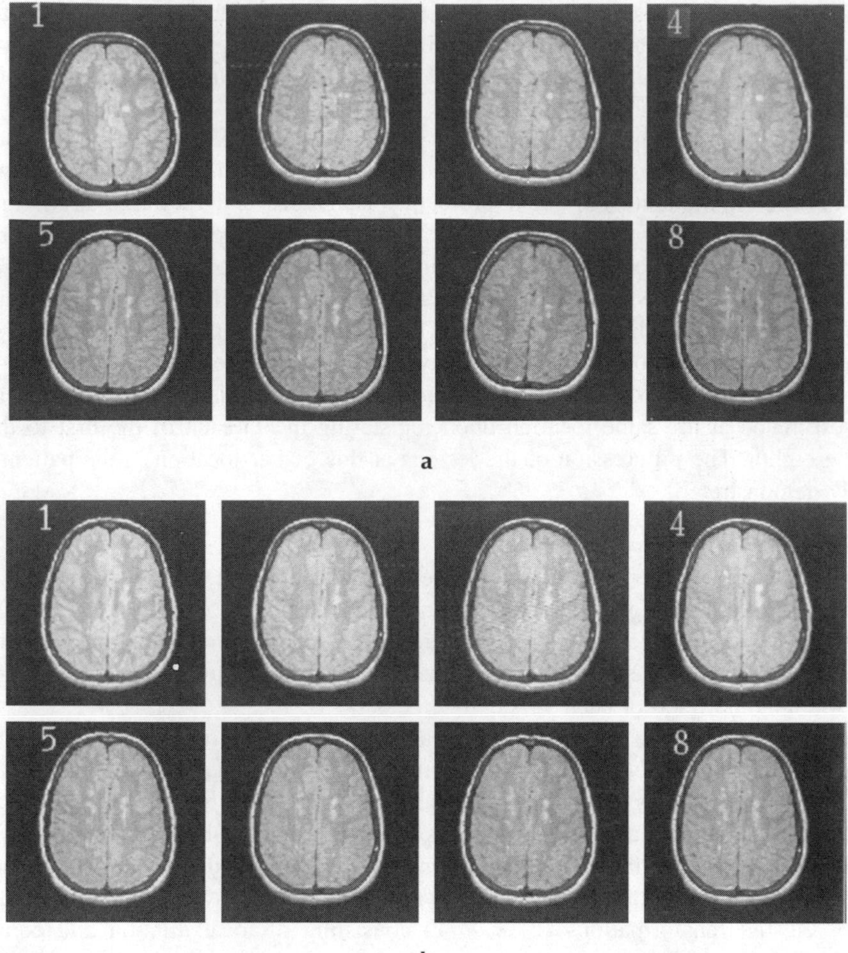

FIGURE 1.12 (a) An MR PD slice roughly at the same level of an MS patient's brain. The eight images represent eight longitudinal time instances, with several months between successive instances. Since the scenes are not registered, the slices are not exactly at the same level, and therefore, it is difficult to see the progression of the MS lesions (appearing as hyper-intense blobs). (b) Slices at the same level after the scenes have been registered. Now it is readily seen (at least on these slices) that the lesions are increasing in number and size.

1.2.5.2.1 Rigid

A majority of the existing registration methods[60–69] are of the object-based rigid type. The process underlying these methods can be generically described as follows:

1. Choose a criterion function G for determining the degree of match/mismatch between ST_2 and ST_1.
2. Choose a stopping criterion S.
3. Do an initial translation and rotation of ST_2 to roughly align it with ST_1.
4. Compute $G(P)$ for the current pose P of ST_2.
5. If S is satisfied, stop. Otherwise, go to Step 6.
6. Modify P incrementally; say, by one voxel translation and/or 1° rotation using partial derivatives of $G(P)$ Go to Step 4.

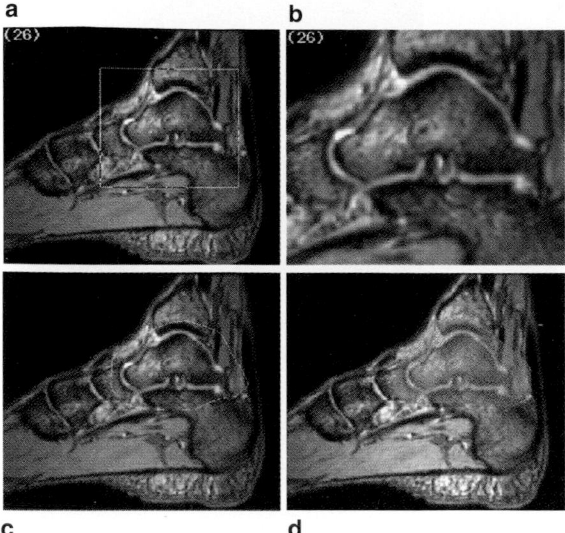

FIGURE 1.5 A region of interest specified by a rectangular box in the scene (a). The output scene is shown in (b). Regions of arbitrary shape are indicated by drawing (c) and painting (d).

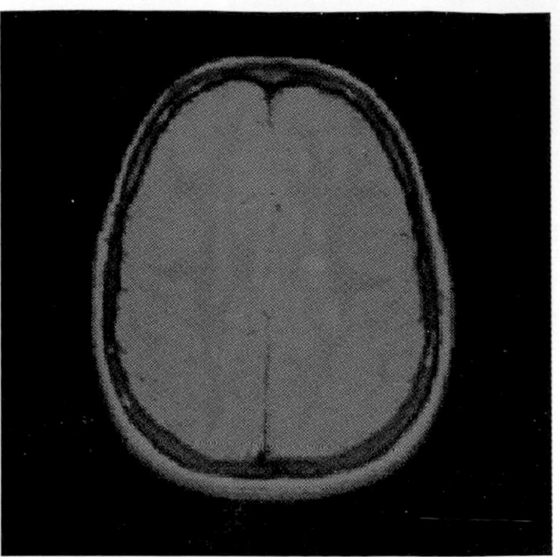

FIGURE 1.27 A pseudocolor display of two MR PD slices corresponding to the same location of the head of an MS patient. The slices are obtained from two scenes that were acquired several months apart and that have been subsequently registered. The older acquisition is displayed in green and the other is displayed in red.

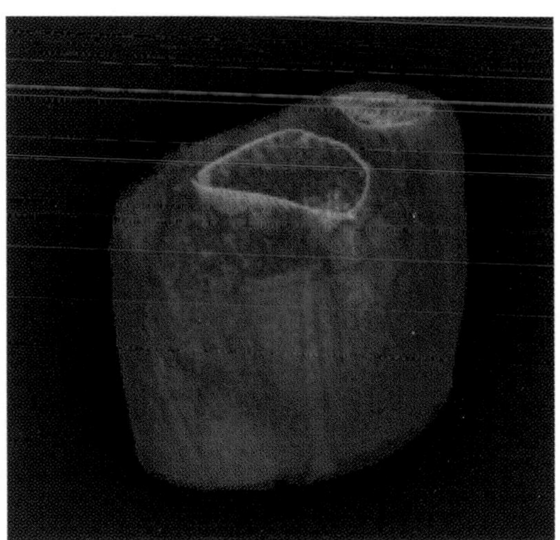

FIGURE 1.38 A volume rendition of bone and soft tissue from a CT scene of a human knee. Two overlapping opacity functions, one for soft tissue and one for bone, were used to assign opacities to the two materials.

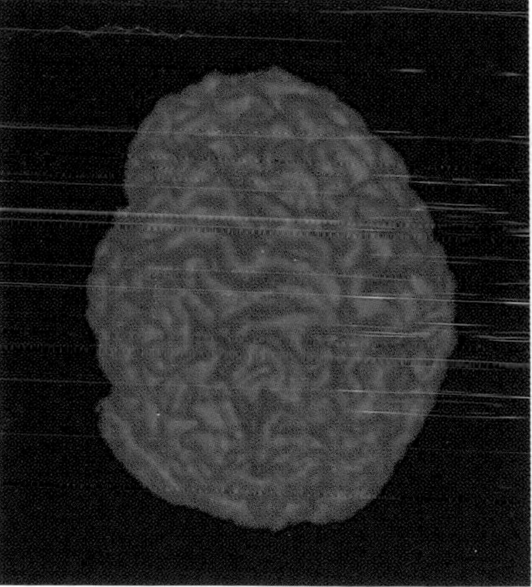

FIGURE 1.39 An example of object-based surface rendition. The T2 and PD scene pair of an MS patient's head was segmented to define the brain as a fuzzy connected object. An isointensity surface of the resulting connectivity scene was defined and rendered using the surface normals derived from the connectivity scene.

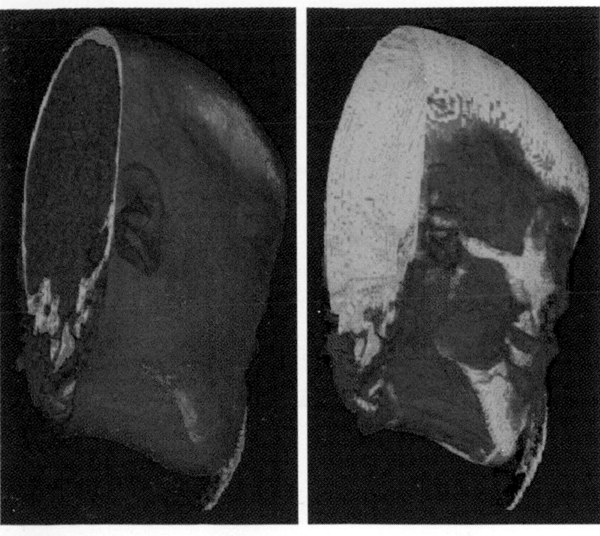

FIGURE 1.40 Object-based volume rendering (right) of craniofacial bone and soft-tissue structures from CT data. For comparison, scene-based volume rendering (via fuzzy thresholding) of the same data is shown on the left. The bone and soft-tissue structures are defined as separate fuzzy-connected objects on the right. Note how the skin has been effectively peeled to show clearly the muscles and even some of the neurovascular structures.

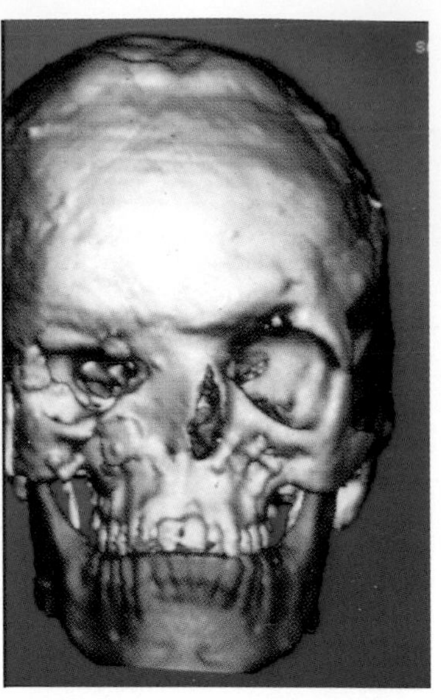

FIGURE 2.1 Male patient, aged 20, with right-sided anopthalmia and heminasal aplasia. Status after reconstruction of the right nasal half and an attempt to enlarge the right orbit. Note that the total overview of the asymmetry can be appreciated only on the 3D image.

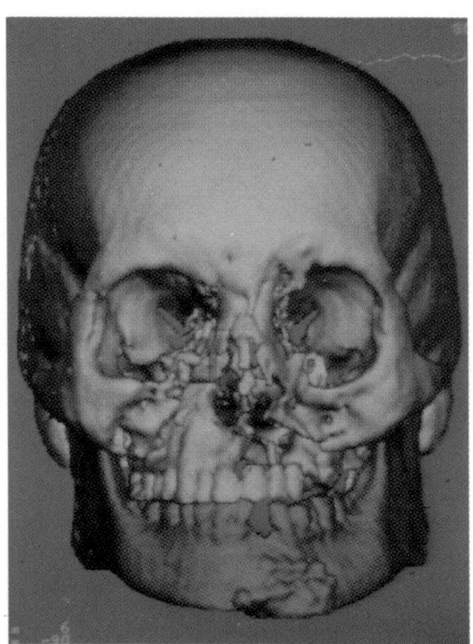

FIGURE 2.3 Severe facial trauma in a 20-year-old male who sustained a motor vehicle accident. Conservative treatment has led to a severely disfiguring condition that is difficult to treat. The 3D image is especially helpful to assess the comminuted midfacial skeleton.

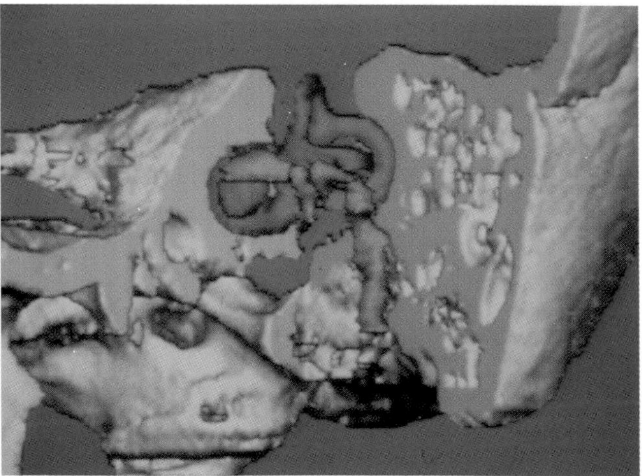

FIGURE 2.5 Antero-lateral view of the left temporal bone in a cadaveric specimen. A cutaway view shows the labyrinth (green), ossicles (yellow), and facial nerve (yellow).

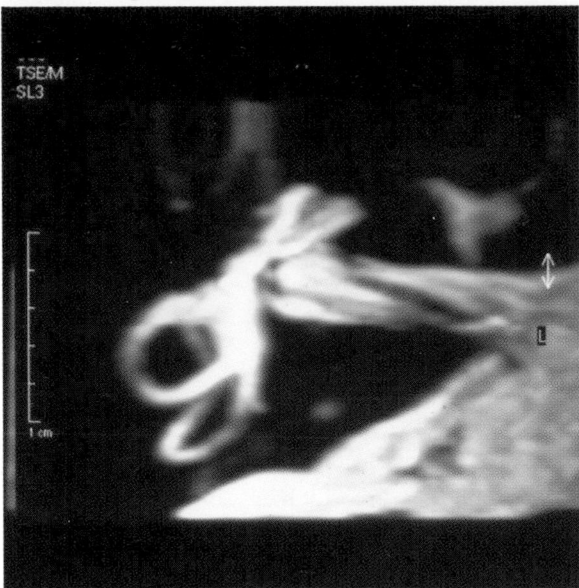

FIGURE 2.6 Maximum intensity projection (MIP) of the normal temporal bone based on a high-resolution T2-weighted MR sequence. Note the spiral lamina in the cochlea and the nerves in the internal auditory meatus.

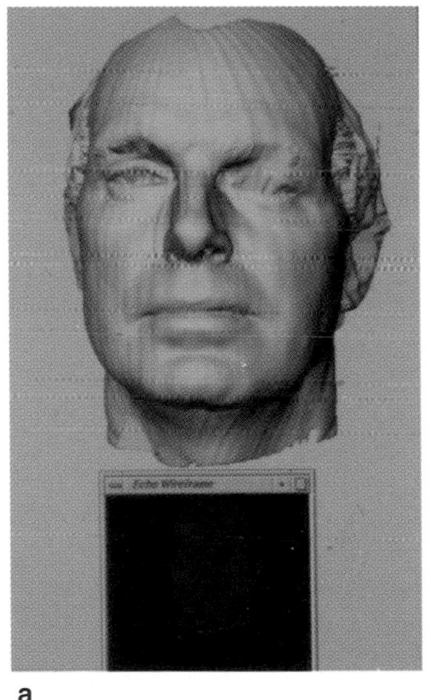

a

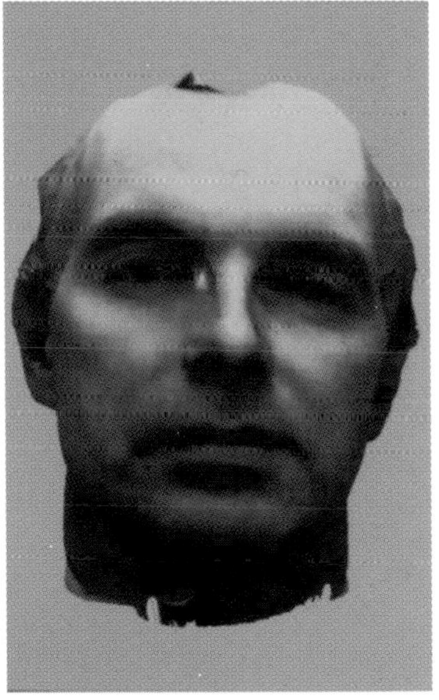

b

FIGURE 2.7 Laser scan of the author's face (Cyberware, Monterey, CA). (Courtesy of A.H. Joel, Image Technologies Int., Norcross, GA.) (a) 3D reconstruction of the surface only. (b) 3D reconstruction after adding color in the form of texture mapping.

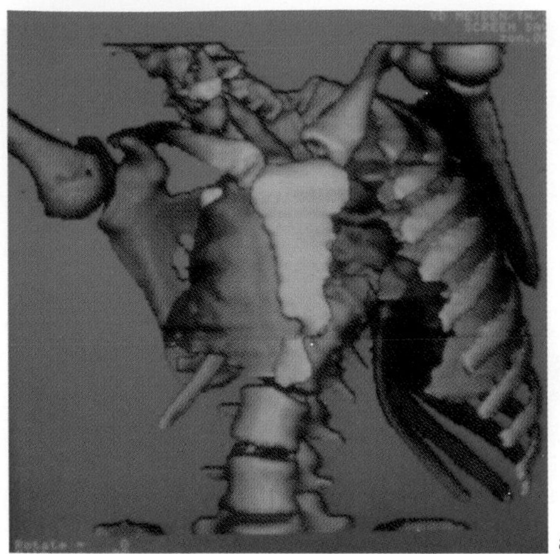

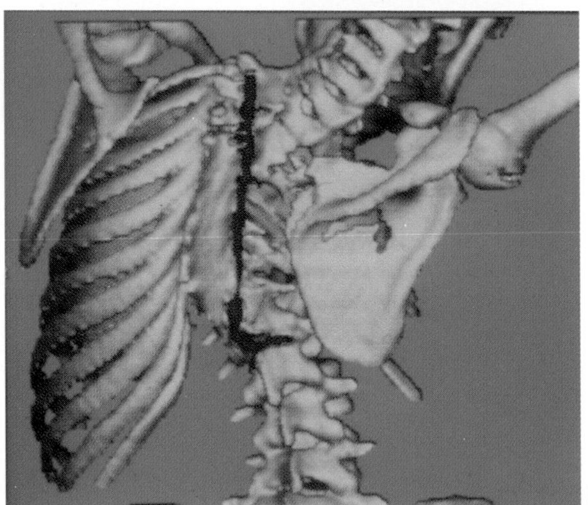

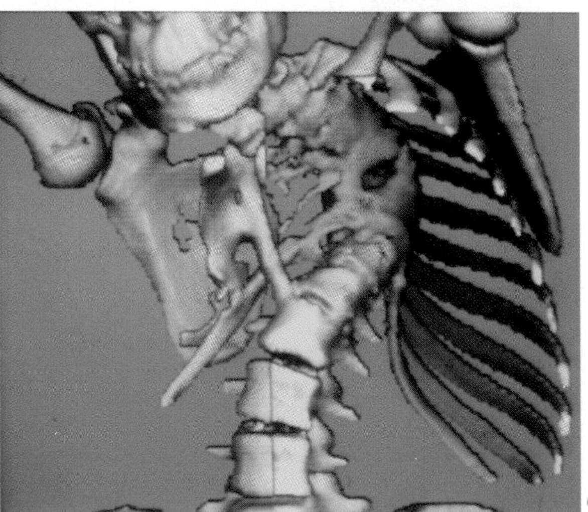

FIGURE 2.9 A 13-year-old female patient with severe right costal agenesis that has resulted in severe scoliosis. (a) Antero-posterior (AP) view showing the reduction of the right lung volume. (b) Posterior view showing a metal splint to suppport the spine. (c) AP cutaway view showing a fibula graft that has been placed as a strut between the lumbar spine and the cervical spine.

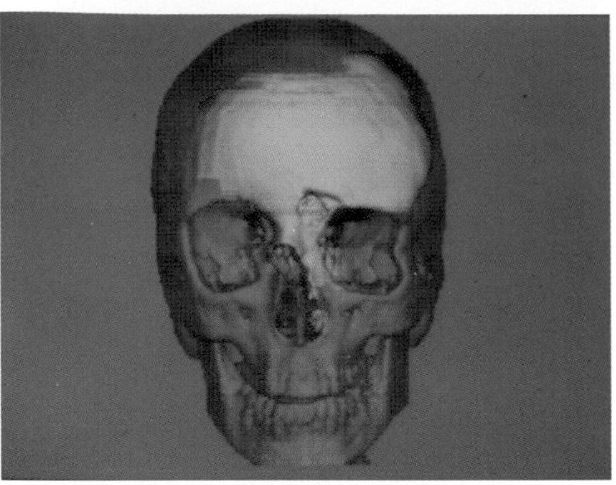

FIGURE 2.10 A 19-year-old female patient with fibrous dysplasia. This image shows the value of disarticulating the pathologic bone and displaying the remainder of the skull in a transparent fashion.

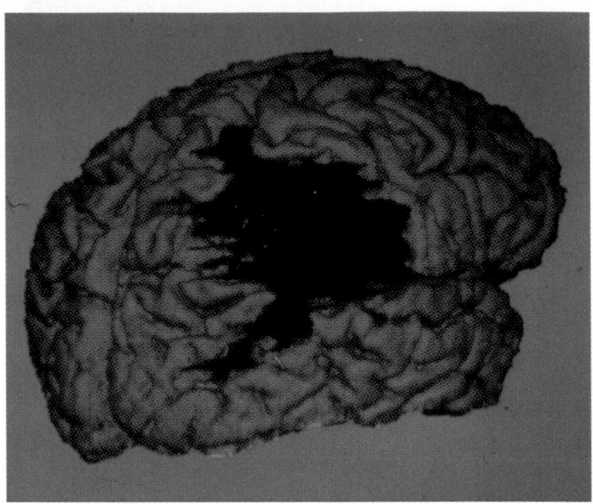

FIGURE 2.12 Disarticulation of infarcted brain tissue in a patient who had a minute embolus that passed the trifurcation of the middle cerebral artery and stranded at the level of the posterior parietal arterial branch, thus causing a small infarct that was associated with unusual neurologic findings.

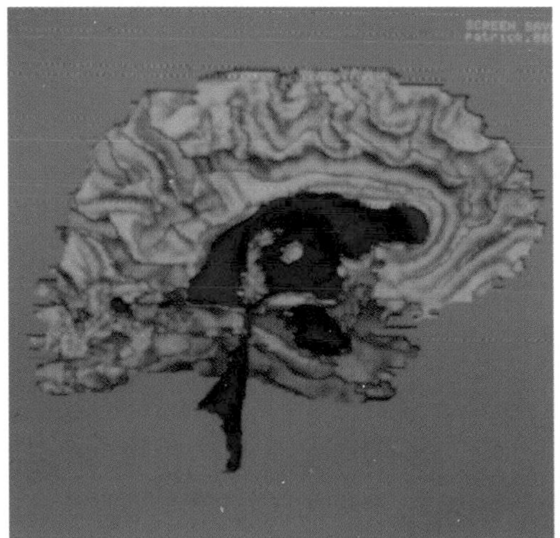

FIGURE 2.13 Segmentation of the ventricular system in combination with the left hemispheric white matter that was disarticulated from the gray matter. This image shows the potential of a T1-weighted data set with thin 1-mm slices.

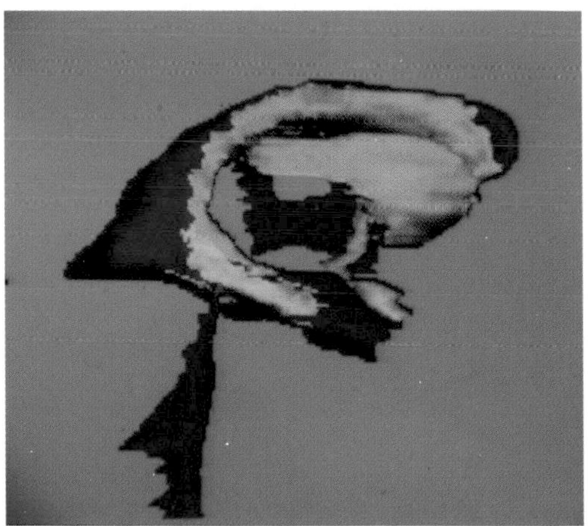

FIGURE 2.14 Segmentation of the ventricular system (blue) in combination with the caudate nucleus (yellow), lentiform nucleus (yellow), and the fornix and hippocampus (white). (Same patient as in Figure 2.13.)

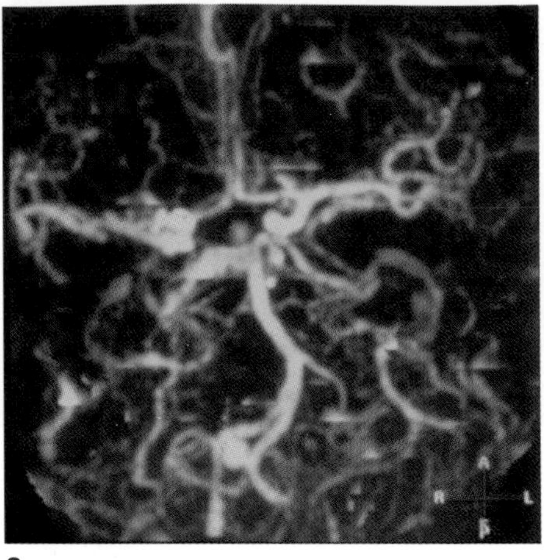

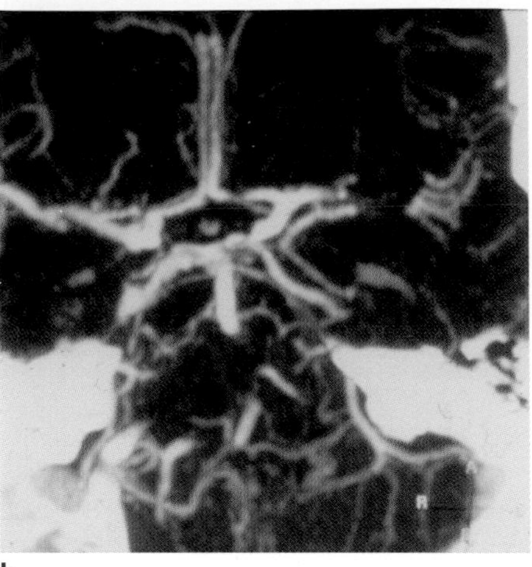

a b

FIGURE 2.15 MIP of the circle of Willis. (Courtesy of A.M.H. Huitema, Philips Medical Systems, Best, the Netherlands.) (a) In CT, the bone must be edited out to obtain images of the vessels only. (b) To avoid this process, a slab of tissue can be imaged with little risk of bone superimpositioning (slab MIP).

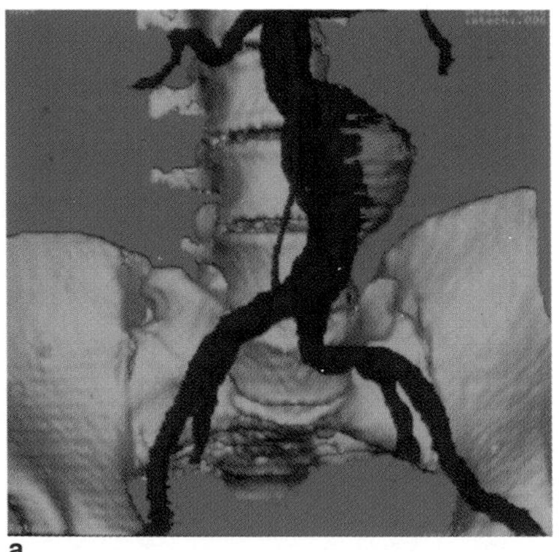

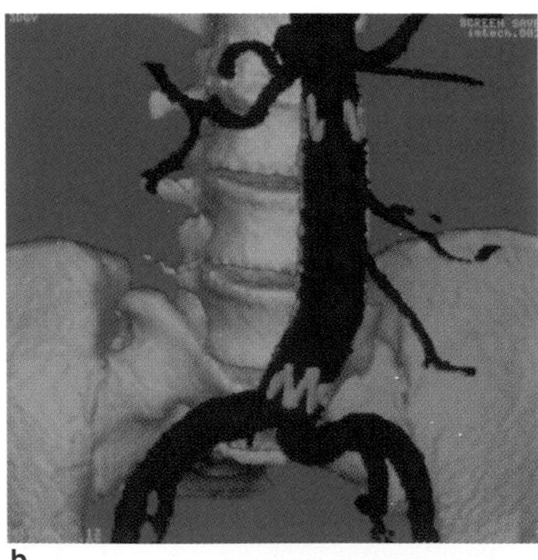

a b

FIGURE 2.16 Patient with an abdominal aneurysm that was treated with an endovascular stent. (a) Pre-operative situation with the thrombus shown in yellow. The dimensions of the required stent are taken from this reconstruction. (b) Post-operative situation showing the metallic struts of the endovascular stent graft in green.

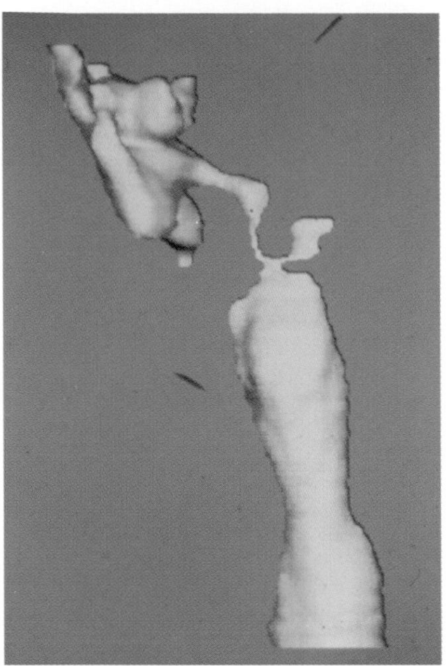

FIGURE 2.17 3D image of a subglottic tracheal stenosis in a patient with Morbus Wegner (female patient, aged 53 years).

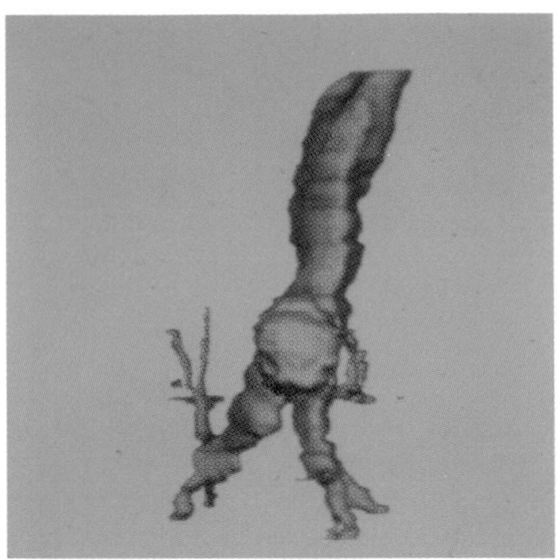

FIGURE 2.18 Tracheal compression by a local tumor (bronchus carcinoma) at the carina (male, 61 years of age).

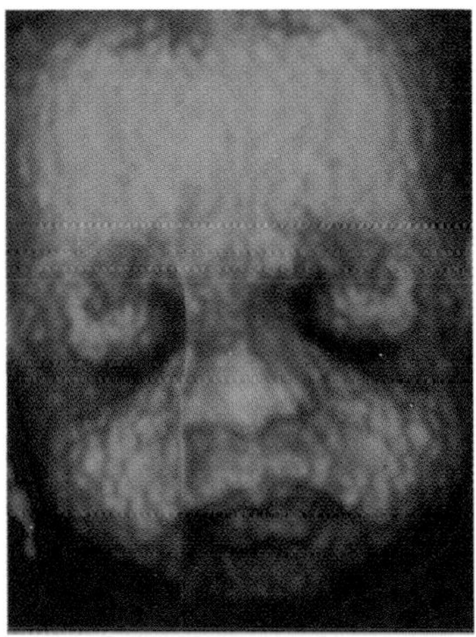

FIGURE 2.20 3D ultrasound image of a fetus at 18 weeks gestation with a bilateral cheilognathopalatoschisis. (Courtesy of R. Gombergh, Centre d'Imagerie Médicale Numerisée, Paris, France.)

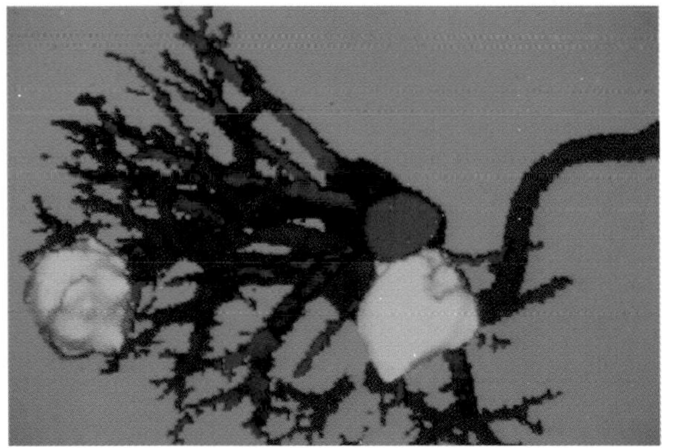

FIGURE 2.19 Superior view of a segmentation of the portal vascular system (red), the venous system (blue), and two colorectal metastases (white). This type of image shows the relationship between the individual vascular tree and the lesions to allow for local resection. (Courtesy of M.S. Van Leeuwen, Dept. of Radiology, Utrecht University Hospital, Utrecht, the Netherlands.)

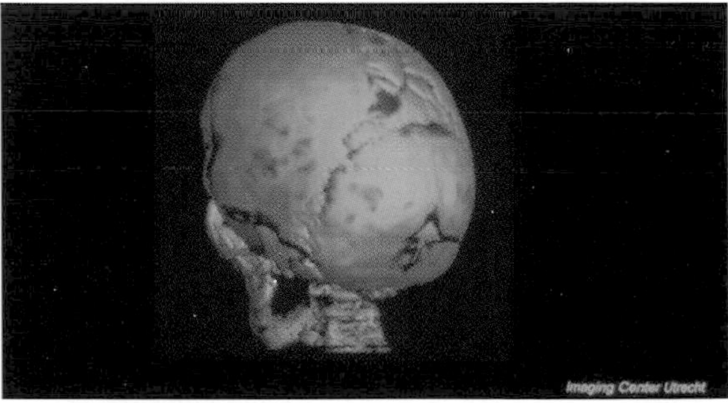

FIGURE 2.21 Skull thickness encoding in color on a 3D image of the skull. All measurements are done in a direction perpendicular to the external cranial surface. (Courtesy of K. Zuiderveld, Computer Vision Dept., Utrecht University Hospital, Utrecht, the Netherlands.)

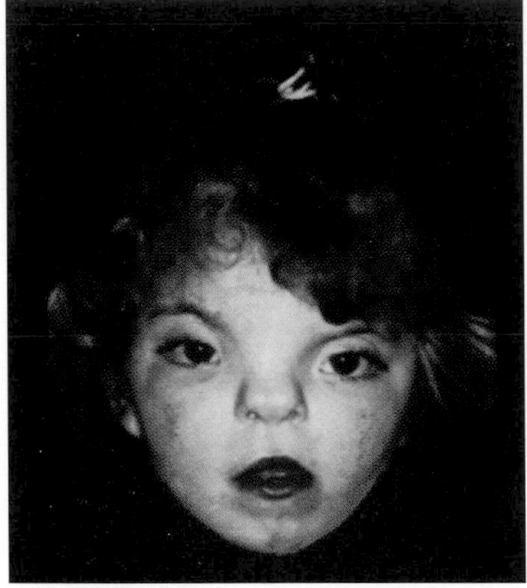

a

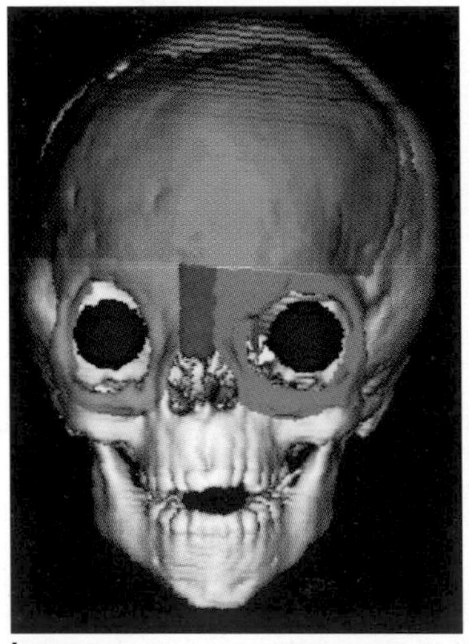

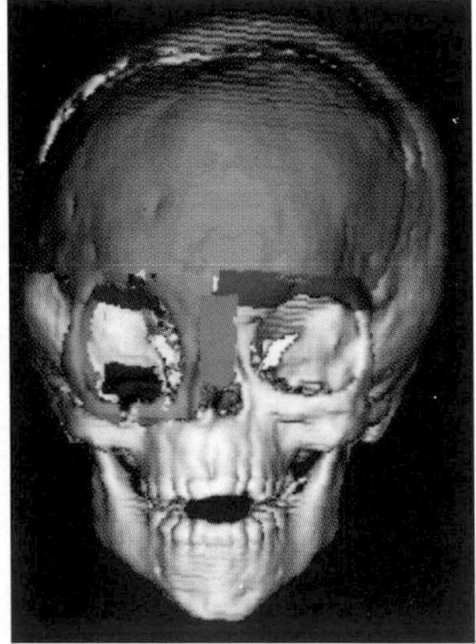

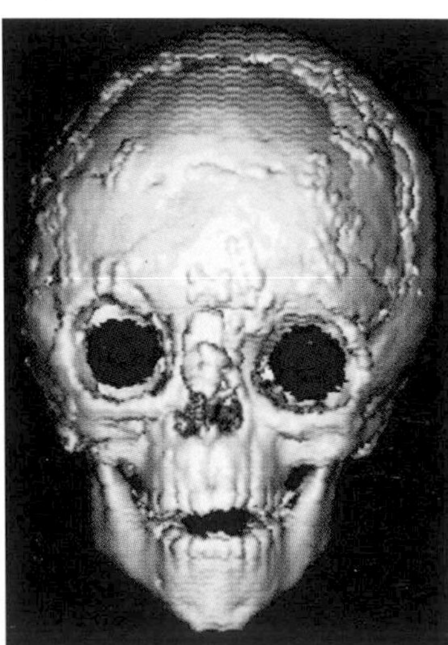

b c d

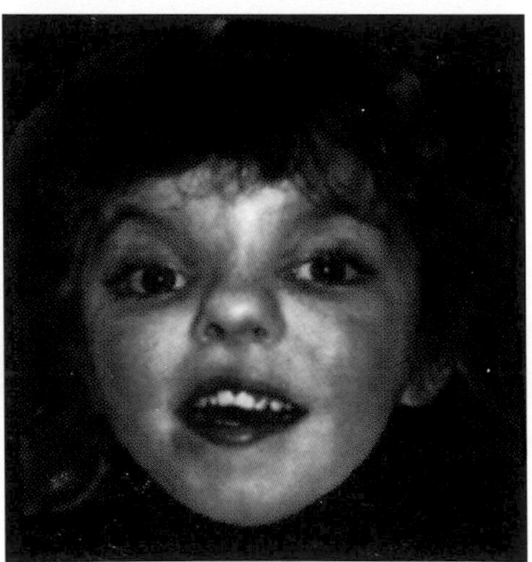

e

FIGURE 2.23 Validation of surgical simulation and consequent surgery. (Courtesy of J.L. Marsh and V.V. Patel, Mallinckrodt Institute of Radiology, St. Louis, MO.) (a) 3D pre-operative image of a 4-year-old girl with asymmetric hypertelorism secondary to craniofrontonasal dysplasia. Status after the release of the right unicoronal synostosis at 3 months of age. (b) The standard Tessier "useful orbit" orbital segments are indicated in green and yellow and the median ostectomy in orange on the unaltered pre-operative frontal surface 3D CT image. (c) Dissatisfied with the simulated outcome of mesial movement of both "useful" orbits, an asymmetrical segmented movement of the entire right ventral orbit (green) and the left superial orbital rim (orange) with onlay bone grafts (yellow) to the nasal dorsum and right orbit (purple). (d) The actual state of the patient 1 week post-operatively. (e) The appearance of the patient 1 year following correction of the hypertelorism and associated craniofacial anomalies.

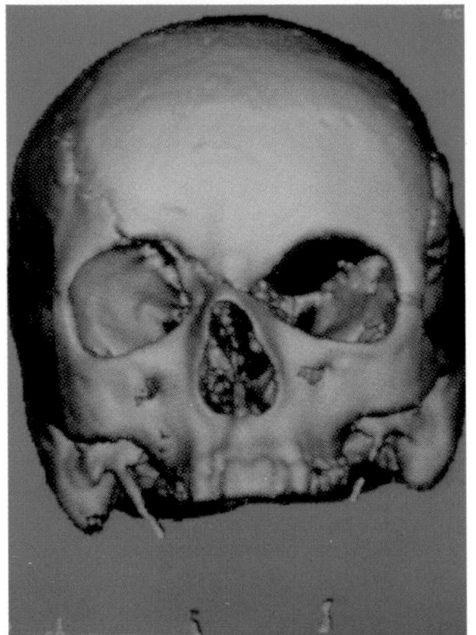

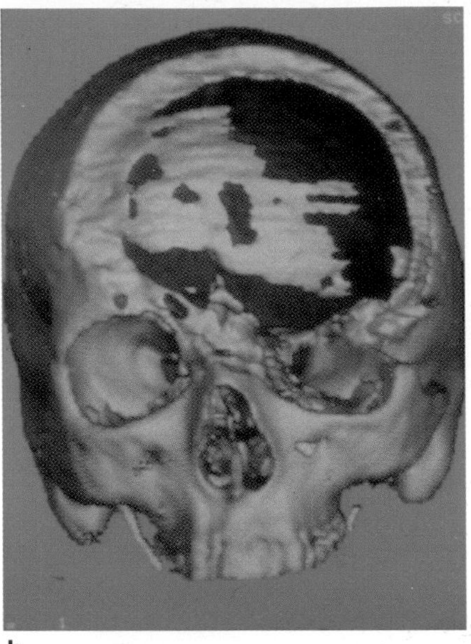

a b

FIGURE 2.25 Post-operative view of same patient as in Figure 2.10. (a) This image shows the position of the glass ionomer implant that was manufactured using a physical model. (b) In this image the implant is not shown. Now the new bone that has formed between the dura and the implant can be appreciated.

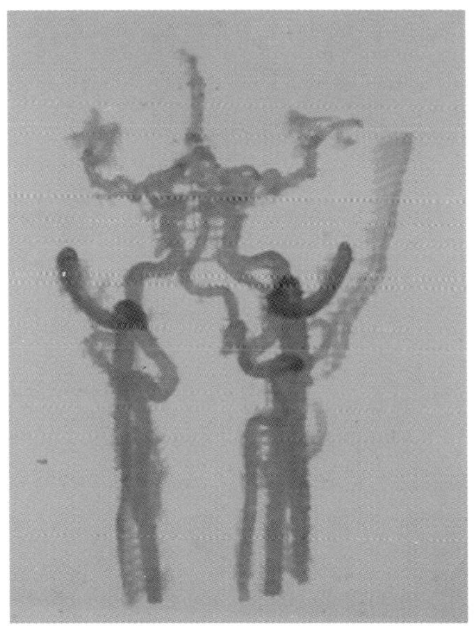

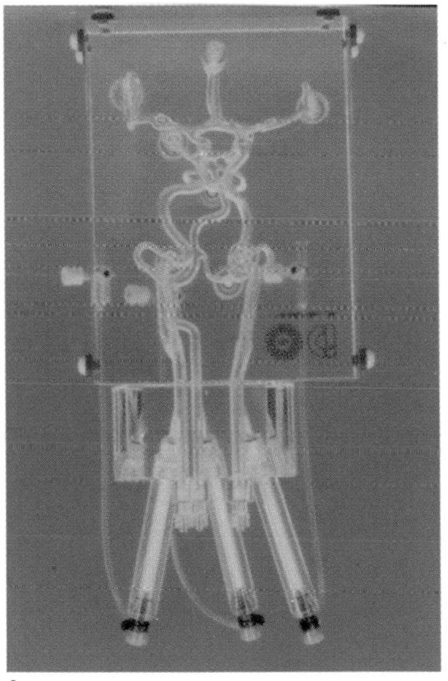

a b

FIGURE 2.26 Use of stereolithography to manufacture physical models of vascular structures, in this case the circle of Willis and the carotid and vertebral arteries. (a) Stereolithographic model (Materialise, Heverlee, Belgium) after removal of the support structures. (b) Plexiglas flow phantom for MRI made with the use of the stereolithographic model. This model was copied by a skillful glass blower. The result was cast in Plexiglas and then the glass was etched away. (Courtesy of W.P.Th.M. Mali, Department of Radiology, Utrecht University Hospital, Utrecht, the Netherlands.)

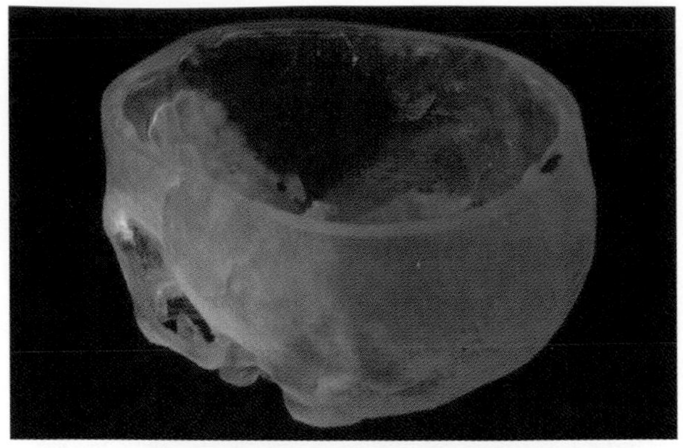

FIGURE 2.27 Use of color to highlight specific parts in the stereolithographic model. The resin contains a dope chemical that turns to a specific color as soon as the ultraviolet light reaches a critical energy. In this case the bony involvement of a hyperostotic meningioma is colored in red after the radiologist prepared a separate segmentation of the tumor extent. (Courtesy of B. Swaelens, Materialise, Heverlee, Belgium.)

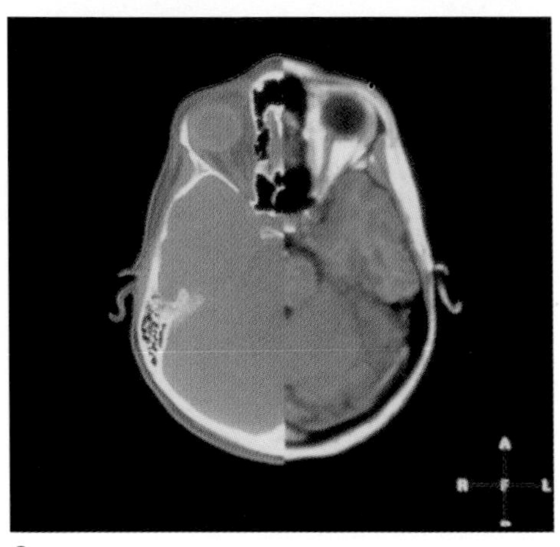

a

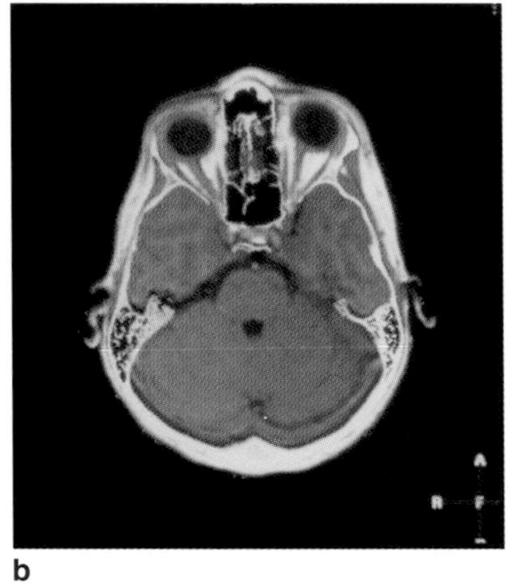

b

FIGURE 2.28 2D display of matched data sets from different imaging modalities. This case represents a patient with Romberg syndrome. A combination of CT and MRI is shown. (Courtesy of A.M.H. Huitema, Philips Medical Systems, Best, the Netherlands.) (a) Use of split image to display a multimodality matching. The transition can be moved interactively. (b) MRI image with bone replaced by CT data (yellow).

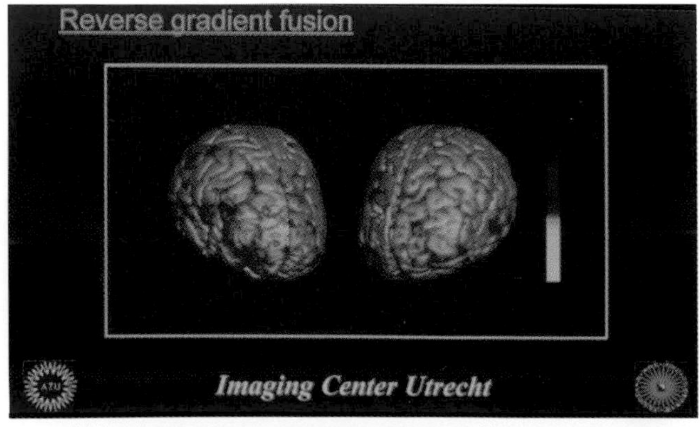

FIGURE 2.29 Multimodality matching between MRI and SPECT in a patient with a low-grade astrocytoma. The SPECT data are shown as a color wash on top of the MRI data showing a blood concentration surrounding the tumor. (Courtesy of R. Stokking, Computer Vision Dept., Utrecht University Hospital, Utrecht, the Netherlands.)

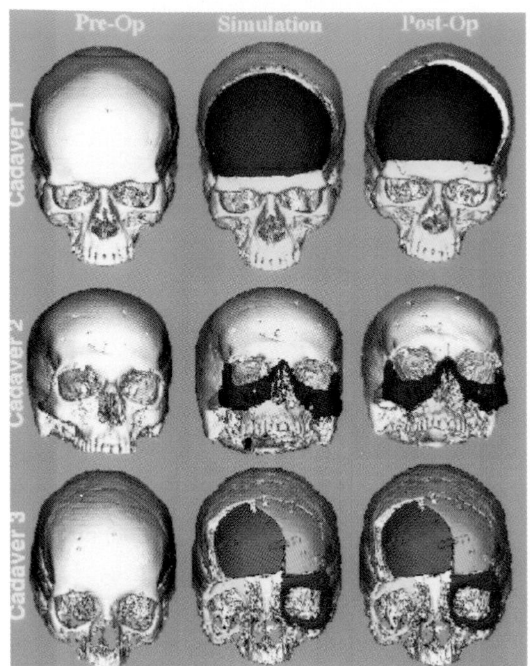

FIGURE 4.5 Cadaver study. Three cadaver skulls are shown, one in each row. The three columns depict: (1) a baseline pre-operative view, (2) a computer-generated surgical simulation which resulted from interaction with the pre-operative scan at the workstation, and (3) a post-operative view obtained upon rescanning after the surgery. The surgical procedures and methods used to assess the differences among the three volumetric data sets are explained in the text. (From Patel VV, Vannier MW, Marsh JL, Lo L-J. Assessing craniofacial surgical simulation. *IEEE Comp Graph Appl* 16 (1):46, 1996. With permission.)

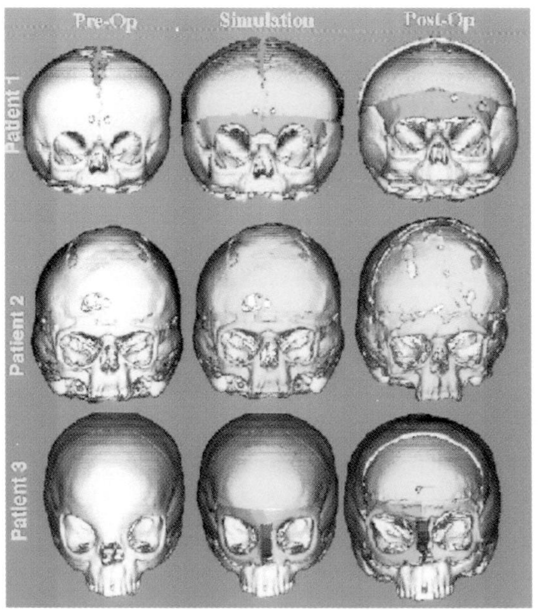

FIGURE 4.6 Patient study. Three patient skulls are shown, one in each row. These are based upon archived CT scan data sets where both pre- and post-operative scans were available *a priori*. There are three columns: (1) a baseline pre-operative view, (2) a computer-generated surgical simulation which resulted from interaction with the pre-operative scan at the workstation, and (3) a post-operative view obtained after the surgical procedure and rescanning. The surgical procedures and methods used to assess the differences among the three volumetric data sets are explained in the text. Patient 1: Female aged 4 years 1.5 months (pre-operative and simulation), with the post-operative scan at 4 years 5.8 months (7 days after surgery). Patient 2: Female aged 1.8 months (pre-operative and simulation), with the post-operative scan at 4.0 months (6 days after surgery). Patient 3: Female aged 4 years 9.7 months old (pre-operative and simulation), with the post-operative scan at 4 years 10.5 months (7 days after surgery). (From Patel VV, Vannier MW, Marsh JL, Lo L-J. Assessing craniofacial surgical simulation. *IEEE Comp Graph Appl* 16(1):46, 1996. With permission.)

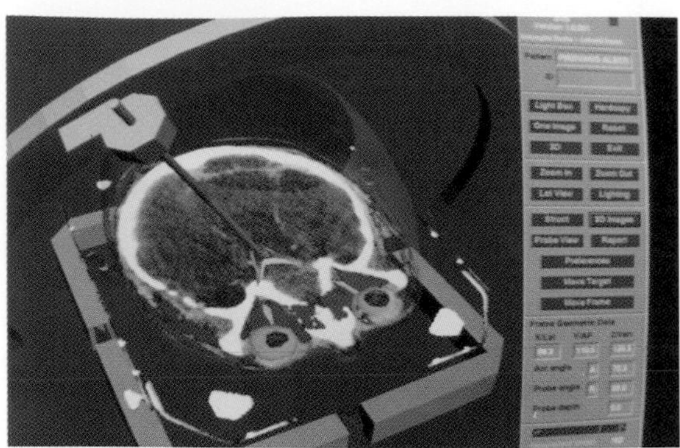

FIGURE 5.1 Interactive stereotactic neurosurgery: positioning of a probe on pre-operative CT images using an articulated stereotactic frame. (With courtesy of Dr. Cesare Giorgi, Istituto Nazionale Neurologico C. Besta, Milano, Italy.)

a 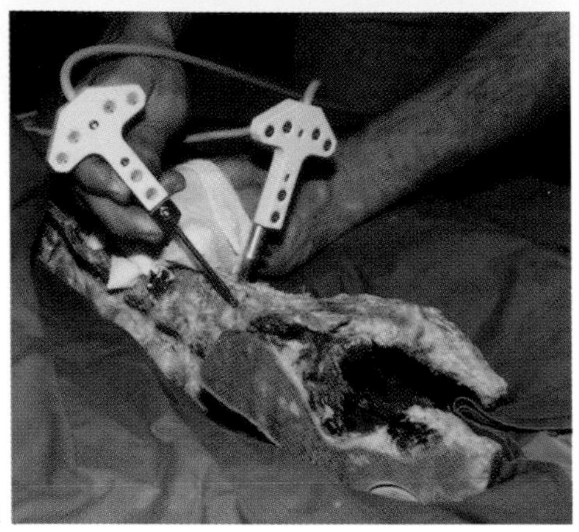

b 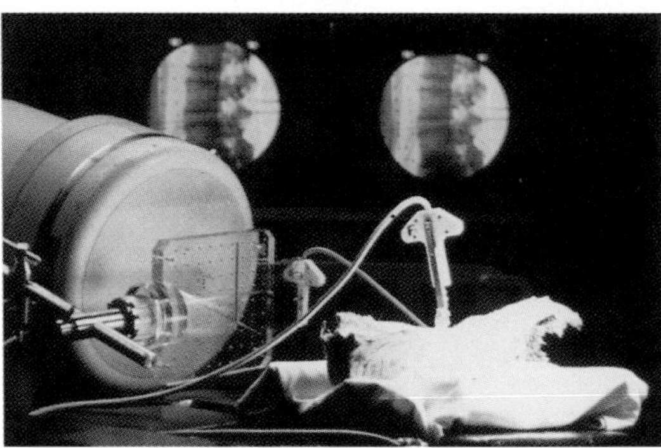

FIGURE 5.4 Multiple use of 3D localizers in computer-integrated surgery. (a) Digitization of 3D points with a pointer in a relative coordinate system attached to a bone (*in vitro* experiment on spine). (b) X-ray C arms.

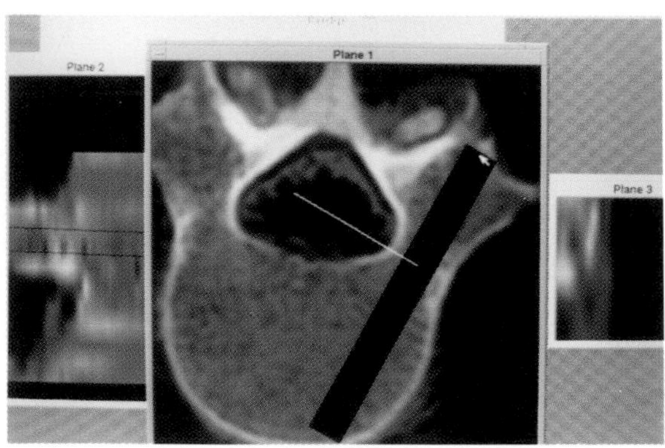

FIGURE 5.6 Interactive selection of a screw position on pre-operative CT images of a vertebra. By reslicing the volume of CT images, the surgeon first selects an oblique slice and then defines a line in this plane. A second slice passing through the selected line and a third slice orthogonal to the line are also computed and displayed. The size of the screw is made to materialize by a cylinder around the selected axis.

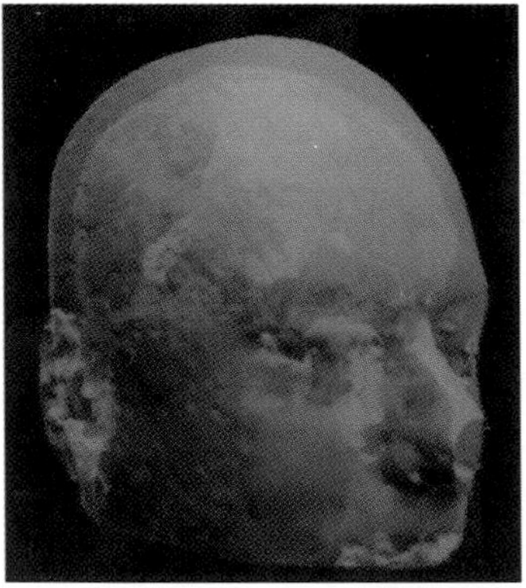

FIGURE 5.8 Registration of multimodality images using entropy-based methods. (With courtesy of S. Wells from Brigham and Women Hospital, Boston, MA. With permission of reprint from *MEDIA Journal*, Oxford University Press [WVA+96]. A rendering of the 3D models constructed from different MR acquisitions that were registered together: anatomic information (the skin, the brain, the vessels, the ventricles) was generated from the post-contrast gradient echo (SPGR) MR images, whereas the tumor was segmented from the registered and reformatted T2-weighted MR images.

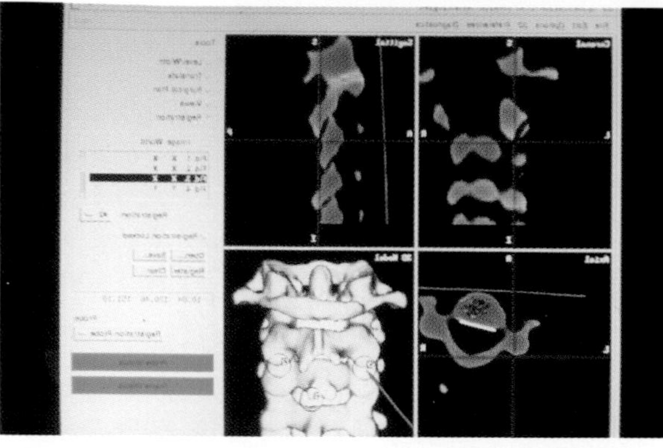

FIGURE 5.15 Standard interface for passive navigation: three reformatted slices passing through the tool tip are displayed in real time. This user interface is used for spine surgery on the Stealth workstation. (Courtesy of Sofamor-Danek.)

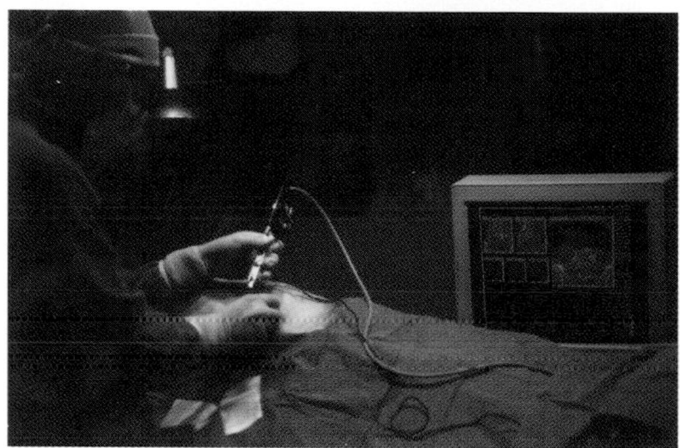

FIGURE 5.16 Computer-assisted retroperitoneoscopy. The position of a rigid endoscope is tracked in real time in pre-operative CT images. Three orthogonal CT slices passing through the tip of the endoscope are computed and displayed at a frequency of 1 Hz. It was found that using the original CT orientation (axial, sagittal, frontal) was the most acceptable for the surgeon. This method has been validated on cadavers. (Courtesy of Dr. Chaffanjon and Pr. Sarrazin, General Thoracic and Infantile Surgery Department, Grenoble Hospital.)

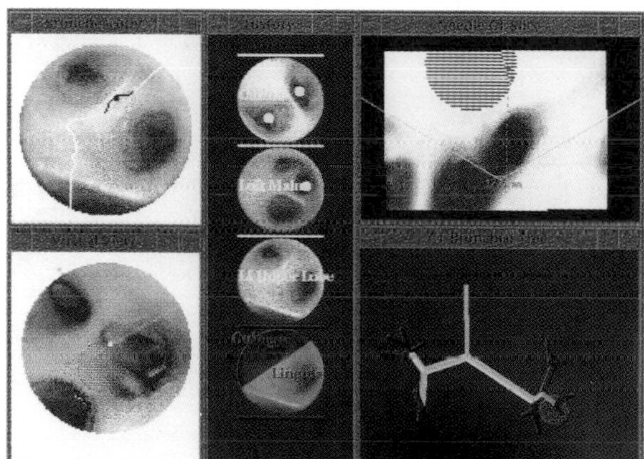

FIGURE 5.17 Computer-assisted bronchoscopy. The system achieves an automatic matching between real and virtual bronchoscopy. This permits a guidance to transbronchial needle biopsy. In the upper left window, the real bronchoscopic video sequence is analyzed in quasi real time by the computer. In the current subdivision image, we see the automatic segmentation of the wall that split both bronchi. In the middle column, the computer is able to recognize the different explored bronchi. From top to bottom, each subdivision level encountered is extracted. The bottom view identifies both current bronchi (culmen and lingula). In the bottom right window, the computer tracks the trajectory of the flexible endoscope inside a 3D geometrical model of the bronchial tree. Both current bronchi are located by specific colors. We can see a spherical target defined in the model for transbronchial needle biopsy. In the bottom left window, the system can synthesize a virtual view from CT scan data. The target appears in transparency. Using specific image processing algorithms, bronchoscopic camera position is automatically computed, so that the virtual view follows the actual camera movements and automatically matches the real view. In the upper right window, the computer shows the CT slice containing the bronchoscopic center of view and the expected biopsy needle trajectory. (Courtesy of Dr. Ferretti, Pr. Coulomb, Radiology Department, Grenoble Hospital.)

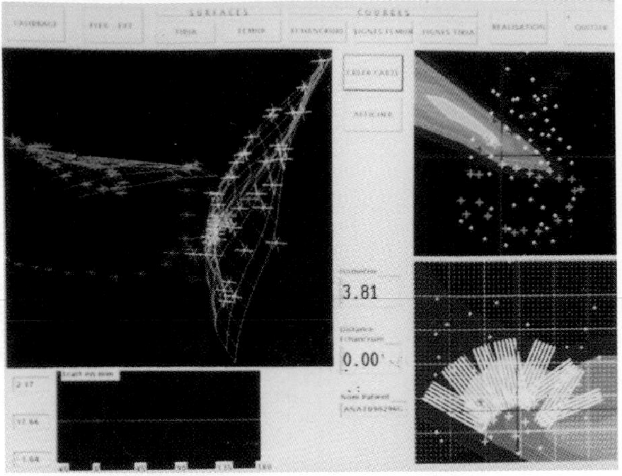

FIGURE 5.18 User interface for passive help to optimal knee ACL placement. Left part of the screen shows a 3D view of the tibial surface trajectory with respect to the femoral surface. Right part shows pseudocolor representations of the anisometry criterion on both femur and tibia surfaces, with representations of notch impingement. The surgeon locates the projection of a drilling tool tip on those images by watching the cross-hairs positions. (Courtesy of Dr. Julliard, Orthopedics Department at Cliniquie Mutualiste de Grenoble.)

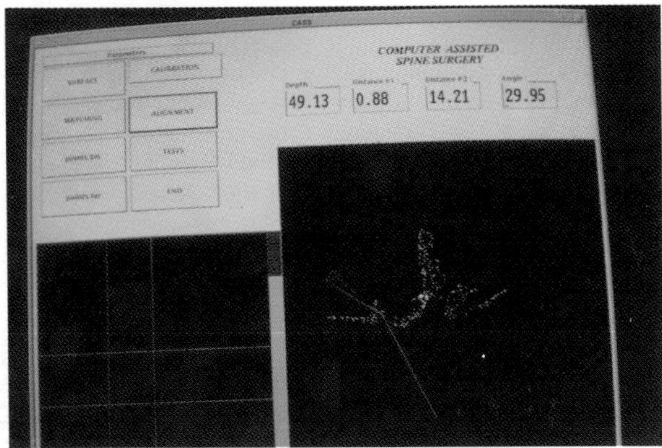

FIGURE 5.19 Passive alignment for pedicle screw insertion in spine surgery. An aiming system helps the surgeon to drill inside the vertebra pedicle according to a 3D line defined on CT images. The drill is equipped with a rigid body and its position is compared with the optimal position using cross-hairs superimposition for two points. A color bar indicates the depth of tool penetration. Graphics data are also displayed in 3D and as distances in millimeters. (Courtesy of Pr. Merloz, Orthopedics Department, Grenoble Hospital.)

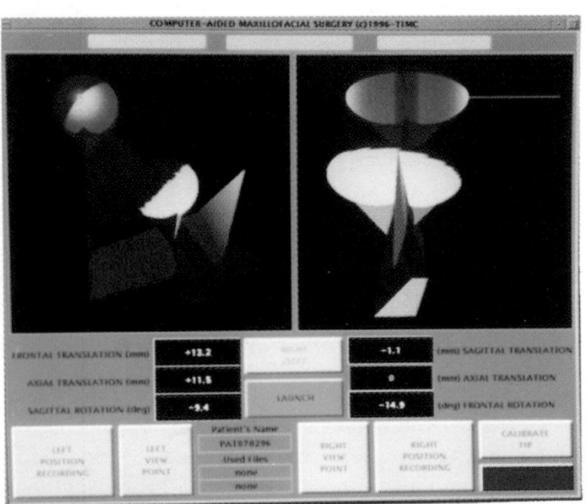

FIGURE 5.20 Interactive bone positioning in craniofacial surgery. The surgeon manipulates the condyle fragment and looks at this screen in order to superimpose the current condyle position with the reference position obtained before mandible osteotomy. Two orthogonal 3D views are presented. (Courtesy of Dr. Bettega and Pr. Raphael, Cranio-facial Department, Grenoble Hospital.)

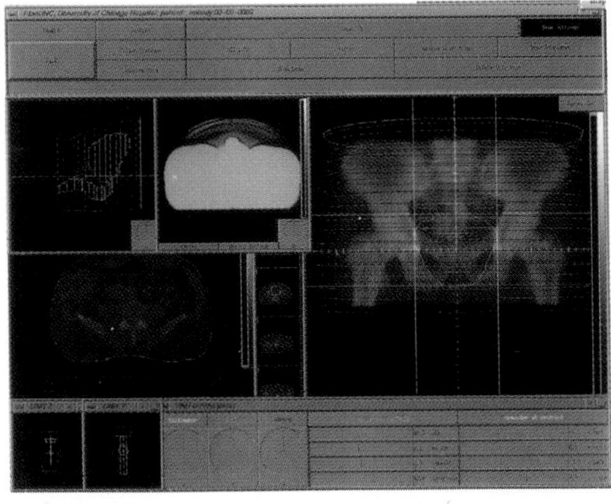

FIGURE 7.3 Main screen of the University of North Carolina radiation treatment planning system, PlanUNC. This is the control panel for the original virtual simulator. On the right, a beam aperture has been drawn by enclosing the prostate and seminal vesicle contours from each CT slice with a user-specified margin, as seen from the point of view of an anterior field. A digitally reconstructed radiograph is also included as a backdrop to the beam's-eye view.

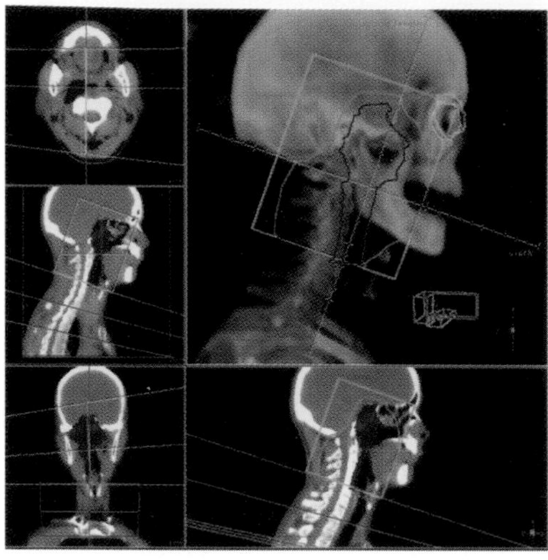

FIGURE 7.4 Example of non-coplanar field matching in the Picker AcQSim CT simulator. In the lower right window, a lateral field is shown to have its lower border matching the superior plane of an anterior supraclavicular field. (upper right) Computed radiograph from the lateral beam's perspective. (other panels) Multiplanar reformations of the 3D CT data.

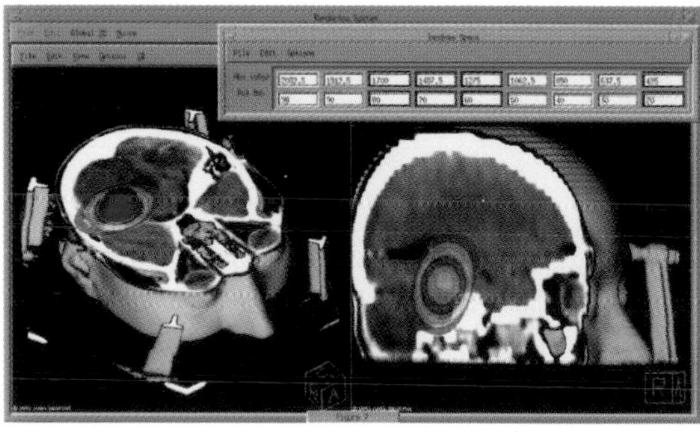

FIGURE 7.5 Visualization of idealized high dose region, calculated dose distribution, CT data, and patient surface from the University of Wisconsin stereotactic radiosurgery planning program of Gehring and colleagues.

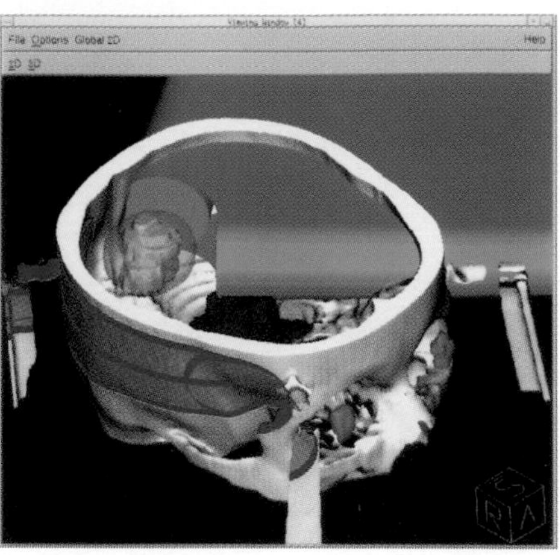

FIGURE 7.6 Example of visualization of several radiosurgery fields from the ADAC Pinnacle^3 treatment planning program (see text).

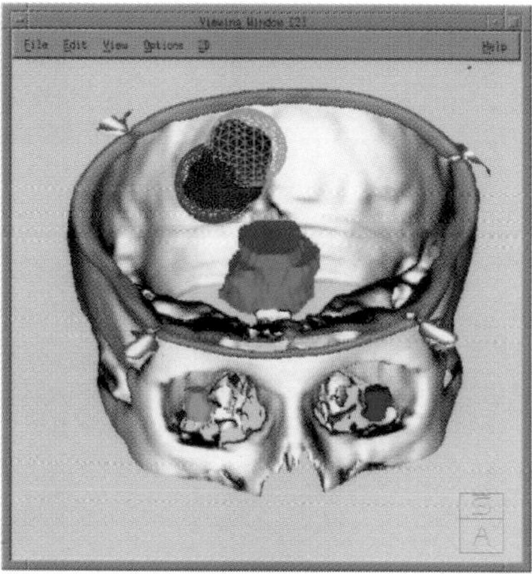

FIGURE 7.7 Visualization from Pinnacle^3 for a radiosurgery case incorporating both geometrically and volumetrically rendered components.

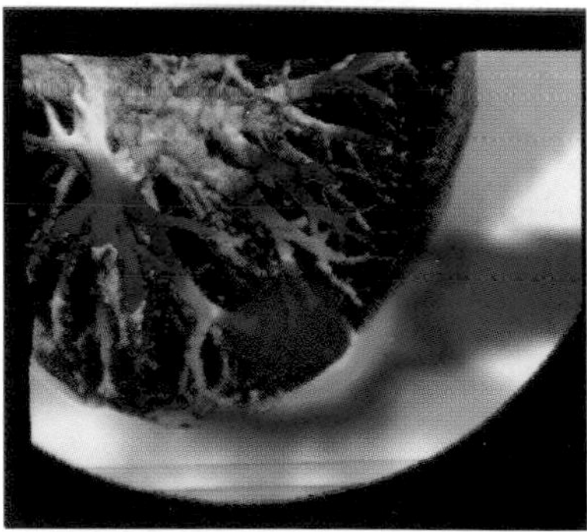

FIGURE 7.10 Volume-rendered view of a lung tumor from an inferior viewpoint. Using a z-buffer to retain 3D coordinates, color has been mapped onto each pixel according to calculated radiation dose for a five-field plan, from high (red) to low (blue).

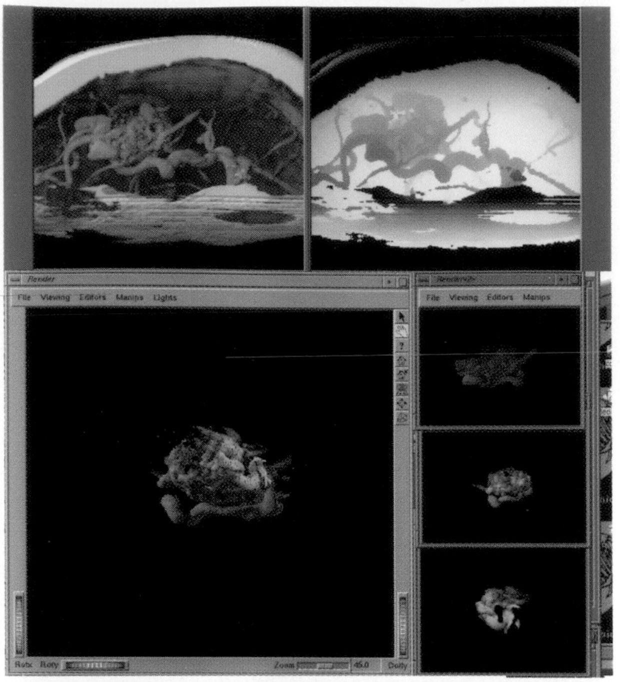

FIGURE 7.11 Example of 3D aided segmentation for a cerebral AVM. Rendered view (upper left) and corresponding z-buffer (upper right, darker = closer to viewpoint). Partial surfaces of the AVM (lower right) from the top view and two others have been combined into a single 3D target volume (lower left).

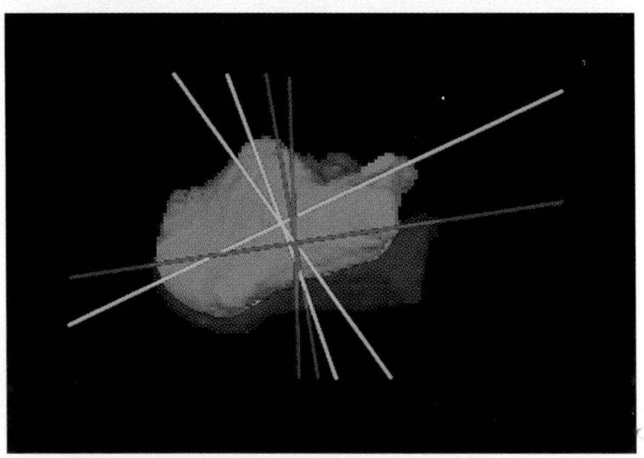

FIGURE 9.5 A calcaneus is shown in two positions: pronated (lighter gray) and supinated. The principal axes of the bone in each position are also shown; in the pronated position they are green, and in the supinated position they are red.

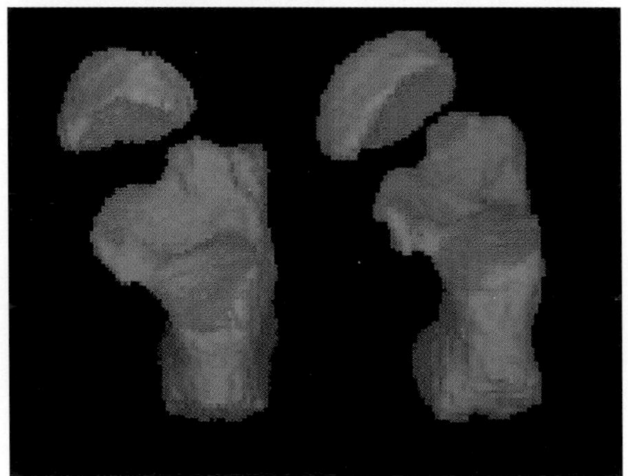

FIGURE 9.14 This dorsal view of the calcaneus and navicular in pronation (left) and supination (right) illustrates the areas where the talus was close to those bones. In this example, the areas where the talus was 4.0 mm or less from the other bones is colored pink and can be considered indicative of joint contact areas. In this example, the joint was not loaded, so the contact areas do not necessarily represent the areas of weight transmission.

The essential differences in the methods come from what ST_1 and ST_2 constitute and how they are represented and from Steps 1, 2, and 6. ST_1 and ST_2 may correspond to intrinsic objects intentionally attached to the body region for observing a common object in the two acquired scenes.[70,71] Most of the time, they correspond to intrinsic objects in the body region under investigation. ST_1 and ST_2 may represent a set of points corresponding to landmarks or features,[60,62,66,68] edges,[64,69] surfaces,[61,65,72,73] or regions.[74] In all cases, these entities should represent nearly the same geometric aspects of the same objects imaged in the two scenes.

Examples of the criterion function and the stopping criterion commonly used are given below.

$$\begin{aligned}
&G_{2,1}(P) = \sum_{v \in ST_2} \left(\text{distance of } v \text{ to } ST_1\right)^2 \\
&G(P) = G_{2,1}(P) \\
&G(P) = \max\left(G_{2,1}(P), G_{1,2}(P)\right) \\
&G(P) = \sqrt{G_{2,1}(P)G_{1,2}(P)} \\
&G(P) = \frac{1}{2}\left(G_{2,1}(P) + G_{1,2}(P)\right) \\
&S(P): G(P) \le \text{a threshold.}
\end{aligned} \tag{1.13}$$

Various definitions of distance have been used by different methods. To speed up the search for P, commonly a multiresolution approach is taken. In this approach, several representations of the structures are created first corresponding to different levels of discretization going from very coarse to fine. P is found first using the coarsest representation, and subsequently refined, stepwise using finer representations. This usually saves a considerable amount of search which otherwise has to be carried out using representations at high levels of discretization.

The simplest among object-based (rigid) approaches is the principal axes method,[75] also known as the method of principal component analysis, inertia axes method, and singular value decomposition. Let $\{Q_1^i, \ldots, Q_{n_i}^i\}$, be the set of points representing ST_i for $i = 1, 2$, where each Q_j^i is a three-component vector, representing the coordinates of Q_j^i with respect to the structure coordinate system of ST_i. Then the centroid O_i of ST_i is given by

$$O_i = \frac{1}{n_i}\sum_j Q_j^i. \tag{1.14}$$

The 3×3 covariance (or inertia) matrix M_i of ST_i is given by

$$M_i = \left[Q_1^i - O_i, \ldots, Q_{n_i}^i - O_i\right]\left[Q_1^i - O_i, \ldots, Q_{n_i}^i - O_i\right]^T. \tag{1.15}$$

The eigenvectors of M_i define the directions of the principal axes of ST_i. The axes system defined by O_i and these eigenvectors is called the principal axes system of ST_i. If ST_1 and ST_2 are similar in shape, then to match ST_2 to ST_1, O_2 is translated to O_1 and the principal axes of ST_2 are rotated to match with those of ST_1. Note that if $\boldsymbol{x}$ is an eigenvector of M_i, then so is $-\boldsymbol{x}$. Hence, the positive and negative directions of the principal axes cannot be ascertained. If the rotations are known to

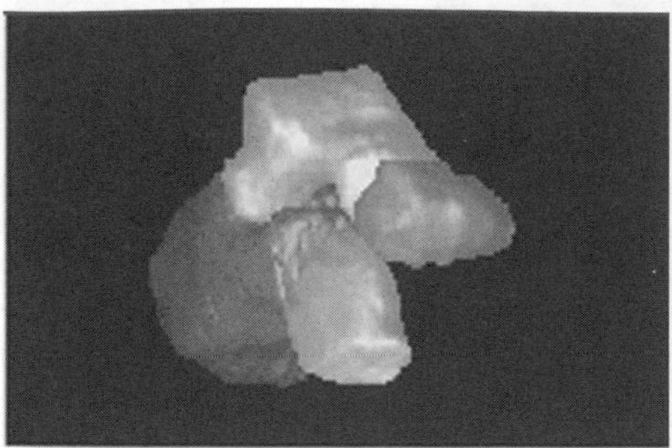
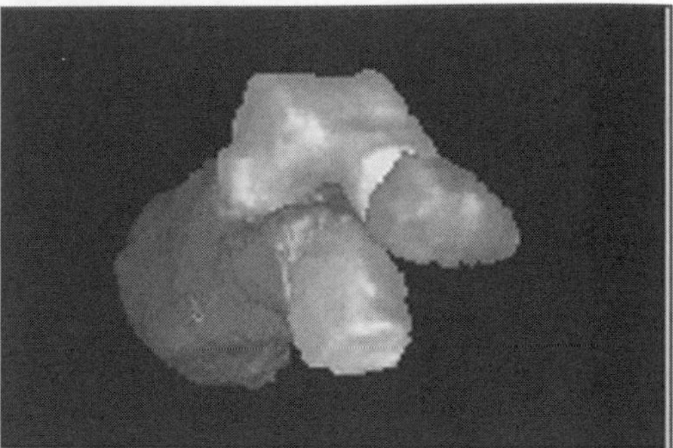

FIGURE 1.13 Illustration of an application of an approach to object-based registration. The two pictures show renditions of the four bones in the peritalar joint complex of the foot obtained from MRI for two different positions of the joint. By registering the same bone in two positions, the motion (translation and rotation) of the bone from one position to the next can be determined.

be less than 90°, this knowledge can be utilized in estimating correctly the rotations. Otherwise, additional information becomes necessary to select one among the several solutions provided by this method.

Figure 1.13 illustrates the use of this method in the analysis of the kinematics of the midtarsal joints of the foot.[76,77] 3D scenes are acquired corresponding to different positions of the joints. In each position, the surfaces of the bones are constructed from the scenes and their principal axes system is determined. The motion of a given bone is quantified by matching its principal axes system from one position to the next. The method has also been applied to the *in vivo* analysis of kinematics of the glenohumeral joints.[78]

1.2.5.2.2 Deformable

These approaches are far fewer in the literature than rigid object-based techniques. Two groups of methods may be identified — point (or landmark) based[79,80] and atlas based.[81–83]

In point-based methods, homologous landmarks are identified on the two structures ST_1 and ST_2. The optimum deformation needed to match the points in ST_2 with those in ST_1 is then computed.

In atlas-based methods, a topographical standard atlas is first created. For the human brain, several established techniques are available[84,85] for this purpose. Such an atlas constitutes ST_1. From an acquired scene for the same body region as that for the atlas, features such as landmarks, ridges, and boundary contours are identified. These are then matched with homologous features in the atlas by deforming ST_2.

Using the rigid transformation resulting from matching carefully implanted extrinsic markers as a gold standard in a neurosurgical application,[73] the accuracy of a variety of scene-based and object-based rigid registration techniques has been evaluated.[86] The modalities tested included CT to MR and MR to PET. Generally, the errors for the latter task were greater than for the former. In the former, the best results were obtained by scene-based techniques.

The effectiveness of a registration method, scene based or object based, rigid or deformable, depends on accurately identifying the same object information in the two given scenes. Object information in images is inherently fuzzy. As observed in Ref. 86, when object gradation information is utilized (as in scene-based methods), registration may become more accurate. Given these factors, fuzzy object-based registration may combine the best of the current (hard) object- and scene-based methods. Considering the fact that deformation becomes necessary in dealing with most soft-tissue objects, fuzzy mechanics theories and algorithms may be needed for effectively registering soft object information in acquired scenes. Clearly, as in other preprocessing operations, segmentation is needed for registration.

An object-based and a scene-based registration method are available in 3DVIEWNIX under PREPROCESS → StructureOperations → Register and PREPROCESS → SceneOperations → Register.

1.2.6 Segmentation

The purpose of these operations is to extract object information from given scenes and to output this as a structure system. In many situations, the structure system consists of a single structure. As we observed in previous sections, and as we will see in later sections, segmentation is needed for most of the 3D imaging operations. It is also the most difficult of all operations.

Segmentation may be thought of as consisting of two related tasks — recognition and delineation. *Recognition* is the high-level task of determining roughly the whereabouts of the object in the scene. *Delineation* is the low-level task of determining the precise spatial extent of the object and its graded composition. In most recognition tasks, trained human operators outperform any computer algorithms. On the contrary, computer algorithms exist that are more precise, accurate, and efficient than human delineation of object regions. Human delineation that specifies graded objectness is impossible at present. As we will see below, recognition and delineation are not completely disparate steps in segmentation. It is helpful to follow this conceptual division to study segmentation methods systematically and to understand their strengths and weaknesses.

Approaches to recognition may be broadly classified into two groups: automatic and human assisted. In automatic methods, one of two approaches is taken. In the *knowledge-based* approach, artificial intelligence techniques are used to represent knowledge of objects in the body region of interest.[87–90] Usually, a preliminary delineation of objects is done first and then object hypotheses are formed and tested. This loop may be executed several times before an acceptable solution is found. For the *atlas-based* approach, an atlas representing the geometry and topological relationships of the objects in the body region is constructed first.[81,82,84,91–94] Subsequently, certain geometric entities, such as points, ridges, contours, and anatomic planes, identified in the given scene (delineation step) for the same body region are mapped to match with homologous entities in the atlas. This mapping is then applied to the whole scene to recognize object regions/boundaries in the scene from such information stored in the atlas.

In automatic recognition methods, a question arises as to what to do in case of failures. Completely automatic methods that are fool-proof and that have been demonstrated to work correctly routinely in trials involving a large number of patient studies do not seem to have been constructed yet. The premise in human-assisted methods then is that often a simple help from an operator (on a per-study basis) is sufficient as a recognition aid. Therefore, if we can make this process efficient, then the uncertainties of the automatic methods can be overcome, and we have a solution that is practical. This help may be in the form of (1) specification of a few "seed" points in the object region or on its boundary, (2) indication of a box enclosing the object, or (3) clicking of a mouse button to accept a real object that has been delineated or to reject a false object.

It is important to distinguish between two types of recognition tasks, the first for identifying pathological growths such as lesions in the breast and lungs via X-ray projection images,[95–98] and the second for identifying the anatomic organs in scenes. The former is currently an active area of research, commonly referred to as computer-aided diagnosis. The pathologies are detected commonly via the classical two-stage pattern recognition approach: scene-intensity-based feature extraction and pattern classification. Unfortunately, this paradigm is ineffective for the second task of recognizing anatomic organs. As such, approaches that consider shape of and relationship among objects have been investigated.[87–94] However, such (automatic) recognition strategies that have been demonstrated to work routinely on a large number of patient studies for any body region are yet to be developed.

Approaches to delineation, on the other hand, are studied far more extensively than those for recognition. In fact, usually delineation itself is considered to be the total segmentation problem. That is, whatever is output by the delineation method is considered to represent the object of interest. Two classes of methods exist for delineation: boundary based, in which the output structure represents the boundary of the object, and region based, in which the output structure represents the region occupied by the object. In both groups, the output structure may be hard (crisp) or fuzzy. In the hard case, the structure is a hard set of certain elements, each with a membership value in the structure of either 0 or 1. This representation does not allow capturing graded composition of objects. In the fuzzy case, the structure is a fuzzy set with a degree of membership (between 0 and 1) associated with each element.

If we combine the two strategies of recognition — automatic and human assisted — with the four groups of delineation approaches, there are eight classes of segmentation strategies possible, as listed below.

1. Hard, boundary-based, automatic.
2. Fuzzy, boundary-based, automatic.
3. Hard, boundary-based, assisted.
4. Fuzzy, boundary-based, assisted.
5. Hard, region-based, automatic.
6. Fuzzy, region-based, automatic.
7. Hard, region-based, assisted.
8. Fuzzy, region-based, assisted.

In the rest of this section, we will study these strategies systematically, focusing mainly on the most common approaches.

1.2.6.1 Hard, Boundary-Based, Automatic Methods

There are mainly two classes of approaches for creating hard boundary representations of objects from scenes of their body region. In the first group, it is assumed that an object surface is specifiable via a fixed scene intensity threshold value.[99–116] That is, the surface in the scene domain on which the scene intensity is the specified value is taken to be the structure representing the object. This group of approaches is commonly referred to as *iso-surfacing*. In the second group, the rate of change of scene intensity (scene intensity gradient) is used to locate and form the boundaries.[117–124] We will refer to these methods as gradient based.

1.2.6.1.1 Iso-surfacing methods

Among currently popular iso-surfacing methods, there are two distinct groups.

The first, which we will call digital surface methods, output a digital representation of the object surface. "Digital" here means that the representation consists of basic elements, which have one of a small number of possible shapes and orientations. For the 3D case, for example, the basic elements may be voxels or the faces of voxels. If the slice spacing is the same between all slices of the given scene, then all voxels of the scene are of identical size. There are six types of voxel faces based on their orientation. They are all rectangular, and their size depends on the relationship between pixel size and slice spacing of the scene.

The second group of methods output the object surface as a set of triangular or other polygonal elements. These are usually not digital in the sense described above. We will refer to these as polygonal surface methods.

Digital surfaces — These methods[99–105] start with a formal mathematical definition of a digital surface as the boundary between a digital object — a connected component of voxels whose intensities are at or above the specified intensity threshold T — and a digital co-object — a connected

0	20	30	10	15
20	50	80	20	10
30	70	40	10	20
16	15	20	60	15
10	15	20	30	20

FIGURE 1.14 Digital boundary definition for a threshold of 50. There are two digital objects — the set of three pixels with intensities 50, 70, and 80 and the set of one pixel with value 60. There is one digital co-object — the set of all remaining pixels in the scene domain. The two digital boundaries are shown in bold.

component of voxels whose intensities are below T. In a scene $\mathscr{V} = (V,g)$, the common face between two voxels v_1 and v_2 (that differ in exactly one coordinate by 1) is a boundary element if $g(v_1) \geq T$ and $g(v_2) < T$. The orientation of this element is specified by the unit vector in the direction from the center of v_1 to the center of v_2. The six possible boundary element orientations correspond to the unit vectors in the six principal directions of the scene coordinate axes. Figure 1.14 shows an example for the 2D case, with two digital objects and one digital co-object and two boundaries between them. Boundary elements in this case are oriented pixel edges. We will refer to the oriented boundary element between v_1 and v_2 by the ordered pair (v_1,v_2), where it is clear that v_1 is inside the boundary and v_2 is outside.

The subject of digital surfaces is well studied in the literature.[99–105,125–133] The definitions are designed to ensure that the surfaces satisfy the following three properties:

Closure: The surface partitions the scene domain into two sets, an interior and an exterior, such that any path taken starting from a voxel in the interior to a voxel in the exterior meets the surface.

Orientedness: The surface itself has an inside and an outside. The boundary element orientation indicates the surface orientation locally.

Connectedness: Any boundary element in the surface can be reached from any other boundary element going from one element to the adjacent without leaving the surface.

These are all desirable properties and the surfaces of (real) objects in the body region possess them. The digital iso-surfacing algorithms guarantee that what they output indeed satisfies these properties. Below we present, as an example, one such algorithm,[101,102] which is one of the most efficient among algorithms for finding closed, oriented, and connected iso-surfaces.

1. Find an initial face and place it in a queue Q.
2. If Q is empty, stop. Else, take out a face F from Q, output F, and find its unique adjacent face F' in each direction that is assigned to F. The direction(s) assigned to a face and how to find the adjacent face are illustrated in Figure 1.15.
3. For each F' found in Step 2, if it was not found previously, put it in Q. Go to Step 2.

Note that, in any boundary surface, as per the model described in Figure 1.15, only those faces that are orthogonal to the z axis of the scene coordinate system have two directions associated with them and the rest have only one. This implies that most of the time the algorithm goes from a face to a unique adjacent face and once in a while branches off to two adjacent faces to ensure that all faces on the closed, connected surface are found. If the level of discretization (determined by the

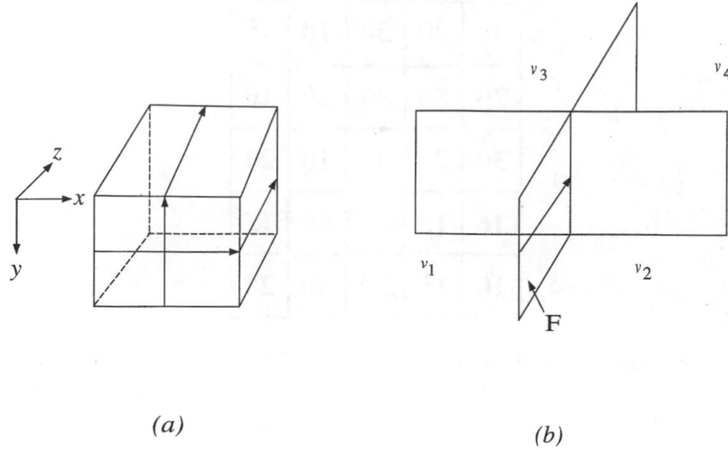

FIGURE 1.15 (a) A voxel with two sequences of arrows drawn around it. The arrows on the invisible faces are not shown but are determined by continuing the sequence. To determine the direction assigned to a face with orientation (v_1,v_2) (say, $v_1 = (x,y,z)$ and $v_2 = (x+1,y,z)$), fix v_1 to be the voxel shown, locate the face (v_1,v_2) (in this case the visible face orthogonal to the x axis), and find the direction (in this case, it points in $+z$ direction). (b) To find the face adjacent to a face $F = (v_1,v_2)$ in the direction shown, locate the other two voxels v_3 and v_4 sharing the edge pointed to by the arrow indicating the direction. The adjacent face $F' = (v_4,v_2)$ if $g(v_3) \geq T$ and $g(v_4) \geq T$, $F' = (v_1,v_3)$ if $g(v_3) < T$, otherwise $F' = (v_3,v_4)$.

size of the output faces) desired for the output surface is different from that of the input scene, then this is easily incorporated[102] into Step 2 (Figure 1.15) wherein the intensities of v_3 and v_4 are estimated via a local interpolation operation such as trilinear (see Section 1.2.4.1). For ease of understanding, we eliminated several optimizing computational steps in the above algorithm. See Refs. 101–103 for such details including parallelization,[103] and see Refs. 99, 100, and 126 for predecessors of this type of algorithm.

The above iso-surfacing algorithm is a 3D version of a general algorithm that works for any finite two- and higher dimensional scene.[131] Theories and algorithms for defining closed, connected, oriented digital surfaces using voxels as the boundary elements,[100,132,133] as well as for other non-rectilinear digitization grids,[104] have also been developed. There is a related topic of constructing digital surfaces from continuous parametric descriptions of mathematical surfaces. This has applications in and is an active area of computer-aided design and graphics. See Refs. 134–136 for examples.

Iso-surfacing methods based on voxels and voxel faces are available in 3DVIEWNIX under PREPROCESS → Segment → Threshold.

Polygonal surfaces — The most popular among these methods are undoubtedly those that use triangles as the basic surface elements. The main reason for the emphasis on triangular elements is the availability of standard software libraries such as Open GL and hardware accelerators and rendering engines from workstation vendors such as Silicon Graphics, Inc. and Sun Microsystems to rapidly generate renditions of such surfaces. We will examine this and other aspects for comparing digital and polygonal iso-surfacing methods in Section 1.3.

The most popular triangulated iso-surfacing methods are the so-called "marching cubes" approaches[106,107] and its descendents.[108–110,113–116] The basic idea underlying this approach[107] can be explained with reference to Figure 1.16 as follows. Let $\mathcal{V} = (V,g)$ be a given scene and let T be the specified threshold. Consider a $2 \times 2 \times 2$ block of voxels as in Figure 1.16, wherein $v_1, v_2, \ldots, v_8$ represent the centers of these eight voxels. For clarity, the voxels themselves are not shown. Each of these voxels v_i may be inside or outside the boundary surface we wish to construct, depending

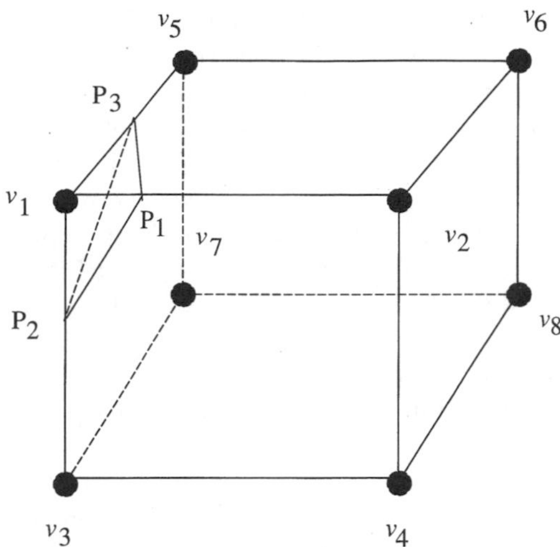

FIGURE 1.16 Illustration of surface construction by the marching cubes family of methods. $v_1, \ldots, v_8$ are centers of voxels in a $2 \times 2 \times 2$ block. There are 2^8 possible configurations of v_i inside or outside the boundary. In the configuration shown, v_1 is assumed to be inside and the rest of the voxels in this block to be outside the boundary.

on if $g(v_i) \geq T$ or $g(v_i) < T$. One such configuration is illustrated in Figure 1.16 corresponding to $g(v_1) > T$ and $g(v_i) < T$ for $2 \leq i \leq 8$. In this case, only v_1 within this $2 \times 2 \times 2$ block is inside the surface. We construct the surface locally with one triangle as shown in the figure. Here the location of P_1 along the line connecting (the centers of) v_1 and v_2 is determined by linear interpolation. Since $g(v_1) > T$ and $g(v_2) < T$, there exists P_1 along this line at which the intensity equals T. The locations of P_2 and P_3 are determined analogously. Clearly, for any other configuration, the triangular arrangement can be determined in a similar fashion. In fact, there are only 15 distinct configurations (taking into account rotation and symmetry) of triangular arrangements. These can be stored in a table, and surface construction can then be done by examining each $2 \times 2 \times 2$ block of voxels and table lookup.

In the above method, in its original form,[107] there is no guarantee that the resulting surface will have any of the three properties we described previously. Connectedness is not considered in the design of the algorithm. However, examples can be easily created to show when the resulting surfaces are not closed.[108] Many subsequent papers have proposed solutions to overcome these problems. However, a systematic theoretical framework that guarantees the satisfaction of the three properties is still lacking. A recent attempt to provide such a framework through the established results from digital surfaces can be found in Ref. 137.

There exists a separate class of approaches[138–143] to create triangulated (and other polygonal) surfaces. These early attempts to create surfaces in 3D imaging were motivated by the problem of creating surfaces that "tile" contours given on a stack of slices. If these are iso-intensity contours, then the resulting surfaces can be thought of as iso-surfaces. One unsolved problem in these approaches is to create "correct" surfaces in situations where an object branches and/or merges from one slice to the next.

1.2.6.1.2 Gradient-based methods

The basic premise in these methods[117–124] is that in the vicinity of the object boundary, the magnitude of the scene intensity gradient is much higher than at points far away from the boundary. Therefore, the set of all boundary elements — pixels/voxels/pixel edges/voxel faces — at which the intensity gradient magnitude is sufficiently high, should represent the object boundary we are seeking. Unfortunately, in practice, this set contains elements that do not belong to the structure and/or it lacks elements that really belong to the structure. To overcome this problem, a variety of optimization strategies are devised with the hope of minimizing missing and false boundary segments.[118,119,121–124,144–151] One possible approach is to assign a cost to every boundary element and to find a boundary whose total cost is the smallest among all possible boundaries. Unfortunately, the computations associated with this approach are prohibitive. More importantly, the boundary so found may not agree with the object boundary we are seeking. This problem is usually simplified considerably by making assumptions about the nature of the boundaries and by offering some simple recognition help. For example, in the 2D case, a point is specified inside the structure and it is assumed that any line emanating from this point intersects the boundary at exactly one point. The problem then is to find that boundary whose interior contains the specified point and which has the total minimum cost among the boundaries that intersect a finite set of equally spaced radial lines emanating from the point.[148] This problem is solved via dynamic programming.

Instead of attempting to find the optimum solutions, greedy strategies have also been used.[118,119,144,145] These approaches start from a boundary element and keep adding that neighboring boundary element that is best qualified for inclusion among all the neighbors. The inclusion criteria consist of gradient magnitude and any other intensity-based constraints as well as topological constraints such as closure of the surface.

Automatic algorithms cannot be guaranteed to be fail-safe for routine execution in large applications. Although this is very true of iso-surfacing methods, they are perhaps the most commonly used among segmentation methods. The main reason for this is that, even on inexpensive platforms such as a 300-MHz Pentium PC, it is possible to create and render iso-surfaces in a fraction of a second from scenes with domain $256 \times 256 \times 200$ (VISUALIZE → Slice → Reslice in 3DVIEWNIX). This allows one to check quickly and roughly the object of study. Other methods do not enjoy this speed advantage.

1.2.6.2 Fuzzy, Boundary-Based, Automatic Methods

The mathematical concepts of closure, orientedness, and connectedness have not been developed in a fuzzy setting for defining boundaries, unlike in the hard setting discussed in Section 1.2.6.1. Computational methods, however, have been proposed that are used in volume visualization.[152] The basic idea is to somehow assign a degree of boundariness to every voxel in the scene without worrying about connectedness, orientedness, or closure properties. A simple way of making this assignment is to make boundariness some (usually linear) function of gradient magnitude $|\nabla g(v)|$ within a specified interval of $|\nabla g(v)|$. Below and above this interval, the boundariness may be set to a fixed low and high value, respectively. Often scene intensity $g(v)$ and $|\nabla g(v)|$ are used[152] for specifying boundariness. This can be done, for example, by specifying two nested rectangles in a 2D histogram of $g(v)$ and $|\nabla g(v)|$ as in Figure 1.17. The boundariness is 1 inside the inner rectangle and 0 outside the outer rectangle, and it varies bilinearly in between.

It is not possible to guarantee that, even for a fixed application based on a fixed imaging protocol, a fixed arrangement of the rectangles will always yield acceptable results.

This method is implemented in 3DVIEWNIX under PREPROCESSING → SceneOperations → Classify → 2Features.

1.2.6.3 Hard, Boundary-Based, Assisted Methods

Clearly, the simplest of these methods is the slice-by-slice manual outlining of object boundaries. When the object regions have multiple contours and/or holes in the slices, even this simple idea poses challenges to implement, especially if we need to obtain a binary scene representation of the segmented structure.[27]

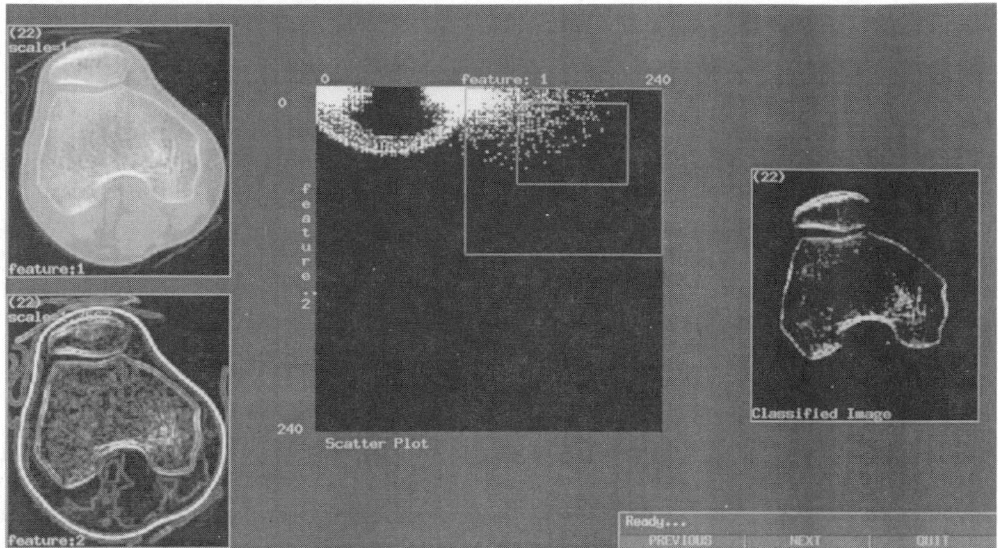

FIGURE 1.17 A CT slice of a knee (left), a 2D histogram of $g(v)$ (horizontal axis) and $|\nabla g(v)|$ (vertical axis) with two nested rectangles (middle), and the boundariness image (right). Boundariness is 1 for a voxel v if $g(v)$ and $|\nabla g(v)|$ fall inside the inner rectangle, 0 if they are outside the outer rectangle, and in [0, 1] if they fall in between.

1.2.6.3.1 Active contours

A class of more sophisticated assisted methods has evolved during the past 10 years whose aim is to minimize the degree of assistance needed. These are referred to by names such as active contour, active boundary, snakes, active surface, and deformable boundary methods.[153–162] The basic idea in these approaches can be described as follows. Although methods for the 3D case also have been developed, we confine our discussion to the 2D case. First, an initial contour is specified which lies in the vicinity of the boundary of interest. Subsequently this contour is deformed algorithmically to make it drawn toward edges in the image. A mechanical system is set up wherein the contour is assumed to have certain stiffness properties, and forces are exerted on the contour by image feature points, typically edges. The contour's final shape is estimated by minimizing an energy functional. This functional is considered to consist of an internal as well as an external energy component. The internal energy imposes smoothness and continuity constraints on the contour. The external energy pulls the contour toward image edges. The contour is represented by a parametric curve $v(s) = [x(s), y(s)]$, where s is the arc length. The energy functional is defined by

$$E = \int_0^1 \{E_{\text{int}}[v(s)] + E_{\text{ext}}[v(s)]\} ds \tag{1.16}$$

where E_{int} and E_{ext} are the internal and external energy components, respectively. E is minimized to determine the curve. The differences in the methods in this family come from how (1) the initial contour is specified, (2) edges are defined, (3) E_{int} and E_{ext} are set up, and (4) the minimum of E is found. Typically, E_{int} contains terms that regulate the elasticity and rigidity of the contour and E_{ext} consists of terms to regulate image forces and constraints specified by the user.

Since it is difficult to guarantee that the optimization process finds the global minimum of E, usually the contour shape corresponding to a local minimum is found and accepted. This fact is really beside the point. The more important considerations are (1) accuracy—the degree to which the contour found agrees with the true boundary, (2) precision—the extent of repeatability of the method, and (3) efficiency—the extent of operator help taken by the method, especially compared to manual boundary tracing. Although these methods are used in a variety of applications, their precision, accuracy, and efficiency do not seem to have been evaluated carefully.

1.2.6.3.2 Live wire/lane

There is no guarantee in the active boundary methods that the boundary found corresponding to a (local) minimum of the energy functional is acceptable. Consequently, some manual examination and/or correction after the contour is found becomes necessary on a per-study basis. To avoid this, a different paradigm has been developed recently, called live wire/lane methods.[163–167] In these, an operator offers a continuous recognition help to a delineation algorithm that is automatic. In this fashion, the superior ability of the human operator in recognition is combined optimally with the superior ability of the computer algorithm in delineation. This results in a continuous spectrum of methods within the live paradigm over a considerable range of the degree of automation for recognition and delineation. In addition, with this fundamental departure from active boundary methods, the live wire methods differ significantly from the former in the optimization model as described below.

The basic idea in live wire methods is to do the delineation correctly the first time without requiring correction afterwards. This is achieved by providing a tight control to the user on the segmentation process while it is underway. The user initially selects a point on the boundary of interest on a slice display. At this time a live wire segment — an optimal digital curve — from the initial point to any subsequent point indicated by the cursor is computed and displayed in real time. If the cursor is close to the boundary and not too far from the initial point, the live wire segment snaps onto the boundary. If the live wire segment delineates the boundary accurately, the cursor is deposited at this location. This now becomes a new starting point and the live wire process continues. In practical segmentation, two to five points specified in this fashion are adequate to segment a complete 2D boundary.

The optimal digital curves are specified and computed through a graph model. In the approach described in Ref. 166, the graph model used consists of pixel vertices as its nodes. Each pixel edge is represented by two directed arcs in the graph corresponding to the two possible orientations of the pixel edge, as illustrated in Figure 1.18. Each directed arc is assigned a cost that reflects how unlikely it is for the corresponding oriented pixel edge to be a part of the oriented boundary. The cost is assigned based on several features evaluated at the oriented edge. Each feature gives rise to a cost value. Cost values coming from various features for the same oriented edge are combined into a single cost value. As an example, let us assume without loss of generality that the boundary is oriented counterclockwise. Consider two features: scene intensity $g(v_\ell)$ of the pixel v_ℓ to the left of each directed edge e and scene intensity gradient magnitude $|\nabla g(e)|$ evaluated at edge e using an appropriate digital approximation of the gradient operator. Suppose we assign costs to e as a (inverted) Gaussian function of $g(v_\ell)$ and $|\nabla g(e)|$. The mean and covariances for this function are set up via training by an operator tracing typical boundary segments. This cost function is set up so as to have the smallest cost value (0) corresponding to the mean value of the features. This form of training is not required for each study. It is done for a given application only once. Typically, tracing is required only on a couple of slices in one study.[166] Based on segmenting over 15,000 slices in two applications,[168,169] it has been found that this form of training and cost assignment works effectively without having to modify the cost function once it has been set by training initially in an application. The method actually finds (very rapidly) that path (a sequence of connected, oriented pixel edges) whose total cost is the smallest of all possible paths between the two specified points (pixel vertices). In other words, the path found is the best-oriented (in our case, counterclockwise) boundary segment between two points. Figure 1.19 illustrates live wire tracing and the advantage of the boundary orientedness consideration in defining optimum boundaries. The MR images pertain to the joints of the foot of a human subject. The orientedness-based model of Figure 1.18 can effectively resolve different boundaries that are closely situated and that have identical boundary features.

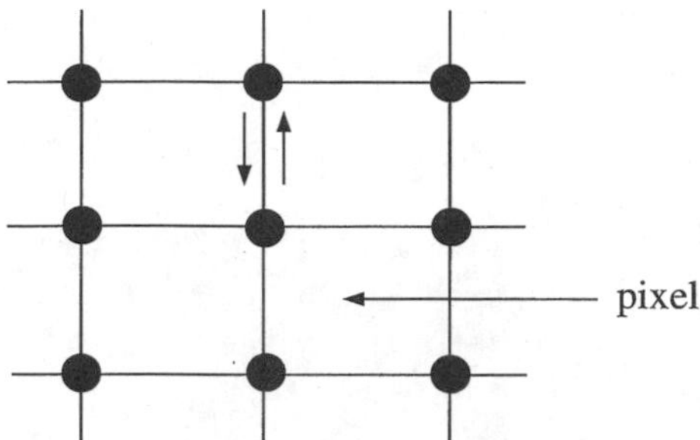

FIGURE 1.18 The graph model used in the live wire method. Pixel vertices represent the nodes in the graph and each pixel edge is represented by two directed arcs. A boundary is represented as a closed, oriented, connected digital curve.

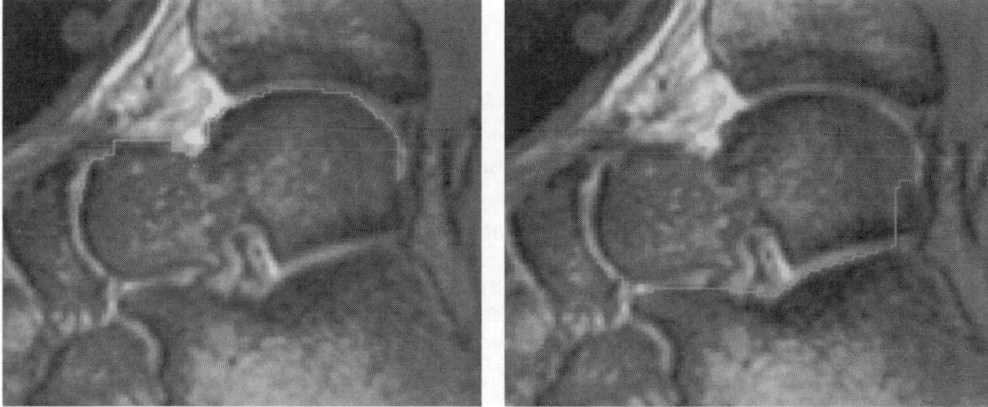

FIGURE 1.19 Illustration of orientedness of the boundary traced by the live wire method. An MR slice of a human foot is shown. The boundary of interest is that of the bone called talus. (left) The orientedness that is incorporated in this implementation is such that the interior (the darker region) of the bone is to the left of the contour. The live wire segment begins on the right and ends on the left end. (right) If we force the optimum path to go clockwise, it will not snap onto the correct boundary of the talus because this orientation is not the correct orientation for the boundary. Note also that in the image on the left, for exactly the same reasons, the live wire segment does not snap onto the boundary of the tibia just above the talus.

In the live lane method, the operator initially selects a point on the boundary and subsequently steers the cursor roughly in the vicinity of the boundary of interest within a lane of a specified width. Points are selected within this lane intermittently automatically. Optimum paths are found between each pair of successive points so selected. Since these computations are done in real time, from the operator's point of view, the rough steering action results in the operator-traced path automatically modified and attracted to the real boundary. The lane width is modified depending on the speed and acceleration of cursor motion, the width increasing with speed. Live lane thus offers within a single framework a continuum from manual tracing (width = 1 pixel) to live wire tracing (large width). Based on 2000 tracings in one application,[166] the live wire and live lane methods have been found to take two to three times less time than manual tracing for segmentation. They are also statistically significantly more repeatable than manual tracing and have about 97% agreement with the latter in terms of segmented region overlap.[166] If the boundary of interest has fairly well-defined segments, then live wire is more effective than live lane. If the boundary is mostly poorly defined, then live lane is more efficient than live wire.

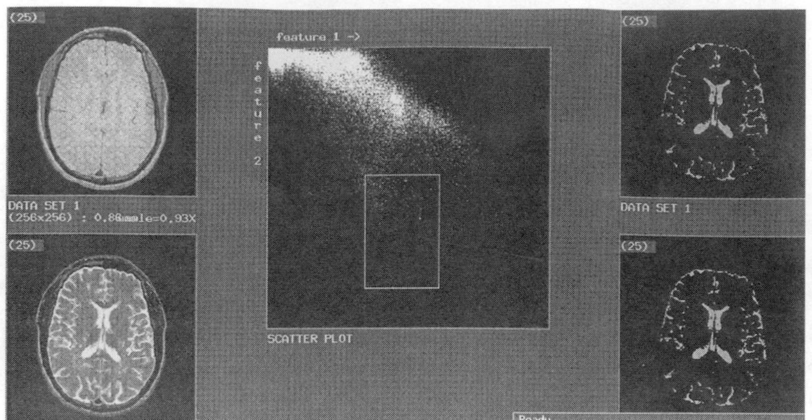

FIGURE 1.20 Illustration of interval thresholding. (left) PD and T2 images of a patient's head. (middle) A 2D histogram of PD (horizontal) and T2 (vertical) values in the slice. A rectangle is superimposed to indicate the two threshold intervals for PD and T2. (right) The segmented binary images (top and bottom are same).

Several live wire/lane and interactive methods are available for segmentation in 3DVIEWNIX under PREPROCESS → SceneOperations → Segment → Interactive2D.

We are not aware of any published fuzzy, boundary-based, assisted methods.

1.2.6.4 Hard, Region-Based, Automatic Methods

These methods can be considered to output a binary scene $\mathcal{V}_o = (V_o, g_o)$ in which the voxels with intensity 1 represent the region occupied by the structure. The input is a set of scenes $\mathcal{V}_{ij} = (V_{ij}, g_{ij})$, for $1 \le j \le s$, representing the same body region (e.g., a T2 and a PD MR scene of a patient's head). Two classes of methods may be identified: thresholding and clustering.

1.2.6.4.1 Thresholding

In these methods,[170–173] a threshold interval $[t_{j1}, t_{j2}]$ is specified for each input scene with the idea that the structure can be specified entirely by the voxels whose intensities lie in this interval. The output binary scene is thus defined as follows:

$$V_o = V_{i1} = V_{i2} = \cdots = V_{is}$$

and for any $v \in V_o$,

$$g_o(v) = \begin{cases} 1, & \text{if } g_{ij}(v) \in \left[t_{j1}, t_{j2}\right] \text{ for all } 1 \le j \le s \\ 0, & \text{otherwise.} \end{cases} \tag{1.17}$$

Figure 1.20 illustrates thresholding of a set of two input T2 and PD MR scenes of a patient's head. The two intervals are indicated by a rectangle in the 2D histogram (also known as a scatter plot) shown in the center, which represents the number of voxels in the input scenes corresponding to each possible combination of T2 and PD values. In this figure, an attempt was made to segment the CSF region. Note that, in most situations where thresholding is utilized, $s = 1$, and only t_{j1} is specified since t_{j2} is assumed to be the highest intensity value in the scene.

Thresholding rarely ever produces perfect results. Note in Figure 1.20 the non-CSF regions that have been included and the CSF regions that have been missed in the segmentation. However, because of its simplicity and efficiency, thresholding is perhaps the most commonly used method. Determination of "optimal" threshold intervals for given scenes is widely studied in the literature.[171–173]

Thresholding is available under PREPROCESS → SceneOperations → Segment → Threshold in 3DVIEWNIX.

1.2.6.4.2 Clustering

The basic premise in clustering techniques is that structures manifest themselves as separate clusters of points in a "feature space" of property values. In the example of Figure 1.20, the 2D histogram represents the feature space of two property values, namely T2 and PD. The properties considered may be the original scene intensities, as in this example, or may be those computed from scene intensities (such as gradients). To identify and define structures, the appropriate clusters in the feature space are identified. Thus, the segmentation problem is translated into the problem of identifying and delineating clusters in the feature space. Methods differ in the approaches taken to identify and delineate clusters.[174–186] Note that in Figure 1.20, the cluster representing CSF was specified by a rectangle. Thus, thresholding is a simple approach to clustering.

A more sophisticated approach, perhaps the most commonly used clustering technique in medical application, is the *k* nearest neighbor (*k*NN) method.[174,183–186] Consider the case of one object and one background and *m* input scenes representing different property values in the same body region. The method consists of a "training" phase and a classification phase.

1. Identify two sets of voxels X_o in object region and X_b in background region. This can be done, for example, by an expert painting object regions in a display of the slices of the scenes obtained for the same body region and protocol that are used to acquire the given scenes. This training step needs to be executed only once in the beginning and not for each patient study that is to be analyzed. Choose a value for parameter *k*.
2. For each voxel v in the input scene $\mathcal{V}_{ij} = (V_{ij}, g_{ij})$, $1 \leq j \leq m$, find its location $P(v) = (g_{i1}(v), g_{i2}(v), \ldots, g_{im}(v))$, in the feature space.
3. Find *k* voxels v' from $X_o \cup X_b$ such that $P(v')$ are the closest points in the feature space to $P(v)$.
4. If a majority of these voxels is from X_o, classify v as belonging to the object. Otherwise, consider v as belonging to the background.

All clustering methods have parameters whose values need to be somehow determined. In the *k*NN method, *k* and the sets X_o and X_b constitute these parameters. If these are fixed in an application, the effectiveness of the method in routine processing cannot be guaranteed. Usually some user assistance becomes necessary eventually for each study.

In 3DVIEWNIX, some 2D clustering techniques are available under PREPROCESS → SceneOperations → Segment → 2DScatterPlot.

1.2.6.5 Fuzzy, Region-Based, Automatic Methods

These methods can be thought of as outputting a gray scene $\mathcal{V}_o = (V_o, g_o)$ in which the voxel intensity $g_o(v)$ represents the degree of objectness of v. The input is a set of gray scenes $\mathcal{V}_{ij} = (V_i, g_{ij})$ for $1 \leq j \leq s$, for the same body region.

The simplest among these methods is fuzzy thresholding,[187] as illustrated in Figure 1.21, which is a generalization of hard thresholding. It is commonly used with a single input scene $\mathcal{V}_i = (V_i, g_i)$. In this case, it requires the specification of four intensity thresholds. The output scene is defined as follows:

$$V_o = V_i$$

and for any $v \in V_o$,

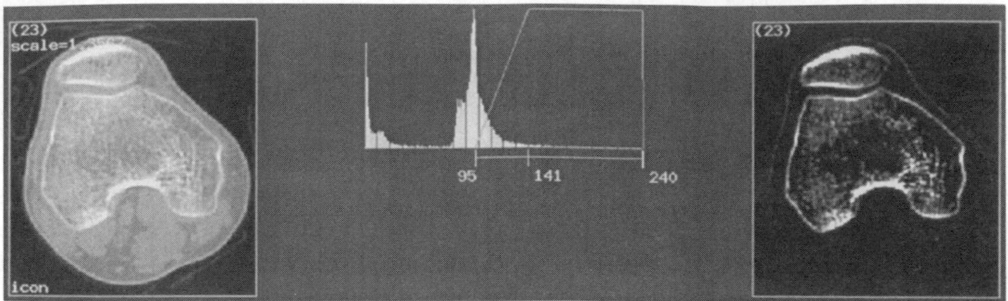

FIGURE 1.21 Fuzzy thresholding. (left) A CT slice of a knee. (middle) An intensity histogram with a superimposed trapezium that is used for fuzzy segmentation. (right) The output slice. Higher intensity indicates denser bone.

$$g_o(v) = \begin{cases} 0, & \text{if } g_i(v) > t_4 \text{ or } g_i(v) < t_1 \\ 1, & \text{if } t_2 \le g_i(v) \le t_3 \\ \dfrac{g_i(v) - t_1}{t_2 - t_1}, & \text{if } t_1 \le g_i(v) \le t_2 \\ \dfrac{t_4 - g_i(v)}{t_4 - t_3}, & \text{if } t_3 \le g_i(v) \le t_4. \end{cases} \tag{1.18}$$

That is, if $g_i(v)$ is within the inner interval $[t_2,t_3]$, v is considered to have 100% objectness. If $g_i(v)$ is outside the outer interval $[t_1,t_4]$, v does not belong to the object. For other intensities of v, objectness takes on values between 0 and 1. Unlike hard thresholding, this strategy allows accounting for graded composition of objects in their representation as a structure. In Figure 1.21, bones of the knee are represented fuzzily in this fashion from CT data. The denser aspects of the bone appear brighter in the output scene (right), indicating higher objectness value. Note that, in this example, $t_3 = t_4$. This is because there are no tissues with higher intensity than bone in this scene. Note that this method is readily generalized to handle multiple input scenes. Functional forms different from that in Equation 1.18 have also been used in fuzzy segmentation.[188,189]

Many of the (hard) clustering methods can be generalized to output fuzzy object information. For example, in the *k*NN method, if m out of k voxels, whose locations $P(v')$ in feature space are closest to $P(v)$, are from the set X_o, then the objectness of v may be considered to be m/k. Note that fuzzy thresholding is a form of fuzzy clustering.

An approach to more generalized fuzzy clustering is the fuzzy c-means method.[190] Its application in segmenting brain tissue components in MR images has been investigated.[191,192] Roughly, the idea is as follows. Suppose that there are two types of tissue regions to be segmented (say, WM and GM) and that we have two input scenes (T2 and PD). We need to consider three classes of materials: WM, GM, and the rest. In the 2D histogram of the input scenes, our task is to define three clusters corresponding to these three classes. The set X of points to which the given scenes map in the feature space can be partitioned into three clusters in a large (although finite) number of ways. The idea in the hard c-means methods is to choose that particular cluster arrangement for which the sum (over all clusters) of the squared distance between points in each cluster and the cluster center is the smallest. In the fuzzy c-means method, each point in X is allowed to have an objectness value that lies between 0 and 1; now the number of cluster arrangements is infinite. The distance in the criterion to be minimized is modified by the objectness value. Algorithms have been described for both methods[190,193] to find clusters that approximately minimize the criterion described above.

As with hard clustering methods, the effectiveness of fuzzy clustering methods in routine applications cannot be guaranteed; as such, some user assistance on a per-scene basis is usually needed.

In 3DVIEWNIX, fuzzy thresholding is available under PREPROCESS → SceneOperations → Classify → 1Feature.

1.2.6.6 Hard, Region-Based, Assisted Methods

The simplest among these techniques is manual painting of regions using a mouse-driven paint brush.[23] This is the region dual of manual boundary tracing. For most medical applications, boundary tracing is perhaps less time consuming than painting of regions.

In contrast to this completely manual recognition and delineation scheme, there are methods in which recognition is manual but delineation is automatic. Region growing is a popular method in this group.[87,194–198] Its general approach can be summarized as follows:

1. A set of criteria for inclusion of a voxel in the structure is specified. Some examples follow: (a) The scene intensity of the voxel should be within an interval $[t_1,t_2]$. (b) The mean intensity of voxels included in the growing region at any time during the growing process should be within an interval $[t_3,t_4]$. (c) The intensity variance of voxels included in the growing region at any time during the growing process should be within an interval $[t_5,t_6]$.
2. The user specifies one or more seed voxels within the object region using a mouse pointer on a slice display. These are placed in a queue and also specially marked.
3. If the queue is empty, stop. Otherwise, remove a voxel v from the queue, and output v.
4. Examine the neighbors (usually the closest 6, 18, or 26 neighbors) of v for inclusion. Those that satisfy the criteria and have not been previously marked are added to the queue (included in the growing region) and specially marked so that they will not be reconsidered later for inclusion. Go to Step 3.

Note that if we use only criterion (a), and if t_1 and t_2 are fixed during the growing process, then the above method outputs the largest set of voxels connected to the seed voxels satisfying the hard threshold interval $[t_1,t_2]$. For any combination of criteria (a) to (c), or if t_1 to t_6 are not fixed, it is not possible to guarantee that the set of voxels $O(v_1)$ obtained with a seed voxel v_1 is the same as the set of voxels $O(v_2)$, obtained with a seed voxel v_2, where $v_2 \neq v_1$ is a voxel in $O(v_1)$. This lack of robustness is a problem with many region-based methods.

1.2.6.7 Fuzzy, Region-Based, Assisted Methods

We pointed out that some of the fuzzy, region-based, automatic methods eventually need human assistance for correct segmentation in large, routine applications. In this sense, therefore, these techniques fall in this category; for example, a *k*NN method (which outputs fuzzy object information), which requires training for each study.

A recently developed method, which by design takes human assistance, is the fuzzy connectedness technique.[199] In this method, recognition is manual and involves pointing at an object in a slice display. Delineation is automatic and takes into account both the characteristics of graded composition and hanging-togetherness. It has been effectively used in several applications including MS lesion quantification via MR imagery,[200–205] MR angiography,[206] and soft-tissue display for craniomaxillofacial surgery planning.[207]

We think of nearby voxels in a scene $\mathcal{V} = (V,g)$ as having a fuzzy affinity relation κ. The strength of this relation μ_κ (varying between 0 and 1) between any two voxels v and u in V is a function of the distance between v and u as well as $g(v)$ and $g(u)$. A simple example of μ_κ is given below.

$$\mu_\kappa(v,u) = \frac{1-|g(v)-g(u)|}{\|v-u\|}. \tag{1.19}$$

Here $||v-u||$ denotes the distance between v and u, and we have assumed that the range of scene intensities is [0, 1]. Affinity expresses the degree to which voxels hang together locally. Voxels that are far apart will have negligible affinity. In the applications mentioned above, the following form of affinity has been used, where $\mu_\kappa(v,u) = 0$ for any distinct v, u that differ in more than one coordinate by one or more.

$$\mu_\kappa(v,u) = w_1 g_1(\mathbf{g}(v),\mathbf{g}(u)) + w_2(1 - g_2(\mathbf{g}(v),\mathbf{g}(u))) \tag{1.20}$$

$$g_1(\mathbf{g}(v),\mathbf{g}(u)) = \frac{1}{(2\pi)^{m/2}|S_1|^{1/2}} e^{-\frac{1}{2}\left[\frac{1}{2}(\mathbf{g}(v)+\mathbf{g}(u))-\mathbf{m_1}\right]^T S_1^{-1}\left[\frac{1}{2}(\mathbf{g}(v)+\mathbf{g}(u))-\mathbf{m_1}\right]} \tag{1.21}$$

$$g_2(\mathbf{g}(v),\mathbf{g}(u)) = \frac{1}{(2\pi)^{m/2}|S_2|^{1/2}} e^{-\frac{1}{2}\left[\frac{1}{2}|\mathbf{g}(v)-\mathbf{g}(u)|-\mathbf{m_2}\right]^T S_2^{-1}\left[\frac{1}{2}|\mathbf{g}(v)-\mathbf{g}(u)|-\mathbf{m_2}\right]} \tag{1.22}$$

In these expressions, g_1 and g_2 are multivariate Gaussian functions, $\mathbf{g}(v)$ and $\mathbf{g}(u)$ are m-component column vectors, $\boldsymbol{m_1}$ and $\boldsymbol{m_2}$ are m-component mean vectors, S_1 and S_2 are $m \times m$ covariance matrices, S_1^{-1} and S_2^{-1} are the inverses of S_1 and S_2, $|S_1|$ and $|S_2|$ are determinants of S_1 and S_2, $|\mathbf{g}(v) - \mathbf{g}(u)|$ denotes componentwise absolute difference between $\mathbf{g}(v)$ and $\mathbf{g}(u)$, and w_1 and w_2 are non-negative weights such that $w_1 + w_2 = 1$. The rationale for this functional form for $\mu_\kappa(v,u)$ is as follows. $\mu_\kappa(v,u)$ as defined in Equations 1.20–1.22 considers affinity between v and u to be greater when they are more adjacent and their average intensity is close to a mean intensity m_1 but their difference (like a gradient magnitude) is not close to a mean m_2 of intensity differences. In other words, affinity expresses how close v and u are spatially and intensity based propertywise. In the MS application[200] $m = 2$ and the two properties are the T2 value and the PD value.

The real hanging-togetherness of voxels in a global sense is captured through a fuzzy relation among voxels called fuzzy connectedness K, defined as follows. To every possible pair (v,u) of voxels in the scene domain, a strength of connectedness $\mu_K(v,u)$ (varying between 0 and 1) is assigned in the following way. There are numerous possible paths between v and u. A path from v to u is a sequence of voxels starting from v and ending on u, the successive voxels being nearby with a certain degree of adjacency. The "strength" of a path is the smallest of the affinities associated with pairs of successive voxels along the path. The strength of connectedness between v and u is simply the largest of the strengths associated with all possible paths between v and u. A fuzzy object is a pool of voxels together with a membership (between 0 and 1) assigned to each voxel that represents its "objectness." The pool is such that the strength of connectedness between any two voxels in the pool is greater than a small threshold value and the strength between any two voxels, one in the pool and the other not in the pool, is less than the threshold value. Obviously, computing fuzzy objects even for the simple affinity relation of Equation 1.19 is computationally impractical if we proceed straight from the definitions. But the theory allows us to simplify the complexity considerably for a wide variety of affinity relations so that fuzzy object computation, which now translates into dynamic programming, can be done in practical time (about 3–5 min for a 1024×1024 16-bit/pixel 2D scene and about 30 min for $256 \times 256 \times 60$ 16-bit/voxel 3D scene on a Sparc20 workstation). It is clear that a wide variety of application-specific knowledge of image characteristics can be incorporated into affinity.

Figure 1.22 shows an example of fuzzy connected segmentation (in 3D) of WM, GM, CSF, and MS lesions in a T2 and PD scene pair. The algorithms are described in detail in Ref. 200. Figure 1.23 shows a (maximum intensity projection) rendering (left) of an MRA data set and a rendition of a fuzzy connected vessel tree (right) obtained for a point specified in the vessel via

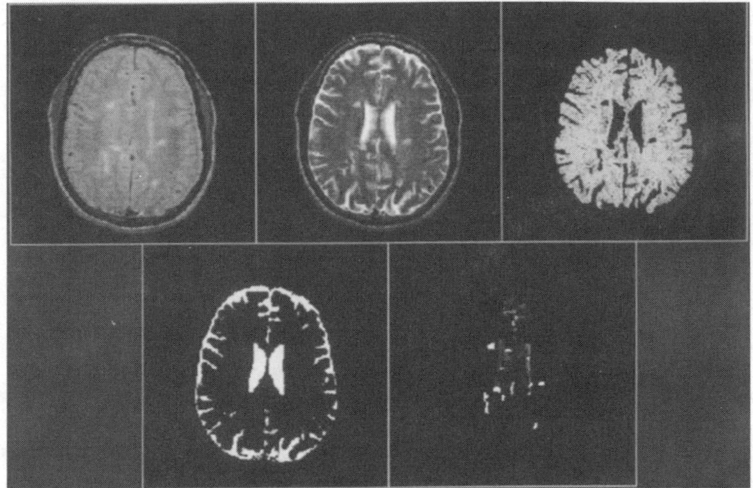

FIGURE 1.22 (top, left to right) PD and T2 MR slices of an MS patient's head; a slice of the union of WM and GM fuzzy objects. (bottom, left to right) A slice of the CSF fuzzy object and a slice of the union of lesion objects.

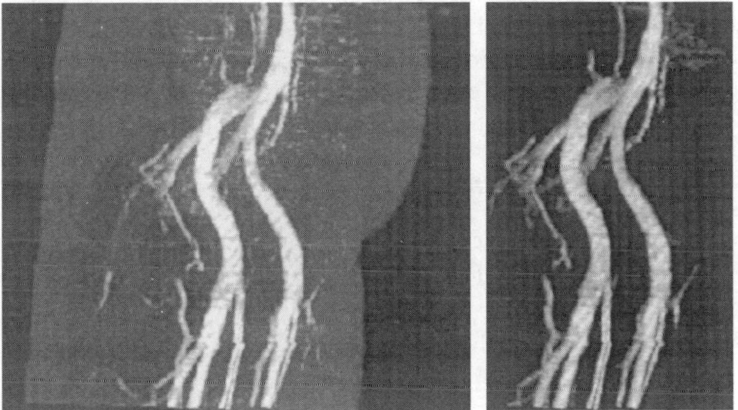

FIGURE 1.23 A (maximum intensity projection) rendition (left) of an MR angiography scene and a rendition of the fuzzy connected vessels segmented from the scene (right).

the rendition on the left. Here fuzzy connectedness is used to remove the clutter that obscures the vessel display.

In 3DVIEWNIX, the fuzzy connectedness approach is implemented under PREPROCESS → SceneOperations → Classify → FuzzyComp.

In spite of nearly four decades of research in segmentation, several key challenges remain: (1) To develop general methods that can be easily adapted to a given application; (2) to keep human assistance required in practical segmentation on a per-scene basis to a minimum; (3) to develop fuzzy methods that can realistically handle uncertainties in data; and (4) to assess the efficacy of segmentation methods. We will come back to this last aspect at the end of this chapter.

1.3 VISUALIZATION

These operations create renditions of given scenes or structures. Their purpose is, given a set of scenes or a structure system, to create renditions that facilitate viewing of object information

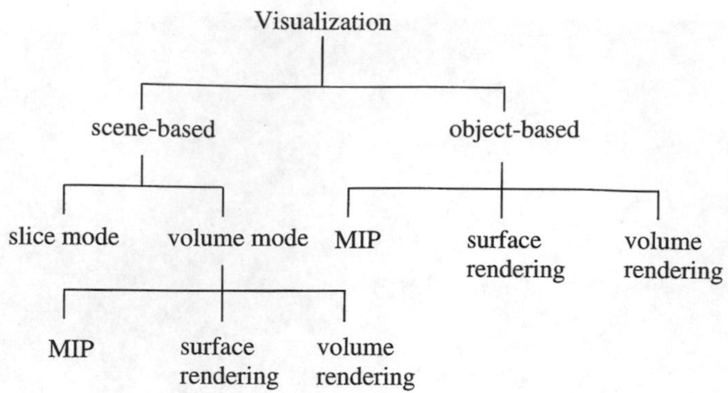

FIGURE 1.24 A classification of visualization methods. (MIP, maximum intensity projection)

contained in the given data. Two classes of approaches may be identified: scene based and object based. In scene-based methods, renditions are created directly from given scenes. In object-based methods, structures (hard or fuzzy) representing object information are explicitly defined first and then rendered. Historically, object-based methods were developed first. Many of the associated techniques were subsequently adopted by scene-based methods. Our description of visualization methods in the rest of this section will follow the classification shown in Figure 1.24. In the literature, there is no consistent and well-accepted meaning associated with the terms used to characterize different classes of visualization techniques. In our classification, *surface rendering* refers to methods in which the object of interest is described as a hard structure, irrespective of whether the approach is scene based or object based. Analogously, *volume rendering* refers to methods in which the object of interest is described as a fuzzy structure.

1.3.1 Scene-Based Visualization Methods

Two further subclasses may be identified: slice mode and volume mode. In slice mode, the given scenes are broken up into 2D scenes (slices) and the 2D scenes are displayed directly on the screen. In volume mode, the 3D object information contained in the scene is directly rendered on the screen by using a variety of rendering techniques.

1.3.1.1 Slice Mode

Methods differ based on what is considered to constitute a slice and how this information is displayed:

What:	natural slices,	*How*:	montage,
	orthogonal slices,		roam through,
	oblique and curved slices.		gray level window,
			pseudocolor.

The natural slices of the given scene are the simplest to obtain since they do not require any computation. Slices that are orthogonal to a scene coordinate axis can be computed easily. If the natural slices of the scene are axial, then the coronal and sagittal slices constitute the two orthogonal sets. Depending on how the images are acquired, especially in MRI, any of the three sets may represent the natural slices and then the remaining two constitute the orthogonal set.

It may be helpful, especially when the object or some aspect of it has a predominant orientation that is not parallel to any of the scene coordinate planes, to obtain slices corresponding to planes at any orientation within the scene domain.[208–210] There are several ways of specifying the orientation

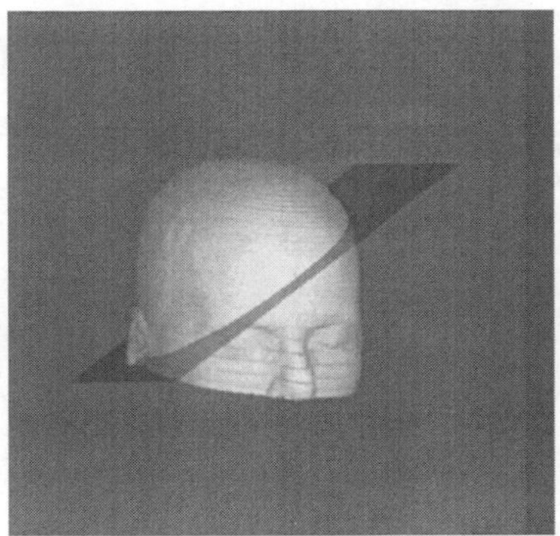

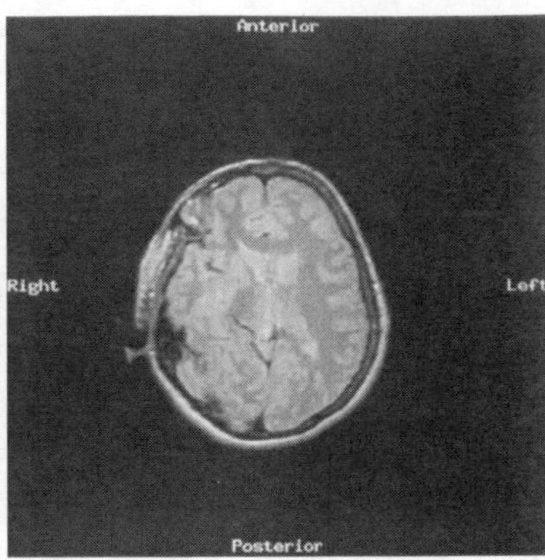

FIGURE 1.25 Specification of oblique slices via a 3D rendition of an MR scene of the head of a patient. The 3D rendition is created by surface rendering the structure resulting from thresholding the scene. The resulting oblique slice is shown on the right.

of the oblique plane. In an interactive viewing situation, this specification must be done with user interaction. Perhaps the most facilitating way of doing this is through some 3D rendition of the given scene that also depicts a translucent plane whose orientation and location can be easily altered by the user through mouse control. The easiest way of creating a 3D rendition that portrays some useful object information in the scene, which guides the user in selecting the plane, is thresholding and surface rendering the resulting binary scene. On PCs such as a 300-MHz Pentium, this can be done at interactive speeds (0.2–5 s) for most of the scenes encountered in clinical use. Figure 1.25 illustrates this for an MR scene of the head of a patient. The threshold can be selected interactively. Once the plane is specified, the computation of the corresponding slice is done through scene interpolation. First, a rectangular region that encloses the scene domain intersected by the plane is determined. Then, this region is divided into pixels of specified size. The scene intensity at the center of each of these pixels is then computed using any of the interpolation methods described in Section 1.2.4.

Attempts have also been made to specify curved slices[211] by drawing curves on natural, orthogonal, or oblique slices, that indicate an orthogonal intersection of the curved surface with the slice, and then to unwarp the surface so indicated and the scene intensities on them into a planar picture.

Once what constitutes slices is specified, they can be displayed in a variety of ways. The slices of a scene can be displayed as a montage (Figure 1.26). This form of display has the advantage that all slices can be visualized simultaneously. Its disadvantage is that small details are usually lost in trying to accommodate all slices within a limited screen space. Another method is the roam-through display. A single slice with full resolution is displayed and all parallel slices are rapidly displayed one after another at the same location. On machines such as a 300-MHz Pentium, the display can be done rapidly enough to give the sensation of continuously and smoothly roaming through the scene domain in one direction and back for commonly encountered scenes. To display a slice on the screen, usually a technique known as windowing is used. This is mainly because the number of gray levels available in the display device is usually smaller than the number of distinct intensities in the given scene. The operation consists of specifying an interval $[L,H]$ of scene intensities. Within this interval, all intensities are mapped linearly to the display device gray levels. The scene intensities less than L and greater than H are mapped to the lowest and highest gray levels, respectively. Pseudocolor display is an alternative to windowing. Instead of the gray levels from a gray scale, colors available in the display device are assigned in some manner to scene intensities. PET and SPECT images are often displayed using this technique. The colors should be chosen carefully with considerations as to how they will be perceived in the rendition. Otherwise, artificial structures and boundaries may become visible in the displayed image. An example of

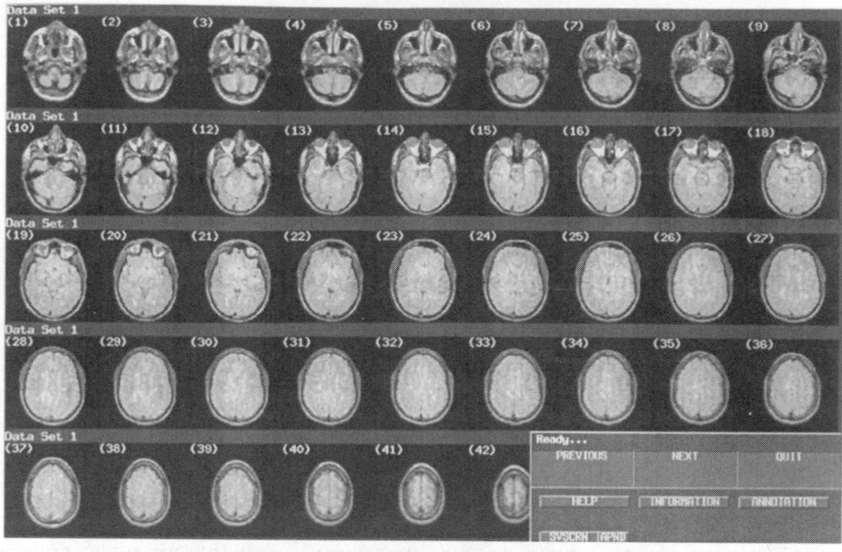

FIGURE 1.26 A montage display of the natural slices of an MR scene of the head of a patient.

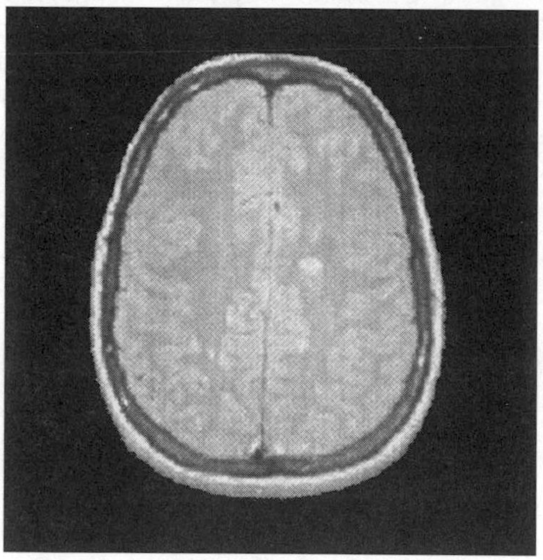

FIGURE 1.27 A pseudocolor display of two MR PD slices corresponding to the same location of the head of an MS patient. The slices are obtained from two scenes that were acquired several months apart and that have been subsequently registered. The older acquisition is displayed in green and the other is displayed in red.

pseudocolor display is illustrated in Figure 1.27. Here, two MR PD slices corresponding to the same location of the head of an MS patient are shown overlaid. The two slices are obtained from two scenes of the patient's head that were acquired at two time instances several months apart and that have been subsequently registered via a scene-based method. The slice from the older data is displayed in green hue and at a brightness proportional to the voxel intensities. The other slice is displayed similarly in red. To give the effect of translucency, pixels are selected from the two slices in a checkerboard fashion. Only odd-numbered pixels from odd-numbered rows and even-numbered pixels from even-numbered rows are displayed for the first slice. For the second, only even-numbered pixels from odd-numbered rows and odd-numbered pixels from even-numbered rows are displayed. Where there is misregistration or where there has been a change (e.g., an old lesion

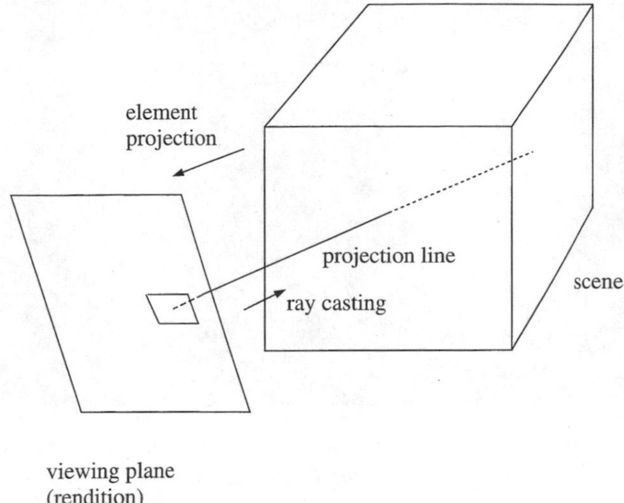

FIGURE 1.28 Two methods of projection are used in converting higher dimensional object information to their 2D renditions. In ray casting, a line orthogonal to the viewing plane is cast into the scene domain for this conversion. In element projection, voxels or other structure elements are projected onto the viewing plane from the scene domain.

disappeared or a new lesion developed), the display would show in either green or red. At other sites, the display appears yellow. This form of display is useful for visualizing change, especially if we allow selectively turning on and off the individual slices with mouse control.

Several slice mode visualization tools are available in 3DVIEWNIX under VISUALIZE → Slice. These are Layout, Montage, Cycle, Reslice, and Overlay.

1.3.1.2 Volume Mode

In this mode, what is displayed and how it is done are as follows:

What:	surfaces,	*How*:	maximum intensity projection,
	interfaces,		surface rendering,
	intensity distributions.		volume rendering.

In any combination of these methods, a projection technique is needed to go from the higher dimensional scene to the 2D rendition. For 4D and higher dimensional scenes, their 3D cross-sections should be determined first before these techniques can be applied. Projections are then applied for going from 3D to 2D. Two approaches are pursued (see Figure 1.28) — ray casting,[152] which consists of tracing a line perpendicular to the viewing plane from every pixel in the viewing plane into the scene domain, and element projection,[212,213] recently also called splatting, which consists of directly projecting voxels or other structure elements encountered along the projection line from the scene onto the viewing plane. Either of these projection methods may be used in the following rendering strategies. Voxel projection is generally considerably faster than ray casting.

Both parallel and perspective projections have been used in 3D imaging. In perspective projection, the projection lines from the different pixels in the viewing plane are not parallel to each as in parallel projection, but converge at a point.[214] This projection gives the effect of making bigger in the rendition those aspects of the structure in the scene that are closer to the viewing plane than those that are farther. In parallel projection, all aspects are presented at the same size in the rendition. When the viewpoint is outside the structure, the difference in the effects seen in the renditions

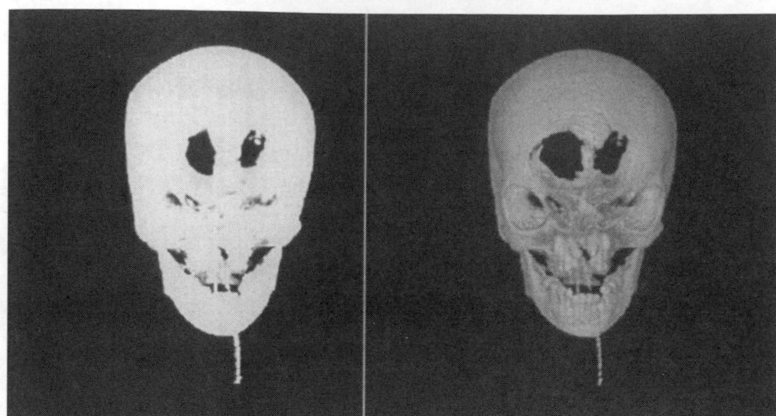

FIGURE 1.29 An MIP rendition (left) of the craniofacial bony structures from a CT data set. A volume rendition of the same structure is shown on the right for comparison.

created by the two methods is not significant. The influence of these effects in actual medical applications has not been studied. However, when the viewpoint is inside the structure, as in virtual endoscopic applications,[215] considering perspective becomes essential. Computationally, parallel projection is considerably less expensive than perspective projection. Our description in this section, will be confined only to parallel projection.

1.3.1.2.1 Maximum intensity projection (MIP)

In these methods,[216–219] the intensity assigned to a pixel in the rendition is simply the maximum of the scene intensity encountered along the projection line within the scene domain. It is the simplest among 3D rendering techniques. It is most effective when the objects of interest are the brightest in the scene, they sparsely fill the scene domain, have a simple 3D morphology, and have minimal gradation of scene intensity. Contrast-enhanced CT angiography and MR angiography (MRA) ideally suit these requirements, and consequently, MIP is commonly used in CTA and MRA.[220–225] Figure 1.23 illustrates an MIP rendition of an MRA scene. Its main advantage is that it does not require segmentation of any sort. However, the conditions mentioned above are frequently not fulfilled. For example, there are often other bright objects such as clutter coming from surface coils in MRA, nearby bony structures in CTA, and other obscuring vessels which may not be of interest to us in both CTA and MRA. For these reasons, some segmentation often becomes necessary even in situations that are suited for MIP. MIP is useless even when the objects are the brightest in the scene but they are not sparse, as illustrated in Figure 1.29, which shows an MIP rendition of bone from a craniofacial CT scene. This figure also illustrates the fact that MIP renditions do not portray geometric relationships among object components and their shape.

MIP rendering is available in 3DVIEWNIX under VISUALIZE → Volume and under MANIPULATE under Cut, Separate, Move, and FuzzyConnect.

1.3.1.2.2 Surface rendering

In these methods,[226–233] object surfaces are portrayed in the rendition directly from the given scene. Usually, thresholding is used to specify the structure of interest in the given scene. Clearly, the speed of rendering is of utmost importance here since the idea is that object renditions are created interactively directly from the scene as the threshold is changed. Instead of thresholding, any automatic, hard, boundary- or region-based method can be used. However, in this case, the parameters of the method will have to be specified interactively and sufficient speed of segmentation and rendition should be possible for this mode of visualization to be practically useful. At present, thresholding can be accomplished in about 0.1–2 s on a 300-MHz Pentium for most 3D scenes using appropriate algorithms in software.[23] However, more sophisticated segmentation methods (such as *k*NN) do not permit interactive speed. Therefore, the only viable segmentation method in scene-based rendering at present is thresholding.

The actual rendering itself by scene-based methods consists of the following three basic steps: projection, hidden part removal, and shading. These are needed to impart a sense of three dimensionality to the rendered image that is created. Additional cues for three dimensionality may be provided by techniques such as stereoscopic display, motion parallax by rotation of the objects, shadowing, and texture mapping.

If ray casting is the method of projection chosen, then points equally spaced along the ray are sampled, and at each such point, the scene intensity is estimated using an appropriate interpolation method. Hidden part removal is then done by stopping at the first sampled point encountered along each ray that satisfies the threshold criterion.[226] The value of shading assigned to the pixel (in the viewing plane) corresponding to the ray is determined as described below. Ray casting is generally computationally far more expensive than element projection for the following reasons: (1) The need to sample points along the ray, (2) the need to interpolate, (3) the need to store the entire scene in the main memory. Note that interpolation becomes necessary irrespective of whether or not the given scene has cubic voxels. Several methods of overcoming these drawbacks have been suggested. Since these were developed in connection with volume rendering, we will discuss them under that topic, although they are applicable for surface rendering as well. In element projection, hidden part removal is done by retaining the shading value associated with the elements belonging to the structure that are closest to the viewing plane. The most commonly used element is a voxel. This is perhaps the most natural and efficient choice, considering the fact that scenes are represented usually as arrays of voxels. Further, in voxel projection, considerable computational savings can be made over ray casting by avoiding the interpolation step required in ray casting altogether. This is made possible by the following elegant property of rectangular voxel arrays:[234,235]

> *The voxels in the domain of a 3D scene projecting onto any given pixel P in the viewing plane are in the strict back-to-front (BTF) or front-to-back (FTB) order if they are projected onto the viewing plane in certain row-by-row, column-by-column, and slice-by-slice orders.*

For illustration of this property, we will use a 2D example as shown in Figure 1.30. The property holds true for any arrays of any (finite) dimensionality. Here, the voxels (actually, pixels) are numbered 1 through 16 for reference in the 4×4 array. For pixel P indicated on the viewing plane, the BTF order of the voxels is 4, 8, 7, 11, 15, 14. This order of projection onto P is achieved if we go through the array in the row-by-row order (of the voxels) 4, 3, 2, 1, 8, 7, …, 13 and project each voxel onto the viewing plane. Note that the BTF order is achieved in this projection for any pixel in the viewing plane. For P, the FTB order of projection is (the opposite of BTF) 13, 14, 15, 16, 9, 10, …, 4. For 3D scenes, there are only eight distinct orders of traversing the array for each of BTF and FTB projection. They correspond to the eight octants of the scene coordinate system in which the viewpoint may be situated. Within an octant, for any position of the viewpoint, the order of traversal remains fixed. Given the viewpoint, the order of traversal can be selected from among the eight using simple calculations. Rendering in the voxel projection method consists of the following steps for BTF projection:

1. Initialize a 2D pixel array R, which will eventually contain the rendition, to a background illumination value.
2. For the viewpoint, determine the order of traversal of the scene domain.
3. For each voxel v visited that satisfies the threshold, do the following (Steps 4–6).
4. Determine the projection of v onto the viewing plane. That is, identify the pixels in rendition R that are covered by the voxel's projection.
5. Determine the shading associated with v (see below).
6. For each pixel in R in the projection of v, replace its value by the shading assigned to v.

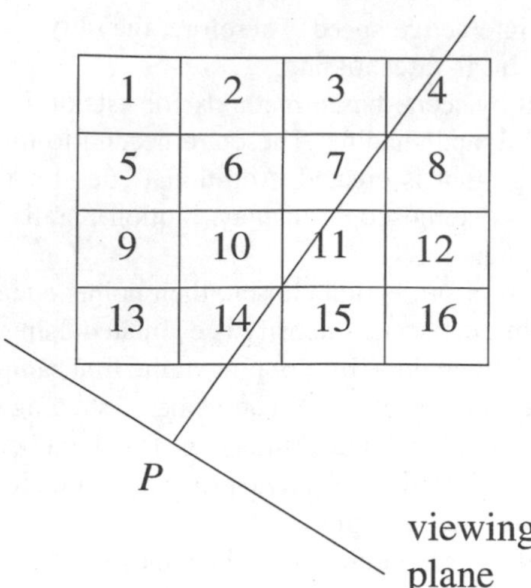

FIGURE 1.30 The back-to-front (BTF) order of voxels in the 2D scene projecting onto pixel P in the 1D rendition is the sequence of voxels numbered 4, 8, 7, 11, 15, 14. The order of traversing voxels to achieve BTF projection is 4, 3, 2, 1, 8, 7, …, 13.

For FTB projection, Step 6 should be modified. Instead of replacing the pixel value unconditionally, it is replaced only if its value is the background value. Thus, in BTF and FTB projection, the shading of the voxel closest to the viewing plane (that satisfies the threshold) will eventually remain in the rendition.

Other elements that are used to represent the structure include voxel faces, triangles, other polygons, and surface patches. The property mentioned above for voxels is not satisfied by these elements except by voxel faces.

The shading value assigned to each voxel v that is projected onto a viewing plane will determine how well the object is portrayed in the rendition. The faithfulness with which this value represents the shape of the object surface around v depends on the object's optical properties in the vicinity of v such as its color, shininess/matteness, and texture. Some of these characteristics (e.g., color), are not usually captured in the scene data pertaining to live body regions, and therefore cannot be determined by any preprocessing operation. Consequently, in 3D imaging systems, the associated parameters are left under user control. One aspect of object shape that is captured reasonably well and that is commonly utilized in depicting shape in the rendition is the surface normal. The faithfulness with which the shading value assigned to v represents the shape of the object surface is more or less entirely determined by how accurately a unit vector N_v orthogonal to the object surface in the vicinity of v is determined.

Two classes of methods are available for surface normal estimation: object based and scene based. In object-based methods,[236–242] N_v is estimated based on the geometry of the arrangement of the structure elements in the vicinity of v. For example, if the element v represents voxel faces, N_v is taken to be the weighted average of the vectors representing the geometric normals of v and of its four adjacent faces in the structure (see Figure 1.31).[236]

In scene-based methods,[33,107,226] the premise is that, in the given scene $\mathcal{V} = (V,g)$, the scene intensity in the vicinity of the structure surface changes most rapidly in the direction orthogonal to the surface. This is true for (iso-intensity) surfaces generated directly from the scene via thresholding. However, if other methods of segmentation are used, this property may not hold. When it holds, the surface normal N_v can be estimated by applying a gradient operator on the scene since the gradient vector indicates the direction in which $g(v)$ changes most rapidly.

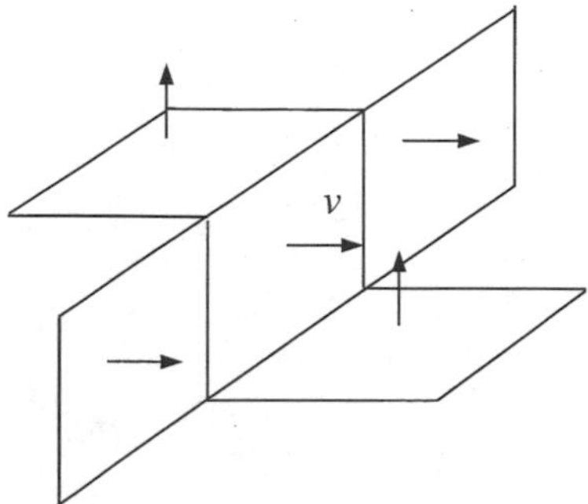

FIGURE 1.31 An example of object-based surface normal estimation. A voxel face v and its four adjacent faces in a structure. The surface normal N_v at v is estimated as the weighted average of the geometric normals of the five faces shown.

$$N_v = \frac{\nabla g(v)}{|\nabla g(v)|}. \tag{1.23}$$

Methods differ in how digital approximations of $\nabla g(v)$ are devised. One commonly used approximation for $\nabla g(v)$ is given in Equation 1.3.

Given the normal vector N_v, the shading assigned to v is determined by using the following formula that computes the light reflected from v toward the viewing plane:

$$\text{shade } (v) = \left[S_d\left(N_v, L\right) + S_S\left(N_v, L, E\right)\right] S_D(v). \tag{1.24}$$

Here L and E are unit vectors indicating the direction of light illuminating the surface and the viewing direction (direction of the line of projection), respectively. S_d, S_s, and S_D are the diffuse, specular, and a distance-dependent component of shading, respectively (see Figure 1.32). The diffuse component represents the matteness of the structure surface. As per this property, the light is scattered from v uniformly in all directions and is independent of the viewing direction (Figure 1.32a). The amount of scattered light is a cosine function of the angle between L and N_v. The specular component represents surface shininess. Here, the reflection is maximum in a direction (**R**) corresponding to the direction of ideal reflection (i.e., as if v were to act like a mirror). It dies off as a cosine function in the vicinity of **R** (Figure 1.32b). The distance-dependent component represents how the reflected light dies off with distance. This component is usually taken to be inversely proportional to the distance of v from the viewing plane. The three components can be weighted in different ways to create different effects.

Figure 1.33 illustrates two scene-based surface renditions, obtained by an object-based (Figure 1.33a)[236] and a scene-based (Figure 1.33b)[226] shading technique. The scene data came from the CT of a dry skull. Figure 1.34 illustrates the effect of varying the diffuse and specular components of reflection in a rendition of a child's skull from a CT scene.

Two important characteristics of scene-based normal estimation must be emphasized. Even if certain fine and subtle features, such as the sutures in the skull, are not explicitly captured (or are represented poorly) in the geometric model of the structures, they are often portrayed well in the rendition if scene-based normal estimation is used. This is because the scenes often contain sufficient intensity discontinuities, although subtle, in the vicinity of these features and the scene-based shading methods capture this information in the estimated normals. Thus, even when the hard structure does not contain the features, the surface normals assigned in the vicinity of the features

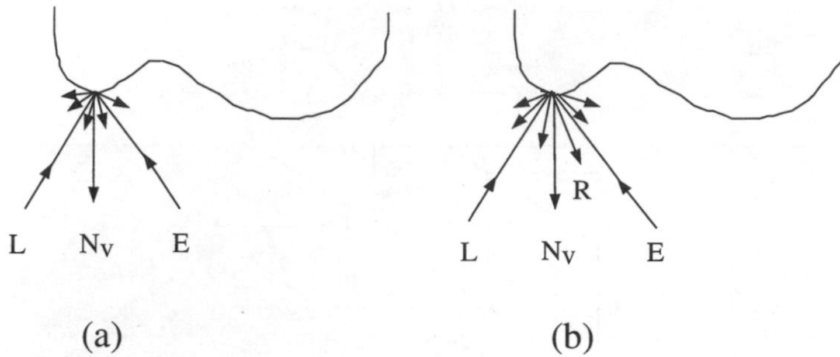

FIGURE 1.32 Illustration of diffuse (a) and specular (b) reflection.

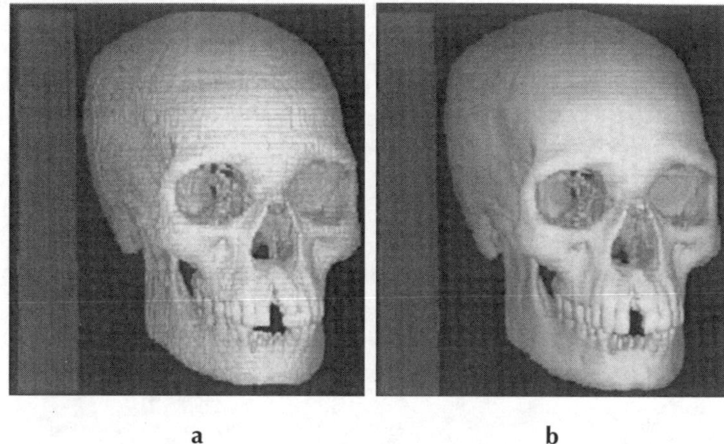

FIGURE 1.33 Scene-based surface rendition of the CT scene of a dry skull via (a) object-based and (b) scene-based shading (surface normal estimation).

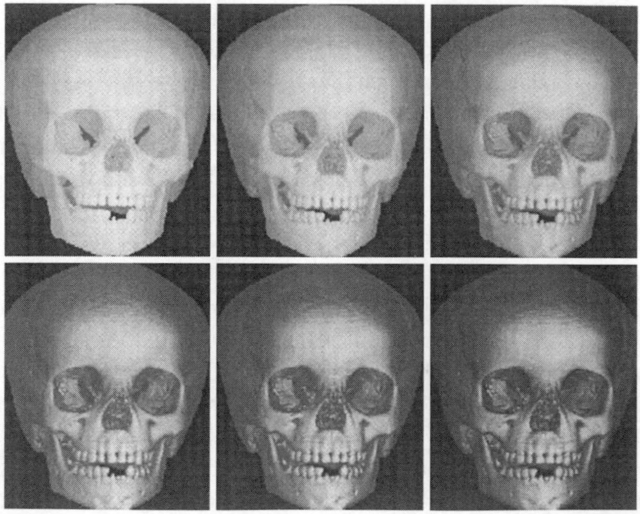

FIGURE 1.34 A scene-based surface rendition of a child's skull from a CT scene using voxels as surface elements and scene-based surface normals. The renditions show (from the beginning of the first row to the end of the second row) the effect of increasing the specular component and decreasing the diffuse component between two extremes.

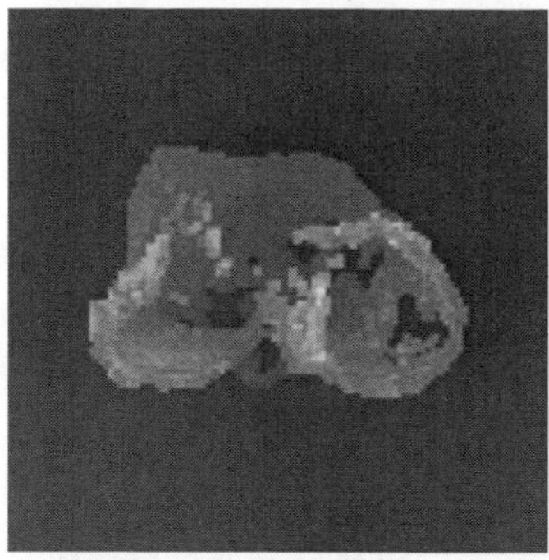 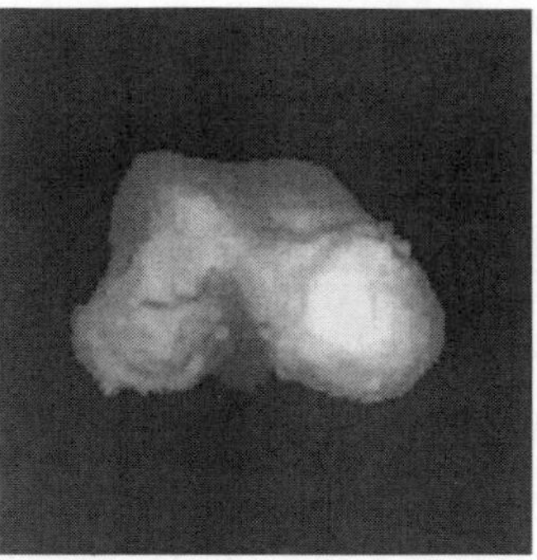

FIGURE 1.35 A bone (talus) of the foot segmented using the live wire method described in Section 1.2.6.3 from an MR scene of a foot. (left) This structure is rendered using (the original MR) scene-based normals. (right) The rendition is based on the scene resulting from filtering the segmented binary scene. The rendition on the left is misleading and wrong.

show their presence in the rendition. This phenomenon may be observed in Figure 1.33 for some of the sutures of the skull.

Conversely, if the structure does not represent an iso-intensity surface, as when manual segmentation is used, scene-based normals may not represent a direction orthogonal to the object surface. The renditions from scene-based normals in this case may be unacceptable (see Figure 1.35). Scene-based shading can still be used in such contexts. Suppose a binary scene $\mathcal{V}_b$ was created by manual segmentation. We apply a suppressing (say, a Gaussian) filter to $\mathcal{V}_b$ to create a gray scene $\mathcal{V}_g$ and then use the scene-based normals estimated from $\mathcal{V}_g$ on an appropriate iso-intensity surface in $\mathcal{V}_g$. This operation has the effect of smoothing digital artifacts in the structure. This idea is illustrated in Figure 1.35. See Ref. 33 for a detailed account of a variety of such approaches and for a quantitative comparison of rendering strategies.

1.3.1.2.3 Volume rendering

In scene-based surface rendering described above, a hard object is implicitly created and rendered on the fly from the given scene. In scene-based volume rendering, a fuzzy object is implicitly created and rendered on the fly from the given scene. Clearly, surface rendering becomes a particular case of volume rendering. Further, volume rendering in this mode is generally much slower than surface rendering, requiring typically 3 to 20 s even on specialized hardware rendering engines.

The central idea in volume rendering[152,187,243,244] is to assign to every voxel in the scene an opacity that can take on any value in the range of 0 to 100%. The opacity value is determined based on the objectness value at the voxel and how prominently we wish to portray this particular grade of objectness in the rendition. This opacity assignment is specified interactively via an opacity function, such as the one shown in Figure 1.21 (center). Here, the vertical axis now indicates percentage opacity. Every voxel is now considered to transmit, emit, and reflect light. Our goal is to determine the light that reaches every pixel in the viewing plane. The amount of transmission depends on the opacity of the voxel. Its emission depends on its objectness and hence on opacity. The greater the objectness, the greater is the emission. Its reflection depends on the strength of the surface that is present. The idea here is that the surface goes through potentially every voxel. The greater this strength the greater is the reflection. Note the generality here compared to surface rendering wherein only reflection from voxels (in the boundary of the structure) is considered. That is, typically all voxels are assumed to be totally opaque (100% opacity), although any other fixed opacity (<100%) can also be used in surface rendering for all voxels. (In the latter case, the shading method will have to take into account the reflected light coming from voxels in the back along each projection line.) Note also that, as in surface rendering, the entire set up is quite artificial. However, what matters is the fact that the methods produce renditions that have been proven to be medically useful.

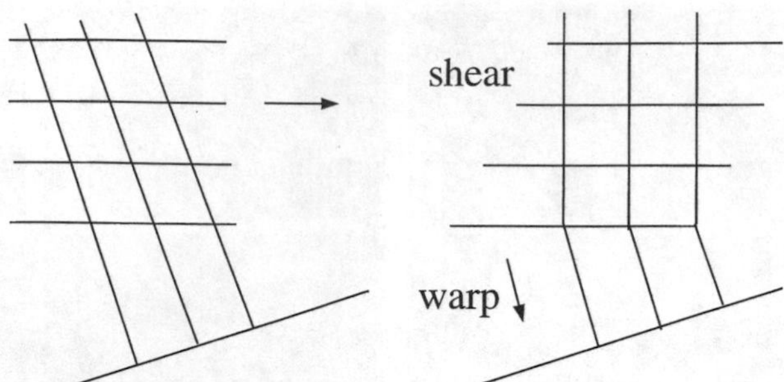

FIGURE 1.36 To facilitate essentially voxel projection in ray casting, first the scene is sheared. In the sheared scene, voxels are aligned along the projection line. After voxel projection and rendering, warping is done to remove the effect of shear in the final rendition.

Just as in surface rendering, there are three basic steps: projection, hidden part removal, and shading or compositing. The principles underlying projection are identical to those described under surface rendering. Hidden part removal is more complicated than for surface rendering. In ray casting, several strategies, as described below, have been used to speed up computation. It would take several minutes per rendition if ray casting were implemented directly.

1. Instead of resampling points along each ray and estimating intensities, perform a shear-warp transformation of the scene[245–248] as follows, so that on the transformed scene a BTF or an FTB voxel projection strategy can be applied. This technique is applicable to ray casting for surface rendering also.
   a. Shear the scene by shifting slices (see Ref. 248 for details) so that the points of intersection of each ray with the slice plane are in rows parallel to one of the scene coordinate axes in the sheared scene. The degree of shear depends on the position of the viewpoint. This transformation can be implemented as a geometric transformation and can be executed in hardware at high speed in workstations that provide hardware-based geometric transformation. This is illustrated in Figure 1.36.
   b. In the sheared scene, voxel centers are aligned in the direction of the projection line. Project this scene as in voxel projection. Shading is computed as described below.
   c. Transform the resulting image (rendition) by warping (Figure 1.36) to remove the effect of shearing.
2. Along each ray, discard all those sampled points (or voxels in the sheared scene) beyond a point at which the "cumulative opacity" is above a high threshold (say 90%).[249,250] The idea here is that if there are points along the ray closer to the viewing plane that have sufficiently high opacity, then points along the same ray that are farther from the viewing plane cannot make any noticeable contribution to the shading assigned to the pixel associated with the ray.
3. Tag all voxels in the scene whose opacity is below a low threshold (say 10%) before commencing rendering. This usually reduces the computation by discarding such voxels while rendering.[249]

In voxel projection, the BTF and FTB strategies of surface rendering are applicable in conjunction with the methods of shading described below. The strategies described in Steps 2 and 3 above are also applicable. Additionally, a voxel can be discarded if the voxels surrounding it in the direction of the projection line have "high" opacity.[250]

The shading operation, which is more appropriately called compositing, is more complicated than for surface rendering. We may start from the voxel/point farthest from the viewing plane and work toward the front along each projection line, calculating for each voxel/point its output light. The input light is the light output from the previous voxel/point. For the farthest voxel/point, the input is the

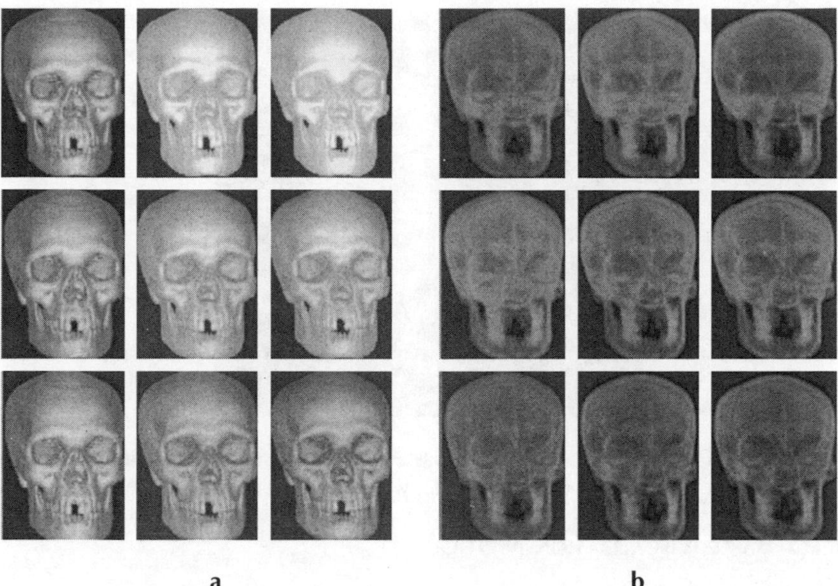

FIGURE 1.37 Volume renditions of an adult skull CT scene for varying degrees of emission, reflection, and (a) low transmission or (b) high transmission. Emission increases from left to right and reflection increases from top to bottom in a and b.

background light. The net light output by the voxel/point closest to the viewing plane is assigned to the pixel associated with the projection line. For a given voxel with input light C_i, transmission, emission, and reflection are accounted for and the output light C_o is calculated as follows:[187]

$$
\begin{aligned}
C_o^B &= C^B + \left(1-\alpha^B\right)C_i \\
C_o^S &= C^S + \left(1-\alpha^S\right)C_o^B \\
C_o^F &= C^F + \left(1-\alpha^F\right)C_o^S = C_o.
\end{aligned}
\tag{1.25}
$$

Every voxel is considered to consist of three parts — the front (F), the surface (S), and the back (B). The first equation computes the light output C_o^B by the back part. The second and the third equations express the outputs C_o^S and C_o^F (=C_o) by the surface and the front part. α^B, α^S, and α^F represent opacities of the three parts. They account for the transmission component. Usually it is assumed that $\alpha^S = \alpha^B$. When dealing with an object with one material (say bone), the front is considered to consist of air and α^F is assumed to be 0. When multiple materials are considered, opacity functions that specify material composition based on scene intensities are used.[187] C^B and C^F represent the emission components of the back and front parts, respectively. They are usually taken to be some monotonic function of α^B and α^F, respectively. C^S represents the reflection component. Usually, this is computed using the shading formula given in Equation 1.24. Finally, the output C_o^F from the front part is considered to be the light output by the voxel under consideration. In these equations, all Cs represent a three-component vector indicating color. When scalars are used instead, the resulting rendition will be a gray-scale picture.

As with surface rendering, voxel projection methods are faster than ray casting. Figure 1.37 shows an adult skull CT scene rendered in gray scale via voxel projection for varying degrees of emission, reflection, and transmission. Figure 1.38 shows a knee CT scene rendered in color via voxel projection wherein bone (light yellowish) and soft tissues (reddish) have been specified using two overlapping trapezoidal functions such as the one shown in Figure 1.21.

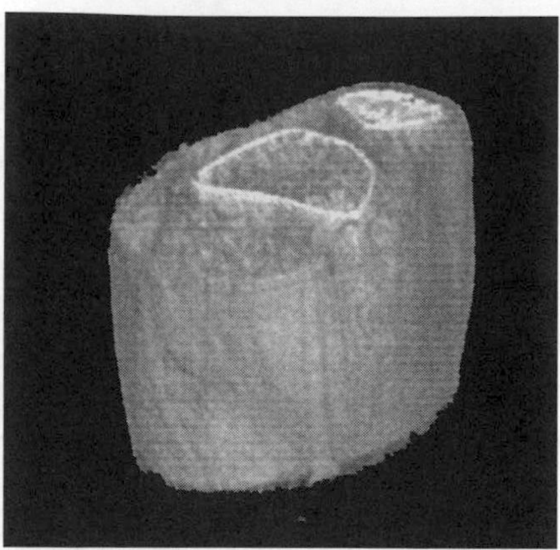

FIGURE 1.38 A volume rendition of bone and soft tissue from a CT scene of a human knee. Two overlapping opacity functions, one for soft tissue and one for bone, were used to assign opacities to the two materials.

1.3.2 Object-Based Visualization Methods

In these methods of visualization, objects (hard or fuzzy) are explicitly defined first and then rendered. In difficult segmentation situations, or when segmentation is time consuming or has too many parameters, it is not practical to do direct scene-based rendering. The intermediate step of completing structure definition first then becomes necessary. Structures defined in a hard fashion are rendered using object-based surface rendering techniques.[212,213,235,251–254] Structures defined in a fuzzy fashion are rendered via object-based MIP or volume rendering techniques.[250,255,256]

1.3.2.1 Maximum Intensity Projection

In these methods,[206,257,258] the given scene $\mathcal{V}_i = (V_i, g_i)$ is first converted into another scene $\mathcal{V}_i' = (V_i, g_i')$ via a fuzzy segmentation method. In $\mathcal{V}_i'$, the scene intensity $g_i'(v)$ indicates the objectness of v. Subsequently $\mathcal{V}_i'$ is rendered via scene-based MIP. When the object regions do not manifest themselves with a higher intensity than other non-object regions in the domain of the given scene, scene-based MIP cannot be used. However, MIP may still be applicable in these situations if we create another scene wherein the requirement of higher intensity for object regions is satisfied. Examples of such situations are the display of vascular tree of the lungs via (unenhanced) CT, and the display of peripheral CSF from MR images of the brain. Figure 1.23 shows an object-based MIP rendition (right) of an MRA data set. The object was defined here using the fuzzy connectedness method.

1.3.2.2 Surface Rendering

These methods[212,213,235,251–254] take as input hard object descriptions and create renditions. The methods of projection, hidden part removal, and shading are similar to those described under scene-based surface rendering. The only difference here is that a variety of surface description methods have been investigated using voxels,[132,134,235,252,253,] voxel faces,[100,102,125,127] triangles,[106,107,116,138–142] and other surface patches. Therefore, projection and hidden part removal methods that are appropriate for the specific surface elements have also been developed. Since the premise here is that object definition is done in a separate step (unlike in scene-based methods), data structures that are optimal for the type of surface element used in structure representation can be devised. With this one-time cost, substantial savings in the actual view-to-view rendering time can be made. For example, if we use oriented voxel faces (see Section 1.2.6.1) as the surface elements, the set of elements constituting any surface can be divided into six groups, each representing one of the six

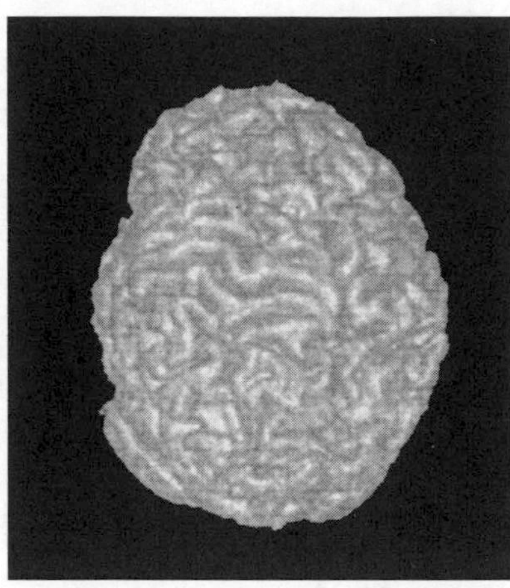

FIGURE 1.39 An example of object-based surface rendition. The T2 and PD scene pair of an MS patient's head was segmented to define the brain as a fuzzy connected object. An iso-intensity surface of the resulting connectivity scene was defined and rendered using the surface normals derived from the connectivity scene.

possible orientations of voxel faces.[259] For any given viewpoint, clearly, faces in at most three of these groups will have an orientation that will face the viewing direction and the rest will face away. Therefore, the latter groups can be simply discarded using trivial calculations. To make use of these properties is usually costly in scene-based methods if the application calls for a frequent change of segmentation parameters (threshold). If sufficient computational power becomes available so that such finer properties can also be incorporated with sufficient speed of rendition directly from the scene, then the difference between scene-based and object-based methods will disappear. Historically, object-based methods emerged first,[143,212] perhaps mainly because of the limited power and RAM capacity of the computers in those days which put severe challenges on methodology and algorithm design. The main aim of early software packages in those days[260] was, therefore, to optimize storage space and computation, and not so much interactability, which was out of the question.

There is a vast body of literature in computer graphics on hidden part removal and rendering of structures represented by triangles and other surface elements. Representations using voxels and their faces have emerged mostly in the context of visualization of multidimensional digital image data, and specifically in medical 3D imaging. The latter representations have substantial geometric advantages over the former. Their implementations entirely in software offer substantial speed advantages over the implementations of the former methods even in specialized hardware rendering engines. Using a particular voxel representation of the structure boundary,[252] we can render most small- and moderate-sized objects in real time (10 to 35 views per second) on a 300-MHz Pentium entirely in software.[23] Using this method, even large objects with about a million voxels in the boundary can be rendered at about 4 views per second on the above platform.

Figure 1.39 shows an object-based surface rendition of an MS patient's brain MR scene data. Segmentation was done using the fuzzy connectedness method described in Section 1.2.6.7.

1.3.2.3 Volume Rendering

These methods take as input fuzzy object descriptions and generate their renditions. Object-based volume rendering becomes necessary when simple segmentation methods, such as fuzzy thresholding, fail, and objectness values cannot be generated on the fly during rendering. Since the object description can be made more compact than the original scene, and since additional information to speed up computation can be stored as part of the object representation (as in object-based surface rendering), object-based volume rendering[250] can be done at speeds of 2 to 40 s per view on machines such as a 300-MHz Pentium. These speeds are comparable to the speed of scene-based volume rendering achievable today using specialized hardware engines.

An example is the shell rendering method described in Ref. 250. A shell is a compact and efficient data structure that attempts to store only those voxels that potentially contribute to the rendering. It consists of a set of voxels — those in the vicinity of boundaries — together with several parameters associated with each voxel. The "thickness" of the shell (i.e., how far from the object boundary the voxels are included in the shell) depends on the fuzziness of the boundary interface. In one extreme, the thickness may be one voxel, in which case we essentially have a binary shell[252] (used for rapid surface rendering). In the other extreme, the thickness considered may be such that the entire body region is represented in the shell. Voxels whose opacities are less than a low threshold or whose six neighbors have opacities greater than a high threshold are not included in the shell. The idea here is that both these groups make a negligible contribution to the rendering. Each voxel v in the shell has a 5-tuple associated with it, as described below:

x_v : the x coordinate of v in the scene domain;
$nbrcode(v)$: a code that indicates which of the six neighbors of v have opacity greater than the high threshold;
$op(v)$: opacity assigned to v;
$gm(v)$: scene gradient magnitude at v that indicates the strength of the surface at v;
N_v : surface normal at v.

The 5-tuples are stored row by row and slice by slice. BTF voxel projection and compositing as described in Section 1.3.1.2 are used in shell rendering. v is not projected, if, in the direction of viewing, v is obstructed by high-opacity voxels as indicated by its neighbor code. An FTB strategy[250] is slightly faster than BTF projection. The method also allows making linear, curvilinear and angular measurements on the fuzzy surface. See Ref. 250 for details.

Figure 1.40 illustrates shell rendering from CT data of craniofacial bone and soft-tissue structures, both of which have been defined separately using the fuzzy connected method described in Section 1.2. Note that if we use direct scene-based volume rendering based on fuzzy thresholding, the skin becomes inseparable from other soft tissues and always obscures the rendition of muscles as illustrated in Figure 1.40. Further, two additional problems in scene-based rendering are effectively overcome by fuzzy-connected object rendering: (1) Although thin bones can be captured via fuzzy thresholding, frequently some aspects of skin and muscles are also segmented with thin bones because of similar CT numbers. In a volume rendition of only bone, the skin and muscles appear as a veil over the bone surface. (2) Analogously, when we try to capture only muscles via fuzzy thresholding, skin is also segmented. Additionally, voxels in the boundary between bone and fat and bone and air are also identified as muscles because of the partial volume effect.

1.3.3 Misconceptions and Challenges in Visualization

Several misleading statements relating to visualization methods appear frequently in the literature. The following occur most frequently:

1. *Surface rendering equated to thresholding*: Clearly, as described in Section 1.2.6, thresholding is only one (actually the simplest) of the many available hard region- and boundary-based segmentation methods, the output of any of which can be surface rendered.
2. *Volume rendering not requiring segmentation*: The phrase "volume rendering" is very general and is used in different senses. This is clarified below. In whatever sense it is taken, the above statement is not true. The only useful volume rendering/visualization technique that does not require segmentation of any sort is MIP. The opacity assignment schemes described in Figure 1.21 and in Section 1.3.1 are clearly fuzzy segmentation

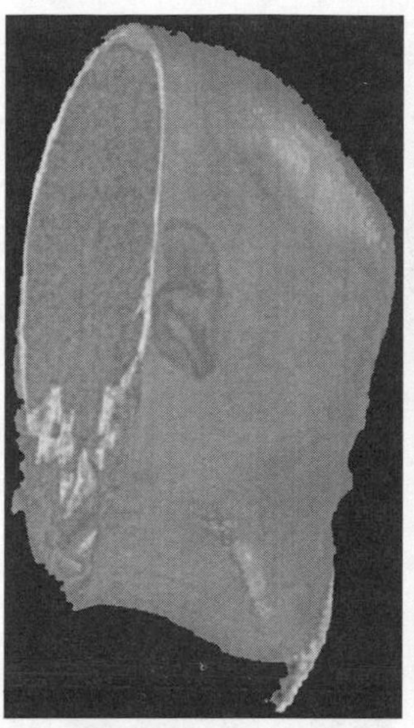
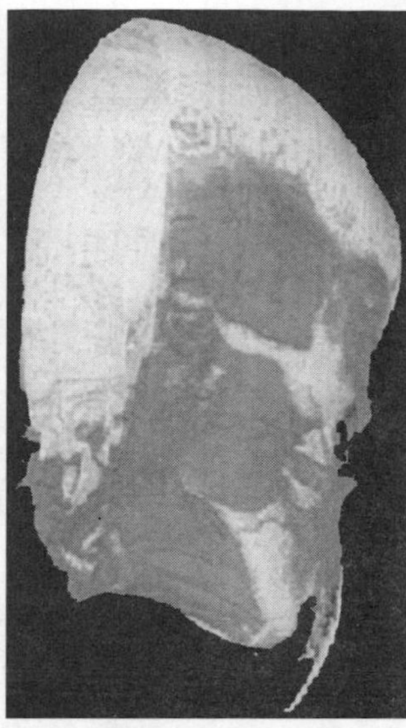

FIGURE 1.40 Object-based volume rendering (right) of craniofacial bone and soft-tissue structures from CT data. For comparison, scene-based volume rendering (via fuzzy thresholding) of the same data is shown on the left. The bone and soft-tissue structures are defined as separate fuzzy-connected objects on the right. Note how the skin has been effectively peeled to show clearly the muscles and even some of the neurovascular structures.

strategies, and they face the same problems that any segmentation method encounters, as illustrated in Figure 1.40. Note how clearly unconvincing it is to call opacity functions such as the one shown in Figure 1.21 not representing segmentation, but its particular manifestation when $t_1 = t_2$ and $t_3 = t_4$, which corresponds to thresholding, indeed segmentation.

3. *The meaning of volume rendering*: The meaning conveyed by this phrase varies considerably in its use in the literature. Frequently, it is used to refer to any scene-based rendering techniques, hard as well as fuzzy. It is also used to refer to object-based rendering techniques. In this general sense, clearly the slice mode of visualization is also captured within this phrase. It is better to reserve this term to refer to only fuzzy object rendering, whether it is done via scene-based or object-based methods, but not to refer to hard object rendering methods.

In spite of the considerable progress made in visualization during the past two decades, several basic issues remain: (1) Note that the preprocessing operations and, subsequently, the visualization operations can be applied in many different sequences to produce the desired end results. The results may vary considerably among different sequences. For example, the sequence filtering → interpolation → segmentation → rendering may produce significantly different renditions from those produced by interpolation → segmentation → filtering → rendering. Considering the different methods for each operation and the parameters associated with each operation, there is a large number of ways of producing the desired end results. Figure 1.41 shows five different sequences of such operations applied to a CT scene of a skull. A systematic study is needed to understand what combination of operations is best for a given application. Usually, whatever fixed combination is provided by the 3D imaging system is taken to be the best for the application. (2) An objective comparison of visualization methods, especially in view of the above comment, becomes a daunting task. (3) Realistic tissue display, including color, texture, and surface properties, is closely tied to proper segmentation and requires further research. (4) Unlike surface rendering, the speed of volume

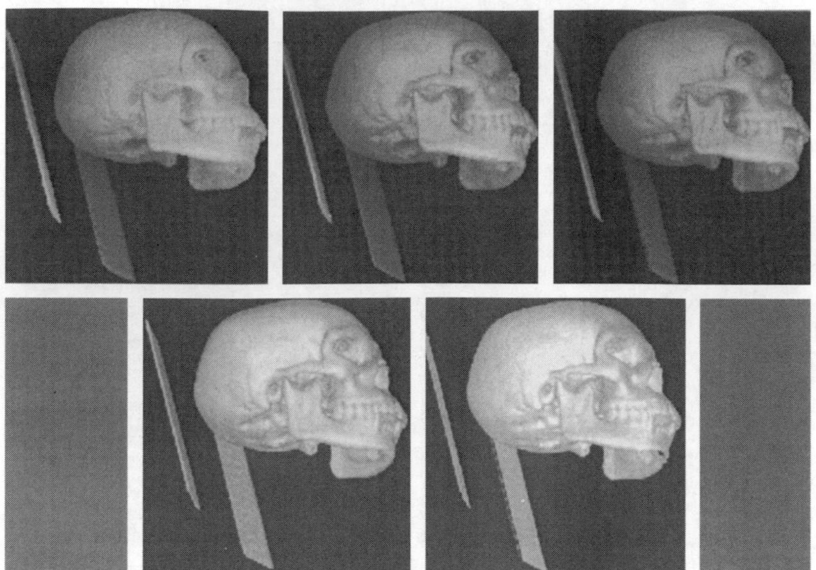

FIGURE 1.41 The five renditions shown of a human skull, derived from a CT scene, are obtained through five different sequences of preprocessing and rendering operations. There is a considerable variation in the appearance of the renditions. Many other renditions can be created for the same scene by changing the sequence, the algorithms used for the individual operations, and their parameters.

rendering is still not in the interactive realm, especially for large data sets. Therefore, there is a need and scope for speeding up both object-based and scene-based volume rendering methods.

1.4 MANIPULATION

The main purpose of these operations is, given a structure system, to create another structure system by modifying structures or their relationship in the system. The main motivation for these operations is to simulate surgery procedures based on patient-specific scene data, and to develop aids for interventional and therapy procedures. They are also useful for removing obscuring structures to facilitate clearer visualization of the structure of interest. Compared to preprocessing and visualization, work on manipulation is in its infancy. Therefore, we will not discuss this topic in detail. Two classes of operations are being developed: rigid and deformable.

1.4.1 RIGID

Operations to cut, separate, add, subtract, move, and mirror objects and their components have been developed, using both hard[252,253,261,262] and fuzzy object definitions.[263] The idea here is that the user directly interacts with an object-based surface or volume rendition of the object system to execute these operations. Clearly, for the operations to be practically useful, they should be executable at interactive speeds. This is indeed possible using both hard as well as fuzzy object definitions[252,263] on a machine such as a 300-MHz Pentium PC.[23]

Figure 1.42 illustrates a craniomaxillofacial osteotomy and segmental movement procedure[264] simulated using a child's skull structure defined via a CT scene by thresholding. Curved cutting, separation of the segment, and movement of the segment have been done to show the simulation of a frontal bone advancement procedure used in correcting deformities of the forehead and of the orbits.[264] Figure 1.43 illustrates the mirror reflection operation, considered to be useful in assessing the extent of deformities that are unilateral. Once the deformity is modeled, existing devices[265] can be used to create physical models of the deformity.

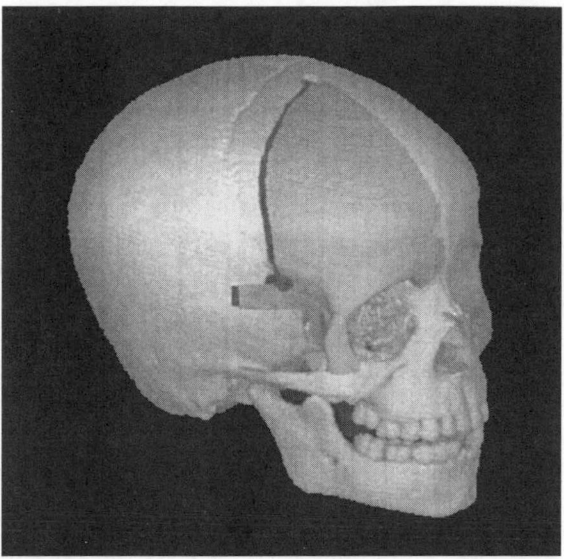

FIGURE 1.42 Illustration of the simulation of a "frontal bone advancement" craniofacial surgery procedure using several manipulation operations. The structure was derived from a CT scene of a child's skull.

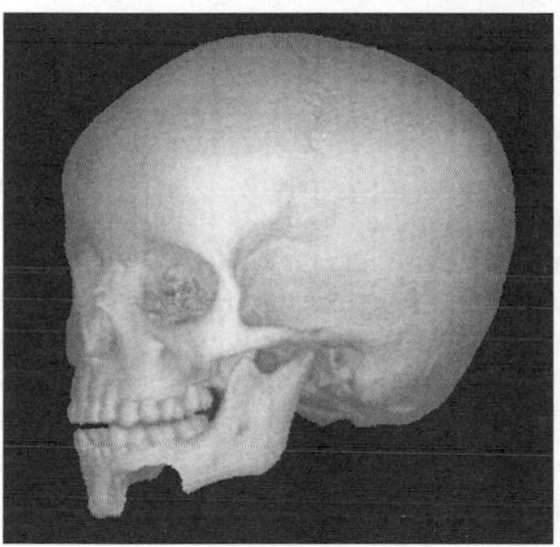

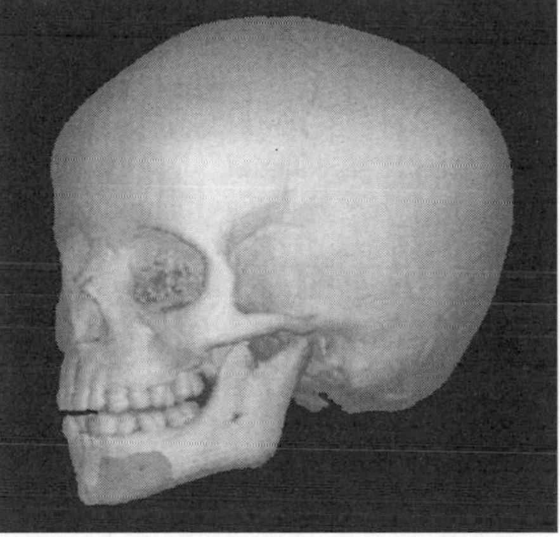

FIGURE 1.43 Illustration of the mirror reflection operation. A deformity was artificially introduced on the mandible on the left side of the skull. Mirror reflection about a central saggital plane of the normal side to the affected side shows the extent of the deformity. A separate structure can be created that represents this reflected piece. Devices exist[265] which can create physical prosthesis models when they are given proper structure data such as that of the reflected piece.

1.4.2 Deformable

Operations to stretch, compress, and bend are being developed. Mechanical modeling of soft-tissue structures including muscles, tendons, ligaments, and capsules is complicated because forces generated by them and their behavior under external forces are difficult to determine, especially in a patient-specific fashion. Therefore, past attempts have considered properties of soft tissues to build generic models. Generic models based on local deformations are used as an aid in facial plastic surgery[266] quite independent of the underlying bone and muscle, but treating only the skin surface. The use of multiple layers — skin, fatty tissue, muscle, and bone, where bone does not move — has been explored in different combinations to model facial expression animation.[267–269]

Although attempts have been made to model soft tissue in this fashion and in capturing their mechanical properties (e.g., how a musculo-tendon actuator functions,[270] or what the force-length function is),[271] no attempt seems to have been made in integrating hard-tissue (bone) changes with the soft-tissue modifications in a model. The reasons for this are the lack of adequate visualization tools, the lack of tools to simulate osteotomy procedures, and the lack of tools to integrate soft-tissue models with hard-tissue changes.

This area is open for further research. Considering that most of the tissues in the body are deformable and movable, and the fact that object information in images is inherently fuzzy, basic fuzzy mechanics theories and algorithms need to be developed to carry out patient-specific object manipulation and analysis.

1.5 ANALYSIS

The main purpose of these operations is, given a set of scenes or a structure system, to generate a quantitative description of the morphology or function of the structure system.

The goal of many 3D imaging applications is analysis of an object system. Although visualization is used as a visual aid, that in itself may not always be the end goal. As such, many of the current application-driven works are in analysis. They tend to be application specific. We will not go into a detailed discussion of analysis methodologies, but we will give an outline of the classes of analysis operations that are common among applications. See Chapters 3 and 9 for a more detailed discussion of particular types of analysis operations. As in other operations, we may classify them into two groups: scene based and object based.

1.5.1 Scene Based

In these methods, the quantitative description is based directly on scene intensities. Examples of measures include ROI statistics, density, activity, perfusion, and velocity. Object structural information derived from a scene from another modality is often used to guide the selection of regions for these measurements. The ROI statistics[272] are measured to study how different anatomic regions differ in these measures based on the particular imaged property. Density measurements[273] are used to assess the material density of an object (such as bone). Measures of activity[274,275] and perfusion[276] are used to assess the degree of enhancement of scene intensities in object regions in response to the administration of certain agents into the body. In flow and velocity analysis,[277,278] the movement of a fluid or of a dynamic organ is studied based on intensity patterns created by a specialized imaging device. Usually, data are acquired in a time sequence in this case.

1.5.2 Object Based

In these methods, a quantitative description is obtained from the structures segmented from scenes based on their morphology and how it changes with time, or on the relationship among objects in the system and how that changes. Examples of measures include distance, length, curvature, area volume, mechanical properties, and mechanics.

Morphologic measures (distance, thickness, length, curvature, area, volume)[279–283] and mechanical properties[284,285] are extensively used in establishing norms for normal populations and studying their variations under disease conditions and in response to therapy. The goal is similar in the study of kinematics and mechanics:[286–289] to study the motions of objects for establishing normal ranges, for characterizing abnormal motions, and for studying how they change in response to therapy. Since a component of time is involved in these, images are acquired for different time instances over the interval of dynamics of the object studied.

Considering the fact that object information in images is fuzzy, fuzzy morphometry and mechanics theories and algorithms are needed to realistically analyze object information in images.

1.6 SOURCES OF DIFFICULTY IN 3D IMAGING

There are mainly two types of difficulties in 3D imaging, those relating to object definition and to validation. Object definition difficulties have already been discussed in detail in Section 1.2. Difficulties in validation are discussed below. There are two types of entities that need to be validated: qualitative and quantitative.

1.6.1 VALIDATION: QUALITATIVE

The purpose of qualitative validation is to assess preprocessing and visualization methods for the improvements they achieve in the visual manifestation of object features in images/renditions. The assessment is usually conducted for a specific task. These are well-established methods of observer studies and receiver operating characteristic (ROC) analysis that can be used for this purpose.[290] A major challenge here, especially in comparing rendering methods,[291] is how to sift through the large number of combinations of operations, methods, and their parameter settings so that a small number of methods can be selected for formal ROC analysis. The main difficulty in this analysis is that truth about the figure of merit employed for evaluation must be known.

1.6.2 VALIDATION: QUANTITATIVE

The purpose of quantitative validation is to assess the precision, accuracy, and efficiency of the measurement process.

Precision: This refers to the reliability of the method. This is usually easy to establish. It consists of repeating the measurement process and assessing variation using standard statistical methods such as coefficient of variation, correlation coefficient, kappa statistic, and analysis of variance.[292] All steps that involve subjectivity have to be repeated (including, for example, how the patient is positioned in the scanner), and the repeatability of the measures can be analyzed.

Accuracy: This refers to how the measurement agrees with truth. We may handle accuracy for recognition and delineation separately. For small objects, establishing recognition accuracy requires histological assessment of object presence/absence. For big (anatomic) objects, an expert reader can provide recognition truth. One can then apply ROC analysis.

Establishing delineation accuracy requires a point-by-point assessment of object presence and its grade within the body region. Since truth is very difficult to establish in this manner, usually the following surrogates are used: physical phantoms, mathematical phantoms, manual (expert) delineation, simulation of mathematical objects and burying them in actual images, and comparison with a process whose accuracy is known. All of these methods have their own problems, and in all cases, their ability to represent truth is questionable.

Efficiency: This refers to the practical viability of the method, say in terms of the number of studies that can be processed per hour. This has two components — computer time and operator time. The former does not matter as long as it is not impractical. The latter however is very crucial in determining whether or not a method is practically viable no matter how precise and accurate it is. The degree of operator help required by 3D imaging operations may vary considerably from study to study. This aspect of validation is usually ignored. Most methods require operator help for acceptable precision and accuracy when a sufficiently large number of studies are analyzed. Therefore, efficiency should be evaluated and its statistical variation should be analyzed for all 3D imaging methods that require operator assistance.

In summary, generally there are two approaches to 3D imaging: scene based and object based. There are mainly two types of difficulties related to object definition and validation of delineation.

There are also numerous challenges for mathematicians, engineers, physicists, and physicians, as outlined throughout this chapter.

ACKNOWLEDGMENTS

This work was supported by NIH grant NS37172 and a grant from the Department of Army, DAMD179717271. The author is grateful to Mary A. Blue for typing the manuscript and preparing the drawings.

REFERENCES

1. I. Sobel, C. Levinthal and E. Macagno, "Special techniques for the automatic computer reconstruction of neuronal structures," *Annual Review of Biophysics and Bioengineering*, 9:347–362, 1980.
2. R. Kruger and T. Cannon, "The application of computerized tomography, boundary detection, and shaded graphics reconstruction to industrial inspection," *Materials Evaluation*, 36:75–80, 1978.
3. C. Lin and M. Cohen, "Quantitative methods for microgenetic modeling," *Journal of Applied Physics*, 53:4152–4165, 1982.
4. R. Grotjahn and R. Chervin, "Animated graphics in meteorological research and presentations," *Bulletin of the American Meteorological Society*, 65:1201–1208, 1984.
5. L. Hesselink, "Digital image processing in flow visualization," *Annual Review of Fluid Mechanics*, 20:421–485, 1988.
6. Z. Cho, J. Jones and M. Singh, *Foundations of Medical Imaging*. New York: John Wiley & Sons, 1993.
7. K. Höhne, H. Fuchs and S. Pizer (eds.), *3D Imaging in Medicine, Algorithms, Systems, Applications*. Berlin: Springer-Verlag, 1990.
8. J. Udupa and G. Herman (eds.), *3D Imaging in Medicine*. Boca Raton, Florida: CRC Press, 1991.
9. C. Roux and J. Coatrieux, *Contemporary Perspectives in Three-Dimensional Biomedical Imaging*. Amsterdam, The Netherlands: IOS Press, 1997.
10. R. Taylor, S. Lavallee, G. Burdea and R. Mosges, *Computer Integrated Surgery*. Cambridge, Massachusetts: MIT Press, 1996.
11. A. Kaufman (ed.), *A Tutorial on Volume Visualization*. Los Alamitos, California: IEEE Computer Society Press, 1990.
12. G. Nielson, S. Shriver and L. Rosenblum, *Visualization in Scientific Computing*. Washington, D.C.: IEEE Computer Society Press, 1990.
13. *Proceedings of Visualization in Biomedical Computing*, Los Alamitos, California: IEEE Computer Society Press, 1990.
14. *Proceedings of Visualization in Biomedical Computing*, 1808, Bellingham, Washington: Society of Photo-Optical Instrumentation Engineers, 1992.
15. *Proceedings of Visualization in Biomedical Computing*, 2359, Bellingham, Washington: Society of Photo-Optical Instrumentation Engineers, 1994.
16. *Proceedings of Visualization in Biomedical Computing*, Institute of Mathematics and Computer Science in Medicine (IMDM), University Hospital Eppendorf, Hamburg, Germany, 1996.
17. M. Dalton, J. Hunter, W. Olan, D. Robertson, S. Wetzner and M. Andre, "Simulation of digital holography images for computer based medical imaging systems," *Radiology*, 205:592, 1997.
18. *Communications of the ACM*, A special issue on "New Technologies in Health Care," 40, 1997.
19. *Proceedings of the IEEE*, A special issue on "Virtual and Augmented Reality in Medicine," 86(3),1998.
20. F. Jolesz, "Image-guided procedures and the operating room of the future," *Radiology*, 204:601–612, 1997.
21. L. Adams, W. Krybus, D. Meyer-Ebrecht, Rueger, J. Gilsbach, R. Mosges and G. Schloendroff, "Computer assisted surgery," *IEEE Computer Graphics and Applications*, 10:43–51, 1990.
22. J. Udupa, J. Tian, D. Hemmy and P. Tessier, "A Pentium PC-based craniofacial 3D imaging and analysis system," *Journal of Craniofacial Surgery*, 8:333–339, 1997.

23. J. Udupa, D. Odhner, S. Samarasekera, R. Goncalves, K. Iyer, K. Venugopal and S. Furuie, "3DVIEWNIX: An open, transportable, multidimensional, multimodality, multiparametric imaging software system," *SPIE Proceedings*, 2164:58–73, 1994.
24. J. Browne, G. Herman and D. Odhner, "SNARK93: A programming system for image reconstruction from projections," Technical Report MIPG198, Medical Image Processing Group, Department of Radiology, University of Pennsylvania, Philadelphia, Pennsylvania, 1993.
25. L. Zusne, *Visual Perception of Form*. New York: Academic Press, 1970.
26. J. Udupa, G. Herman, P. Margasahayam, L. Chen and C. Meyer, "3D98: A turnkey system for the display and analysis of 3D medical objects," *SPIE Proceedings*, 671:154–168, 1986.
27. J. Udupa, "Interactive segmentation and boundary surface formation for 3D digital images," *Computer Graphics and Image Processing*, 18:213–235, 1982.
28. M. Health, S. Sarkar, T. Sanocki and K. Bowyer, "Comparison of edge detectors," *Computer Vision and Image Understanding*, 69:38–54, 1998.
29. O. Monga and S. Benayoun, "Using partial derivatives of 3D images to extract typical surface features," *Computer Vision and Image Understanding*, 61:171–189, 1995.
30. R. Chin and C. Yeh, "Quantitative evaluation of some edge-preserving noise smoothing techniques," *Computer Graphics and Image Processing*, 23:67–91, 1983.
31. P. Perona and J. Malik, "Scale space and edge detection using anisotropic diffusion," *IEEE Transactions on Pattern Analysis and Machine Intelligence*, 12:629–639, 1983.
32. G. Gerig, O. Kubler, R. Kikinis and F. Jolesz, "Nonlinear anisotropic filtering of MRI data," *IEEE Transactions on Medical Imaging*, 11:221–232, 1992.
33. J. Udupa and R. Goncalves, "Imaging transforms for visualizing surfaces and volumes," *Journal of Digital Imaging*, 6:213–236, 1993.
34. W. Pratt, *Digital Image Processing*. New York: Wiley, 1991.
35. J. Foley and A. van Dam, *Fundamentals of Interactive Computer Graphics*. Reading, Massachusetts: Addison-Wesley, 1982.
36. M. Stytz and R. Parrott, "Using kriging for 3D medical imaging," *Computerized Medical Imaging and Graphics*, 17:421–442, 1993.
37. S. Raya and J. Udupa, "Shape-based interpolation of multidimensional objects," *IEEE Transactions on Medical Imaging*, 9:32–42, 1990.
38. W. Higgins, C. Morice and E. Ritman, "Shape-based interpolation of tree-like structures in three-dimensional images," *IEEE Transactions on Medical Imaging*, 12:439–450, 1993.
39. G. Herman, J. Zheng and C. Bucholtz, "Shape-based interpolation," *IEEE Computer Graphics and Applications*, 12:69–79, 1992.
40. R. Lotufo, G. Herman and J. Udupa, "Combining shape-based and gray-level interpolation technique for three-dimensional images," *SPIE Proceedings*, 1808:289–298, 1992.
41. G. Grevera and J. Udupa, "Shape-based interpolation of multidimensional grey-level images," *IEEE Transactions on Medical Imaging*, 15:881–892, 1996.
42. W. Barrett and R. Stringham, "Shape-based interpolation of grayscale serial slice images," *SPIE Proceedings,* 1898:105–115, 1993.
43. W. Barrett and E. Bass, "Interpolation by directed distance morphing," *SPIE Proceedings*, 2359:110–121, 1994.
44. A. Goshtasby, D. Turner and L. Ackerman, "Matching of tomographic slices for interpolation," *IEEE Transactions on Medical Imaging*, 11:507–516, 1992.
45. D. Puff, D. Eberly and S. Pizer, "Object-based interpolation via cores," *SPIE Proceedings*, 2167:104–115, 1994.
46. B. Morse, S. Pizer and D. Fritsch, "Robust object representation through object-relevant use of scale," *SPIE Proceedings*, 2167:143–150, 1994.
47. G. Grevera and J. Udupa, "Objective comparison of interpolation methods," *SPIE Proceedings*, 3031:2–11, 1997.
48. G. Herman, S. Rowland and M.M. Yau, "A comparative study of the use of linear and modified cubic spline interpolation for image reconstruction," *IEEE Transactions on Nuclear Science*, NS-26:2879–2894, 1979.

49. R. Woods, S. Cherry and J. Mazziotta, "Rapid automated algorithm for aligning and reslicing PET images," *Journal of Computer Assisted Tomography*, 16:620–633, 1992.
50. R. Woods, J. Mazziotta and S. Cherry, "MRI-PET registration with automated algorithm," *Journal of Computer Assisted Tomography*, 17:536–546, 1993.
51. K. Chinzei, T. Dohi, T. Horiuchi, Y. Ohta, M. Suzuki, Y. Yamauchi, D. Hashimoto and M. Tsuzuki, "Quantitative integration of multimodality medical images," *SPIE Proceedings*, 1808:187–195, 1992.
52. A. Liu, S. Pizer, D. Eberly, B. Morse, J. Rosenman, E. Chaney, E. Bullitt and V. Carrasco, "Volume registration using the 3D core," *SPIE Proceedings*, 2359:217–226, 1994.
53. P. van den Elsen, E.-J. Pol, T. Sumanaweera, P. Hemler, S. Napel and J. Adler, "Grey value correlation techniques used for automatic matching of CT and MR brain and spine images," *SPIE Proceedings*, 2359:227–237, 1994.
54. D. Hill, C. Studholme and D. Hawkes, "Voxel similarity measures for automated image registration," *SPIE Proceedings*, 2359:205–216, 1994.
55. A. Venot, J. Lebruchec and J. Roucayrol, "A new class of similarity measures for robust image registration," *Computer Vision Graphics and Image Processing*, 28:176–184, 1984.
56. M. Herbin, A. Venot, J. Devaux, E. Walter, J. Lebruchec, L. Dubertret and J. Roucayrol, "Automated registration of dissimilar images: Application to medical imagery," *Computer Vision Graphics and Image Processing*, 47:77–88, 1989.
57. D. Collins, T. Peters and A. Evans, "An automated 3D non-linear image deformation procedure for determination of gross morphometric variability in human brain," *SPIE Proceedings*, 2359:180–190, 1994.
58. M. Miller, G. Christensen, Y. Amit and U. Grenander, "Mathematical textbook of deformable neuroanatomies," *Proceedings of the National Academy of Science*, 90:1944–1948, 1993.
59. U. Grenander, Y. Chow and D. Keenan, *HANDS: A Pattern Theoretic Study of Biological Shapes*. New York: Springer, 1990.
60. K. Arun, T. Huang and S. Blostein, "Least-squares fitting of two 3-D point sets," *IEEE Transactions on Pattern Analysis and Machine Intelligence*, 9:698–700, 1987.
61. C. Pelizzari, G. Chen, D. Spelbring, R. Weichselbaum and C. Chen, "Accurate three-dimensional registration of CT, PET and MR images of the brain," *Journal of Computer Assisted Tomography*, 13:20–26, 1989.
62. K. Toennies, J. Udupa, G. Herman, I. Wornom, III and S. Buchman, "Registration of 3D objects and surfaces," *IEEE Computer Graphics and Applications*, 10:52–62, 1990.
63. P. Gerlot-Chiron and Y. Bizais, "Registration of multimodality medical images using a region overlap criterion," *CVGIP: Graphical Models and Image Processing*, 54:396–406, 1992.
64. J. Maintz, P. van den Elsen and M. Viergever, "Comparison of edge-based and ridge-based registration of CT and MR brain images," *Medical Image Analysis*, 1:151–161, 1996.
65. H. Jiang, K. Holton and R. Robb, "Image registration of multimodality 3-D medical images by chamfer matching," *SPIE Proceedings*, 1660:356–366, 1992.
66. C. Henri, A. Cukiert, D. Collins, A. Olivier and T. Peters, "Towards frameless stereotaxy: Anatomical-vascular correlation and registration," *SPIE Proceedings*, 1808:214–224, 1992.
67. C. Pérault, A. Loboguerrero, J.C. Liehn and F. Batteux, "Automatic superimposition of CT and SPET immunoscintigraphic images in the pelves," *SPIE Proceedings*, 1808:235–240, 1992.
68. G. Maguire, M. Noz and H. Rusinek, "Graphics applied to medical image registration," *IEEE Computer Graphics and Applications*, 11:20–29, 1991.
69. J. Maintz, P. van den Elsen and M. Viergever, "Evaluation of ridge seeking operators for multimodality medical image matching," *IEEE Transactions on Pattern Analysis and Machine Intelligence*, 18:353–365, 1996.
70. M. Wang, C.J. Maurer, J. Fitzpatrick and R. Macinunas, "An automatic technique for finding and localizing externally attached markers in CT and MR volume images of the head," *IEEE Transactions on Biomedical Engineering*, 43:627–637, 1996.
71. J.C.R. Maurer, J. Fitzpatrick, M. Wang, R.J. Galloway, R. Maciunas and G. Allen, "Registration of head volume images using implantable fiducial markers," *IEEE Transactions on Medical Imaging*, 16:447–462, 1997.
72. D. Lemoine, E. Liegeard, D. Lussot and C. Barillot, "Multimodal registration system for the fusion of MRI, CT, MEG and 3D or stereotactic angiographic data," *SPIE Proceedings*, 2164:46–56, 1994.

73. P. Hemler, T. Sumanaweera, P. van den Elsen, S. Napel and J. Adler, "A versatile system for multimodality image fusion," *Journal of Image Guided Surgery*, 1:35–45, 1995.
74. G. Malandain, S. Fernandez-Vidal and J. Rocchisani, "Rigid registration of 3-D objects by motion analysis," *Proceedings of the 12th International Conference on Pattern Recognition*, 579–581, 1994.
75. E. Hall, *Computer Image Processing and Recognition*, pp. 115–123. New York: Academic Press, 1979.
76. J. Udupa, B. Hirsch, S. Samarasekera and R. Goncalves, "Joint kinematics via 3D MR imaging," *SPIE Proceedings*, 1808:664–670, 1992.
77. J. Udupa, B. Hirsch, S. Samarasekera, H. Hillstrom, G. Bauer and B. Kneeland, "Analysis of in vivo 3D internal kinematics of the joints of the foot," *IEEE Transactions on Biomedical Engineering*, 45:1387–1396, 1998.
78. R. Rhoad, J. Klimkiewicz, G. Williams, S. Kesmodel, J. Udupa, J. Kneeland and J. Iannotti, "A new in vivo technique for 3D shoulder kinematics analysis," *Skeletal Radiology*, 27:92–97, 1998.
79. F. Bookstein and W. Green, "Edgewarp: A flexible program package for biometric image warping in two dimensions," *SPIE Proceedings*, 2359:135–147, 1992.
80. J. Peifer, E. Garcia, C. Cooke, J. Klein, R. Folks and N. Ezquerra, "3-D registration and visualization of reconstructed coronary arterial trees on myocardial perfusion distributions," *SPIE Proceedings*, 1808:225–234, 1992.
81. R. Bajcsy and S. Kovacic, "Multiresolution elastic matching," *Computer Vision, Graphics and Image Processing*, 46:1–21, 1989.
82. J. Gee, C. Barillot, L. Le Briquer, D. Haynor and R. Bajcsy, "Matching structural images of the human brain using statistical and geometrical image features," *SPIE Proceedings*, 2359:191–204, 1994.
83. A. Evans, W. Dai, L. Collins, P. Neelin and S. Marrett, "Warping of a computerized 3-D atlas to match brain image volumes for quantitative neuroanatomical and functional analysis," *SPIE Proceedings*, 1445:236–246, 1991.
84. J. Talairach, G. Szikla, P. Tournoux, A. Prossalentis, M. Bordas-Ferrer, L. Covello, M. Jacob, A. Mempel, P. Buser and J. Bancaud, *Co-Planar Stereotaxis Atlas of the Human Brain: 3-Dimensional Proportional System — An Approach to Cerebral Imaging*. New York: Thieme Medical, 1988.
85. G. Schaltenbrand and W. Wahren, *Atlas of Stereotaxy of the Human Brain*. Stuttgart, Germany: Georg Thieme Verlag, 1977.
86. J. West, J. Fitzpatrick, M. Wang et al., "Comparison and evaluation of retrospective intermodality registration techniques," *Journal of Computer Assisted Tomography*, 21:554–566, 1997.
87. S. Raya, "Low-level segmentation of 3-D magnetic resonance brain images — a rule-based system," *IEEE Transactions on Medical Imaging*, 9:327–337, 1990.
88. L. Gong and C. Kulikowski, "Composition of image analysis processes through object-centered hierarchical planning," *IEEE Transactions on Pattern Analysis and Machine Intelligence*, 17:997–1009, 1995.
89. D. Collins and T. Peters, "Model-based segmentation of individual brain structures from MRI data," *SPIE Proceedings*, 1808:10–23, 1992.
90. M. Sonka, S. Tadikonda and S. Collins, "Knowledge-based interpretation of MR brain images," *IEEE Transactions on Medical Imaging*, 15:443–452, 1996.
91. J. Gee, M. Reivich and R. Bajcsy, "Elastically deforming 3D atlas to match anatomical brain images," *Journal of Computer Assisted Tomography*, 17:225–236, 1993.
92. G. Christensen, R. Rabbitt and M. Miller, "3-D brain mapping using a deformable neuroanatomy," *Physics in Medicine and Biology*, 39:609–618, 1994.
93. M. Kamber, R. Shinghal, D. Collins, G. Francis and A. Evans, "Model-based 3D segmentation of multiple sclerosis lesions in magnetic resonance brain images," *IEEE Transactions on Medical Imaging*, 14:442–453, 1995.
94. W. Nowinski, "A dual probabilistic classifier for three-dimensional neuroimaging from MRI data," *SPIE Proceedings*, 2359:373–384, 1994.
95. S.C. Lo, S.-L. Lou, J.-S. Lin, M. Freedman, M. Chien and S. Mun, "Artificial convolution neural network techniques and applications for lung nodule detection," *IEEE Transactions on Medical Imaging*, 14:711–718, 1995.
96. Y. Wu, K. Doi, C. Metz, N. Asada and M. Giger, "Simulation studies of data classification by artificial neural networks: Potential applications in medical imaging and decision making," *Journal of Digital Imaging*, 6:117–125, 1993.

97. D. Wei, H. Chan, M. Helvie, B. Sahiner, N. Petrick, D. Adler and M. Goodsitt, "Classification of mass and normal breast tissue on digital mammograms: Multiresolution texture analysis," *Medical Physics*, 22:1505–1513, 1995.
98. F.F. Yin, M. Giger, K. Doi, R. Schmidt and C. Vyborny, "Computerized detection of masses in digital mammograms: Investigation of feature analysis techniques," *Journal of Digital Imaging*, 7:18–26, 1994.
99. E. Artzy, G. Frieder and G. Herman, "The theory, design, implementation and evaluation of a three-dimensional surface detection algorithm," *Computer Graphics and Image Processing*, 15:1–24, 1981.
100. J. Udupa, S. Srihari and G. Herman, "Boundary detection in multidimensions," *IEEE Transactions on Pattern Analysis and Machine Intelligence*, PAMI-4:41–50, 1982.
101. D. Gordon and J. Udupa, "Fast surface tracking in three-dimensional binary images," *Computer Vision, Graphics, and Image Processing*, 45:196–214, 1989.
102. J. Udupa, H. Hung and K. Chuang, "Surface and volume rendering in 3D imaging: A comparison," *Journal of Digital Imaging*, 4:159–168, 1991.
103. S. Raya, J. Udupa and W. Barrett, "A PC-based 3D imaging system: Algorithms, software, and hardware considerations," *Computerized Medical Imaging and Graphics*, 14:353–370, 1990.
104. G. Herman, *Geometry of Digital Spaces*. Cambridge, Massachusetts: Birkhauser Boston, 1998.
105. A. Rosenfeld, T. Kong and A. Wu, "Digital surfaces," *CVGIP: Graphical Models and Image Processing*, 53:305–312, 1991.
106. G. Wyvill, C. McPheeters and B. Wyvill, "Data structures for soft objects," *The Visual Computer*, 2:227–234, 1986.
107. W. Lorensen and H. Cline, "Marching cubes: A high-resolution 3D surface construction algorithm," *Computer Graphics*, 21:163–169, 1987.
108. M. Dürst, "Additional reference to marching cubes," *Computer Graphics*, 22:72–73, 1988.
109. A. Kalvin, *Segmentation and Surface-Based Modeling of Objects in Three-Dimensional Biomedical Images*. Ph.D. Thesis, Department of Computer Science, New York University: New York, 1991.
110. J. Cox, D. Karron and B. Mishra, "The spiderweb surface rendering algorithm," *Innovation and Technology in Biology and Medicine*, 14:634–655, 1993.
111. H. Baker, "Building, visualizing and computing on surfaces of evolution," *IEEE Computer Graphics and Applications*, 8:31–41, 1988.
112. A. Wallin, "Constructing surfaces from CT data," *IEEE Computer Graphics and Applications*, 11:28–33, 1991.
113. A. van Gelder and J. Wilhelms, "Topological considerations in isosurface generation," *ACM Transactions on Graphics*, 13:337–375, 1994.
114. S. Röll, A. Haase and M. von Kienlin, "Fast generation of leakproof surfaces from well-defined objects by a modified marching cubes algorithm," *Computer Graphics Forum*, 14:127–138, 1995.
115. B. Natarajan, "On generating topologically consistent isosurfaces from uniform samples," *The Visual Computer*, 11:52–62, 1994.
116. H. Müller and M. Stark, "Adaptive generation of surfaces in volume data," *The Visual Computer*, 9:182–199, 1993.
117. J. Canny, "A computational approach to edge detection," *IEEE Transactions on Pattern Analysis and Machine Intelligence*, 8:679–698, 1986.
118. H. Liu, "Two- and three-dimensional boundary detection," *Computer Graphics and Image Processing*, 6:123–134, 1977.
119. G. Herman and H. Liu, "Dynamic boundary surface detection," *Computer Graphics and Image Processing*, 7:130–138, 1978.
120. D. Morgenthaler and A. Rosenfeld, "Multidimensional edge detection by hypersurface fitting," *IEEE Transactions on Pattern Analysis and Machine Intelligence*, PAMI-3:482–486, 1981.
121. D. Pope, D. Parker, D. Gustafson and P. Clayton, "Dynamic search algorithms in left ventricular border recognition and analysis of coronary arteries," *IEEE Proceedings of Computers in Cardiology*, 9:71–75, 1984.
122. M. Fischler, J. Tenenbaum and H. Wolf, "Detection of roads and linear structure in low resolution aerial imagery using a multi-source knowledge integration technique," *Computer Graphics and Image Processing*, 15:201–223, 1981.
123. J. Cappelletti and A. Rosenfeld, "Three-dimensional boundary following," *Computer Vision, Graphics, and Image Processing*, 48:80–92, 1989.

124. A. Amini, T. Weymouth and R. Jain, "Using dynamic programming for solving variational problems in vision," *IEEE Transactions on Pattern Analysis and Machine Intelligence*, 12:855–867, 1990.
125. G. Herman and D. Webster, "A topological proof of a surface tracking algorithm," *Computer Vision, Graphics, and Image Processing*, 23:162–177, 1983.
126. G. Frieder, G. Herman, C. Meyer and J. Udupa, "Large software problems for small computers: An example from medical imaging," *IEEE Software*, 2:37–47, 1985.
127. T. Kong and J. Udupa, "A justification of a fast surface tracking algorithm," *CVGIP: Graphical Models and Image Processing*, 54:162–170, 1992.
128. J. Udupa and V. Ajjanagadde, "Boundary and object labelling in three-dimensional images," *Computer Vision, Graphics, and Image Processing*, 51:355–369, 1990.
129. G. Herman, "Discrete multidimensional Jordan surfaces," *CVGIP: Graphical Models and Image Processing*, 54:507–515, 1992.
130. G. Herman, "Oriented surfaces in digital spaces," *CVGIP: Graphical Models and Image Processing*, 55:381–396, 1993.
131. J. Udupa, "Multidimensional digital boundaries," *CVGIP: Graphical Models and Image Processing*, 50:311–323, 1994.
132. D. Morgenthaler and A. Rosenfeld, "Surfaces in three-dimensional digital images," *Information and Control*, 51:227–247, 1981.
133. A. Rosenfeld, "Three-dimensional digital topology," *Information and Control*, 50:119–127, 1991.
134. R. Yagel, D. Cohen and A. Kaufman, "Discrete ray tracing," *IEEE Computer Graphics and Applications*, 12:19–28, 1992.
135. A. Kaufman, "Efficient algorithms for 3-D scan conversion of parametric curves, surfaces, and volumes," *Computer Graphics*, 21:171–179, 1987.
136. A. Kaufman, D. Cohen and R. Yagel, "Volume graphics," *Computer*, 26:51–64, 1993.
137. J. Lachaud, "Topologically defined isosurfaces," *Proceedings of the 6th International Workshop on Discrete Geometry for Computer Imagery*, pp. 245–256. New York: Springer-Verlag, 1996.
138. E. Keppel, "Approximating complex surfaces by triangulation of contour lines," *IBM Journal of Research and Development*, 19:2–11, 1975.
139. H. Fuchs, Z. Kedem and S. Uselton, "Optimal surface reconstruction for planar contours," *Communications of ACM*, 20:693–702, 1977.
140. L. Cook, S. Dwyer IH, S. Batnitzky and K. Lee, "A three-dimensional display system for diagnostic imaging applications," *IEEE Computer Graphics and Applications*, 3:13–19, 1983.
141. M. Shantz, "Surface definition for branching contour-defined objects," *Computer Graphics*, 15:242–259, 1981.
142. A. Shaw and E. Schwartz, "Construction of polyhedral surfaces from serial sections: Exact and heuristic solutions," *SPIE Proceedings*, 1091:221–233, 1989.
143. H. Huang and R. Ledley, "Three-dimensional image construction from in vivo consecutive transverse axial sections," *Computers in Biology and Medicine*, 5:165–170, 1975.
144. Y. Chien and K. Fu, "A decision function method for boundary detection," *Computer Graphics and Image Processing*, 3:125–140, 1974.
145. W. Barrett, P. Clayton and H. Warner, "Determination of left venticular contours: A probabilistic algorithm derived from angiographic images," *Computers and Biomedical Research*, 13:522–548, 1980.
146. S. Zucker and R. Hummel, "An optimal three-dimensional edge operator," *Proceedings of the IEEE Computer Science Conference on Pattern Recognition and Image Processing*, pp. 162–168, 1978.
147. A. Martelli, "Edge detection using heuristic search methods," *Computer Graphics and Image Processing*, 1:169–182, 1972.
148. A. Martelli, "An application of heuristic search methods to edge and contour detection," *Communications of the ACM*, 19:73–83, 1976.
149. U. Montanari, "On the optimal detection of curves in noisy pictures," *Communications of the ACM*, 14:335–345, 1971.
150. K. Chuang and J. Udupa, "Boundary detection in grey-level scenes," *Proceedings, 10th Annual Conference and Exposition of the National Computer Graphics Association*, I:112–117, 1989.
151. A. Martelli, "Contour detection in noisy pictures using heuristic search methods," *Proceedings of the First International Joint Conference on Pattern Recognition* (Washington), 375–388, 1973.

152. M. Levoy, "Display of surfaces from volume data," *IEEE Computer Graphics and Applications*, 8:29–37, 1988.
153. M. Kass, A. Witkin and D. Terzopoulos, "Snakes: Active contour models," *International Journal of Computer Vision*, 1:321–331, 1987.
154. S. Lobregt and M. Viergever, "A discrete dynamic contour model," *IEEE Transactions on Medical Imaging*, 14:12–24, 1995.
155. L. Cohen, "On active contour models," *Computer Vision, Graphics, and Image Processing: Image Understanding*, 53:211–218, 1991.
156. D. Geiger, A. Gupta, L. Costa and J. Vlontzos, "Dynamic programming for detecting tracking and matching deformable contours," *IEEE Transactions on Pattern Analysis and Machine Intelligence*, 17:294–302, 1995.
157. W. Neuenschwander, P. Fua, G. Szekely and O. Kubler, "Initializing snakes," *Proceedings of IEEE Computer Society Conference on Computer Vision and Pattern Recognition (CVPR'94)*, 658–663, 1994.
158. L. Cohen and R. Kimmel, "Global minimum for active contour models: A minimum path approach," *Proceedings of IEEE Computer Society Conference on Computer Vision and Pattern Recognition (CVPR'96)*, San Francisco, California, 1996.
159. L. Cohen, L. Cohen and N. Ayache, "Using deformable surfaces to segment 3-D images and infer differential structures," *Computer Vision, Graphics, and Image Processing: Image Understanding*, 56:242–263, 1991.
160. T. McInerney and D. Terzopoulos, "A dynamic finite element surface model for segmentation and tracking in multidimensional medical images with application to cardiac 4D image analysis," *Computerized Medical Imaging and Graphics*, 19:69–83, 1995.
161. T. McInerney and D. Terzopoulos, "Deformable models in medical image analysis: A survey," *Medical Image Analysis*, 1:91–108, 1996.
162. T. McInerney, *Topologically Adaptable Deformable Models*. Ph.D. Thesis, University of Toronto, 1997.
163. J. Udupa, S. Samarasekera and W. Barrett, "Boundary detection via dynamic programming," *SPIE Proceedings*, 1808:33–37, 1992.
164. E. Mortensen, B. Morse, W. Barrett and J. Udupa, "Adaptive boundary detection using live-wire two dimensional dynamic programming," *IEEE Proceedings of Computers in Cardiology*, 635–638, 1992.
165. E. Mortensen and W. Barrett, "Intelligent scissors for image composition," *Proceedings of Computer Graphics (SIGGRAPH'95)*, 191–198, 1995.
166. A. Falcao, J. Udupa, S. Samarasekera, S. Sharma, B. Hirsch and R. Lotufo, "User-steered image segmentation paradigms: Live wire and live lane," *Graphical Models and Image Processing*, 60:233–260, 1998.
167. A. Falcao and J. Udupa, "Segmentation of 3D objects using live wire," *SPIE Proceedings*, 3034:228–239, 1997.
168. B. Hirsch, J. Udupa and S. Samarasekera, "A new method of studying joint kinematics from 3D reconstruction of MRI data," *Journal of the American Podiatric Medical Association*, 86:4–15, 1996.
169. G. Bauer, H. Hillstrom, J. Udupa and B. Hirsch, "Clinical applications of 3D MR analysis of the joints of the foot," *Journal of the American Podiatric Medical Association*, 86:33–37, 1996.
170. J. Prewitt and M. Mendelsohn, "The analysis of cell images," *Annals of the New York Academy of Science*, 128:1035–1053, 1966.
171. C. Chow and T. Kaneko, "Automatic boundary detection of the left ventricle from cine angiograms," *Computer and Biomedical Research*, 15:388–410, 1972.
172. N. Otsu, "A threshold selection method from gray-level histogram," *IEEE Transactions on Systems, Man and Cybernetics*, 9:62–66, 1979.
173. P. Sahoo, S. Soltani and A. Wong, "A survey of thresholding techniques," *Computer Vision, Graphics, and Image Processing*, 41:233–260, 1988.
174. R. Duda and P. Hart, *Pattern Classification and Scene Analysis*. New York: John Wiley & Sons, 1973.
175. J. Bezdek, L. Hall and L. Clarke, "Review of MR image segmentation techniques using pattern recognition," *Medical Physics*, 20:1033–1048, 1993.
176. M. Vannier, R. Butterfield, D. Jordan and W. Murphy, "Multi-spectral analysis of magnetic resonance images," *Radiology*, 154:221–224, 1985.

177. H. Cline, W. Lorensen, R. Kikinis and F. Jolesz, "Three-dimensional segmentation of MR images of the head using probability and connectivity," *Journal of Computer Assisted Tomography*, 14:1037–1045, 1990.
178. R. Kikinis, M. Shenton, F. Jolesz, G. Gerig, J. Martin, M. Anderson, D. Metcalf, C. Guttmann, R. McCarley, W. Lorensen and H. Cline, "Quantitative analysis of brain and cerebrospinal fluid spaces with MR imaging," *Journal of Magnetic Resonance Imaging*, 2:619–629, 1992.
179. M. Kohn, N. Tanna, G. Herman, S. Resnick, P. Mozley, R. Gur, A. Alavi, R. Zimmerman and R. Gur, "Analysis of brain and cerebrospinal fluid volumes with MR imaging. Part 1. Methods, reliability and validation," *Radiology*, 178:115–122, 1991.
180. H. Rusinek, M. de Leon, A. George, L. Stylopoulos, R. Chandra, G. Smith, T. Rand, M. Mowrino and H. Kowalski, "Alzheimer's disease: Measuring loss of cerebral gray matter with MR imaging," *Radiology*, 178:109–114, 1991.
181. M. Kamber, D. Collins, R. Shinghal, G. Francis and A. Evans, "Model-based 3D segmentation of multiple sclerosis lesions in dual-echo MRI data," *SPIE Proceedings*, 1808:590–600, 1992.
182. H. Soltanian-Zadeh, J. Windham and D. Peck, "A comparative analysis of several transformations for enhancement and segmentation of magnetic resonance images," *IEEE Transactions on Medical Imaging*, 11:302–318, 1992.
183. J. Mitchell, S. Karlick, D. Lee and A. Fenster, "Computer-assisted identification and quantification of multiple sclerosis lesions in MR imaging volumes in the brain," *Journal of Magnetic Resonance Imaging*, 4:197–208, 1994.
184. L. Clarke, R. Velthuizen, S. Phuphanich, J. Schellenberg, J. Arrington and M. Silbiger, "MRI: Stability of three supervised segmentation techniques," *Magnetic Resonance Imaging*, 11:95–106, 1993.
185. M. Vaidyanathan, L. Clarke, R. Velthuizen, S. Phuphanich, A. Bensaid, L. Hall, J. Bezdek, H. Greenberg, A. Trotti and M. Silbiger, "Comparison of supervised MRI segmentation methods for tumor volume determination during therapy," *Magnetic Resonance Imaging*, 13:719–728, 1995.
186. M. Vaidyanathan, L. Clarke, C. Heidman, R. Velthuizen and L. Hall, "Normal brain volume measurement using multispectral MRI segmentation," *Magnetic Resonance Imaging*, 15:87–97, 1997.
187. R. Drebin, L. Carpenter and P. Hanrahan, "Volume rendering," *Computer Graphics*, 22:65–74, 1988.
188. N. Max, "Optical models for direct volume rendering," *IEEE Transactions on Visualization and Computer Graphics*, 1:99–108, 1995.
189. T. He, LichanHong, A. Kaufman and H. Pfister, "Generation of transfer functions with stochastic search techniques," *IEEE Visualization*, 96:227–234, 1996.
190. R. Cannon, J. Dave and J. Bezdek, "Efficient implementation of the fuzzy *c*-means clustering algorithms," *IEEE Transactions on Pattern Analysis and Machine Intelligence*, PAMI-8:248–255, 1986.
191. L. Hall, A. Bensaid, L. Clarke, R. Velthuizen, M. Silbiger and J. Bezdek, "A comparison of neural networks and fuzzy clustering techniques in segmenting magnetic resonance images of the brain," *IEEE Transactions on Neural Networks*, 3:672–683, 1992.
192. W. Menhardt and K. Schmidt, "Computer vision on magnetic resonance images," *Pattern Recognition Letters*, 8:73–95, 1988.
193. J. Bezdek, *Pattern Recognition with Fuzzy Objective Function Algorithms*. New York: Plenum Press, 1981.
194. M. Rhodes, "An algorithmic approach to controlling search in three-dimensional image data," *SIGGRAPH'79 Proceedings* (Chicago, Illinois), pp. 134–142, 1979.
195. P. Burt, T. Hong and A. Rosenfeld, "Segmentation and estimation of region properties through cooperative hierarchical computation," *IEEE Transactions on Systems, Man and Cybernetics*, SMC-11:802–809, 1981.
196. T. Hong and A. Rosenfeld, "Compact region extraction using weighted pixel linking in a pyramid," *IEEE Transactions on Pattern Analysis and Machine Intelligence*, PAMI-6:222–229, 1984.
197. S. Dellepiane and F. Fontana, "Extraction of intensity connectedness for image processing," *Pattern Recognition Letters*, 16:313–324, 1995.
198. N. Pal and S. Pal, "A review on image segmentation techniques," *Pattern Recognition*, 26:1277–1294, 1993.
199. J. Udupa and S. Samarasekera, "Fuzzy connectedness and object definition: Theory, algorithms and applications in image segmentation," *Graphical Models and Image Processing*, 58:246–261, 1996.

200. J. Udupa, L. Wei, S. Samarasekera, Y. Miki, M. van Buchem and R. Grossman, "Multiple sclerosis lesion quantification using fuzzy connectedness principles," *IEEE Transactions on Medical Imaging*, 16:598–609, 1997.
201. S. Samarasekera, J. Udupa, Y. Miki and R. Grossman, "A new computer-assisted method for enhancing lesion quantification in multiple sclerosis," *Journal of Computer Assisted Tomography*, 21:145–151, 1997.
202. Y. Miki, R. Grossman, J. Udupa, S. Samarasekera, M. van Buchen, B. Cooney, S. Pollack, D. Kolson, C. Constantinescu, M. Polansky and L. Mannon, "Computer-assisted quantitation of enhancing lesions in multiple sclerosis: Correlation with clinical classification," *American Journal of Neuroradiology*, 18:705–710, 1997.
203. Y. Miki, R. Grossman, J. Udupa, L. Wei, D. Kolson and L. Mannon, "Isolated U-fiber involvement in MS: Preliminary observations," *Neurology*, 50:1301–1306, 1998.
204. A. Kumar, Z. Jin, W. Bilker, J. Udupa and G. Gottlieb, "Late onset minor and major depression: Early evidence for common neuroanatomical substrates detected by using MRI," *Proceedings of the National Academy of Science*, 95:7654–7658, 1998.
205. M. Phillips, R. Grossman, Y. Miki, L. Wei, D. Kolson, M. van Buchem, M. Polansky, J. McGowan and J. Udupa, "Comparison of T2 lesion volume and magnetization transfer ratio histogram analysis and atrophy and measures of lesion burden in patients with multiple sclerosis," *American Journal of Neuroradiology*, 19:1055–1060, 1998.
206. J. Udupa, D. Odhner, J. Tian, G. Holland and L. Axel, "Automatic clutter-tree volume rendering for MR angiography by using fuzzy connectedness," *SPIE Proceedings*, 3034:114–119, 1997.
207. J. Udupa and D. Hemmy, "Fuzzy connected object rendering," *SPIE Proceedings*, 3335:454–461, 1998.
208. G. Herman and H. Liu, "Display of three-dimensional information in computed tomography," *Journal of Computer Assisted Tomography*, 1:155–160, 1977.
209. M. Rhodes, W. Glenn, Jr. and V. Azzawi, "Extracting oblique planes from serial CT sections," *Journal of Computer Assisted Tomography*, 4:649–657, 1980.
210. K. Maravilla, "Computer reconstructed sagittal and coronal computed tomography head scans: Clinical applications," *Journal of Computer Assisted Tomography*, 2:120–123, 1978.
211. S. Rothman, G. Dobben, M. Rhodes, W. Glenn and Y.M. Azzawi, "Computerized tomography of the spline: Curved coronal reformation from serial images," *Radiology*, 150:185–190, 1984.
212. G. Herman and H. Liu, "Three-dimensional display of human organs from computed tomograms," *Computer Graphics and Image Processing*, 9:1–29, 1979.
213. G. Frieder, D. Gordon and R. Reynolds, "Back-to-front display of voxel-based objects," *IEEE Computer Graphics and Applications*, 5:52–60, 1985.
214. J. Foley, A. Van Dam, S. Feiner and J. Hughes, *Computer Graphics*. Reading, Massachusetts: Addison-Wesley, 1990.
215. G. Rubin, C. Beaulieu, V. Argiro, H. Ringl, A. Norbash, J. Feller, M. Dake, R. Jeffrey Jr. and S. Napel, "Perspective volume rendering of CT and MR images: Applications for endoscopic viewing," *Radiology*, 199:321–330, 1996.
216. P. Keller, B. Drayer, E. Fram, K. Williams, C. Dumoulin and S. Souza, "MR angiography with two-dimensional display," *Radiology*, 173:527–532, 1989.
217. D. Brown and S. Riederer, "Contrast-to-noise ratios in maximum intensity projection images," *Magnetic Resonance in Medicine*, 130–137, 1992.
218. S. Schreiner, C. Paschal and R. Galloway, "Comparison of projection algorithms used for the construction of maximum intensity projection images," *Journal of Computer Assisted Tomography*, 20:56–67, 1996.
219. S. Schreiner, B. Dawant, C. Paschal and R. Galloway, "The importance of ray pathlengths when measuring objects in maximum intensity projection images," *IEEE Transactions on Medical Imaging*, 15:568–579, 1996.
220. M. Prince, D. Narasimhan, J. Stanley, T. Chenevert, D. Williams, M. Marx and K. Cho, "Breathhold gadolinium-enhanced MR angiography of the abdominal aorta and its major branches," *Radiology*, 197:785–792, 1995.
221. T. Grist, F. Korosec, D. Peters, S. Witte, R. Walovitch, R. Dolan, W. Bridson, E. Yucel and C. Mistretta, "Steady-state and dynamic MR angiography with MS-325: Initial experiences in humans," *Radiology*, 207:539–544, 1998.

222. J. Goldfarb and R. Edelman, "Coronary arteries: Breath-hold gadolinium-enhanced, three-dimensional MR angiography," *Radiology*, 206:830–834, 1998.
223. G. Rubin, P. Walker, M. Dake, S. Napel, R. Jeffery, C. McDonnell, R. Mitchell and D. Miller, "Three-dimensional spiral computed tomographic angiography: An alternative imaging modality for the abdominal aorta and its branches," *Journal of Vascular Surgery*, 18:656–664, 1993.
224. S. Napel, M. Marks and G. Rubin, "CT angiography with spiral CT and maximum intensity projection," *Radiology*, 185:607–610, 1992.
225. M. Marks, S. Napel, J. Jordan and D. Enzmann, "Diagnosis of carotid artery disease: Preliminary experience with maximum-intensity-projection spiral CT angiography," *American Journal of Roentgenology*, 160:1267–1271, 1993.
226. K. Höhne and R. Bernstein, "Shading 3D images from CT using gray-level gradients," *IEEE Transactions on Medical Imaging*, MI-5:45–47, 1986.
227. R. Reynolds, *Fast Methods for 3D Display of Medical Objects*. Ph.D. Thesis, Department of Computer and Information Sciences, University of Pennsylvania, Philadelphia, Pennsylvania, 1985.
228. D. Schlusselburg, W. Smith, D. Woodward and R. Parkey, "Use of computed tomography for a three-dimensional treatment planning system," *Computerized Medical Imaging and Graphics,* 12:25–32, 1988.
229. R. Lenz, "Processing and presentation of 3D images," *Proceedings of the IEEE Computer Society International Symposium on Medical Images and Icons* (Arlington, Virginia), pp. 298–303, 1984.
230. E. Farrell, W. Yang and R. Zapulla, "Animated 3D CT imaging," *IEEE Computer Graphics and Applications*, 5:26–32, 1985.
231. H. Tuy and L. Tuy, "Direct 2D display of 3D objects," *IEEE Computer Graphics and Applications*, 4:29–33, 1984.
232. J. Ylä-Jääski, F. Klein and O. Kübler, "Fast direct display of volume data for medical diagnosis," *CVGIP: Graphical Models and Image Processing,* 53:7–18, 1991.
233. D. Meagher, "Geometric modeling using octree encoding," *Computer Graphics and Image Processing*, 19:129–147, 1982.
234. S. Goldwasser, R. Reynolds, T. Bapty, D. Baraff, J. Summers, D. Talton and E. Walsh, "Physician's workstation with real-time performance," *IEEE Computer Graphics and Applications*, 5:44–57, 1985.
235. R. Reynolds, D. Gordon and L. Chen, "A dynamic screen technique for shaded graphics display of slice-represented objects," *Computer Vision, Graphics, and Image Processing*, 38:275–298, 1987.
236. L. Chen, G. Herman, R. Reynolds and J. Udupa, "Surface rendering in the cuberille environment," *IEEE Computer Graphics and Applications*, 5:33–43, 1985.
237. D. Gordon and R. Reynolds, "Image-space shading of three-dimensional objects," *Computer Vision, Graphics, and Image Processing*, 29:361–376, 1985.
238. U. Tiede, K. Hohne, M. Bomans, A. Pommert, M. Riemer and G. Wiebecke, "Investigation of medical 3D rendering algorithms," *IEEE Computer Graphics and Applications*, 10:41–53, 1990.
239. A. Kaufman, "The CUBE workstation: A 3D voxel-based graphics environment," *The Visual Computer*, 4:210–221, 1988.
240. D. Cohen, A. Kaufman, B. Bakalash and S. Bergman, "Real-time discrete shading," *The Visual Computer*, 6:16–27, 1990.
241. S. Bright and S. Laflin, "Shading of solid voxel models," *Computer Graphics Form*, 5:131–137, 1986.
242. T. Ohashi, T. Uchiki and M. Tokoro, "A three-dimensional shaded display method for voxel based representation," *Proceedings, EUROGRAPHICS'85*, 221–232, 1985.
243. C. Upson and M. Keeler, "V-buffer: Visible volume rendering," *Computer Graphics*, 22:59–64, 1988.
244. P. Sabella, "A rendering algorithm for visualizing 3D scalar fields," *Computer Graphics*, 22:51–58, 1988.
245. F. Klein and O. Kübler, "A prebuffer algorithm for instant display of volume data," *SPIE Proceedings*, 596:54–58, 1986.
246. F. Klein and O. Kübler, "Fast direct display of discrete volume data," *Proceedings of the 8th International Conference on Pattern Recognition*, 633–635, 1986.
247. R. Yagel and A. Kaufman, "Template-based volume viewing," Cambridge, United Kingdom: *EUROGRAPHICS'93*, 153–167, 1992.
248. P. Lacroute, "Fast volume rendering using a shear-warp factorization of the viewing transformation," Technical Report CSL-TR-i5-678 and Ph.D. Thesis, Stanford University, Departments of Electrical Engineering and Computer Science, Stanford, California, 1995.

249. M. Levoy, "Efficient ray tracing of volume data," *ACM Transactions on Graphics*, 9:245–261, 1990.
250. J. Udupa and D. Odhner, "Shell rendering," *IEEE Computer Graphics and Applications*, 13:58–67, 1993.
251. R. Ledley and C. Park, "Molded picture representation of whole body organs generated from CT scan sequences," *IEEE Proceedings of the First Annual Symposium of Computer Applications in Medical Care* (Washington, D.C.), 363–367, 1977.
252. J. Udupa and D. Odhner, "Fast visualization, manipulation, and analysis of binary volumetric objects," *IEEE Computer Graphics and Applications*, 11:53–62, 1991.
253. S. Trivedi, "Interactive manipulation of three-dimensional binary scanners," *The Visual Computer*, 2:209–218, 1986.
254. R. Webber, "Ray tracing voxel data via biquadratic local surface interpolation," *The Visual Computer*, 8–15, 1990.
255. T. Biddlecome, S. Fang, K. Dunn and M. Tuceryan, "Image guided interactive volume visualization for confocal microscopy data exploration," *SPIE Proceedings*, 3335:130–140, 1998.
256. S. Fang, R. Srinivasan, and R. Raghavan, "Deformable volume-rendering by 3D texture mapping and octree encoding," *Proceeding of IEEE Visualization'96*, San Francisco, California, 73–80, 1996.
257. V. Raptopoulos, P. Prassopoulos, R. Chuttani, M. McNicholas, J. McKee and H. Kressel, "Multiplanar CT pancreatography and distal cholangiography with minimum intensity projections," *Radiology*, 207:317–324, 1998.
258. S. Shiffman, G. Rubin and S. Napel, "Semiautomated editing of computed tomography sections for visualization of vasculature," *SPIE Proceedings*, 2707:140–151, 1996.
259. E. Artzy, "Display of three-dimensional information in computed tomography," *Computer Graphics and Image Processing*, 9:196–198, 1979.
260. J. Udupa, "DISPLAY: A system of programs for two- and three-dimensional display of medical objects from CT data," Technical Report MIPG41, Medical Image Processing Group, Department of Computer Science, SUNY at Buffalo, Buffalo, New York, 1980.
261. C. Cutting, B. Grayson, F. Bookstein, L. Fellingham and J. McCarthy, "Computer-aided planning and evaluation of facial and orthognathic surgery," *Computers in Plastic Surgery*, 13:449–461, 1986.
262. V. Patel, M. Vannier, J. Marsh and L.-J. Lo, "Assessing craniofacial surgical simulation," *IEEE Computer Graphics and Applications*, 16:46–54, 1996.
263. D. Odhner and J. Udupa, "Shell-manipulation: Alteration of multiple material fuzzy structures," *SPIE Proceedings*, 2431:35–42, 1995.
264. I. Jackson, I. Munro, K. Salyer and L. Whitaker, *Atlas of Craniomaxillofacial Surgery*. St. Louis, Missouri: The C.V. Mosby Company, 1982.
265. E. Rose, M. Norris and J. Rosen, "Application of high-tech three-dimensional imaging and computer-generated models in complex facial reconstructions with vascularized bone grafts," *Plastic and Reconstructive Surgery*, 91:252–264, 1992.
266. A. Paouri and N. Thalmann, "Creating realistic three-dimensional human shape characters for computer-generated films," *Proceedings of Computer Animation '91* (Tokyo), pp. 89–100. Springer-Verlag, 1991.
267. K. Waters, "A muscle model for animating three dimensional facial expression," *Proceedings of SIGGRAPH'87*, 21:17–24, 1987.
268. S. Platt and N. Badler, "Animating facial expressions," *Proceedings of SIGGRAPH'81*, 245–252, 1981.
269. D. Terzopoulos and K. Waters, "Techniques for realistic facial modeling and animation," *Proceedings of Computer Animation '91* (Tokyo), pp. 59–74, Springer-Verlag, 1991.
270. F. Zajac, T.E.L. and P. Stevenson, "A 'dimensionless' musculotendon model," *Proceedings of IEEE Engineering in Medicine and Biology*, 1:601–606, 1986.
271. S. Jianhua, T.M.N. and D. Thalmann, "Muscle-based human body deformations," *Proceedings of CAD/Graphics '93*, 95–100, 1993.
272. G. Wang, N. Volkow, A. Levy, J. Fowler, J. Logan, D. Alexoff, R. Hitzemann and D. Schyuler, "MR-PET image coregistration for quantitation of striatal dopamine D2 receptors," *Journal of Computer Assisted Tomography*, 20:423–428, 1996.
273. M. Ciarelli, S. Goldstein, J. Kuhn, D. Cody and M. Brown, "Evaluation of orthogonal mechanical properties and density of human trabecular bone from the major metaphyseal regions with materials testing and computed tomography," *Journal of Orthopaedic Research*, 9:674–682, 1991.

274. R. Carson, Y. Yan, B. Chodkowski, T. Yap and M. Daube-Witherspoon, "Precision and accuracy of regional radioactivity quantitation using the maximum likelihood EM reconstruction algorithm," *IEEE Transactions on Medical Imaging*, 13:526–537, 1994.
275. J. Poline and B. Mazoyer, "Analysis of individual brain activation maps using hierarchical description and multiscale detection," *IEEE Transactions on Medical Imaging*, 13:702–710, 1994.
276. M. Jerosch-Herold, N. Wilke and A. Stillman, "Magnetic resonance quantification of the myocardial perfusion reserve with a fermi function model for constrained deconvolution," *Medical Physics*, 25:73–84, 1998.
277. S. Song, R. Leahy, D. Boyd, B. Brundage and S. Nape, "Determining cardiac velocity fields and intraventricular pressure distribution from a sequence of ultrafast CT cardiac images," *IEEE Transactions on Medical Imaging*, 13:386–397, 1994.
278. M. Chwiaklowski, Y. Ibrahim, H. Li and R. Peshock, "A method for fully automated quantitative analysis of arterial flow using flow-sensitized MR images," *Computerized Medical Imaging and Graphics*, 20:365–378, 1996.
279. K. Hamano, N. Iwasaki, T. Takeya and H. Takita, "A comparative study of linear measurement of the brain and three-dimensional measurement of brain volume using CT scans," *Pediatric Radiology*, 23:165–168, 1993.
280. F. Bookstein, *Morphometric Tools for Landmark Data: Geometry and Biology*. Cambridge University Press, Cambridge, U.K.: 1–435, 1991.
281. J. Kulynych, K. Vladar, D. Jones and D. Weinberger, "Three-dimensional surface rendering in MRI morphometry: A study of the planum temporals," *Journal of Computer Assisted Tomography*, 17:529–535, 1993.
282. K. Lin, S. Bartlett, M. Yaremchuk, R. Grossman, J. Udupa and L. Whitaker, "An experimental study on the effect of rigid fixation on the developing craniofacial skeleton," *Plastic and Reconstructive Surgery*, 87:229–235, 1991.
283. M. Dulce, G. Mostbeck, K. Friese, G. Caputo and C. Higgins, "Quantification of the left ventricular volumes and function with cine MR imaging: Comparison of geometric models with three-dimensional data," *Radiology*, 188:371–376, 1993.
284. S. Hwang and F. Wehrli, "Probability-based structural parameters from three-dimensional nuclear magnetic resonance images as predictors of trabecular bone strength," *Medical Physics*, 24:1255–1262, 1997.
285. C. Korstjens, R. Spmijt, W. Geraets, L. Mosekilde and P. van der Stelt, "Reliability of an image analysis system for quantifying the radiographic trabecular pattern," *IEEE Transactions on Medical Imaging*, 16:230–234, 1997.
286. B. Hirsch, J. Udupa and S. Samarasekera, "Kinematics of the tarsal joints via 3D MR imaging," *SPIE Proceedings*, 2359:672–679, 1994.
287. D. Kraitchman, A. Young, C.N. Chang and L. Axel, "Semi-automatic tracking of myocardial motion in MR tagged images," *IEEE Transactions on Medical Imaging*, 14:422–433, 1995.
288. J.T.S. Denney and J. Price, "Reconstruction of 3-D left ventricular motion from planar tagged cardiac MR images: An estimation theoretic approach," *IEEE Transactions on Medical Imaging*, 14:625–635, 1995.
289. F. Meyer, R. Constable, A. Sinusas and J. Duncan, "Tracking myocardial deformation using phase contrast MRI velocity fields: A stochastic approach," *IEEE Transactions on Medical Imaging*, 15:453–465, 1996.
290. J. Swets, *Signal Detection and Recognition by Human Observers*. Los Altos, California: Peninsula Publishing, 1988.
291. M.W. Vannier, C.F. Hildebolt, J.L Marsh et al., "Cranio-synostosis: Diagnostic value of three-dimensional CT reconstruction," *Radiology*, 173:669–673, 1989.
292. B. Rosner, *Fundamentals of Biostatistics*. New York: Duxbury Press, 1995.

2 3D Imaging and Its Derivatives in Clinical Research and Practice

Frans W. Zonneveld

CONTENTS

0-8493-3179-X/00/$0.00+$.50

2.1 CLINICAL APPLICATIONS AND RESEARCH MAKING USE OF 3D IMAGING

2.1.1 INTRODUCTION

3D imaging has now been used clinically for almost 15 years. The first edition of this book[1] reflected the situation in November 1989 when the second meeting on Three-Dimensional Imaging in Medicine in San Diego was organized by the Department of Radiology of the Hospital of the University of Pennsylvania (HUP). This second edition reflects the current situation. Important improvements have been established in the acquisition of volumetric data sets. In CT this was done by the introduction of helical scanning,[2,3] which led to CT angiography (CTA),[4,5] and by added functionality in electron-beam CT.[6] In MRI it was the introduction of new sequences such as fast field echo (FFE), turbo spin echo (TSE), echoplanar imaging (EPI),[7] and gradient spin echo (GRASE). The time of flight (TOF) and phase contrast angiography (PCA) led to magnetic resonance angiography (MRA) and stimulated the development of a quasi-volume-rendering type of 3D imaging known as maximum intensity projection (MIP) which was later also applied to CT.[8] A special new method of MRI is functional MRI (fMRI), which requires gated patient activity and then highlights the brain regions involved in that particular activity. In ultrasound imaging, new 3D transducers were introduced as well as linear translation devices for standard transducers.[9,10] A new intravascular transducer mounted on a catheter produces endovascular volumetric data. In general, one can state that all tomographic imaging modalities can easily acquire volumetric data sets, thus increasing the need for 3D imaging as a means to analyze these data and extract medically relevant information and to support and guide therapy.

The quality of rendering of 3D images has been significantly improved in terms of using better lighting models and avoiding rendering artifacts. Some institutions have done dedicated studies on this topic[11,12] and, fortunately, the discussion about whether volume rendering (a technique using a "fuzzy" segmentation) was better than surface rendering[13,14] (a technique using a binary segmentation), or vice versa,[15] has died out because it was realized that, when the correct parameters are used, their quality is comparable,[16] that different types of cases need different types of rendering, and, in some cases, new algorithms have been developed that can be considered as a hybrid form resulting from the use of very flexible opacity curves.[17]

Another vital improvement is the rendering speed.[18] It has improved to such a degree over the past few years that real-time rendering has become possible on specialized graphical parallel computers that are coined "reality engines." In the near future we will see this capability becoming possible in the mid- and low-end workstations as well.

The application of 3D imaging was, in 1989, primarily limited to craniofacial surgery,[19–21] orthopedic surgery, neurosurgery, and radiotherapy.[22] Now, it has spread to many additional areas[23] such as otolaryngology, vascular surgery,[24] thorax surgery,[25] general surgery, obstetrics, urology, and even to more remote fields such as anatomy,[26,27] microscopic pathology[28] and cell biology,[29,30] dermatology,[31] archeology,[32–34] physical anthropology,[35–37] and forensic medicine.[38] Such topics are beyond the scope of this chapter. The imaging of soft tissues and vascular structures has matured and new applications such as surgical simulation and navigation, manufacturing of physical models,[39] and virtual and augmented reality, respectively, for presurgical training and intrasurgical reference have been developed and are in the process of maturing. We will not focus on the history of 3D imaging,[40] nor will we discuss surgical navigation, but instead try to demonstrate and discuss recent achievements from a clinical perspective. When useful, however, the technical literature will be referenced as well. We will discuss the major systems of the body (craniomaxillofacial complex including the head and neck, the central nervous system, musculoskeletal system, cardiovascular system, pulmonary system, gastrointestinal system, and genitourinary system) separately, indicate the contribution of each applicable imaging modality, and the value of 3D imaging to radiation therapy planning. Finally, we will discuss issues related to the derivatives of 3D imaging.

2.1.2 Craniomaxillofacial Complex Including the Head and Neck

2.1.2.1 Computed Tomography

The role of CT in 3D imaging of the craniomaxillofacial complex has been extensively covered in the literature, both from its craniofacial[19,41–43] as well as its maxillofacial aspect.[44–47] Its primary value is the visualization (qualitative aspect) and quantitative assessment of bony pathology. This qualitative aspect involves the comprehension of the shape of a deformed skull[48,49] (Figure 2.1) and the extent of disease such as suture ossification in craniosynostosis[50] (Figure 2.2), which are also possible in a panoramic fashion called "cylindrical surface map,"[51] the course of fractures and associated deformity in trauma[52–56] (Figure 2.3), and the extent of tumor destruction in oncology.[57] The quantitavive aspects will be discussed in Section 2.2.2.

In addition to providing an overview image which can be used to classify the severity of the disease,[58,59] 3D imaging can also create views that are impossible with direct imaging modalities. Examples of cutaway views are endocranial views of the skull base.[60–64] Inferior views of the skull base with the mandible and cervical spine removed,[65] a technique known as "disarticulation," can also facilitate, when removing the cranium, the assessment of the mandibular condyles[66] which otherwise cannot be studied from all directions[67] (Figure 2.4). In the same fashion, the temporomandibular meniscus can be disarticulated and visualized.[68] The same disarticulation technique can be applied to soft-tissue tumors and bony tumors (e.g., hyperostotic meningioma, osteoma, and fibrous dysplasia) to separate them from the surrounding healthy bone.[69]

Some investigators, however, feel that disarticulation is too time consuming and prefer cutaway imaging as has been demonstrated in the assessment of subcondylar fractures of the mandible.[70]

In the temporal bone, the combination of submillimeter resolution, 1 to 1.5 mm slice thickness, and submillimeter slice indexing have made 3D imaging of the labyrinth[71] possible, including details such as the aperture of the vestibular aqueduct[72] and the ossicles[73,74] (Figure 2.5). The use of overlapping thin slices without increasing the radiation dose as compared to contiguous scanning is a virtue of the helical scanning technique. In the future, this technique may be applied in the cochlea for the assessment of electrode position in cochlear implants.[75]

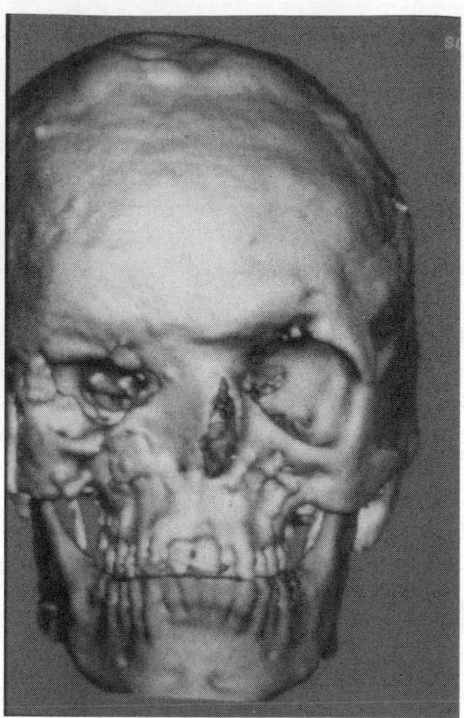

FIGURE 2.1 Male patient, aged 20, with right-sided anopthalmia and heminasal aplasia. Status after reconstruction of the right nasal half and an attempt to enlarge the right orbit. Note that the total overview of the asymmetry can be appreciated only on the 3D image.

3D visualization of air spaces is perfectly possible as we will see in Section 2.1.6. This means that 3D imaging of the paranasal sinuses is possible but will require some skill to disarticulate them from the nasopharynx.[76]

In the oropharynx, electron-beam CT has been used to assess the dynamic aspects of the swallowing process.[77] It is expected that this procedure is valuable for the study of dysphagic conditions and potential compensatory strategies.

In the parapharyngeal space, soft-tissue imaging has been used to image tumors in relationship to the carotid artery (see Section 2.1.5). Cutaway views are necessary to remove the mandible.[78]

In the larynx, it is possible to image the cartilage only when it is calcified[79,80] since normal cartilage has the same density on CT as muscle. 3D imaging is useful for visualization of tumor extent.[81] For reconstructions of the airway, see Section 2.1.6.

2.1.2.2 Magnetic Resonance Imaging

Magnetic resonance imaging presents the problem that segmentation (isolation of the structure of interest from the data volume) is much more difficult than in CT. As a result a technique has been applied that combines surface rendering of the skin, which is easy, with cutaway imaging of the tissues inside of the skin in the form of mapping MR images on the cutting planes. In this way tumors of the head and neck have been visualized.[82–84]

In the temporal bone, the labyrinth can be imaged by T2-weighted sequences followed by a maximum intensity projection (MIP) reconstruction, which can be considered as a special form of volume rendering[85] (Figure 2.6).

MRI has also been applied to the 3D animation of the temporomandibular joint by combining a 3D reconstruction of this area with opto-electronically recorded motion data.[86]

Finally, MRI has been applied to the imaging of tumor extent into the parapharyngeal space.[78]

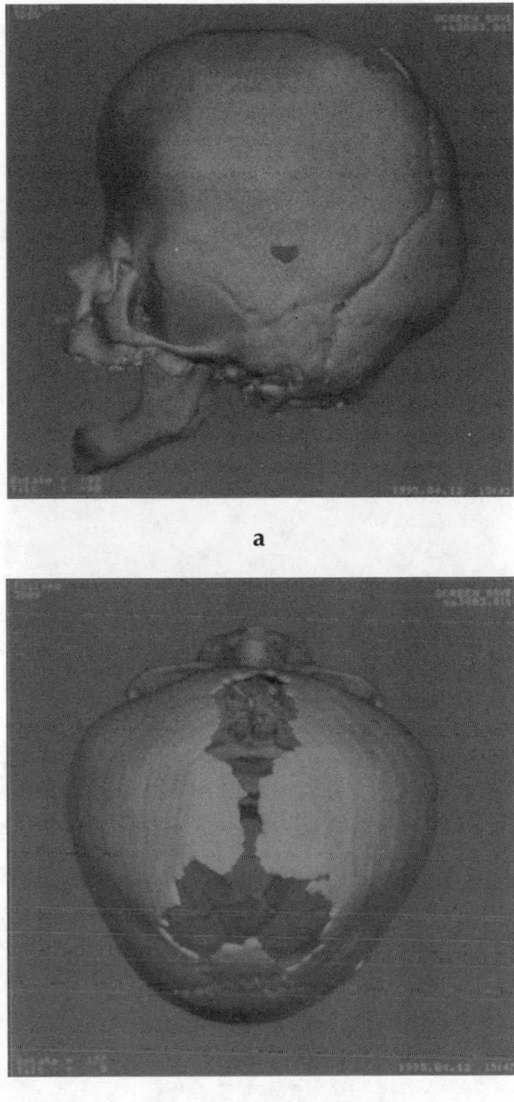

a

b

FIGURE 2.2 Four-month-old female with Saethre-Chotzen syndrome. (a) This left lateral view demonstrates the fusion of the coronal suture and the facial retrusion that has resulted from it. (b) This superior view shows the flattened forehead and the agenesis of the metopic suture. It also shows that the coronal synostosis is bilateral.

2.1.2.3 Sonographic Imaging

Although sonographic imaging is not routinely applied to the craniofacial system, except for its potential value in imaging of the fetal face (see Section 2.1.8), it has been capable of imaging the sternocleidomastoid muscle, underlying lymph nodes, jugular vein, and carotid artery.[87] A special case is 3D sonographic imaging of the eye which is capable of imaging a tumor of the iris.[88]

2.1.2.4 Facial Skin Digitization

There are various technical possibilities to digitize the facial skin such as used in laser scanning[89–92] (Figure 2.7) and stereophotogrammetry.[93] Although the skin can also be extracted from CT scans,

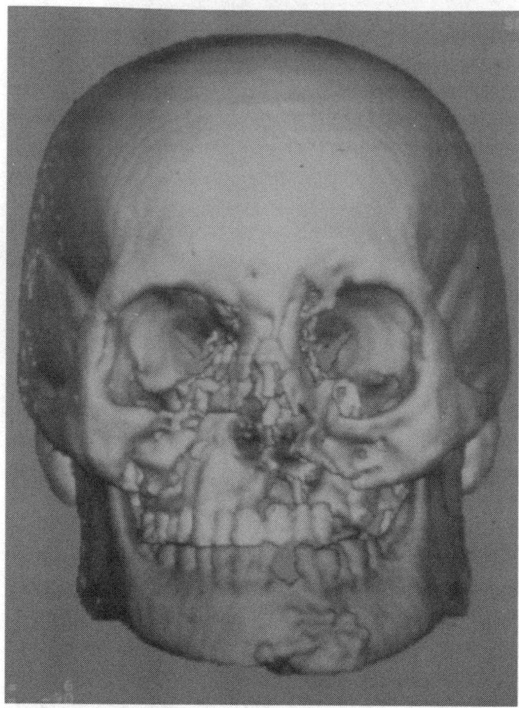

FIGURE 2.3 Severe facial trauma in a 20-year-old male who sustained a motor vehicle accident. Conservative treatment has led to a severely disfiguring condition that is difficult to treat. The 3D image is especially helpful to assess the comminuted midfacial skeleton.

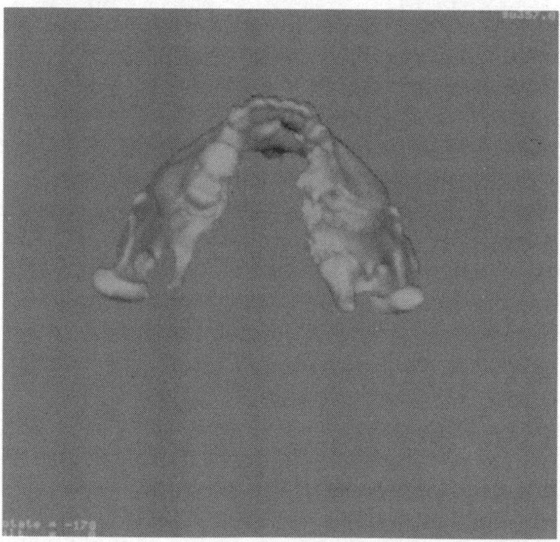

FIGURE 2.4 Posterior view of a 17-year-old male patient with Oral-facial-digital syndrome type II (Mohr syndrome). Note the atrophic condyles of the underdeveloped second mandible. For reasons of clarity, the mandible has been disarticulated.

digitization techniques are applicable, if the internal bony information is not required, for biostereometrical evaluation of facial skin asymmetry.[94,95] This is of special help to assess necessary skin corrections after craniofacial reconstructive surgery.[96] A pitfall in facial skin digitization, however, is the difference between the skin shape in upright and supine positions.[97]

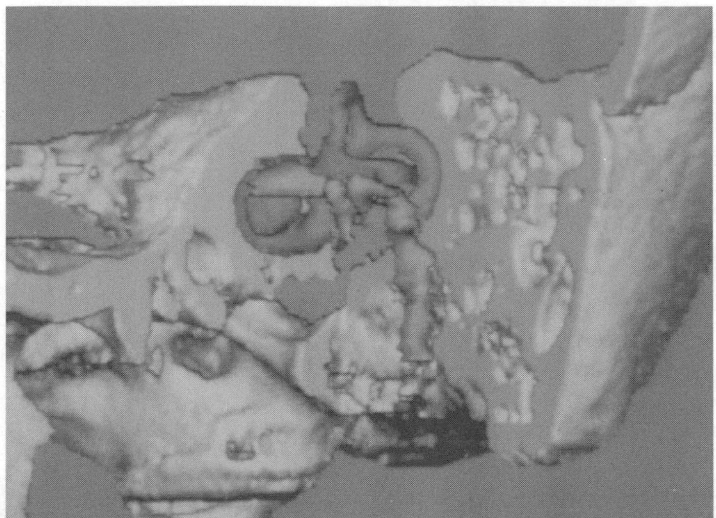

FIGURE 2.5 Antero-lateral view of the left temporal bone in a cadaveric specimen. A cutaway view shows the labyrinth (green), ossicles (yellow), and facial nerve (yellow).

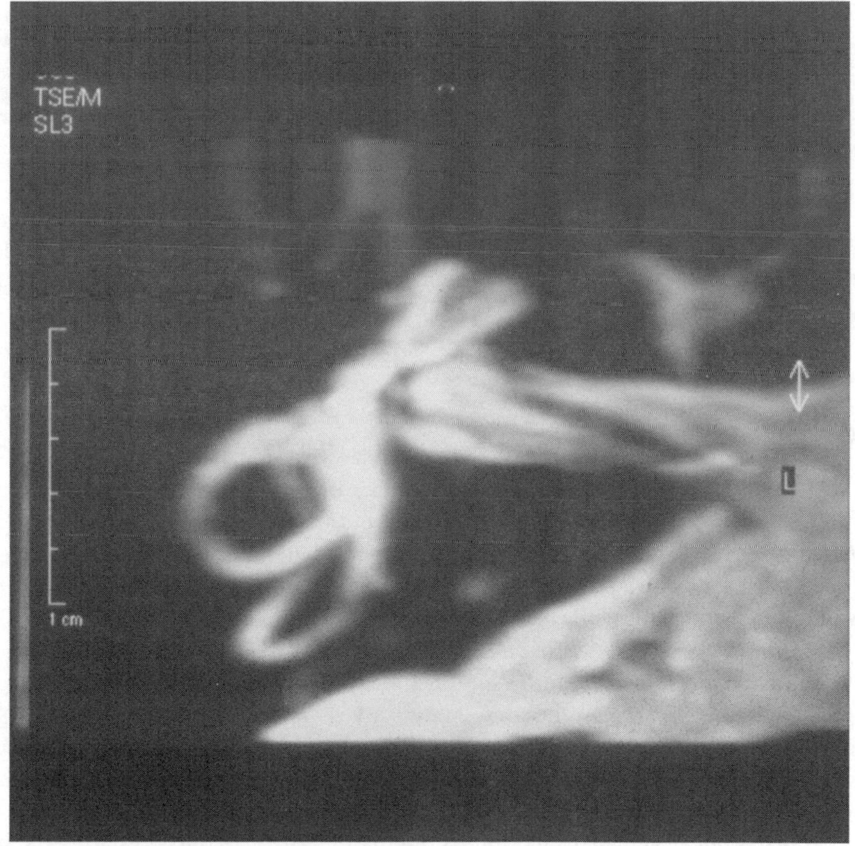

FIGURE 2.6 Maximum intensity projection (MIP) of the normal temporal bone based on a high-resolution T2-weighted MR sequence. Note the spiral lamina in the cochlea and the nerves in the internal auditory meatus.

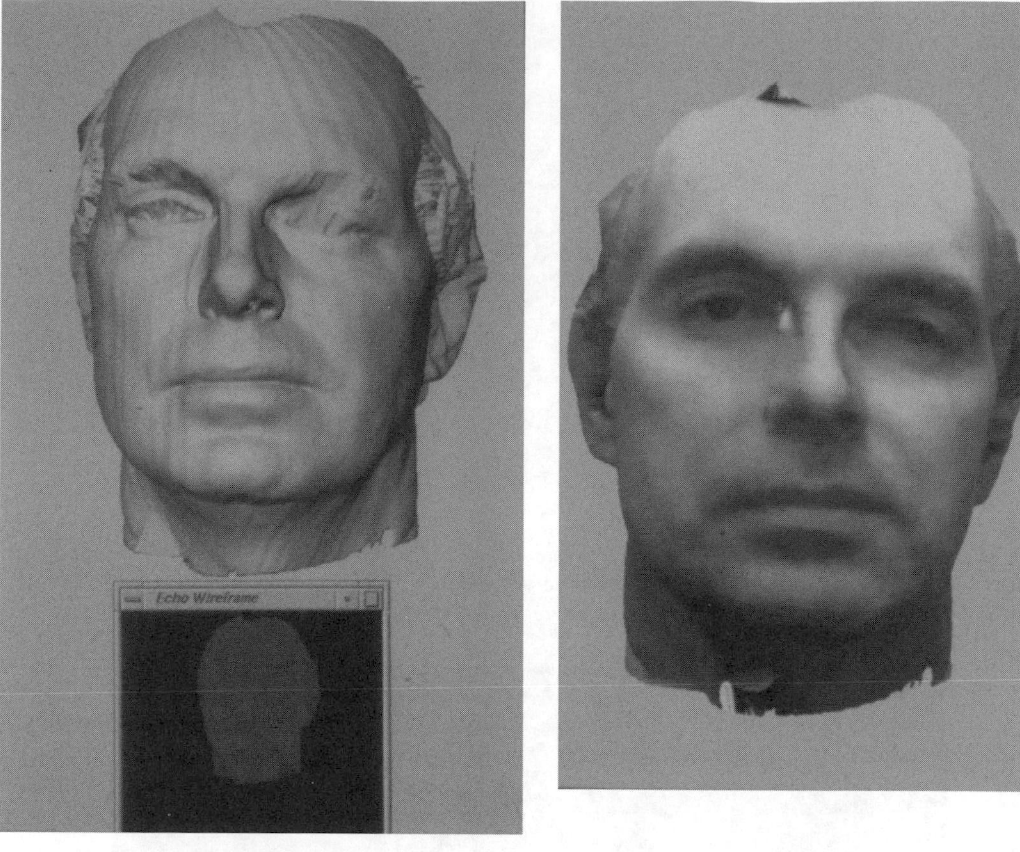

FIGURE 2.7 Laser scan of the author's face (Cyberware, Monterey, CA). (Courtesy of A.H. Joel, Image Technologies Int., Norcross, GA.) (a) 3D reconstruction of the surface only. (b) 3D reconstruction after adding color in the form of texture mapping.

2.1.3 Musculoskeletal System

2.1.3.1 Computed Tomography

The musculoskeletal system is a classic application area of 3D imaging.[98,99] Much effort has been spent on the pros and cons of surface rendering and volume rendering.[100] One group in particular made extensive use of volume rendering using a Pixar computer that was developed especially for use by George Lucas for motion picture image synthesis.[101–105] It was claimed that volume rendering uses all available information while surface rendering preserves only the surface and discards everything else. In fact, volume rendering assigns overlapping ranges of voxel values with gradually changing weighting factors to different tissue opaquenesses thus applying a "fuzzy" type of segmentation,[106,107] whereas in surface rendering there is a yes–no decision concerning the assignment of a particular voxel to the object of interest thus applying a "binary" type of segmentation which is often referred to as thresholding as it is the most popular segmentation technique. More sophisticated ways of finding the object contours, however, do exist.[108] In the 1980s, volume rendering was still very transparent and caused superimpositioning of structures thus obscuring the pathology. The concept of depth was apprehended only when rotating the image around a horizontal or vertical axis thus introducing parallax, but this precluded the study of small details. Surface rendering allows the electronic removal of a plaster cast while preserving the bone tissue[109] and disarticulation

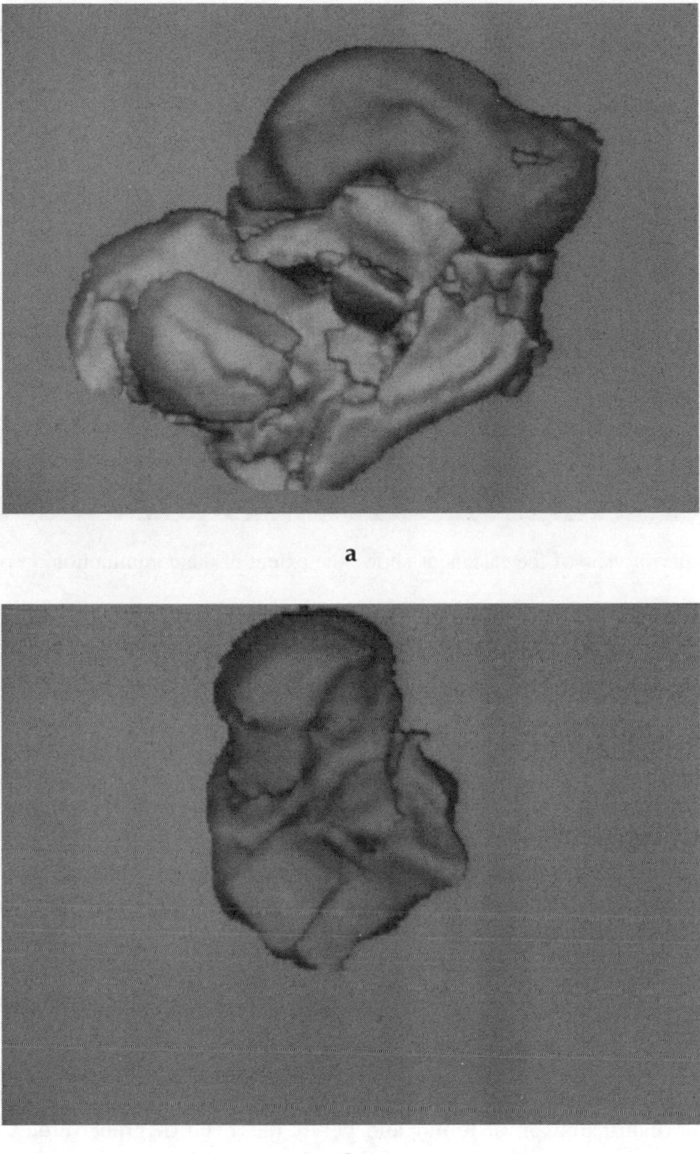

FIGURE 2.8 Disarticulation of talus and calcaneus in severe trauma of the left foot. This is the type of disarticulation that most radiologists find too time consuming. (a) Combined medial view showing the relationship between talus and calcaneus. (b) Inferior view of the talus shows an intra-articular fracture.

of intra-articular surfaces[110] (Figure 2.8) and tumor volumes, thus clearly visualizing them. Also for volume rendering, tools have been devised for interactive disarticulation.[111] The fabrication of models (see Section 2.2.4) also requires binary segmentation. However, surface rendering has difficulties in areas with details smaller than the resolution of the CT scanner, causing non-displaced fractures to be obscured[13] and pseudoforamina to form in thin cortical bone layers. In such situations and for the visualization of soft-tissue interfaces such as muscle and fat,[101,112] volume rendering may be the method of choice to obtain a better tissue representation in the rendered image. However, in other instances, such as in the assessment of fracture stability, fragment presence or absence in the joint space, comminution, and the number of fragments, when measured with receiver operating characteristic (ROC) analysis,[113] surface rendering was better than volume rendering. Since then,

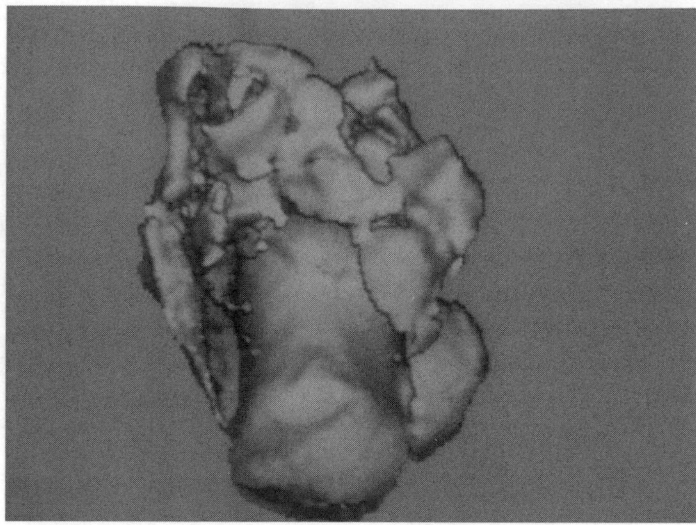

FIGURE 2.8c Superior view of the calcaneus shows the extent of the comminution, in particular that of the articular surface.

volume rendering algorithms have improved to the point that they use a "fuzzy" object segmentation but combine this with the advantages of binary segmentation[106,107] such as surface shading[114] and the definition of landmarks used for morphometric analysis.[18]

This means that the rendering method can be adapted to the specific visualization needs. Other improvements are the use of smaller slice increments (0.1–2 mm) without increasing patient radiation dose with the use of spiral CT.[115] This drastically improves the quality of the 3D image and the mapping of reformatted images on cutaway planes in the z direction. The possibility of the acquisition of isotropic image data is now a subject of speculation.[116]

In the musculoskeletal system, 3D CT imaging has been applied to the chest, spine, hip,[117] knee, ankle, foot,[117] shoulder, elbow, and wrist.[110]

In the chest, evaluation of congenital deformities such as Poland's syndrome[118] or similar types of costal agenesis (Figure 2.9) has been of great value. This also applies to the spine which can be scoliotic in this deformity. Other spine applications are focused on herniation of the nucleus pulposis,[119] plasmacytoma,[120] compression fractures,[120,121] pseudarthrosis in posterior lumbar fusion,[122] post-surgical "failed back" syndrome,[123] and post-operative evaluation of a sacral metastasis resection.[100]

In the hip, the disarticulation of femur and pelvis has been of great value for the assessment and classification of acetabular fractures[124-126,317] and hip dysplasia.[127,128] In the knee, it has been used to assess trauma, such as in tibial plateau fractures[100,120,317] and osteoarthritis.[129]

In the foot, much attention is paid to the classification of calcaneus fractures[130,131] (Figure 2.8) while, in the shoulder, trauma is also the main field of application, in primary complex trauma,[120] as well as in chronic unreduced dislocations of the joint.[132]

A special application is the assessment of the microstructure of bone trabeculae. This requires a high resolution of 0.25 mm or better, and thin slices of 0.5 mm or less, and is only possible with dedicated CT equipment.[133]

2.1.3.2 Magnetic Resonance Imaging

3D MR imaging of the musculoskeletal system is not as much focused on bone pathology as in 3D CT imaging, but the first focus is cartilage for the assessment of meniscal tears,[134,135] including calculation of cartilage volume,[136] and congenital hip luxation.[137] The second focus is connective tissue for the assessment of the disruption of ligaments and tendons such as the cruciate ligaments[138]

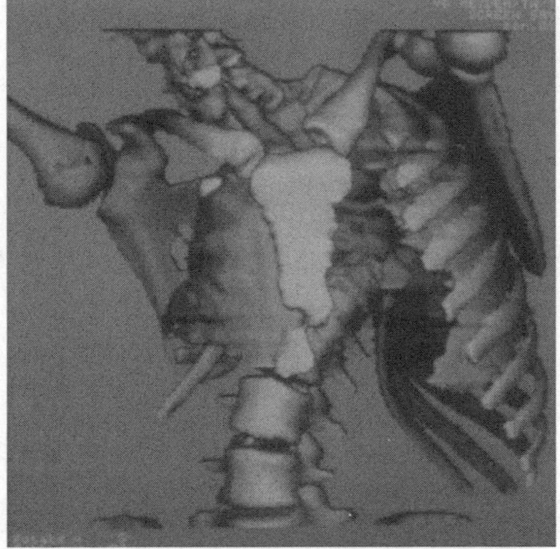

a

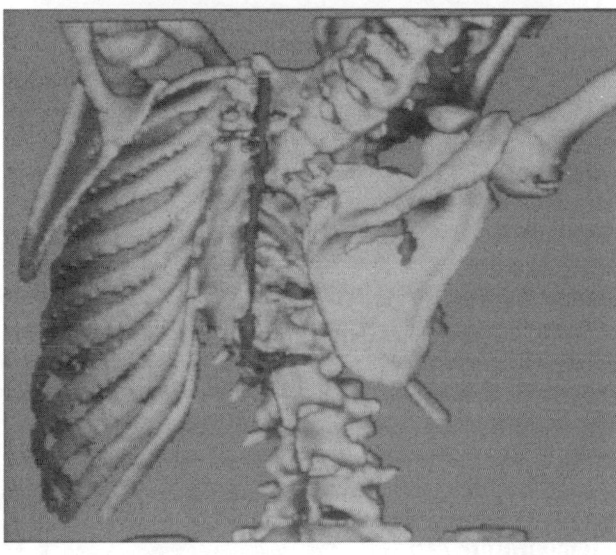

b

FIGURE 2.9 A 13-year-old female patient with severe right costal agenesis that has resulted in severe scoliosis. (a) Antero-posterior (AP) view showing the reduction of the right lung volume. (b) Posterior view showing a metal splint to suppport the spine.

and the tendons of the foot and ankle.[139] But imaging of cortical bone and the fat content of trabecular bone is possible. It is even possible to animate joint motion.[140] MRI, by the use of different sequences with or without fat suppression, also allows for large contrasts between tissues or fluids that, on CT, are known to have only minimal contrast. In some cases, special normalizing filters are useful to decrease the inhomogeneity that is so typical for MRI.[141] Examples of these contrasting tissues are the distribution of joint fluid,[142] assessment of the extent of femoral head necrosis,[142] and pannus formation as well as joint effusion in rheumatoid arthritis of the wrist.[143]

Using high-field (9.4 T) MRI, researchers have determined the 3D trabecular bone architecture in *in vitro* experiments on excised tibial, calcaneal, and vertebral bone samples.[144]

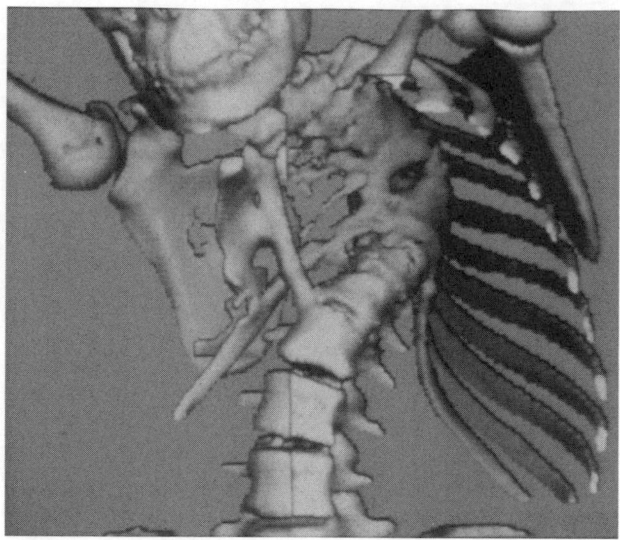

FIGURE 2.9c AP cutaway view showing a fibula graft that has been placed as a strut between the lumbar spine and the cervical spine.

Because the segmentation of MRI images for the isolation of relevant structures is time consuming, it is not yet used in clinical practice but limited to research.

2.1.3.3 Sonographic Imaging

In the musculoskeletal system, a primitive form of sonographic 3D imaging (wire frames) has been used to assess the acetabular depth and femoral head position in babies[145] with suspected hip luxation. Multiplanar sonographic imaging, however, appears to be equally helpful in the classification of the degree of luxation.[146] Only in veterinary medicine have we found a sonographic application in the assessment of hemorrhage, edema, and granulation tissue formation in an injured tendon which was, in essence, also limited to multiplanar imaging.[147] This means that 3D sonographic imaging in the musculoskeletal system is virtually non-existent.

2.1.4 Central Nervous System

2.1.4.1 Computed Tomography

When using CT, the emphasis is primarily on imaging bony detail, and in this respect 3D imaging can be very useful in assessing the extent and complexity of the pathology. In the skull this has been applied to fractures of the skull base[148,149] and the assessment of bony destruction by tumors such as meningioma,[149,150] chondroblastoma,[150] metastasis,[151] and epidermoid,[149] or the post-operative evaluation of bone resection[149] or subsequent osteoplasty[150] after tumor removal. When tumors affect the bone such that its density changes, as in hyperostotic meningioma, osteoma, and fibrous dysplasia, it is possible to segment the pathologic bone separately and display it in a different color[60] (Figure 2.10). In the cervical spine, CT is also excellent to diagnose rotatory subluxation of C1–C2[152] (Figure 2.11) in torticollis and to assess hemi- and block vertebrae[153] as well as the complexity of a craniocervical dysplasia.[165] It has even been demonstrated that the cervical spine can be imaged in flexion and in extension to analyze the stability in a neglected luxation fracture of the atlas.[149]

In the lumbar spine, 3D CT perfectly shows spinal canal stenosis and the vertebral dislocation in spondylolisthesis.[23,154]

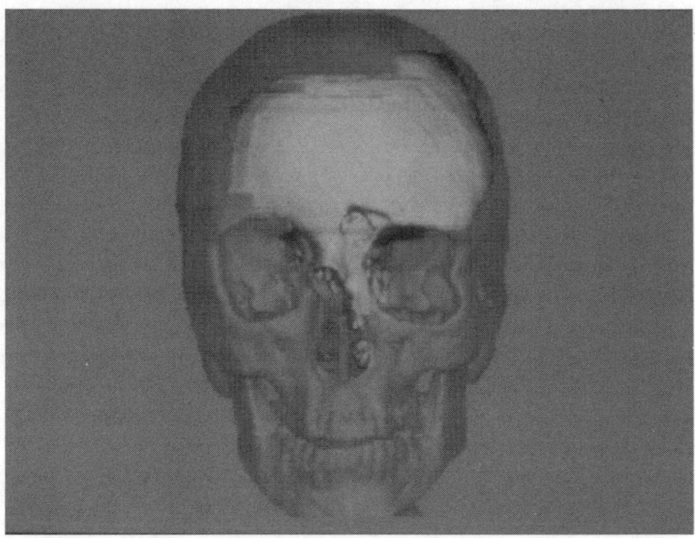

FIGURE 2.10 A 19-year-old female patient with fibrous dysplasia. This image shows the value of disarticulating the pathologic bone and displaying the remainder of the skull in a transparent fashion.

The first attempts to show tissues other than bone made use of large contrast differences induced by contrast that was administered intravenously for tumor[155,156] or vessel enhancement[157,158] (see paragraph on the neurovascular system), or intrathecally for imaging the cord tethered by a lipomatous mass in rachischisis,[159,160] the thecal sac in lumbar trauma,[161] or in ventriculography.[160]

Today, the much smaller contrast between brain and cerebrospinal fluid (CSF) can be visualized, resulting in images of the non-contrast-enhanced ventricular system[162] or the cisterns. This has allowed 3D visualization of pathologies such as hydrocephalus, ventricular asymmetry, callosal agenesis, Dandy-Walker malformation, and CSF distribution in meningoceles. It is even possible to use edge-preserving smoothing of the CT scans which further facilitates imaging of minimally contrasting tissues. In the segmentation of CSF spaces, one problem remains: interactive separation between different spaces is still required (e.g., between the ventricular system and basal cisterns). Because computers still don't have the anatomical knowledge required for automatic segmentations, the best results are obtained with manual editing, which is time consuming.[163]

Another problem is 3D imaging of the cortex. Beam-hardening artifacts caused by the calvarium are not always completely compensated for and cause a gradual density change from bone to brain. This means that the small CSF spaces in the sulci are lost and the segmentation therefore results in an endocast instead of a brain surface. There is, however, one method to avoid this problem, at least partially. This is the hybrid combination of thresholding and volume rendering, in the sense that all bone is removed from the data volume by setting a bone threshold and then the remaining soft tissue is volume rendered. This results in 3D images that clearly show the sulci and gyri and that can demonstrate the location of small infarctions.[164] The best images of the cortex, however, require MR imaging (Figure 2.12).

2.1.4.2 Magnetic Resonance Imaging

In T1-weigted MR images, both cortical bone and CSF are black and thus make clear delineation of the brain surface possible. The only high signal surrounding the brain is the fat signal from the trabecular bone in the diploë and the subcutaneous fat, but this can easily be excluded from the segmentation of the brain tissue[165] by region growing or by fat suppression. The ventricular system can also be easily segmented on both T1- and T2-weighted images. This possibility was recognized very early by Herman et al.[166] (Figure 2.13).

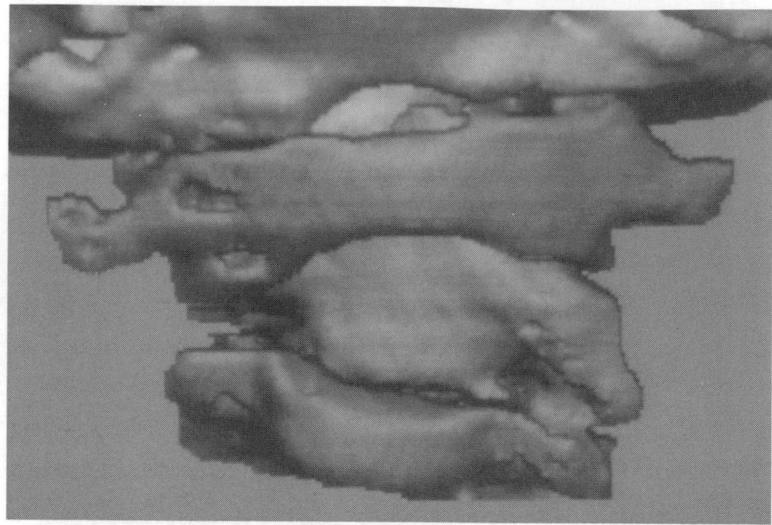

a

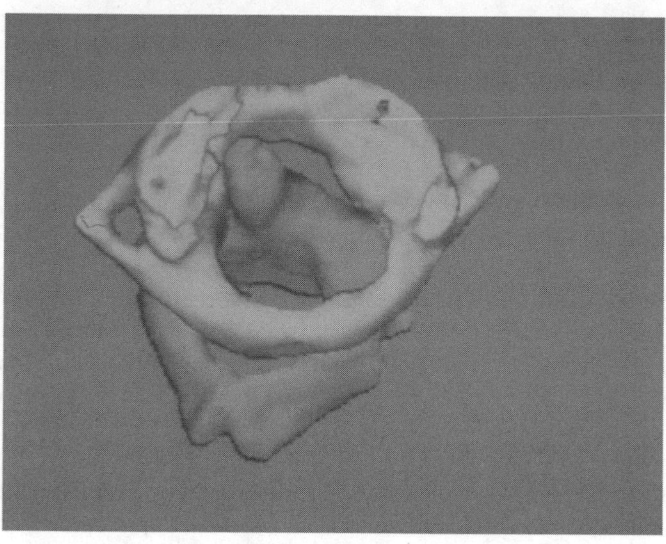

b

FIGURE 2.11 Possiblities of disarticulating separate vertebrae to demonstrate the traumatic dislocation of the proximal cervical spine in a 5-year-old girl. (a) Anterior view showing the relative displacement of the vertebrae with respect to each other and to the skull base. Note the compression fracture of the left occipital condyle. (b) Superior view of C1 and C2 demonstrates their relative rotation.

Good quality cortex reconstruction requires slices no thicker than 2 mm, preferably acquired in the coronal plane.[167] Fine-tuning of segmentation and rendering has resulted in excellent image quality.[168] On cortical 3D images, various important landmarks can be recognized such as the central sulcus, and the relationship of motor, premotor, and sensory areas can be evaluated[167] and compared to atlases.[169] These areas can later be used in multimodality matching with functional imaging modalities (see Section 2.2.5) or can be used to plan surgical approaches that avoid vital cortical regions such as the precentral (movement), postcentral (sensation), left superior temporal (hearing), and left inferior frontal (speech) gyri.[170] Detection of pachygyria can be used to diagnose Fukuyama-type congenital muscular dystrophy,[171] and gyral effacement is a sign of an underlying superficial tumor.

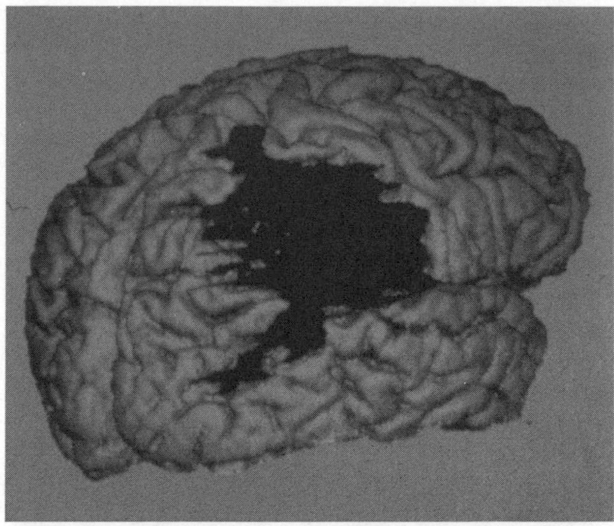

FIGURE 2.12 Disarticulation of infarcted brain tissue in a patient who had a minute embolus that passed the trifurcation of the middle cerebral artery and stranded at the level of the posterior parietal arterial branch, thus causing a small infarct that was associated with unusual neurologic findings.

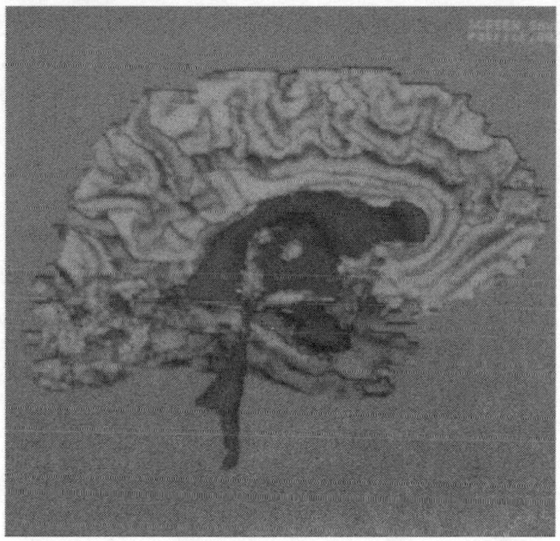

FIGURE 2.13 Segmentation of the ventricular system in combination with the left hemispheric white matter that was disarticulated from the gray matter. This image shows the potential of a T1-weighted data set with thin 1-mm slices.

Segmentation of internal structures in the brain, such as white matter, basal ganglia, and tumors, presents with more difficulty. This can be done by tedious manual segmentation, which takes too long for clinical use (Figure 2.14), but attempts have been made to automate the segmentation process to some degree by using scale-space theory,[172] fractal analysis,[173] spectral tissue classification,[174,175] deformable geometric models,[176] and transformation (warping) of an atlas template.[177]

2.1.4.3 Nuclear Medicine

The application of 3D imaging in nuclear medicine[178] is relatively rare. However, it has been used in single-photon emission CT (SPECT) and in positron emission tomography (PET) in the form of surface rendering as well as volume rendering.[179] Volume rendering is a basic projection image

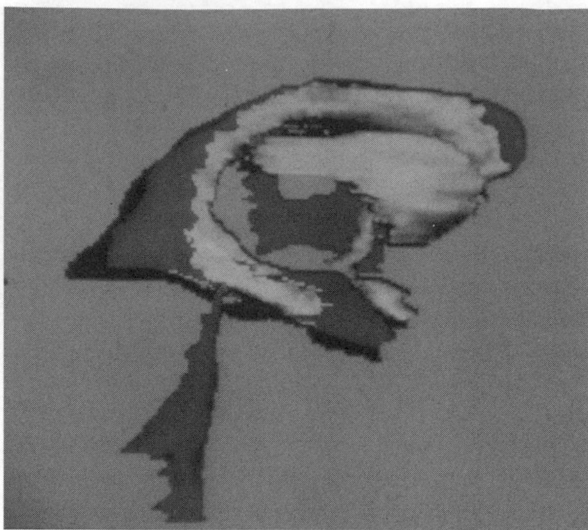

FIGURE 2.14 Segmentation of the ventricular system (blue) in combination with the caudate nucleus (yellow), lentiform nucleus (yellow), and the fornix and hippocampus (white). (Same patient as in Figure 2.13.)

that shows “hot spots” but only derives its 3D effect by rotation of the data volume thus producing parallax. In a simplified form, it is possible to acquire only 2D views in all directions and rotate these around. The surface used for surface rendering is basically an “iso-count” surface in a spatial activity distribution expressing the threshold level as a percentage of the maximum count in the data volume.[180] Different disease entities and different parts of the brain require different thresholds to show the perfusion defect in an optimum fashion.[181,182]

Surface imaging does not show internal perfusion defects but when the volume is slowly stripped, these defects become visible.[183] 3D imaging has been applied in the assessment of epilepsy, acute stroke, and Alzheimer’s and Parkinson’s disease.[181,182] It has been shown that, in Alzheimer’s disease, defects in the 3D SPECT image correlate well with cognitive deficits,[184] but the 3D image only enhances the more easy comprehension of anatomical relationships.

2.1.4.4 Sonographic Imaging

3D sonographic imaging of the brain may thrive in the future as an intra-operative navigation tool but is currently only being tested in animals such as dogs and rabbits.[185] Human application has been limited to assessment of the development of the brain cavities in embryos between 8 and 11 weeks of gestation (13 to 40 mm crown–rump length, respectively).[186]

2.1.5 Neuro- and Cardiovascular Systems

2.1.5.1 Computed Tomography

Segmentation and 3D rendering of vascular structures requires sufficient contrast by means of rapid contrast infusion. Early on, this resulted in imaging a small tissue volume, usually a slab of 10 to 15 scans, that could be scanned during the phase of maximum contrast enhancement before the contrast started to decrease significantly by means of kidney excretion. This technique acquired the name computed tomographic angiography (CTA) and has been applied to arteriovenous malformations[165,187] and cerebral aneurysms.[188] However, with the advent of spiral (helical) CT,[3,189,190] this tissue volume increased enormously and could contain overlapping slices at a radiation dose equal to that belonging to contiguous slices and thus image a wide variety of vascular lesions[24,191] while preserving bony morphology for anatomic reference.

In the neurovascular system, this has facilitated the assessment of aneurysms at the cranial base and stenoses of the proximal internal carotid artery at the carotid bifurcation. Aneurysms can be clearly depicted, provided that the scans are done with a slice thickness of 1 or 1.5 mm. Thin vessels, such as the anterior cerebral arteries, suffer from partial volume averaging, and can therefore be better delineated on an MIP rendition.[24] Usually, MIP reconstruction requires the manual removal of the bony tissue before projecting the data volume[192] (Figure 2.15a). However, a new technique, developed at Philips Medical Systems (Best, the Netherlands) creates an MIP of a small slab-shaped volume, called "slab MIP," that can be rotated. This usually prevents the bone tissue from obscuring the vessels (Figure 2.15b).

3D imaging has also been used to check the embolization of a carotid-cavernous sinus fistula.[150] In case of large aneurysms, cutaway images, also denoted as "3D CT endoscopy"[193] allow assessment of the vascular orifice and the configuration of thrombus formation. CT of aneurysms does not suffer from flow artifacts as in MRA, but reliable 3D imaging requires a correct segmentation.[194]

3D imaging of the carotid artery suffers from the same problem,[24] which can under- or overestimate the stenosis, but it has many advantages.[195] The prescence of calcified plaques can impair the visualization of the stenosis. However, this can be avoided by a separate segmentation of the plaque.[8,196] The plaque can thus also be rendered transparently.[197] Partial volume averaging of short stenoses can be avoided by the use of 1.5 mm slice thickness or less.

In the extracranial vascular system, excluding the cardiac vascular system, 3D imaging and MIP reconstructions have been applied to all major arteries.[198] Examples are aorta, pulmonary trunk[199] and arteries,[200] celiac trunc, hepatic arteries, splenic artery, gastroduodenal artery, superior mesenteric artery, renal arteries, and iliac arteries.

The primary application of 3D imaging in the aorta is assessment of abdominal aortic aneurysm (AAA). In some cases no effort was made to segment and visualize the thrombus.[201] If this effort is made, however, the extent of the thrombus and the involvement of the renal arteries and iliac bifurcation can be assessed and visualized[24,317] (Figure 2.16a). In patients where these arteries are not involved, an endovascular stent[202] can be prepared according to the diameter of the aortic lumen and the length of the aneurysm. Post-interventional imaging documents the stent position (Figure 2.16b). This is also possible using MIP.[203] Another aortic application is the assessment of aortic dissecting aneurysms, for instance in the case of more than one false lumen.[204] Volume rendering has been applied to visualize the geometry of the intimal flap.[205]

In the arterial visceral vasculature, 3D imaging has been used to demonstrate congenital vascular variants such as hepatic arteries arising from the superior mesenteric artery instead of the celiac trunc.[206]

The main application in the renal arteries is assessment of stenoses although detection of accessory renal arteries is also done. As in the carotid artery, calcified atheroma can impair this detection.[198]

Imaging of the liver vasculature will be discussed in Section 2.1.7.

The cardiac vascular system is different from the previously described vascular systems in the sense that it is subjected to rapid cardiac contractile motion. This has required special solutions to freeze the heart motion and avoid motion artifacts. The first dedicated experimental heart scanner was the dynamic spatial reconstructor (DSR).[23,207] It could acquire dynamic 3D images of the complete beating heart.[208]

Routine clinical use of ultrafast CT became available in the form of the Imatron C-100 cine-CT scanner (Imatron, Inc., South San Francisco, CA),[209] which was later upgraded to the C-150. This scanner has been successfully applied to the assessment of anomalous coronary artery origin,[210] the extent of coronary artery calcification,[211] coronary artery stenosis and post-PTCA (percutaneous transluminal coronary angioplasty) follow-up,[212] and the relationship between ventricular function and shape.[213,214] To some degree, it has been possible to study gross pathology, such as pulmonary artery stenosis and aberrant left subclavian artery, also by means of classic rapid CT scanning.[215]

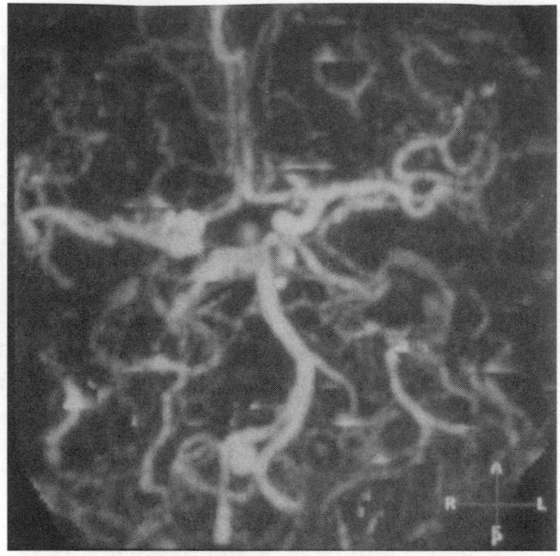

a

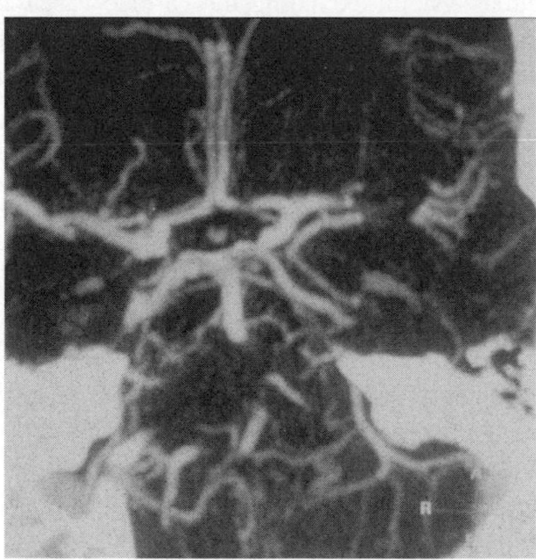

b

FIGURE 2.15 MIP of the circle of Willis. (Courtesy of A.M.H. Huitema, Philips Medical Systems, Best, the Netherlands.) (a) In CT, the bone must be edited out to obtain images of the vessels only. (b) To avoid this process, a slab of tissue can be imaged with little risk of bone superimpositioning (slab MIP).

2.1.5.2 Magnetic Resonance Imaging

MRI has always been especially suited for vascular imaging. This was first made possible by the "flow-void" phenomenon[216] and later by special vascular sequences known as "in-flow" or "time-of-flight" (TOF) imaging and "phase-contrast" (PCA) imaging. This led to the term magnetic resonance angiography (MRA). The signal dependence in MRA of the blood flow velocity led, on the one hand, to its quantitative use[217,218] but, on the other hand, it also had inherent drawbacks in areas of increased flow (stenosis)[219] and of reduced or complex flow (aneurysm).[220] Because MRA only demonstrates signal in flowing blood, vessel segmentation becomes very simple.[221] However, small vessels suffer from partial volume averaging and low noisy signals that may require special noise reduction operations.[222] These problems can be avoided by the use of the MIP technique,[223]

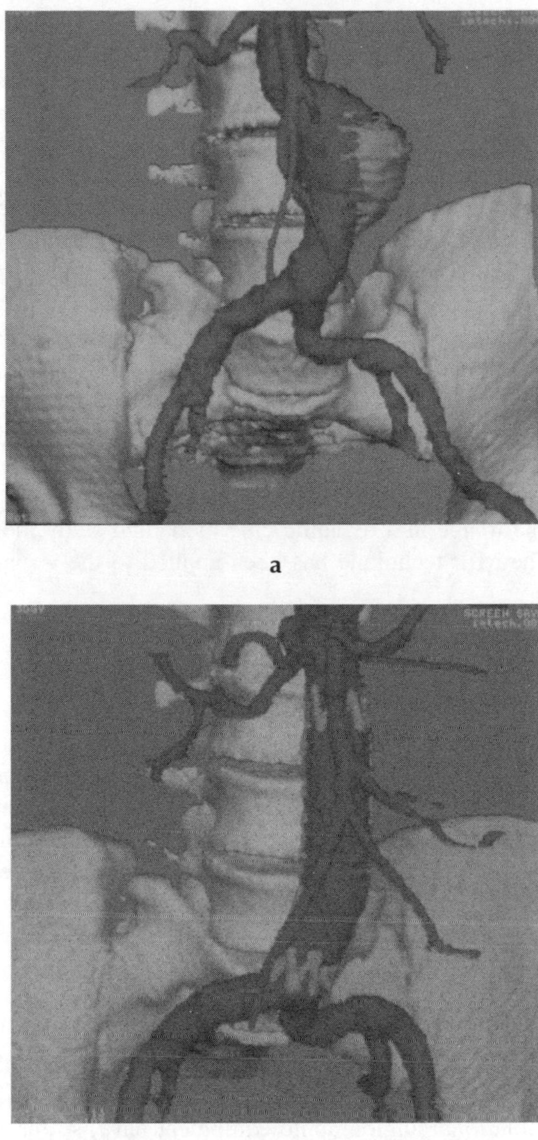

a

b

FIGURE 2.16 Patient with an abdominal aneurysm that was treated with an endovascular stent. (a) Pre-operative situation with the thrombus shown in yellow. The dimensions of the required stent are taken from this reconstruction. (b) Post-operative situation showing the metallic struts of the endovascular stent graft in green.

but lack of signal also fades the vessels on an MIP, and bright vessels in the background will overpower smaller, darker vessels in the foreground. Therefore, a special technique was developed that preserves the smaller vessels in the foreground. It is called closest vessel projection (CVP).[39,224] A special case of lack-of-signal occurs in in-flow MRA when the flow is inverted in a syphon-shaped tortuous vascular deformity. When sequences are used that highlight surrounding tissues in addition to the blood vessels, MIPs of pulmonary vasculature are still possible, either by eliminating the surrounding tissues[225] or by the use of slab MIPs.

With regard to the neurovascular system, in the assessment of endocranial aneurysms, MRA has a distinct advantage over angiography in that the vascular tree can be observed from all possible angles. For assessment of the aneurysm orientation, the same 3D endoscopy technique as described above for CT has been applied to MRA.[226] MRA TOF assessment of intracranial aneurysms, however, can also be impaired by the presence of subacute thrombus, a sizable hematoma, clips, or coils.[220]

Some investigators have not accepted the poor quality of vessel surfaces in 3D rendering of a vascular tree, and have devised dedicated modeling techniques to create a symbolic description of the vascular system. This leads to a more realistic vascular model that can then be used for simulation of a bolus injection or introduction of catheters such as has been applied to the cerebral vascular system.[227] It has thus become feasible to estimate vessel diameter and orientation,[228] and to reconstruct the integrity of the vessel in case of interruptions by the use of different MIP projections.[229]

In the extracranial vascular system, excluding the cardiac system, MRA is still in a developmental phase but has been applied to the renal arteries.[230]

In the cardiac vascular system MRA has been applied to the aortic arch, heart, and coronary arteries. This application usually requires both cardiac as well as respiratory gating to avoid motion artifacts[231,232] and can be used for the assessment of congenital heart disease in pediatric[233–235] as well as adult[236] patients. By making use of the data acquisition in different phases of the heart cycle it is possible to display the image in a dynamic cine mode and study motion disturbances of the left ventricular wall.[237] The MIP technique has been applied to the visualization of the coronary arteries.[238]

2.1.5.3 Angiography

Before the use of volumetric imaging modalities, which could acquire the image data quickly and could identify the vessel wall with or without the administration of contrast medium, and today, with the advent of rotational angiography, attempts have been made to reconstruct vascular trees from multiple 2D projection views. In this process, it is, strictly mathematically speaking, not possible to reconstruct a vascular tree from two projections. However, with the assumption that the vessels are elliptic in cross-section, and with the help of anatomic knowledge about the course of the vessels,[239] such reconstructions have been made[240] (e.g., for the assessment of coronary artery stenoses[241] and diffuse coronary artery disease[242]). Good reconstructions are possible with 25 to 35 angiographic views,[243] but even with the ideal number of 2D projections (angiograms from a rotational angiography apparatus) being available, special algorithms are required to reconstruct a 3D image of a vascular tree[244] and preprocessing of the angiographic projections may be required.[245] Such algorithms are also referred to as "cone-beam reconstruction algorithms,"[246] but before they can be used, one must first correct for the pin cushion distortion of the image intensifier tube.[247] Most attempts to design rotational angiographic equipment have, so far, used a rigid CT type of gantry, usually with one X-ray tube and one image intensifier tube,[248] but sometimes with two such combinations (perpendicular central axes).[249] When using standard angiographic equipment, however, it is necessary to also compensate for deviations of the X-ray tube and detector from an ideal circular path due to mechanical sagging.[250]

2.1.5.4 Sonographic Imaging

The same primitive wire frame images, as mentioned above, under the musculoskeletal system have also been applied to the heart for the assessment of cardiac wall motion.[251] The difference is the use of the speed of sonographic imaging, which allows for assessing dynamic aspects.[252] Therefore this technique has also been called 4D sonography.

For studying the heart, a wide variety of imaging modes has been developed.[253] There is an external precordial approach with a rotating probe[254] which allows for different probe orientations (e.g., parasternal and apical). A technique that deserves special attention is the transesophageal approach for echocardiography (TEE). The classic 3D approach using rotating or sweeping arrays has been implemented in these esophageal probes;[255] however, a special array has been devised that looks like a chain of beads, each one of which is a separate 2D transducer. By pulling so-called "Bowden cables" this chain of transducers can be straigtened such that parallel slices of the heart can be acquired.[256] This TEE technique has primarily been focused on imaging of congenital heart disease[257] and on pathology associated with the valves[256] such as mitral stenosis and valve prolapse.[258] TEE has also been used for the assessment of masses such as vegetation, tumors (e.g., atrial mixoma[258]), abscesses,[259] and mobile aortic debris.[252] 3D images of cardiac morphology have been combined with 3D rendering of color Doppler-based blood flow phenomena such as flow through an atrial septum defect[255] or a mitral regurgitant jet.[252] Vascular areas have first been studied with 3D sonographic imaging by rendering the echo-free vascular lumen as, for example, applied to the carotid arteries.[260] Now it is also possible to base the 3D rendering on the Doppler or color velocity imaging (CVI)[261] signals alone, which can discriminate between arterial and venous structures,[262] or on the combination of flow-based 3D images with cross-sectional images of the surrounding tissues.[263] This will, in the future, be facilitated by the development of power Doppler imaging[264] and color velocity angiography, which no longer suffer from signal dependency of the transducer angle with respect to the blood flow direction, as well as the use of harmonic imaging in combination with sonographic contrast agents,[265] which produces only images of the contrast medium distribution. Power Doppler has already been used to reconstruct endoscopic views of blood vessels.[266]

Finally, there is also an intravascular sonographic acquisition mode using a transducer at the tip of a catheter which is retracted slowly through an artery while recording its position and a series of cross-sectional images, such that a 3D data volume is generated that can be segmented and rendered.[267] However, the noise and the backscatter of the blood requires special processing[268] prior to segmentation. Endovascular 3D sonography has been used to assess an AAA[201] and has been advantageous, as compared to CT, in demonstrating the transmural wall characteristics. A drawback is that the transducer can freely move within the artery while its path is reconstructed as a straight line. However, if this path can be recorded in space, it has been demonstrated that reconstructions of curved vessels are possible.[269] In order to image the correct section of the vessel, external guidance control monitoring systems are helpful.[270] After segmentation and rendering the lumen and plaque, it is possible to extract numerical data such as the cross-sectional area of the lumen and stenotic index.[271]

2.1.5.5 Nuclear Medicine

Nuclear medicine, in the form of SPECT, is used in a variety of ways in cardiac imaging (e.g., cardiac function, myocardial motion, and perfusion). How it is used depends on the type of radionuclide-labeled agents used and the type of imaging.

When red blood cells are labeled with technetium-99m (^{99m}Tc) it is possible, when applying cardiac gating, to image the ventricles as a function of time, and display the different cardiac phases[272] or the beating heart in a dynamic fashion.[273]

Myocardial perfusion can be assessed with thallium-201 (^{201}Tl) and displayed three dimensionally either as an iso-count surface showing perfusion defects or as a color mapping on a unified elipsoidal model.[274] In assessing acute myocardial infarction, use has also been made of ^{99m}Tc-pyrophosphate in combination with volume rendering[275] or mapping of ^{99m}Tc-sestamibi concentration on epicardial surfaces extracted from cardiac MRI.[276] To highlight an infarct, the original (^{201}Tl) scan can be matched with a ^{111}In-antimyosin scan.[277,278] It is even possible to subtract images acquired during stress from the ones acquired during rest.[279]

Myocardial wall motion can be studied directly, as was done by using radiolabeled microspheres in a dog.[25] However, with all phases of the heart cycle available, it has also been possible to color-code wall motion and thus make hypokinetic or akinetic areas more conspicuous.[280]

2.1.6 Pulmonary System

2.1.6.1 Computed Tomography

The earliest attempts to image the pulmonary system using CT were very crude.[281] This was followed, however, by the pioneering work using the DSR, a rapid experimental CT scanner with 14 X-ray tubes.[282]

Although good 3D images of the trachea and lung surface were possible using slice-to-slice scanning combined with superficial breathing,[283] image quality is greatly enhanced using spiral CT, but extremely detailed images of the complete bronchial system are only possible using electron-beam CT.[284] Both volume rendering[285] as well as surface rendering have been applied.

The majority of 3D imaging applications of air-containing structures focus on deformities of the main airway including hypopharynx, larynx (3D laryngogram), trachea, and main stem bronchi. Anatomical details shown are vallecula, piriform sinus, airway narrowing by the true vocal cords, and carina. The pathology includes tumors involving the larynx,[286] laryngeal compression by oral floor tumors,[287] subglottic stenosis in Morbus Wegner (Figure 2.17), congenital tracheal stenosis,[288] tracheal compression by a dilated pulmonary artery[289] or by a local tumor[290] (Figure 2.18), deformities associated with stent placement,[290] and bronchus stenosis following bronchus re-implantation associated with lobectomy.[291] Detailed intraluminal morphology can be visualized using endoscopic cutaway views of 3D reconstructions of the wall of the airway, which has proven to be valuable in patients with intubation problems.[287] In the lung itself, the inherent contrast between the pulmonary vasculature and the surrounding lung tissue has led to 3D imaging of focal lung disease in relation to the blood vessels.[290,292,293] This can be a basis for deciding between lobectomy and pneumectomy,[294] provided that central pulmonary arterial or bronchial tumor invasion can be detected on the axial scans. This is possible when using fast scanning and thin slices, combined with intravenous contrast administration. Combination of vascular and airway morphology in a single 3D image can further clarify the pathologic topography.[291]

Another approach to lung imaging is to outline the lung volume in an automatic[295] or semi-automatic fashion and then image that volume by means of volume rendering or MIP. Volume rendering is a perfect way to detect pulmonary infarcts and nodules and visualize them topographically,[296] while the use of MIP can be advantageous in detecting calcifications in the pulmonary nodules.[297] The use of minimum intensity projection (MIP), however, yields a perfect image of the airways without the need to first outline the lung volume.[298]

2.1.6.2 Magnetic Resonance Imaging

Magnetic resonance imaging has, so far, been little used for 3D imaging of the tracheobronchial system. However, it has been demonstrated that ECG-gated spin-echo images can be used to assess tracheal and bronchial stenoses and even allows for simultaneous display of the pulmovascular system to assess vascular strictures.[299]

2.1.6.3 Nuclear Medicine

3D nuclear medicine imaging has been applied to the pulmonary system in two different ways, namely in the form of perfusion scintigraphy and ventilation scintigraphy. In perfusion SPECT, ^{99m}Tc-macro-aggregated albumin (^{99m}Tc-MAA) is used to show perfusion defects in patients with thoracic masses.[300] The affected lung segment can be better recognized on the 3D image. In ventilation scintigraphy, nebulized aerosols, such as human serum albumin, that are labeled with ^{99m}Tc-MMAD are used).[301] This method is excellent for the differential diagnosis of pulmonary embolism and ventilation defects.[302]

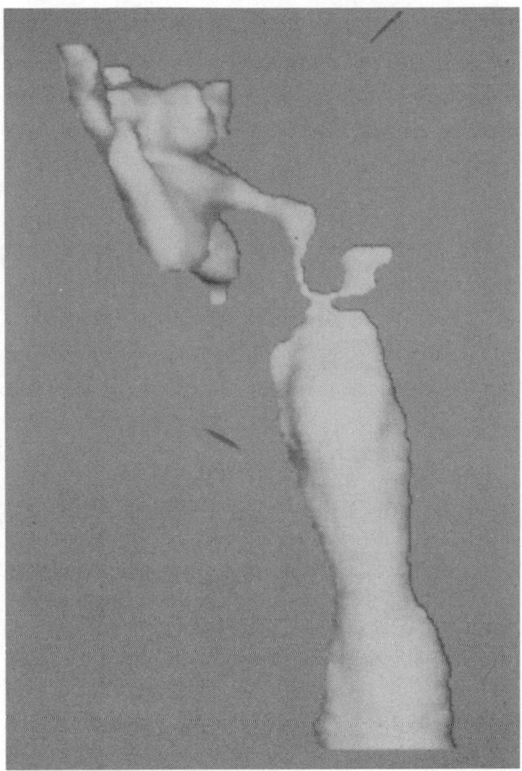

FIGURE 2.17 3D image of a subglottic tracheal stenosis in a patient with Morbus Wegner (female patient, aged 53 years).

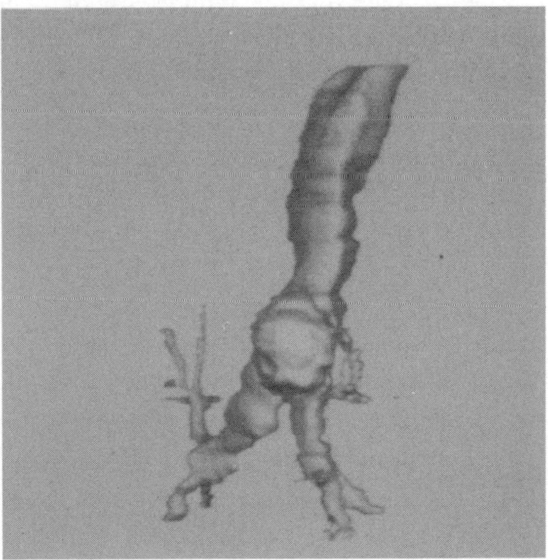

FIGURE 2.18 Tracheal compression by a local tumor (bronchus carcinoma) at the carina (male, 61 years of age).

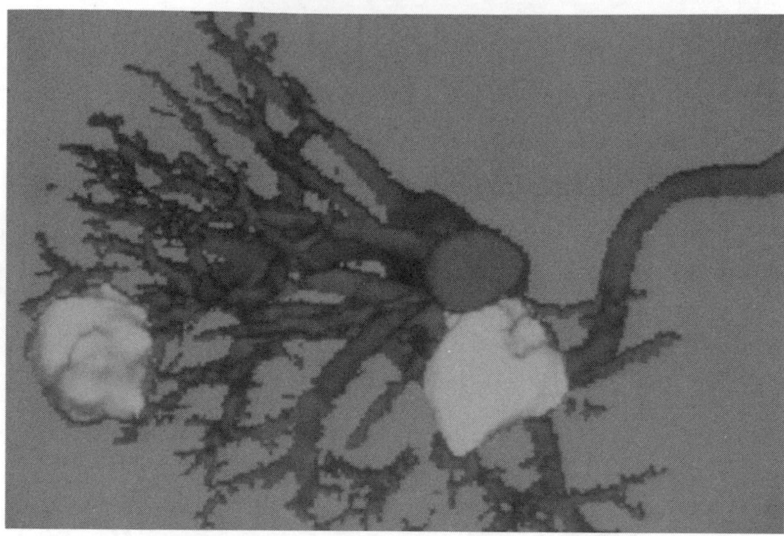

FIGURE 2.19 Superior view of a segmentation of the portal vascular system (red), the venous system (blue), and two colorectal metastases (white). This type of image shows the relationship between the individual vascular tree and the lesions to allow for local resection. (Courtesy of M.S. Van Leeuwen, Dept. of Radiology, Utrecht University Hospital, Utrecht, the Netherlands.)

2.1.7 Gastrointestinal System

2.1.7.1 Computed Tomography

In the gastrointestinal system, most 3D imaging efforts have been focused on the liver. The outlining of the liver and the separation of low contrasting liver and tumor tissues was addressed by some investigators by manual segmentation,[303,304] while others used histograms.[305] These early attempts demonstrated the location of focal liver lesions, the extent of liver atrophy or hypertrophy, and the topographic relationship between liver and spleen.[23] With the use of sequential arterial portography it became possible to segment the five separate liver lobes (left lateral, left medial, right anterior, right posterior, and caudate) and image them in conjunction with the venous and portal vascular system.[306] To minimize the time spent on manual segmentations, computer vision techniques have been applied to obtain smooth liver contours.[307]

With the advent of spiral CT, selective administration of contrast medium to the hepatic artery was no longer necessary and multiple volumetric data acquisitions of the entire liver as a function of time became possible and is known as "multiphasic" liver scanning: preferably in the arterial, portal, and equilibrium phases. Visualization of the liver vasculature has been achieved using volume rendering,[308] simple thresholding,[309] and MIP,[309] but the best results are obtained by manual segmentation[310] because this allows separation of the venous and portal systems, including display in different colors,[311,312,317] and the combined visualization of portal system and focal lesions enables planning of local resections[313] (Figure 2.19) as the liver vasculature varies significantly between individuals.[314] Alternatives for such resections or for lobectomies have been studied by 3D simulation of post-operative liver tissue regeneration.[315]

In a similar fashion as in vascular imaging, 3D cholangiography has been used to plan the resection of hilar cholangiocarcinoma.[316]

A special type of 3D imaging that has been applied to the colon is endoscopic 3D, also called perspective volume rendering.[17] It is a non-invasive technique for finding carcinomas and polyps by rendering a "fly-through" inside of the colon that has been scanned in a clean and air-insufflated condition.

2.1.7.2 Magnetic Resonance Imaging

MR imaging of the liver can provide 3D images of the parenchyma[318] as well as the vasculature[319] without the use of contrast media, although the latter improves imaging of the parenchyma. MRI is expected to display larger contrast between lesions and parenchyma. This led to the use of MRI in the 3D assessment of liver metastases in relation to the liver vasculature.[320] Computer-generated separation of the liver lobes is of additional help.[321]

3D MR cholangiography, using a sequence that produces high signal in the bile, has been used to assess biliary obstruction, the site of which is also clearly visible on an MIP display.[322]

2.1.7.3 Sonographic Imaging

In the gastrointestinal system, 3D sonographic imaging has not been frequently used.[323]

2.1.8 Genitourinary System

2.1.8.1 Computed Tomography

In the genitourinary system, 3D CT imaging has so far been limited to the kidneys. It is as difficult as imaging of the liver and spleen. We have applied it to the assessment of the relationship between polycystic kidneys and the abdominal/retroperitoneal space and as a basis for volume determination. Since nephrectomy is, surgically speaking, a much simpler procedure than segmental liver surgery, the clinical need for renal 3D imaging is limited to pre-operative assessment of the renal vessels, except for the case of organ-sparing partial nephrectomy in a single kidney.[324,325]

2.1.8.2 Magnetic Resonance Imaging

3D MR imaging of the kidney has become feasible with the use of contrast media and has been used for the determination of renal volume.[326]

2.1.8.3 Sonographic Imaging

3D sonographic imaging has been minimally applied to urology, primarily in an introital fashion (intra-urethrally or transrectally). In this way, it has been used to assess urethral sphincter incompetence,[327] benign prosthetic hyperplasia,[328] and kidney volume.[326]

In contrast, its use in obstetrics, for the evaluation of the fetus, has been extensive. This application started to develop in 1992.[329,330] Even early detection (before 10 weeks gestation) of abnormal fetal growth, using transvaginal ultrasound, has become possible.[331] Transabdominal 3D imaging first focused on the fetal surface, which was difficult to extract from its noisy surroundings,[332] but the quality of the data allowed assessment of the fetal head and face,[333] resulting in reasonable 3D image quality[334] (Figure 2.20). A change in the tissue opaqueness used for volume rendering allowed the assessment of the fetal skeleton,[334] which is difficult to analyze on 2D images.[335] 3D imaging has even been used to study the changes in shape of the developing fetal stomach[336] and, with the use of power Doppler, for the assessment of the fetal circle of Willis and aortic arch as well as the placental circulation.[337] We expect this to be an area where 3D sonographic imaging will still significantly grow in the near future.

2.1.8.4 Nuclear Medicine

3D SPECT imaging has been applied to the kidney to assess renal cortical scarring. It appears that this method is more reliable than simple planar imaging.[338]

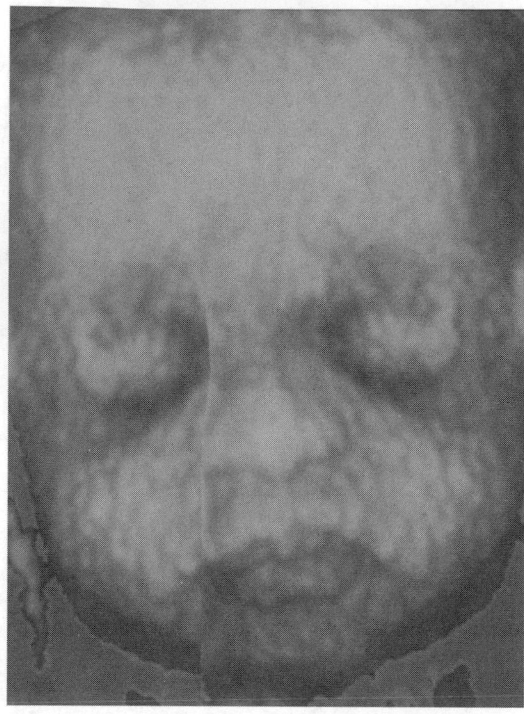

FIGURE 2.20 3D ultrasound image of a fetus at 18 weeks gestation with a bilateral cheilognathopalatoschisis. (Courtesy of R. Gombergh, Centre d'Imagerie Médicale Numerisée, Paris, France.)

2.1.9 Radiation Therapy

2.1.9.1 Computed Tomography

Since the early use of CT image data as a basis for radiation therapy planning (RTP),[339,340] which improved the determination of the planning target volume (PTV) and the 3D dose calculation,[341] a wide variety of improvements (e.g., beam's-eye view [BEV], multileaf collimator, dose–volume histogram [DVH], digitally reconstructed radiograph [DRR], dynamic wedges, computer-controlled machine settings and motions,[342] and intra-operative radiation therapy[343]) gradually turned RTP from a 2D into a 3D procedure.[344] This caused an ongoing urge for more accuracy in tumor and critical tissue localization to deliver highly individualized 3D conformal therapy.[345] After first combining original CT scans or reformatted image planes with dose calculations,[346] the use of 3D renderings[347,348] of anatomical surfaces and the PTV spurred the reconstruction of dose surface displays in the form of wire frame cages[349] surrounding the PTV, to be followed by iso-dose surfaces,[350] or the mapping of dose distributions on such surfaces[351] to judge underdosage of the PTV or overdosage of the tissues at risk.[352] It was also customary to image the radiation beams themselves.[353] It has also been suggested to combine 3D images with 2D CT cross-sections[354] or to bring perpendicular 2D CT images into a 3D setting.[355] As computers become faster, the need grows for real-time interactive planning systems, also coined "virtual simulators."[356] These systems are meant to interactively calculate the dose distribution,[357] display this distribution in combination with the patient's 3D representation,[358] calculate the DVHs[355] of the tissues at risk and the PTV, and even display a real-time DRR which now becomes digitally reconstructed fluoroscopy (DRF).[359] Further improvements can be expected from finding the best irradiation direction by classifying all possible directions in a spherical display[360] and displaying all different image types together on the same display screen.[361] As the planning becomes more accurate, CT simulators are starting to become more popular,[362] although cost is still a concern.[363] For treatment precision, computerized patient position verification systems[364] are under investigation. The next step will be monitoring organ motion between and during treatments and adapting the treatment accordingly.

In the meantime, 3D image display is also being applied to hyperthermia planning.[365]

2.1.9.2 Magnetic Resonance Imaging

Because magnetic resonance images are not directly suitable for the calculation of radiation dose, MRI is directly used for RTP only when matched to CT data[366,367] (see Section 2.2.5). However, MRI is being used for dosimetry in gel phantoms that simulate body shape and contain ferrous sulfate, as the post-irradiation T1 measurement correlates with radiation dose.[368]

2.2 DERIVATIVES OF 3D IMAGING

2.2.1 Introduction

While 3D imaging was a new way of imaging, it was first used for obtaining a topographic view of the area of interest, in the view of diagnostic visualization, communication between radiologist and referring physician, and surgical planning. However, as time passed, it merely became a tool to fully assess the three-dimensionality of the patient and the morphologic aspect of the pathology. And thus it became instrumental in morphologic analysis (distance, volume), surgical simulation, manufacturing of physical models including the design of implants, multimodality imaging, and surgical navigation (which is beyond the scope of this review). We will discuss recent developments in these derivatives of 3D imaging and will finally discuss the possibilities to display 3D images in a stereoscopic fashion. This will enable 3D images to be perceived three dimensionally and not as a shaded 2D image (which has led some investigators to refer to 3D images as "2.5D images").

2.2.2 Image Analysis

Image analysis is the collection of tools used to extract from the 3D data set, with or without 3D image reconstruction, the necessary quantitative information required for diagnosis, treatment, or research. It includes the measurement and interpretation of distances, angles, areas, and volumes, and can thus lead to analysis of shapes and patterns. Most image analysis, so far, has been performed using 2D images (radiographs, CT scans), and has created complete scientific fields such as morphometric analysis of landmark data.[369] With the advent of 3D image data and 3D image reconstructions, it has been shown that landmarks can be identified more accurately, resulting, for example, in more accurate distance measurements. In one study,[370] using 2-mm contiguous scan data of a dry skull, it was found that, averaged over 26 different cranial measurements, the mean difference between caliper and CT slice measurement was 2.31 mm with a range of 0.63 to 4.61 mm for the mean of the minimum and maximum values in the 26 measurements. The respective results for the difference between caliper and 3D CT measurements was a mean of 1.52 mm and a range of 0.57 to 2.73 mm. In comparison, the precision of the caliper measurements was about 1 mm. This demonstrates the improved accuracy of 3D image-based measurements. In the mean time the quality of 3D image rendering has further improved, bringing the accuracy to the same order of magnitude as the precision of caliper measurements.

Linear distance measurements have been used as a basis for shape analysis, as a basis for the design of endovascular stents via an optimally selected reformatted image plane,[371] and in combination with volume measurements.[372] More interesting is automatic thickness determination perpendicular to the outer surface and encoding this in a color wash superimposed on the 3D image, as a form of functional imaging. This method has been applied to MRI of the patellar articular cartilage[373] and CT of the skull in craniosynostosis[374] (Figure 2.21). It has also been used to visualize

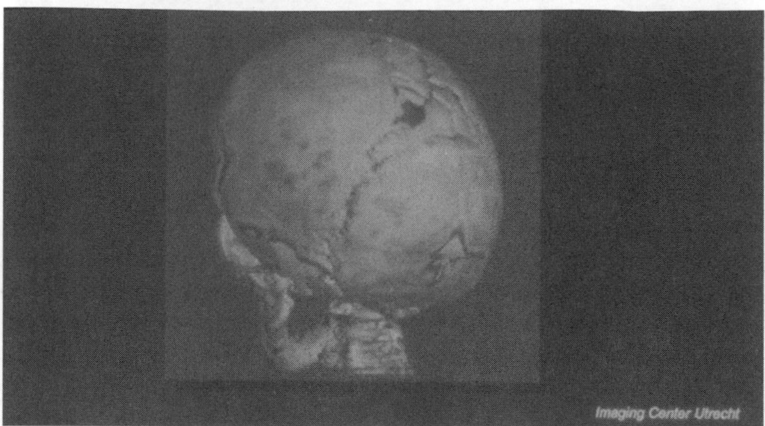

FIGURE 2.21 Skull thickness encoding in color on a 3D image of the skull. All measurements are done in a direction perpendicular to the external cranial surface. (Courtesy of K. Zuiderveld, Computer Vision Dept., Utrecht University Hospital, Utrecht, the Netherlands.)

the thickness of the air gap between an implant and the surrounding bone as in the case of the femoral stem of a hip implant.[375] Distance measurements are not necessarily done along straight lines. An example is the measurement of cortical sulcal lengths.[376]

The measurement of angles has been used to assess deformities as in craniosynostosis in an attempt to quantify distortion (e.g., trigonocephaly)[377] and asymmetry (e.g., plagiocephaly).[378]

3D images have also been used as a reference to determine the location where an area measurement should be taken such as in the case of the planum temporale in the brain.[379]

Extensive use has been made of 3D image data for volume measurements by segmentation of the morphologic entity of interest, followed by voxel summation.[380] The accuracy of this type of measurement depends on the coarseness of the scan data and the accuracy of the segmentation. 3D imaging of this segmentation serves as a check on the correctness of the segmentation. This advantage is not available in the classic approach of addition of slicewise planimetric measurements multiplied by the slice index.[381] Volumetric analysis has been applied to a wide variety of cases such as the cranial vault and ventricles,[382] frontal sinus,[383] left cardiac ventricle,[384] orbital soft tissues,[385] and masticatory muscles (Figure 2.22). Recently, volumetric analysis of gray and white matter of specific brain regions such as the prefrontal lobe, temporal lobe, precentral gyrus, and postcentral gyrus has been carried out to assess potential local relative volume differences between normals and patients with schizophrenia or bipolar disease.[386,387] The differences encountered, however, are still in the same order of magnitude as the measurement accuracy, which implies that the measurement techniques require further refinement.

Shape analysis has primarily been based on connecting landmarks, extracted from CT slices,[388] 3D images,[389,390] skin digitizations,[391] or stereophotogrammetric analysis of 3D-image stereo pairs,[392,393] into a wire frame model known as a "skeletogram."[389,394,395] Such models are subsequently used for morphometric analysis (e.g., finite element scaling[396] and Euclidean distance matrix analysis[397]) for deformity analysis, asymmetry studies that cannot make use of mirror imaging,[398] and growth studies. In the future, the selection of landmarks may be replaced by automatic ridge detection algorithms.[399]

Shape can be used, in combination with tissue properties and a finite element approximation, for the prediction of stress/strain and strength. In case the volume acquisition is repeated multiple times as a function of time, motion analysis of rigid or deformable structures is also possible.

Many other analysis tools are available, such as surface convexity/concavity analysis for the detection of brain sulci and assessment of brain atrophy[400] or irregularities on the surface of blood vessels.[401]

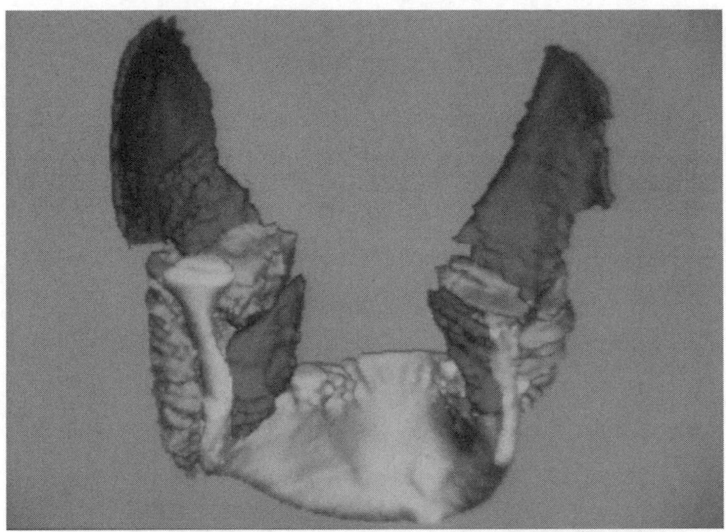

FIGURE 2.22 Segmentation of the masseter, temporalis, and medial and lateral pterygoid muscles in a 16-year-old male patient with Goldenhar syndrome. This enables quantification of the asymmetry of the muscular volumes.

Some of the well-known tool boxes are Analyze (Mayo Clinic),[402–404] 3DVIEWNIX (University of Pennsylvania),[405] VIDA (University of Iowa),[406] Osiris (University of Geneva),[407] Voxel-man (University of Hamburg),[408] and VROOM (University of Utrecht).[409]

2.2.3 Surgical Simulation

During his inaugural address at the first meeting of the International Society for Computer Aided Surgery (Tokyo, December 9–11, 1992), Michael Vannier stated that "computers are used more frequently today for surgery than any time in the past, and we predict that its future role will increase such that the contribution of computers to the success of many procedures is essential."[410]

The first step was to create the ideal end result without simulating the surgery itself. This was usually done using mirror imaging.[411,412]

Early attempts to use the wealth of 3D image data to really simulate a surgical plan were limited to cases with symmetric osteotomies, thus limiting the surgical simulation to a 2D cut-move-and-paste task in the lateral aspect to reposition the osseous parts.[413–417]

Complex 3D simulations were difficult to perform with the help of dedicated software only and were first carried out using physical models. This application, however, will be described in Section 2.2.4.

First, surgical simulation was based on wire frames constructed by connecting landmarks that had been extracted from anterior–posterior and lateral cephalograms.[394] Later on, the more complex task of 3D simulation on a display screen was addressed by defining different types of cutting operations that could work in 3D while the user was only watching the 2D display of the 3D image. A first possibility is to draw a cutting line onto the CT-based 3D image[394,415,418,419] or onto simplified derived 3D representations called polygon solid models.[420] It may occur, however, that the complete cutting line is not visible on a single 3D image. In that case, the vantage point of the 3D image may be adapted and cutting continued in another viewing direction of the same 3D scene. Final refinements are possible in the slice-by-slice editing mode.[421] Another method is to move a wire frame grid, which intersects the 3D object, into place and remove the tissues on one side of the plane defined by this grid. Most frequently, flat[422] and spherical[375,423,424] cutting planes are used. Even if objects are defined in a "fuzzy" fashion, as in volume rendering, such manipulations are still possible.[425,426]

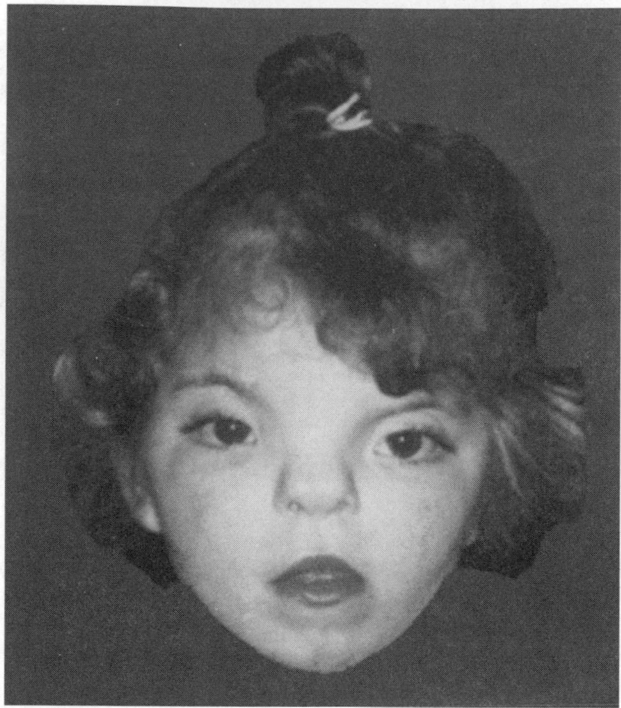

FIGURE 2.23a Validation of surgical simulation and consequent surgery. (Courtesy of J.L. Marsh and V.V. Patel, Mallinckrodt Institute of Radiology, St. Louis, MO.) (a) 3D pre-operative image of a 4-year-old girl with asymmetric hypertelorism secondary to craniofrontonasal dysplasia. Status after the release of the right unicoronal synostosis at 3 months of age.

In many patients, there is a lack of bone tissue that needs to be supplemented by a tissue reconstruction (e.g., trauma, hemifacial microsomia, Romberg's disease, neurofibromatosis, tumor resection). Simulating this surgical reconstruction and then analyzing the dimensions of the missing tissue can be done using a subtraction of the affected side from the mirror-imaged normal side and then displaying the difference. Studies using this technique have been carried out using the Analyze software package.[412,427] This technique can be perfectly combined with robotized milling of autografts.[428]

Another use of surgical simulation is the fitting of a standard implant, such as a middle ear transducer,[429] into the individual anatomy of the patient.

Surgical simulation has been primarily applied to the skull and face, but there are examples in the musculoskeletal system applying simulation to the planning of corrective scoliosis surgery,[430] planning femoral neck rotation in case of avascular necrosis of the femoral head,[431] and fitting of a femoral prosthetic stem[432] thus demonstrating that individualized stems are better than off-the-shelf stems.[433]

Until now, we have only discussed surgical simulation of rigid bone tissue. Simulation of soft tissues is much more complicated but has been attempted on the basis of CT data[415] or the combination of CT and skin digitizations.[434] In craniofacial surgical simulation, the first attempts[415] used filling in of the soft tissues missing in the surgically created diastasis followed by smoothing eventual steps in the transition. This method is not suitable for predicting post-operative facial features and requires more complex procedures.[418,434,435]

The quality of surgical simulation has been recently validated by comparing the surgical simulation with a post-operative 3D reconstruction (Figure 2.23). This has been tested on cadaver heads[436,437] as well as in patients.[437–439] To assess the difference between the pre-operative and post-

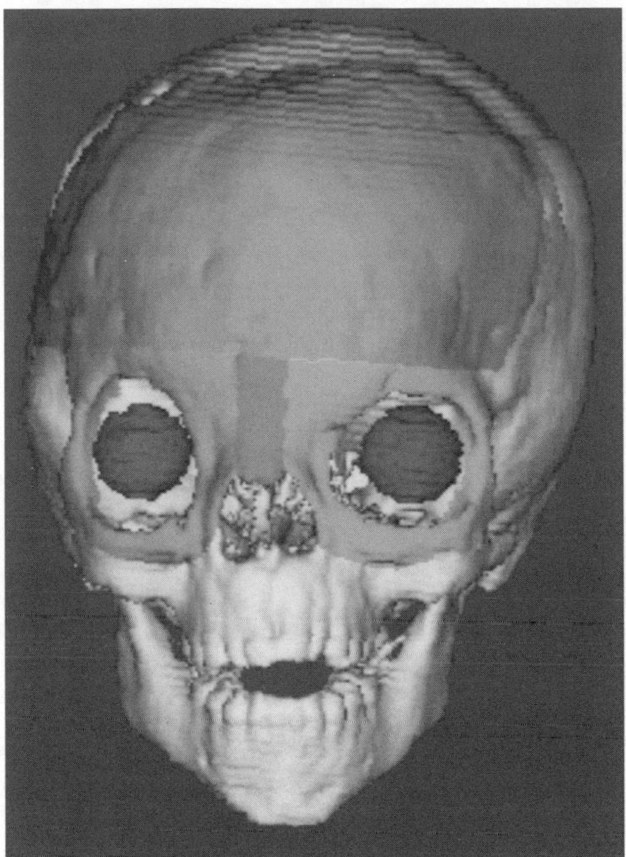

FIGURE 2.23b The standard Tessier "useful orbit" orbital segments are indicated in green and yellow and the median ostectomy in orange on the unaltered pre-operative frontal surface 3D CT image.

operative situation, matching of the two scans has been applied.[440] This method would also be feasible for comparing the surgical simulation and the post-operative result.

In simulation of surgery involving bones, which are submitted to forces (e.g., weight-bearing, chewing), a technique has been developed that can predict the strain and pressure forces applied to the bone after surgery, known as finite element analysis. This method subdivides the tissue into mass elements that are interconnected with force elements.[441] Then it calculates the forces and superimposes these as a color wash onto the 3D image of the surgical simulation.[442] Finite element analysis can even be used to mimic trauma, by simulating impact forces applied to different impact locations on a skull model.[443]

A special type of simulation is used in the design of missing dental elements. The surface of the new dental element cannot be freely chosen but depends on the anatomical shape of its antagonist in combination with all possible chewing motions. The result is a functional surface of the antagonist that can be derived via simulation.[444]

All surgical simulation techniques discussed above are more or less off-line procedures that take considerable time, and if the outcome is not correct, the process has to be repeated. Therefore, the trend is now to devise real-time interactive surgical simulation techniques that can be used both for surgical simulation as well as for training surgeons, just like the flight simulators used for training pilots. Since this process is a virtual surgery, it is related to the computer graphics techniques associated with virtual reality.[445] Virtual reality (VR) simulation tries, by the use of head-mounted displays (HMDs) and tracking of hand and instrument motion using a data glove or other interactive devices,[446] to create a simulation that is as realistic as possible.[447,448] In some

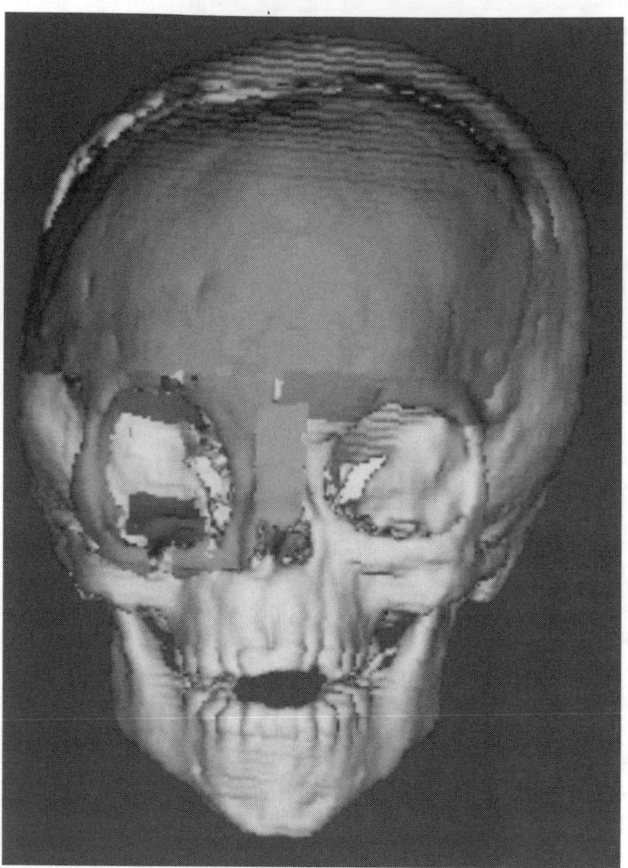

FIGURE 2.23c Dissatisfied with the simulated outcome of mesial movement of both "useful" orbits, an asymmetrical segmented movement of the entire right ventral orbit (green) and the left superial orbital rim (orange) with onlay bone grafts (yellow) to the nasal dorsum and right orbit (purple).

cases, there also is sound feedback,[449] and the ultimate form of feedback (important for surgeons) is tactile or haptic feedback.[450] The most difficult part, again, is the soft-tissue simulation (fidelity, deformation, bleeding after cutting).[451] A preliminary system for laparoscopic surgical simulation is addressing this issue[452] and will be followed by other systems in the market.[453] Improvement of these systems is expected when they are based on detailed data sets such as that of the visible human project[454,455] or the synthesized virtual human,[456] but individualized surgery will have to be based on data sets from medical imaging modalities. In case these modalities still provide too much data for real-time interaction, techniques are availble to drastically reduce the amount of data without significantly violating the morphologic accuracy.[457] The VR technology is only emerging and is expected to support, in addition to surgical simulation, many other fields in medicine such as interactive anatomy education and telepresence surgery. These applications are expected to become essential building blocks of the digital tools used by the physician of the 21st century.[458]

There also are other, less immersive, systems that have some but not all the properties of VR. Völter has given them the following names: desktop VR (computer screen instead of HMD; a system suitable for endoscopic simulation), pseudo VR (interactively controlled animation), and inverse VR (integration of the computer into the real world to help disabled people — e.g., eye-controlled cursor allows a tetraplegic person to communicate).[459]

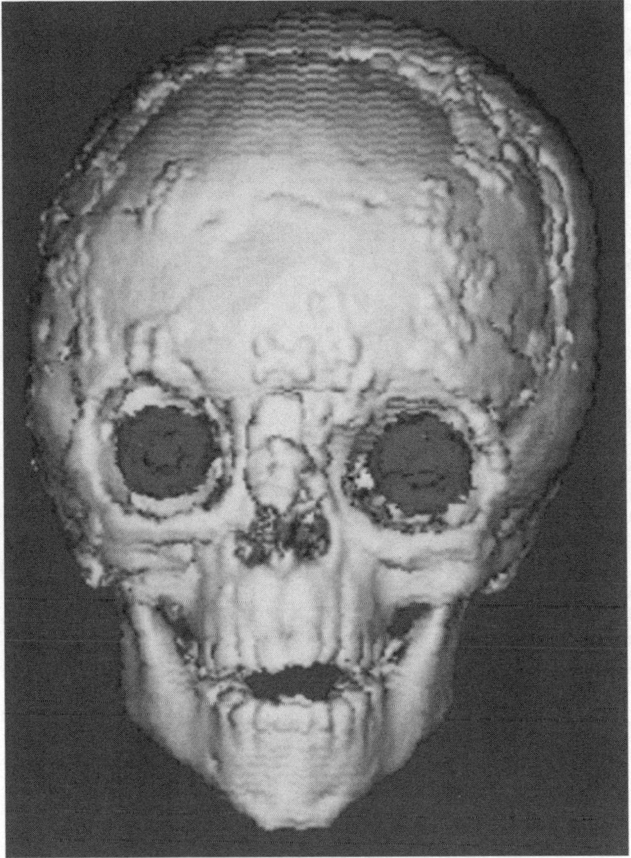

FIGURE 2.23d The actual state of the patient 1 week post-operatively.

2.2.4 Image-Based Physical Model Manufacturing and Implant Design

In 1979, right in the pioneering time of 3D imaging, Alberti annouced his idea to make physical models on the basis of CT scans.[460] However, no company that he contacted was willing to develop his idea. Independent of Alberti, Altschuler and Herman[461] also developed the same idea and even suggested the use of mirror imaging in combination with physical model manufacturing.

2.2.4.1 Plate Stacking

The earliest clinical use of a physical model was in a pelvis that was disrupted by a fibrosarcoma. The model was formed by stacking 15-mm-thick foam plates and supported the design of a custom-made metal implant.[462]

In the early 1980s, Marsh and Vannier started to stack aluminum plates that were cut according to contours extracted from CT scans, and thus pioneered the first craniofacial models.[463] Stacked models always remained coarse due to their straight edges, even when the thickness of the plates was reduced to 2 mm.[20] We have tested the use of computer-controlled laser cutting of 1-mm cardboard plates, however, with a similar coarse result.

This initial type of physical model was followed by a wide variety of model types and manufacturing methods[464,465] (Table 2.1).

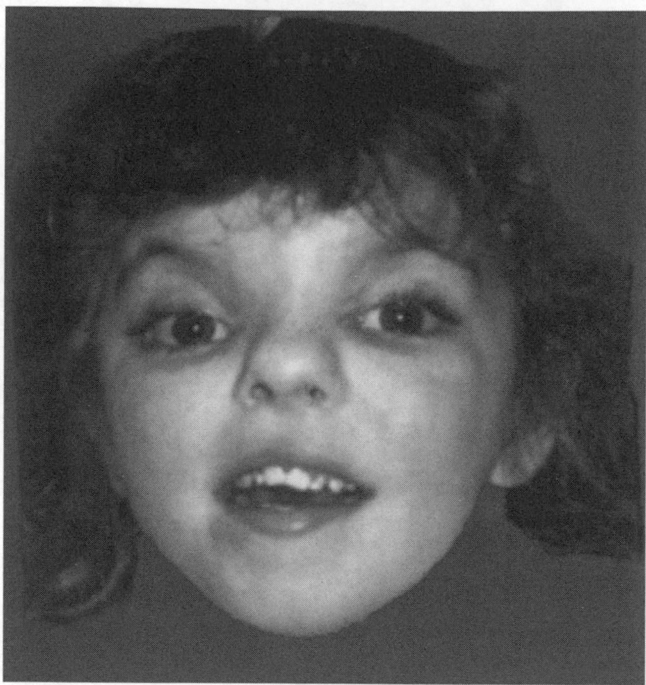

FIGURE 2.23e The appearance of the patient 1 year following correction of the hypertelorism and associated craniofacial anomalies.

TABLE 2.1.
Methods for Image-Based Physical Model Manufacturing

Plate stacking (polystyrene foam, aluminum, polymethylmethacrylate, cardboard)
CNC mold milling and resin casting (wax, polysulfone; also used for implant manufacturing using hydroxy apatite and collagen as implant material and polysulfone as mold)
CNC (four- and five-axis) model milling (polystyrene foam, wax, polyurethane foam)
CNC implant milling (hydroxyapatite, bone graft, titanium)
Stereolithography (laser and mask stereolithography)
Computer-controlled material deposition
Laser sintering (wax, nylon, polycarbonate)
Laminated object manufacturing (LOM) (paper)
Fused deposition modeling (FDM) (acrylonitril-butadiene-styrene-copolymer, wax)

2.2.4.2 Mold Milling Combined with Model Casting

In 1982, David N. White, a plastic surgeon, patented a method to cast models after milling a mold.[466] He founded a company (Contour Medical Systems, later renamed Cemax Medical Systems, Fremont, CA) that pioneered the 1500X 3D workstation, one of the first of its kind. White explained that he saw 3D imaging and physical models as tools that could do away with the "fitting and chipping" that was so common and consumed so much time during reconstructive surgery.[467] The models were accurate within ±3 mm; sufficient for surgical purposes[99,468,469] including the possibility to rehearse surgery.[470] It was even possible to integrate dental casts with these models and to place them in a specially developed articulator to plan orthognathic surgery.[471]

The three-axis milling of the mold shells and the requirement of removing the model without damaging the mold limited the use of these models to simple geometries such as edentate mandibles

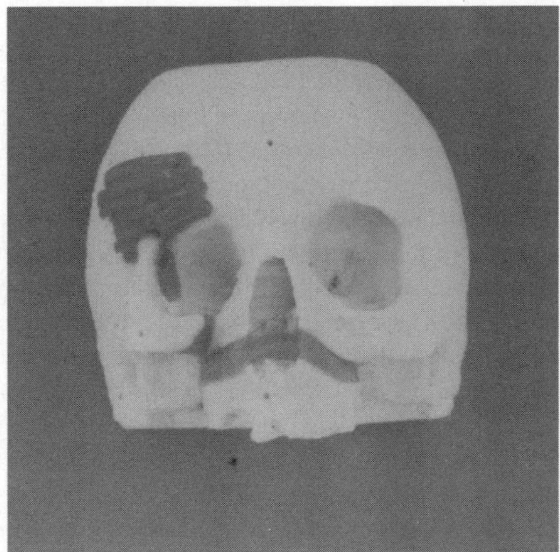

FIGURE 2.24 Use of a physical (milled foam) model to rehearse surgery (female patient, 8 years of age). The simulated surgery involves reduction of facial asymmetry induced by growth retardation due to radiation treatment in childhood for right-sided retinoblastoma. (Courtesy of A.R.M. Wittkampf, Department of Maxillofacial Surgery, Utrecht University Hospital, Utrecht, the Netherlands.)

for the design of subperiosteal implants used for fixing a dental prosthesis.[472] By slightly adapting the model manufacturing procedure, it was possible to make implants. Instead of wax, the mold was milled from polysulfone because this material could be sterilized. Then, instead of resin, a mixture of hydroxyapatite powder and collagen was molded and dried to form implants for cranial defects and zygoma and chin enhancement in patients with mandibulofacial dysostosis (Treacher Collins disease).[473]

2.2.4.3 Computerized Numerically Controlled (CNC) Model Milling

Direct milling of models was a more promising technique for manufacturing of complex models than mold milling followed by casting, although both techniques were developed at the same time — the casting technique in the United States and the milling technique in Germany.[474] The milling technique was originated by the need of radiotherapists to create compensation filters based on density measurements in a thorax radiograph. The lower the density the higher the compensation, and thus the deeper the styrofoam filter that was to be filled with a radiation-absorbing material.[475] Removal of foam material by the use of a heated wire loop did not produce accurate models,[474,476] and therefore, the technique progressed via three-axis milling, four-axis milling, to five-axis milling[477] while the styrofoam[478] was gradually replaced by polyurethane foam. Between 1988 and 1993, the models used for clinical applications primarily were milled models. They were mainly used in orthognathic surgery,[477,479,480] craniofacial surgery,[477,481] and orthopedic surgery[482] for simulation of the surgical approach[483–485] (Figure 2.24) (training, demonstration) and for the design of implants.[486] Dental casts were integrated[487] and osteosynthesis materials applied and bent in the right shape.[474] The accuracy of the milled models was on the order of 1.6 mm[488] and thus about twice as accurate as the cast models. This accuracy also required a good interpolation between thin CT slices and a lack of motion and dental artifacts.[489]

The implants have been designed in different ways. It was possible to mold the implant from wax, using the model as a template, and then copy the wax implant into a biocompatible material such as glass ionomer cement.[39,490] The molding of the wax implant can be done manually or by milling the mirror image of the normal side, then making a wax cast and then modifying that cast such that it fits in the defect.[69] The advantages of glass ionomer cement are that it was much more biocompatible than other types of acrylic materials, and that the same material, in its fluid form, could be used to glue the implant to the bone — a connection that could hold a force of 10 kg/cm^2. The disadvantage, however, is that this fluid material is not allowed to make contact with the cerebrospinal fluid because it may induce aluminum intoxication. Unfortunately this occurred several times, causing mortality. The result was that glass ionomer cement for craniofacial applications was removed from the market. Other implant materials are hydroxyapatite,[491] which also can be milled directly;[492] a combination of hydroxyapatite and tricalcium phosphate;[493] autolyzed, antigen-extracted, allogenic bone of human organ donors;[494] biocompatible resins such as polymethylmethacrylate,[495] and biodegradable materials such as amorphous polylactic acid doped with bone morphogenetic proteins (BMPs) for bone regeneration.[496] This process is called osteoinduction.[497] In case an autograft is preferred, it has been shown that the shape of the defect can be calculated by subtracting the affected side from the mirror-imaged normal side[412] followed by milling of the bone graft itself.[498] Implants also can be milled directly in the same fashion. This often means that the voxel-based geometry of the desired implant has to be translated into a CAD/CAM environment, which usually is a triangulation-based geometry. This translation can create problems because the new data sets tend to be too large for standard CAD/CAM systems[499] and thus require adaptations. The advantage of the CAD/CAM approach is that the desired shape of the implant edge can be determined, that flanges for fixation can be added,[500] surface shape can be adapted to compensate for soft-tissue hypotrophy,[501] and, in the case of titanium implants, the implant thickness can be reduced to 1.5 mm to allow for follow-up CT and MRI investigations.[502] For the design of dental inlays, CT is too coarse and optical scanning techniques must be used to assess the 3D shape of the tooth cavity.[503]

After implantation, 3D imaging can be used to monitor formation of new bone. It is even possible to register the post-operative scan with the pre-operative scan and subtract the pre-operative bone from the post-operative bone to show the difference.[504] We have carried out post-operative follow-up scans and have demonstrated where the new bone had been formed adjacent to the implant (Figure 2.25).

2.2.4.4 Stereolithography

During the second half of the 1980s, a new model manufacturing technique emerged called stereolithography.[505] The principle is that a fluid photoresin (monomer) is locally solidified under computer control by applying ultraviolet light to those parts that belong to the model volume. This means that the complexity of the models can further increase and internal cavities, such as the paranasal sinuses, that could not be reached by the mill can now be faithfully reproduced.[506] So far, two different types of stereolithography have evolved. The older approach uses an ultraviolet laser (3D Systems, Sylmar, CA) that scans the surface of the vat containing the monomer.[507–509] After a layer is finished, the model is lowered into the vat, a new layer of monomer forms above the model, this new layer is distributed evenly, and the next layer is solidified. The power of the laser is insufficient to cure the resin throughout, meaning that, after being finished, the model requires cleaning and postcuring in an oven. A more recent approach that unfortunately has been minimally used for medical models is the technique that uses a computer-generated mask in combination with an ultraviolet floodlight (Cubital, Raanana, Israel).[510,511] This floodlight is so powerful that postcuring is not required and due to the lack of shrinkage, thicker models can be manufactured. This technique replaces the monomer, which is not solidified, by wax, whereas the laser method requires the generation of support structures to prevent substructures, which are not yet connected to the main structure, from drifting away. Recent developments of new photopolymers have resolved many of the early shortcomings of stereolithography. Shrinkage (only a problem in laser systems) has been reduced, polymerization has been improved (leaving no more smelling and toxic monomers), and improved mechanical properties create less brittle and, if desired, even elastic

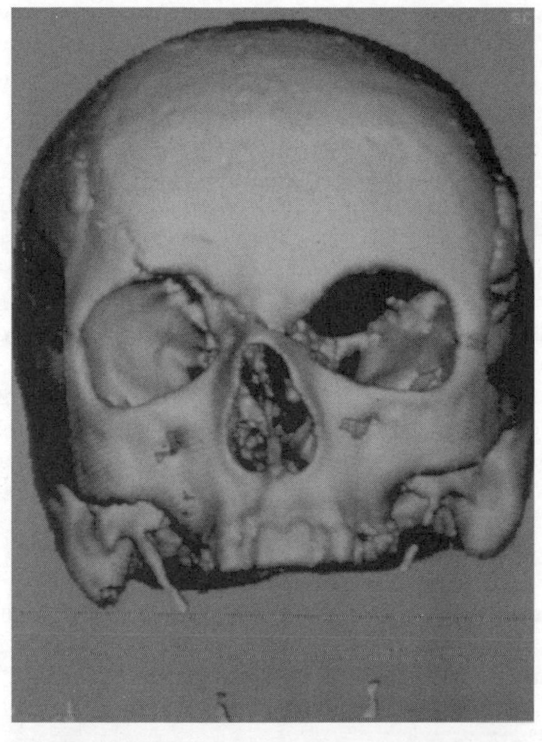

a

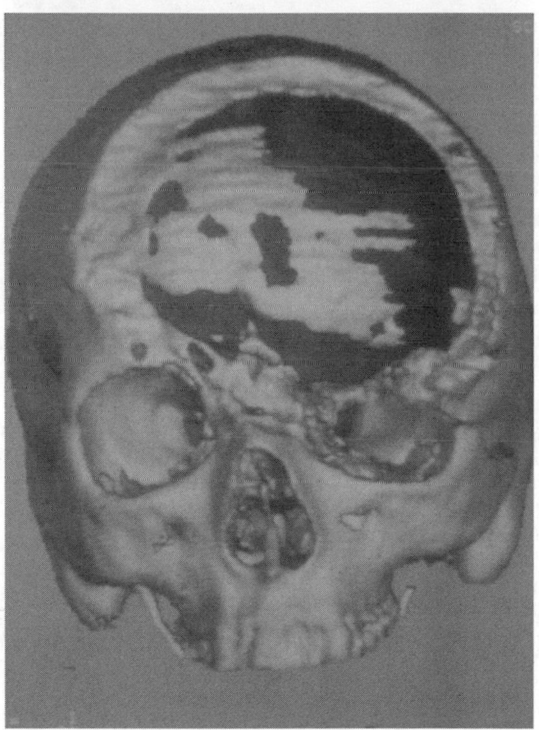

b

FIGURE 2.25 Post-operative view of same patient as in Figure 2.10. (a) This image shows the position of the glass ionomer implant that was manufactured using a physical model. (b) In this image the implant is not shown. Now the new bone that has formed between the dura and the implant can be appreciated.

models. Sometimes the transparency of the model is regarded as an advantage to see internal structures, but at the same time it impairs the quality of the comprehension of shape upon viewing. Today, a resin can be selected that is either transparent or opaque. The end result is a very accurate model, almost as accurate as the CT data themselves. This has led to taking care of using the exact segmentation threshold,[512] to avoid the use of edge-enhancing convolution filters,[513] to avoid rough model surfaces[514] by performing subvoxel interpolation,[515] and the use of thin slices and helical CT aquisition allowing sub-slice-thickness slice reconstruction indices.[516] Since 1993, we have seen a tendency that most models used clinically are of the stereolithography type[517,518] including surgical simulation,[519–521] implant design, and osteodystraction planning.[522] But the minute detail of stereolithographic models has extended its use to vascular trees[523] (Figure 2.26a). On the basis of these, we have been able to create realistic vascular flow phantoms for MR research (Figure 2.26b). The process of laser stereolithography has been sped up by more powerful lasers and a rapid technique to apply the new monomer layer by a moving "waterfall" type of curtain that sprays the new layer onto the model,[524] a technique called curtain recoating.[525] The latest in stereolithography is selective use of color.[526,527] A dope is added to the resin that changes color (red or blue) as soon as the energy transferred by the ultraviolet light per cubic millimeter reaches a certain level (Figure 2.27).

2.2.4.5 Material Deposition Techniques

Only recently, computer-controlled material deposition techniques such as laser sintering have been applied to model manufacturing. Although this creates models with a rough surface,[528] the use of materials such as nylon and polycarbonate, which have better mechanical properties than photopolymers, is considered a great advantage when, for example, using the model for shaping implants from thin titanium plate.[529]

Other material deposition techniques used for rapid prototyping such as LOM and FDM are in a prototype phase and were introduced at the 1996 Annual Meeting of the Radiological Society of North America (Baxter Healthcare Corp., Round Lake, IL, USA).

2.2.4.6 Template Design

Three-dimensional imaging can be a good basis for the design of templates. Templates are individual guides for drilling holes in a precise location and direction or for cutting bone according to a precise edge that is to match with a prepared implant. A good example is the 3D planning of dental implants[530] where a template can guide the drilling of the holes in the mandible.[531] Other examples are the drilling of holes in vertebrae for the introduction of pedicle screws[532,533] or drilling of a hole in the femoral neck.[533]

Templates can also be created in the shape of an implant to be used as an example for the implant that is to be shaped manually from a bone graft[534] or from donor autolyzed, antigen-extracted, allogenic bone.[497]

2.2.5 Intra- and Multimodality Matching

Each imaging modality can provide different tissue-dependent signals that can enhance understanding when combined in a single image. In 2D imaging this has led to sumperimpositioning different image types such as digital radiography and scintigraphy.[535] Similar techniques have also been used for tomographic 2D images after matching the 3D image volumes and reslicing one of the two volumes to obtain matching slice pairs. These pairs can simply be compared, with[536] or without[537] using an interactive pointer (as in comparing pre-operative MRI with intra-operative ultrasound)[538] or be blended,[539] or shown as a split image[540] whereby the transition from one imaging modality to the other can be interactively moved (Figure 2.28a). However, it is also possible to superimpose a contour of interest from one image on top of the other. Examples are an MR contour on top of a CT slice[541] or a PET slice,[537] a vessel cross-section from angiography on top of a CT image,[542]

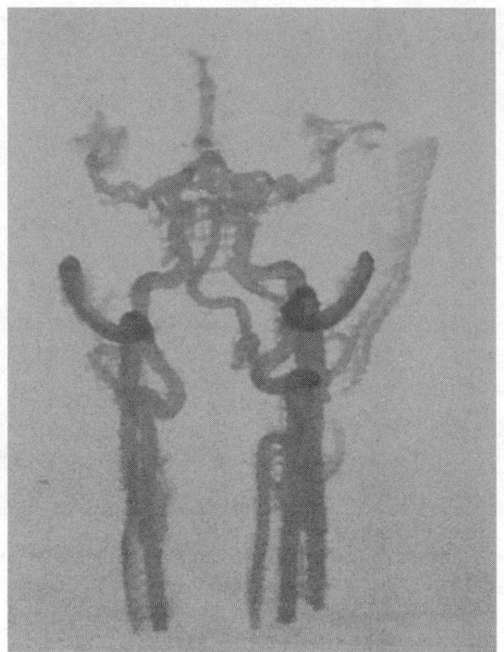

a

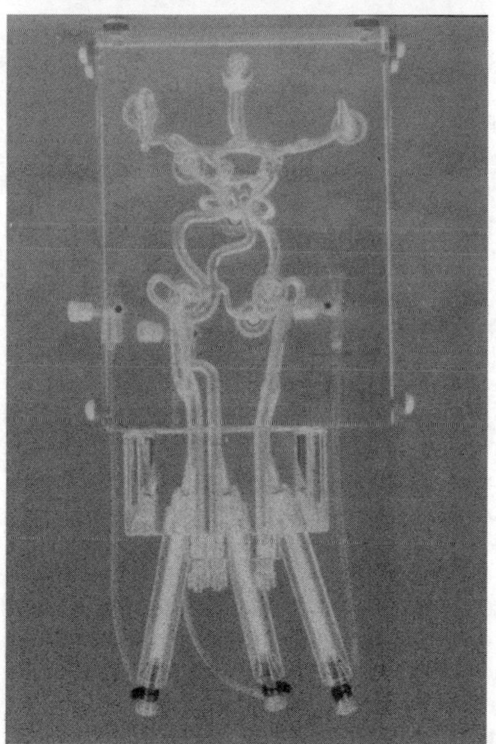

b

FIGURE 2.26 Use of stereolithography to manufacture physical models of vascular structures, in this case the circle of Willis and the carotid and vertebral arteries. (a) Stereolithographic model (Materialise, Heverlee, Belgium) after removal of the support structures. (b) Plexiglas flow phantom for MRI made with the use of the stereolithographic model. This model was copied by a skillful glass blower. The result was cast in Plexiglas and then the glass was etched away. (Courtesy of W.P.Th.M. Mali, Department of Radiology, Utrecht University Hospital, Utrecht, the Netherlands.)

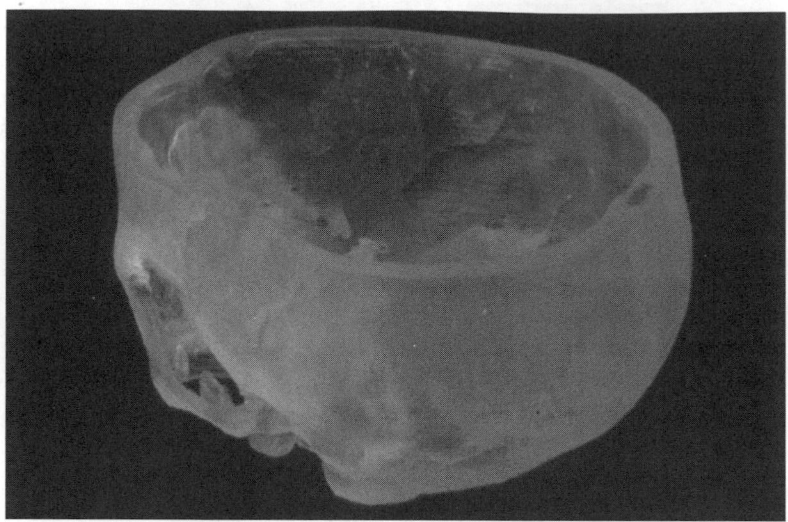

FIGURE 2.27 Use of color to highlight specific parts in the stereolithographic model. The resin contains a dope chemical that turns to a specific color as soon as the ultraviolet light reaches a critical energy. In this case the bony involvement of a hyperostotic meningioma is colored in red after the radiologist prepared a separate segmentation of the tumor extent. (Courtesy of B. Swaelens, Materialise, Heverlee, Belgium.)

a PET contour on top of an MR slice,[537] a CT contour on an angiogram,[543] or a location of MEG activity mapped onto an MR slice.[150,544] In planning radiotherapy, it is useful to have matched CT and MR slices side by side, draw tumor volumes on each, and then combine them in a Boolean "OR" operation to find the final tumor volume definition.[545]

Some imaging modalities, such as EEG, PET, SPECT, and magneto-encephalography (MEG), are of a functional nature and require matching with a high-resolution morphologic image for interpretation of the topographic basis of functional differences. This is often done by mapping the functional image in the form of a color wash on top of the high-resolution image such as PET signal intensities mapped as a color wash on CT[546] or MRI.[547] Multimodality imaging is particularly suitable for imaging specific tissue interfaces with modality-inherent large contrasts. As a result, segmentation of these tissue interfaces is relatively simple, without much manual interaction. Examples for CT are skin, bone, fat, and air-containing cavities. Examples for MRI are skin, nerve tissue, tendons, cartilage, and blood vessels. Most often, the bone is segmented using the CT images and then, wherever there is bone in the CT image, the MR pixels are replaced by CT pixels[540,547,548] (Figure 2.28b). Matching of surfaces does not necessarily mean matching of different image modalities because it is also possible that a modality must be matched with itself to make comparisons in time, in longitudinal studies,[549] or to make sure that radiation treatment is corrected for changes in patient position between treatment sessions.[364] It is, however, also possible to match different modes within the same modality such as MRA and standard MRI[536,550] to show the brain together with the vascular tree;[551,552] to match the functional information acquired with fMRI with MRI to map out specific functional brain centers such as the visual cortex, auditory cortex, Broca's area (speech), and the motor cortex; or to match a donor site for a graft with the receiving defect, both using the same modality (CT).[553]

The best way to make use of multimodality imaging is combining different tissue interfaces from multiple modalities in the form of 3D renderings in a single topographic image by matching (mapping, registration) the corresponding data sets. The best known combination is CT with MRI,[547] for instance to image subarachnoid electrodes (CT) together with the brain surface (MRI).[39,554] But it is also possible to match a CT scan with a laser scan of the skin.[555] The earliest 3D multimodality matching was performed matching a color wash from a PET data set with a 3D image of the brain

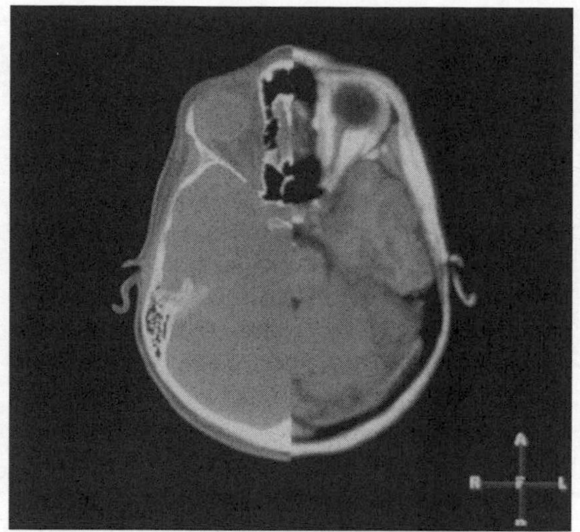

a

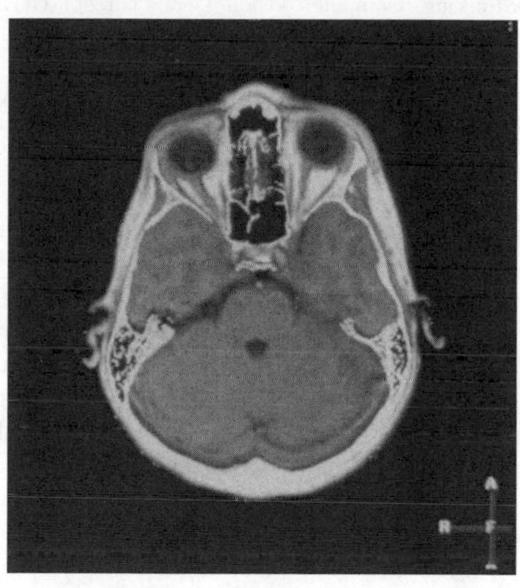

b

FIGURE 2.28 2D display of matched data sets from different imaging modalities. This case represents a patient with Romberg syndrome. A combination of CT and MRI is shown. (Courtesy of A.M.H. Huitema, Philips Medical Systems, Best, the Netherlands.) (a) Use of split image to display a multimodality matching. The transition can be moved interactively. (b) MRI image with bone replaced by CT data (yellow).

surface.[556,557] Other examples of functional images combined with MRI are MEG dipole data in epileptic patients,[558] SPECT[374] (Figure 2.29), and EEG.

Instead of matching different 3D data sets from the same patient, it is also possible to match a 2D image (e.g., radiograph, DSA) with a 2D aspect of a rendering of a 3D data set reconstructed in the same projection direction as the 2D radiographic image. This approach, in a more primitive form without 3D rendering, started 10 years ago as a tool to plan stereotactic approaches to deep targets in the brain while avoiding the risk of rupturing large arteries.[559–561] Such a system enabled the reconstruction of reformatted cross-sectional images perpendicular to the planned needle trajectory,[562] and it was commercialized (Compass, Stereotactic Medical Systems Inc., New Hartford,

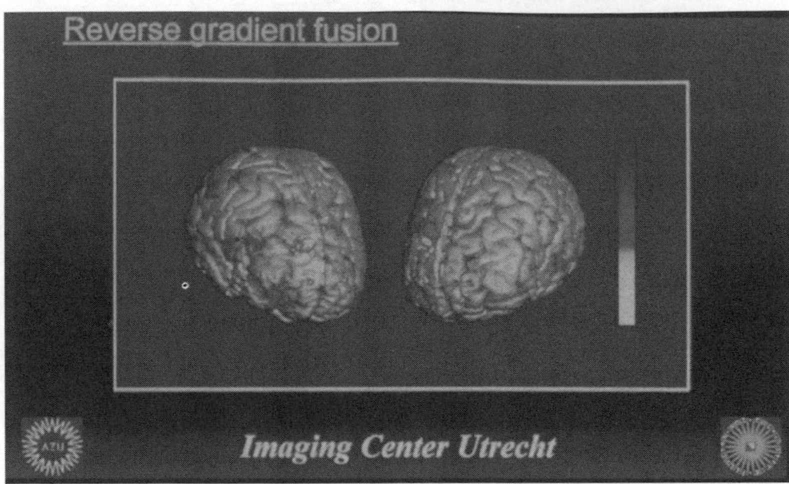

FIGURE 2.29 Multimodality matching between MRI and SPECT in a patient with a low-grade astrocytoma. The SPECT data are shown as a color wash on top of the MRI data showing a blood concentration surrounding the tumor. (Courtesy of R. Stokking, Computer Vision Dept., Utrecht University Hospital, Utrecht, the Netherlands.)

NY).[563] Another example is the matching of an angiogram of the coronary arteries with a myocardial nuclear perfusion study.[564] If desired, stereoangiograms can be used.[536,565]

Different techniques have been developed to achieve the best possible fusion of data sets. The most common situation occurs when both data sets are rigid and the matching is global instead of local. In that situation at least three different matching techniques have been applied: matching the centers of gravity and then aligning the principal axes of inertia,[548] the matching of fiducial points[566] such as landmarks or the use of markers attached to the patient during both scans, and matching of skin surfaces in the two data sets.[540] When applied to the calvarium, this last method is also known as the fitting of the "hat" to the "head."[567] For other kinds of multimodality matching, both global and local, four different matching types have been defined: rigid, affine, projective, and curved.[568] The rigid matching we have discussed above. However, when the structures to be matched cannot be superimposed because of geometric distortion, the differences can be bridged by the affine, projective, and curved matching techniques. The distortions that require affine and projective matching do not frequently occur in medical applications. We therefore concentrate on the free curved matching, using non-linear distortions also known as "warping." Warping is a complex mathematical procedure that can be applied to 2D contours,[569] to 2D contours including the encompassed surfaces[570] (also known as the morphing technique[571]), to complex surfaces in 3D such as that of the liver,[572] and finally to such surfaces including the tissue volume it contains.[573] Applied in 2D this will enable smooth transitions between slices for sub-slice-thickness interpolations and in 3D it will enable interpolations between discrete renderings to create smooth transitions for animations.[574] The warping procedure is usually driven by specific landmarks that must coincide after the warping[369,575] such as anatomic landmarks.

Warping can be used to correct for geometric distortion in an imaging modality such as in MRI,[576] to correct for patient motion between scans, or to match atlas data with patient data. Examples are a functional neuroanatomy atlas such as the Schaltenbrand-Wahren brain atlas[577] or the standardized Talairach and Tournoux stereotactic coordinate system,[578] which is subdivided into functional volumes of interest,[579] a schematic brain atlas of the ventricular system and the basal ganglia,[580] a normal textbook data set representing standard anatomy in a specific imaging modality,[573] and a specific computerized atlas based on CT and MRI including segmentation and labeling of functional areas.[581] Matching of patient data with these atlases can be valuable in the assessment of diseases such as Alzheimer's disease and schizophrenia. Matching, including warping, will have to become more automatic for clinical use, but will have to make use of feature extraction to find the necessary landmarks for matching.[582,583] This will enable the warping technique to be extended to the extracranial parts of the body; for instance, by using the databases acquired in the visible human project[454] as a reference atlas.

2.2.6 Stereoscopic and Volumetric Image Display

The presentation of 3D images to the user has primarily been in a 2D fashion, either as a hard copy or as a CRT display. The lack of stereoscopic cues has often been compensated for by the use of motion parallax, which is as strong a cue as stereopsis. This involves the creation of a series of rendered views covering the full circle of 360° with increments of 1 to 3°. This series is then displayed in the form of a cine loop. A disadvantage of this method is that small details cannot be studied because they are quickly disappearing by the time they have been spotted. Another disadvantage is that motion parallax is a weak depth cue when the image is transparent,[584] as is often the case with volume rendering. Because the use of stereopsis is a recognized strong depth cue,[585] many attempts have been made to create stereoscopic viewing.

The simplest method of all is the use of two hard copies representing two rendered views in directions that are 3 to 7° apart. They are placed side by side with the right-eye image on the left and vice versa. Cross-eye viewing is then the simplest method to create a stereoscopic view.[586] It has been applied to 3D images[374,587] as well as to angiograms.[536] It is also possible to view the images via a stereoscope, but the image position must then be reversed (right-eye image on the right). The stereoscope was invented by Wheatstone in 1838 and was used to view vascular structures in cadaveric specimens that were injected with contrast medium early in this century.[490,588] Later on, the more popular View-master™ stereoscope was used.[589] Other techniques to separate the two views of the two eyes are the anaglyph technique, using red and green color encoding, and the polarization-encoding technique.[590]

Stereoscopic techniques that do not require any type of special glasses are called autostereoscopic and the type that is best known in this category is holography. The best results are obtained by printing a hologram of a surface-rendered 3D image as a cylindric or multiplex hologram[423] or as a rainbow hologram[591,592] but unfortunately, this is too costly for clinical use. Therefore, a technique was developed that avoids segmentation and only integrates individual slices into a hologram.[593] It requires a special lightbox, and, when placing a small projection screen in front of the hologram, a cross-sectional image can be obtained that can be interactively moved through the image data volume.[594] The disadvantage of this type of hologram is that the slice superimpositioning reduces the image contrast. Another disadvantage of holograms is that it is still difficult to reproduce vivid colors. There are several alternative types of hard copy that also make use of the position of the eyes to select the appropriate image for each eye. There is one system that makes use of the venetian blind principle to select the proper image detail that can be computer encoded on a film at a certain distance from the raster pattern. This system is called barrier-strip autostereography.[595] The barrier structure is usually visible and gives a coarse impression. This method also requires special procedures to align the raster with the image carrier. Another type of hard copy is the lenticular system.[596] It makes use of a raster of cylindrical microlenses that allows different parts of the underlying photo-emulsion to be seen by the different eyes and is thus capable of producing stereopairs.[597] The lenticular system can reproduce full color but it can be viewed only from a limited angle and not from a wide angle as in holograms. With the recent development of a printer,[598] the lenticular system can become cost effective for clinical use. It is felt that surgeons can especially gain from stereoscopic vison in cases of complex trauma[599] and in vascular disease.[600]

In order not to be limited by stereoscopic visualization of hard copy images only, it has been attempted as well to create stereoscopic and autostereoscopic electronic display systems that can combine stereopsis with motion parallax.[601] The simplest form is a passive system using a semitransparent mirror combined with polarizing filters and two CRT screens that display the two views for the two eyes.[602] More popular and less bulky, however, are the active stereo displays. Basically two types of active display systems have been developed to achieve stereopsis. The first type makes use of a polarizing liquid crystal stereo shutter screen[603] in front of the CRT. This CRT alternatingly displays the left-eye and the right-eye views in synchrony with switching the polarization direction of the shutter screen. The observer is required to wear glasses with a clockwise- and a counter-clockwise polarized lens. The second type of display makes use of infrared-driven electro-optical liquid crystal shutter glasses.[604] This is currently the most frequently used system and is ideal in combination with real-time volume rendering[605] and for VR-oriented interactive displays.[449,491] A disadvantage is that the image repetition frequency is often too low and causes flicker,[606] which, in turn, may cause headaches. A new alternative is the lenticular screen-based flat CRT display[607] that can also be used in a form suitable for video projection.[608,609]

Recent developments are focused on truly three-dimensional displays in the sense that one can walk around the image while it remains autostereoscopic and consistent with the viewing direction. Such display systems are called direct volume display devices (DVDD) and instead of depth cues, they provide true depth. The simplest of its kind is the vibrating (varifocal) mirror.[610] This display is most suitable to display wire frame images. Other concepts use a rotating helical screen that can be illuminated passively by a laser[611] or actively by a photodiode array embedded in the screen.[612] It is also possible to use volumetric holographic techniques.[613] The most complicated concept we have encountered uses an optical three-dimensional exponential Radon transform and tries to optically reconstruct the 3D image in the display volume.[614]

2.3 DISCUSSION

In 1987, Vannier wrote, "Despite its limitations, three-dimensional imaging is here to stay."[615] Today we know that he was right. When reviewing the references of this chapter, note the tremendous amount of literature that has been published since 1993, as compared to all previous years. In 1991, in the previous edition of this book, Hemmy presented his views on future directions in 3D imaging.[616] We know that the majority of items on his wants list have been accomplished in research environments but have not been able to penetrate to routine clinical practice except for a relatively small number of academic centers. The only item that still has not been solved is the automation of the time-consuming soft-tissue segmentation. Probably, this is the main reason for 3D imaging not becoming a routine daily tool. The combination of investment of specialist time in slice-by-slice manual editing with limited possibilities for reimbursement of these efforts is just not feasible. Another limiting factor is the lack of standardization of image formats and data archival media, which impairs the exchange of image data between radiologist and physician, but also between institutions. The new DICOM format[617] is now being made available as the new standard for the exchange of medical images, but it still lacks a format for object descriptions that result from segmentation. As a result, there are two proposals for such a data format[618,619] that also can be applied to manufacturing of physical models and the printing of autostereographic hard copies. At the same time, however, the Internet is developing as a potential network to exchange such image data in the future, but it makes use of different graphics standards. This means another data conversion.

The consequence of this is that most companies that were dedicated to 3D imaging[620] have either moved to other businesses or simply disappeared. This means that 3D imaging can thrive only if a good infrastructure for image data communication is established in conjunction with tools that facilitate segmentation. Some years ago, there was the feeling that segmentation might not be necessary at all, and in some cases this may still be true if the structure of interest inherently has a high contrast. However, many new applications have been added that do require segmentation, such as physical models, surgical simulation, surgical navigation, and VR-based surgical training.[621,622] We hope that the interest in these new applications will fuel the efforts to solve the segmentation problem. Many of these new applications still sound futuristic but, just as Hemmy's predictions in 1991 are possible today, planning a case using 3D imaging and physical multicolor models, including rubber-like soft tissues, training on that case using VR surgical simulation tools on the "visible human" data warped to the individual patient's morphology, including haptic feedback, followed by telesurgery using augmented reality and intra-operative updates will probably be used in academic centers in another decade. Prerequisites for such a development are knowledge-based[623,624] or atlas-based[177] segmentation, faster medical imaging using thinner slices, faster computer architectures,[625] more sophisticated and more intelligent algorithms[626] (both for segmentation[627] as well as for image rendering[628] and interactive manipulation), user interfaces for the less computer-literate physician, and faster data networks including standards for archival and transmission using feature-based indexing.[629] Only then can we expect to quickly copy the patient's morphology in the form of a volumetric data set that can be rapidly analyzed offline and the results communicated to other physicians using networks, as well as being used to plan and perform complicated treatment procedures.

With the current cost-containment drive, however, it is also possible that this process of advancing technologies is being slowed down, in spite of the proven value of 3D imaging.[547] This means that technology assessment must provide proof of the positive benefit-to-cost balance of 3D imaging and its derivatives and that more cost-effective alternatives are used, when appropriate, such as, for example, a facial moulage instead of a computer-generated facial mask.[630] It may also mean a shift in using less invasive and more cost-effective imaging modalities such as ultrasound.[631] Another cost-saving trend is that simple 3D imaging and image analysis will be carried out on PC-based systems.[632] This may also mean that workstations will have a performance that is now reserved for the so-called "graphics reality engines" without becoming more expensive. We also hope that the sophisticated graphics capabilities that are currently applied to the entertainment industry to create motion picture animations such as *Jurassic Park*[633] and *Toy Story*[634] will become available for 3D medical imaging, but at much more moderate prices.

It remains difficult to predict future developments in medical 3D imaging, and this chapter, therefore, will only be a snapshot in time. But in due time, we will learn if, and how, our expectations take form and become daily routine to the generations of radiologists, physicians, and computer scientists of generations yet to come.

ACKNOWLEDGMENTS

The author is grateful to Drs. A.R.M. Wittkampf (Figures 2.1, 2.10, 2.24, and 2.25), T.F.J.M.C. Specken (Figure 2.2), L. Koornneef (Figure 2.3), R. Koole (Figures 2.4 and 2.22), P.F.G.M. Van Waes (Figures 2.6, 2.17, and 2.18), I. Van Riet (Figure 2.8), G.H. Slot (Figure 2.9), I. Jacobson (Figure 2.11), L.M.P. Ramos (Figure 2.12), B.K. Velthuis (Figure 2.15), R. Balm (Figure 2.16), W.P.Th.M. Mali (Figure 2.26), F.R. Carls (Figure 2.28), and H.E. Hulshoff-Pol (Figure 2.29) for contributing the case material used in the figures. The help in searching the literature by Inger-Janine Mesman and Hok Tjiang Kwee and the support by Philips Medical Systems are greatly acknowledged.

REFERENCES

1. Udupa, J.K. and G.T. Herman, eds. *3D imaging in medicine* (Boca Raton, FL: CRC Press, 1991), pp. 1–347.
2. Kalender, W., W. Seissler, and P. Vock. Single-breath-hold spiral volumetric CT by continuous patient translation and scanner rotation, *Radiology* 173(P):414 (1989).
3. Kalender, W.A., W. Seissler, E. Klotz, and P. Vock. Spiral volumetric CT with single-breath-hold technique, continuous transport, and continuous scanner rotation, *Radiology* 176:181–183 (1990).

4. Wilting, J. and F.W. Zonneveld. Computed tomographic angiography. In: Lanzer, P., ed. *Technique of spiral CT* (Berlin, Germany: Springer-Verlag, 1996), in press.
5. Kalender, W.A. Computed tomographic angiography. In: Udupa, J.K. and G.T. Herman, eds. *3-D imaging in medicine* (2nd ed.) (Boca Raton, FL: CRC Press, 2000).
6. Christiansen, N. Differences between electron beam tomography and conventional CT, *Electromedica* 63:63 (1995).
7. Abduljalil, A.M., A.H. Aletras, and P.-M.L. Robitaille. 3D echoplanar imaging: application to the human head, *Magn. Reson. Med.* 34:144–148 (1995).
8. Napel, S., M.P. Marks, G.D. Rubin, M.D. Drake, C.H. McDonnell, S.M. Song, et al. CT angiography with spiral CT and maximum intensity projection, *Radiology* 185:607–610 (1992).
9. Sohn, Ch. and G. Bastert. *Die dreidimensionale Ultraschall-diagnostik* (Berlin, Germany: Springer-Verlag, 1994), pp. 1–105.
10. Rankin, N., A. Fenster, D.B. Downey, P.L. Munk, M.F. Levin, and A.D. Vellet. Three-dimensional sonographic reconstruction: techniques and diagnostic applications, *AJR* 161:695–702 (1993).
11. Tiede, U., K.-H. Höhne, M. Bomans, A. Pommert, M. Riemer, and G. Wiebecke. Surface rendering: investigation of medical 3D-rendering algorithms. *IEEE Comput. Graph. Appl.* 10(3):41–53 (1990).
12. Huijsmans, D.P. and G.J. Jense. Recent advances in 3D display, *Adv. Electr. Electron Phys.* 85:77–229 (1993).
13. Drebin, R.A., D. Magid, D.D. Robertson, and E.K. Fishman. Fidelity of three-dimensional CT imaging for detecting fracture gaps, *J. Comput. Assist. Tomogr.* 13:487–489 (1989).
14. Rusinek, H., N.S. Karp, and C.B. Cutting. A comparison of two approaches to three-dimensional imaging of craniofacial anomalies, *J. Digital Imaging* 3:81–88 (1990).
15. Udupa, J.K., H.M. Hung, and K.S. Chuang. Surface and volume rendering in three-dimensional imaging: a comparison, *J. Digital Imaging* 4:159–168 (1991).
16. Rusinek, H., M.E. Noz, G.Q. Maguire Jr., C. Cutting, B. Haddad, A. Kalvin, and D. Dean. Quantitative and qualitative comparison of volumetric and surface rendering techniques, *IEEE Eng. Med. Biol.* 90:1531–1534 (1991).
17. Rubin, G.D., C.F. Baulieu, V. Argiro, H. Ringl, A.M. Norbash, J.F. Feller, et al. Perspective volume rendering of CT and MR images: applications for endoscopic imaging, *Radiology* 199:321–330 (1996).
18. Udupa, J.K. and D. Odhner. Shell rendering. *IEEE Comput. Graph. Appl.* 13(6):58–67 (1993).
19. Zonneveld, F.W., S. Lobregt, J.C. Van der Meulen, and J.M. Vaandrager. Three-dimensional imaging in craniofacial surgery, *World J. Surg.* 13:328–342 (1989).
20. Mankovich, N.J., D. Samson, W. Pratt, D. Lew, and J. Beumer III. Surgical planning using three-dimensional imaging and computer modeling, *Otolaryngol. Clin. N. Am.* 27:875–889 (1994).
21. Altobelli, D.E., R. Kikinis, J.B. Mulliken, H. Cline, W. Lorensen, and F. Jolesz. Computer-assisted three-dimensional planning in craniofacial surgery, *Plast. Reconstr. Surg.* 92:576–585 (1993).
22. Fishman E.K., D. Magid, D.R. Ney, E.L. Chaney et al. Three-dimensional imaging, *Radiology* 181:321–337 (1991).
23. Zonneveld, F.W. and K. Fukuta. A decade of clinical three-dimensional imaging: a review. Part 2. Clinical applications, *Invest. Radiol.* 29:574–589 (1994).
24. Van Leeuwen, M.S., L.J. Polman, J. Noordzij, and B. Velthuis. Computed tomographic angiography. In: Lanzer, P. and J. Rösch, eds. *Vascular diagnostics* (Berlin, Germany: Springer-Verlag, 1994), pp. 443–462.
25. Ritman, E.L. Rationale for, and recent progress in, 3D reconstruction of the heart and lungs, *Comput. Med. Imaging Graph.* 17:263–271 (1993).
26. Schubert, S., K.H. Höhne, A. Pommert, M. Riemer, T. Schiemann, U. Tiede, and W. Lierse. A new method for practicing exploration, dissection, and simulation with a complete computerized three-dimensional model of the brain and skull, *Acta Anat.* 150:69–74 (1994).
27. Richter, E., H. Krämer, W. Lierse, R. Maas, and K.H. Höhne. Visualization of neonatal anatomy and pathology with a new computerized three-dimensional model as a basis for teaching, diagnosis and therapy, *Acta Anat.* 150:75–79 (1994).
28. Yoshihara, T., M. Morita, and T. Ishii. Ultrastructure and three-dimensional imaging of epimyoepithelial islands in benign lymphoepithelial lesions, *Eur. Arch. Oto-Rhino-Larynchol.* 252:106–111 (1995).

29. Loew, L.M., R.A. Tuft, W. Carrington, and F.S. Fay. Imaging in five dimensions: time-dependent membrane potentials in individual mitochondria, *Biophys. J.* 65: 2396–2407 (1993).
30. Stevens, J.K., L.R. Mills, and J.E. Trogadis, eds. *Three-dimensional confocal microscopy: volume investigation of biological specimens* (San Diego, CA: Academic Press, 1994), pp. 1–507.
31. Stiller, M.J., J. Driller, J.L. Shupack, C.G. Gropper, et al. Three-dimensional imaging for diagnostic ultrasound in dermatology, *J. Am. Acad. Dermatol.* 29:171–175 (1993).
32. Marx, M. and S.H. D'Auria. Three-dimensional CT reconstructions of an ancient human Egyptian mummy, *AJR* 150:147–149 (1988).
33. Pickering, R.B., D.J. Conces Jr., E.M. Braunstein, and F. Yurco. Three-dimensional computed tomography of the mummy Wenuhotep, *Am. J. Phys. Anthropol.* 83:49–55 (1990).
34. Hughes, S.W., A. Sofat, D. Whitaker, C. Baldock, R. Davis, W. Wong, et al. 3D CT reconstruction of an Egyptian mummy. In: *Proc. CAR'93* (Berlin, Germany: Springer-Verlag, 1993), pp. 395–400.
35. Zonneveld, F.W., C.F. Spoor, and J. Wind. The use of CT in the study of internal morphology of hominid fossils, *Medicamundi* 34:117–128 (1990).
36. Zollikofer, Ch.P.E., M.S. Ponce de León, R.D. Martin, and P. Stucki. Neanderthal computer skulls, *Nature* 375:283–285 (1995).
37. Zur Nedden, D., R. Knapp, K. Wicke, W. Judmaier, W.A. Murphy Jr., H. Seidler, and W. Platzer. Skull of a 5,300-year-old mummy: reproduction and investigation with CT-guided stereolithography, *Radiology* 193:269–272 (1994).
38. Kauczor, H.-U., T. Riepert, B. Wolcke, G. Lasczkowski, and P. Mildenberger. Fatal venous air embolism: proof and volumetry by helical CT, *Eur. J. Radiol.* 21:155–157 (1995).
39. Zonneveld, F.W. A decade of clinical three-dimensional imaging: a review. Part III. Image analysis and interaction, display options, and physical models, *Invest. Radiol.* 29:716–725 (1994).
40. Hemmy, D.C., F.W. Zonneveld, S. Lobregt, and K. Fukuta. A decade of clinical three-dimensional imaging: a review. Part I. Historical development, *Invest. Radiol.* 29:489–496 (1994).
41. David, D.J., D.C. Hemmy, and R.D. Cooter. *Craniofacial deformities. Atlas of three-dimensional reconstruction from computed tomography* (New York, NY: Springer-Verlag, 1990), pp. 1–147.
42. Marsh, J.L. and M.W. Vannier. Three-dimensional surface imaging from CT scans for the study of craniofacial dysmorphology, *J. Craniofacial Genet. Dev. Biol.* 9:61–75 (1989).
43. Lebouq, N., P. Montoya, Y. Martinez, and Ph. Castan. Value of 3D imaging or the study of craniofacial malformations in children, *J. Neuroradiol.* 18:225–239 (1991).
44. Ray, C.E. Jr., M.F. Mafee, M. Friedman, and C.N. Tahmoressi. Applications of three-dimensional imaging in head and neck pathology, *Radiol. Clin. N. Am.* 31:181–194 (1993).
45. Carls, F.R., B. Schuknecht, and H.F. Sailer. Value of three-dimensional computed tomography in craniomaxillofacial surgery, *J. Craniofacial. Surg.* 5:282–288 (1994).
46. Hall, R.K. The role of CT, MRI and 3D imaging in the diagnosis of temporomandibular joint and other orofacial disorders in children, *Aust. Orthodont. J.* 13:86–94 (1994).
47. Zonneveld, F.W., J.C. Van der Meulen, L. Koornneef, J.M. Vaandrager, A.R.M. Wittkampf, and B. Hillen. Three-dimensional CT imaging of the orbit. In: Van der Meulen, J.C. and J. Gruss, eds. *A color atlas and text of ocular plastic surgery* (London: Mosby-Wolf, 1996), pp. 9–30.
48. Zwicker, C., M. Langer, F. Astinet, D. Köhler, et al. Wertigkeit der 3D-CT in der kieferchirurgischen Diagnostik und Therapieplanung, *Fortschr. Röntgenstr.* 152:393–397 (1990).
49. Zinreich, S.J. and M.A. Shermak. Radiologic analysis and visualization of craniofacial anomalies. In: Dufresne, C.R., B.S. Carson, and S.J. Zinreich, eds. *Complex craniofacial problems. A guide to analysis and treatment* (New York, NY: Churchill Livingstone, 1992), pp. 75–95.
50. Parisi, M., H.M. Mehdizadeh, J.C. Hunter, and I.J. Finch. Evaluation of craniosynostosis with three-dimensional CT imaging, *J. Comput. Assist. Tomogr.* 13:1006–1012 (1989).
51. Vannier, M.W., T.K. Pilgram, J.L. Marsh, B.B. Kraemer, S.C. Rayne, M.H. Gado, et al. Craniosynostosis: diagnostic imaging with three-dimensional CT presentation, *Am. J. Neuroradiol.* 15:1861–1869 (1994).
52. Massoud, T., P. Anslow, and A. Molyneux. Three-dimensional computed tomography of complex craniofacial fractures, *Eur. J. Radiol.* 13:233–234 (1991).
53. Brüning, R., R. Quade, V. Keppler, and M. Reiser. 3D-CT-Rekonstruktion bei Frakturen des Schädelbasis und des Gesichtsschädels, *Fortschr. Röntgenstr.* 160:113–117 (1994).

54. Buitrago-Téllez, C.H., R. Wächter, F. Ferstl, P. Stoll, et al. 3-D-CT zur Befunddemonstration bei komplexen Gesichtsschädelverletzungen, *Fortschr. Röntgenstr.* 160:106–112 (1994).
55. Fox, L.A., M.W. Vannier, and R.G. Evens. Three-dimensional CT diagnosis of maxillofacial trauma, *N. Engl. J. Med.* 329:102 (1993).
56. Zonneveld, F.W. The role of medical imaging in the management and diagnostic assessment of trauma, *Medicamundi* 40:134–150 (1995).
57. Friedman, M., M. Mafee, C. Ray, and T.K. Venkatesan. Three-dimensional imaging for evaluation of head and neck tumors, *Arch. Otolaryngol. Head Neck Surg.* 119:601–607 (1993).
58. Marsh, J.L., S.E. Celin, M.V. Vannier, and M. Gado. The skeletal anatomy of mandibulofacial dysostosis (Treacher Collins Syndrome), *Plast. Reconstr. Surg.* 78:460–468 (1986).
59. Marsh, J.L., D. Baca, and M.W. Vannier. Facial musculoskeletal asymmetry in hemifacial microsomia, *Cleft Palate J.* 26:292–302 (1989).
60. Zonneveld, F.W. 3D imaging of the skull base, *Rev. Neuroradiol.* 7:499–502 (1994).
61. Howard, J.D., A.D. Elster, and J.S. May. Temporal bone: three-dimensional CT. Part I. Normal anatomy, techniques, and limitations, *Radiology* 177:421–425 (1990).
62. Howard, J.D., A.D. Elster, and J.S. May. Temporal bone: three-dimensional CT. Part II. Pathologic alterations, *Radiology* 177:427–430 (1990).
63. LaRouere, M.J., J.K. Niparko, S.S. Gebarski, and J.L. Kemink. Three-dimensional x-ray computed tomography of the temporal bone as an aid to surgical planning, *Otolaryngol Head Neck Surg.* 103:740–747 (1990).
64. Tanaka, A., T. Tanaka, Y. Irie, S. Yoshinaga, and M. Tomonaga. Elevation of the petrous bone caused by hyperplasia of the occipital bone presenting as hemifacial spasm: diagnostic values of magnetic resonance imaging and three-dimensional computed tomographic images in a bony anomaly, *Neurosurgery.* 27:1004–1009 (1990).
65. Zonneveld, F.W., J.M. Vaandrager, M.F. Noorman van der Dussen, and J.C. Van der Meulen. Value of disarticulation of the mandible in 3D imaging. In: Lemke, H.U., M.L. Rhodes, C.C. Jaffe, and R. Felix., eds. *Computer assisted radiology. Proc CAR'89* (Berlin, Germany: Springer-Verlag, 1989), pp. 372–377.
66. Tanaka, T., F. Toyofuku, and S. Kanda. Zur drei-dimensionalen CT-Darstellung des Kiefer- und Gesichtsbereichs, *Electromedica* 56:30–37 (1988).
67. Jahrsdoerfer, R.A., E.T. Garcia, J.W. Yeakley, et al. Surface contour three-dimensional imaging in congenitalaural atresia, *Arch. Otolaryngol. Head Neck Surg.* 119:95–99 (1993).
68. Kursunoglu, S., P. Kaplan, D. Resnick, and D.J. Sartorius. Three-dimensional computed tomographic analysis of the normal temporomandibular joint, *J. Oral Maxillofac. Surg.* 44:257–259 (1986).
69. Zonneveld, F.W., J.C. Van der Meulen, L. Koornneef, J.M. Vaandrager, A.R.M. Wittkampf, and B. Hillen. Three-dimensional CT imaging of the orbit. In: Van der Meulen, J.C. and J.S. Gruss, eds. *Color atlas and text of ocular plastic surgery* (London: Mosby-Wolfe, 1996), pp. 9–30.
70. Hamamoto, S., Y. Morita, T. Sato, and T. Noikura. Three-dimensional imaging of subcondylar fractures of the mandible with spiral CT, *Oral Radiol.* 9(2):43–45 (1993).
71. Seldon, H.L. Three-dimensional reconstruction of temporal bone from computed tomographic scans on a personal computer, *Arch. Otolaryngol. Head Neck Surg.* 117:1158–1161 (1991).
72. Yamamoto, E., C. Mizukami, M. Isono, M. Ohmura, and Y. Hyrono. Observation of the external aperture of the vestibular aqueduct using three-dimensional surface reconstruction imaging, *Laryngoscope* 101:480–483 (1991).
73. Hermans, R., G. Marchal, L. Feenstra, and A.L. Baert. Spiral CT of the temporal bone: value of image reconstruction at submillimetric table increments, *Neuroradiol.* 37:150–154 (1995).
74. Ohashi, M. and S. Miyashita. Experience with the helical scan method using the Xpress in ENT examinations, *Toshiba Med. Rev.* 44:30–37 (1993).
75. Skinner, M.W., D.R. Ketten, M.W. Vannier, G.A. Gates, R.L. Yoffie, and W.A. Kalender. Dtermination of the position of nucleus cochlear implant electrodes in the inner ear, *Am. J. Otol.* 15:644–651 (1994).
76. Hillen, B., ed. Paranasal sinuses and anterior skull base (CDi and CD-ROM). In: Hillen, B., ed. *Interactive anatomy, Vol. 1-I* (Amsterdam, the Netherlands: Elsevier, 1993).
77. Kahrilas, P.J., S. Lin, J. Chen, and J.A. Logemann. Three-dimensional modeling of the oropharynx during swallowing, *Radiology* 194:575–579 (1995).

78. Lofchy, N.M., J.K. Stevens, and D.H. Brown. Three-dimensional imaging of the parapharyngeal space, *Arch. Otolaryngol. Head Neck Surg.* 120:333–336 (1994).
79. Zinreich, S.J., D.E. Mattox, D.W. Kennedy, M.E. Johns, J.C. Price, M.J. Holliday, et al. 3-D CT for cranial facial and laryngeal surgery, *Laryngoscope* 98:1212–1219 (1988).
80. Meglin, A.J., J.F. Biedlingmaier, and S.E. Mirvis. Three-dimensional computerized tomography in the evaluation of laryngeal injury. *Laryngoscope* 101:202–207 (1991).
81. Arnould, V., P. Troufleau, J. Stines, and D. Regent. Tumeurs du pharyngo-larynx: apport de la tomodensitometrie en acquisition volumique avec reconstructions tri-dimensionelles, *J. Radiol.* 76:191–199 (1995).
82. Grevers, G., T. Vogl, C. Wilimzig, and G. Laub. Zur Aussagefähigkeit der 3 D-KST-Rekonstruktion am Beispiel eines ausgedehnten Parotisadenoms, *Laryngorhinootologie* 69:389–393 (1990).
83. Grevers, G., J. Assal, T. Vogl, and C. Wilimzig. Three-dimensional magnetic resonance imaging in skull base lesions, *Am. J. Otolaryngol.* 12:139–145 (1991).
84. Vogl, T., C. Wilimzig, J. Assal, G. Grevers, and J. Lissner. 3D MR imaging with Gd-DTPA in head and neck lesions, *Eur. Radiol.* 1:151–157 (1991).
85. Tanioka, H., T. Shirakawa, T. Machida, and Y. Sasaki. Three-dimensional reconstructed MR imaging of the inner ear, *Radiology* 178:141–144 (1991).
86. Krebs, M., L.M. Gallo, R.L. Airoldi, D. Meier, P. Boesiger, and S. Palla. Three-dimensional animation of the temporomandibular joint, *Technol. Health Care* 2(3):193–207 (1994).
87. Hell, B. 3D sonography. *Int. J. Oral Maxillofacial Surg.* 24:84–87 (1995).
88. Silverman, R.H., M.J. Rondeau, F.L. Lizzi, and D.J. Coleman. Three-dimensional high-frequency ultrasonic parameter imaging of anterior segment pathology. *Ophthalmology* 102:837–843 (1995).
89. Addleman, D. and L. Addleman. Rapid 3D digitizing, *Comput. Graph. World* 8(11):41–44 (1985).
90. Arridge, S., J.P. Moss, A.D. Linney, and D.R. James. Three dimensional digitization of the face and skull, *J. Maxillofacial Surg.* 13:136–143 (1985).
91. Uesugi, M. Three-dimensional curved shape measuring system using image encoder, *J. Robotics Megatronics* 3:190–195 (1991).
92. Young, S.T., S.W. Yip, H.C. Cheng, and D.B. Shieh. Three-dimensional surface digitizer for facial contour capture, *IEEE Eng. Med. Biol.* 13:125–128 (1994).
93. Rasse, M., G. Forkert, and P. Waldhäusl. Stereo-photogrammetry of facial soft tissue, *Int. J. Oral Maxillofacial Surg.* 20:163–166 (1992).
94. Savara, B.S., S.H. Miller, R.J. Demuth, and H.K. Kawamoto. Biostereographics and computer graphics for patients with craniofacial malformations: diagnosis and treatment planning, *Plast. Reconstr. Surg.* 75:495–501 (1985).
95. Deacon, A.T., A.G. Anthony, S.N. Bhatia, and J.-P. Muller. Evaluation of a CCD-based facial measurement system, *Med. Inform.* 16:213–228 (1991).
96. Hayashi, A. and Y. Maruyama. Three dimensional measurement of body surface (abstr.), *Comput. Aided Surg.* 1:55 (1994).
97. Kosaka, M. and H. Kamiishi. Importance of the active positioning for the accurate facial contourmetry with laser light scanner. *Proc. CAR'95* (Berlin, Germany: Springer-Verlag, 1995), pp. 1317–1318.
98. Totty, W.G. and M.W. Vannier. Complex musculo-skeletal anatomy: analysis using three-dimensional surface reconstruction, *Radiology* 150:173–177 (1984).
99. Woolson, S.T., L.L. Fellingham, P. Dev, and A. Vassiliadis. Three dimensional image of bone from analysis of computed tomography data, *Orthopedics* 8:1269–1273 (1985).
100. Magid, D. Computed tomographic imaging of the musculoskeletal system. Current status, *Radiol. Clin. N. Am.* 32:255–274 (1994).
101. Fishman, E.K., R. Drebin, D. Magid, W.W. Scott Jr., D.R. Ney, A.F. Brooker Jr., et al. Volumetric rendering techniques: applications for three-dimensional imaging of the hip, *Radiology* 163:737–738.
102. Scott, W.W. Jr., E.K. Fishman, and D. Magid. Acetabular fractures: optimal imaging, *Radiology* 165:537–539 (1987).
103. Fishman, E.K., D. Magid, D.R. Ney, R.A. Drebin, and J.E. Kuhlman. Three-dimensional imaging and display of musculoskeletal anatomy, *J. Comput. Assist. Tomogr.* 12:465–467 (1988).
104. Fishman, E.K., D. Magid, R.A. Drebin, A.F. Brooker Jr., W.W. Scott Jr., and L.H. Riley Jr. Advanced three-dimensional evaluation of acetabular trauma: volumetric image processing, *J. Trauma* 29:214–218 (1989).

105. Magid, D., E.K. Fishman, D.R. Ney, J.E. Kuhlman, and K.M. Frantz. Acetabular and pelvic fractures in the pediatric patient: value of two- and three-dimensional imaging, *J. Pediatr. Orthoped.* 12:621–625 (1992).
106. Udupa, J.K. and S. Samarasekera. Fuzzy connectedness and object definition: theory, algorithms, and applications in image segmentation. *Graph. Models Image Processing* 58:246–261 (1996).
107. Udupa, J.K. and R.J. Gonçalves. Imaging transforms for visualizing surfaces and volumes. *J. Digital Imaging* 6:213–236 (1993).
108. Lobregt, S. and M.A. Viergever. A discrete dynamic contour model. *IEEE Trans. Med. Imaging* 14:12–24 (1995).
109. Tanyü, M.O., P. Vinée, and B. Wimmer. Value of 3D imaging in fractured os calcis, *Comput. Med. Imaging Graph.* 18:137–143 (1994).
110. Ivancevich, S.M., K.A. Buckwalter, E.M. Braunstein, and A.D. Mih. Volumetric data key to wrist evaluation, *Diagn. Imaging* 17(suppl.):CT24–CT27 (Nov. 1995).
111. Ney, D.R. and E.K. Fishman. Editing tools for 3D medical imaging, *IEEE Comput. Graph. Appl.* 11(6):63–71 (1991).
112. Fishman, E.K., D. Magid, D.R. Ney, and J.E. Kuhlman. Three-dimensional imaging: orthopedic applications. In: Udupa, J.K. and G.T. Herman, eds. *3-D imaging in medicine* (Boca Raton, FL: CRC Press, 1991), pp. 223–254.
113. Vannier, M.W., C.F. Hildebolt, L.A. Gilula, T.K. Pilgram, F. Mann, B.S. Monsees et al. Calcaneal and pelvic fractures: diagnostic evaluation by three-dimensional computed tomography scans, *J. Digital Imaging* 4:143–152 (1991).
114. Ney, D.R., E.K. Fishman, D. Magid, and R.A. Drebin. Volumetric rendering of computed tomography data: principles and techniques, *IEEE Comput. Graph. Appl.* 10(3):24–32 (1990).
115. Wilting, J.E. and F.W. Zonneveld. Computed tomographic angiography. In: Lanzer, P. and M. Lipton, eds. *Diagnostics of vascular diseases* (Berlin, Germany: Springer-Verlag, 1996), pp. 135–153.
116. Kalender, W.A. Thin-section three-dimensional spiral CT: is isotropic imaging possible?, *Radiology* 197:578–580 (1995).
117. Zonneveld, F.W. The role of medical imaging in the management and diagnostic assessment of trauma, *Medicamundi* 40:134–150 (1995).
118. Hurwitz, D.J., G. Stofman, and H. Curtin. Three-dimensional imaging of Poland's syndrome, *Plast. Reconstr. Surg.* 94:719–723 (1994).
119. Sartoris, D.J. 3D display of CT data: new aid to preop surgical planning, *Diagn. Imaging* 8(5):74–80 (1986).
120. Pate, D., D. Resnick, M. Andre, D.J. Sartoris, S. Kursunoglu, D. Bielecki, et al. Perspective: three-dimensional imaging of the musculoskeletal system, *AJR* 147:545–551 (1986).
121. Kilcoyne, R.F. and L.A. Mack. Computed tomography of spinal fractures, *Appl. Radiol.* 16(3):40–54 (1987).
122. Lang, Ph., H.K. Genant, N. Chafetz, P. Steiger, and J.M. Morris. Three-dimensional computed tomography and multiplanar reformations in the assessment of pseudarthrosis in posterior lumbar fusion patients, *Spine* 13:69–75 (1988).
123. Zinreich, S.J., D.M. Long, R. Davis, C.B. Quinn, P.C. McAfee, and H. Wang. Three-dimensional CT imaging in postsurgical "failed back" syndrome, *J. Comput. Assist. Tomogr.* 14:574–580 (1990).
124. Böhmer, G., M. Roesgen, and G. Hierholzer. Dreidimensionale Computertomographie in der Unfallchirurgie, *Aktuelle Traumatol.* 22:47–56 (1992)
125. Martinez, C.R., T.G. DiPasquale, D.L. Helfet, A.W. Graham, R.W. Sanders, and L.D. Ray. Evaluation of acetabular fractures with two- and three-dimensional CT, *Radio-Graphics* 12:227–242 (1992).
126. Seebode, Ch., R. Shubert, A. Pommert, M. Riemer, Th. Schiemann, U. Tiede, et al. An interactive 3D-atlas of acetabular fractures, *Proc. CAR'93* (Berlin, Germany: Springer-Verlag, 1993), pp. 716–721.
127. Lafferty, C.M., D.J. Sartoris, R.Tyson, D. Resnick, S. Kursunoglu, D. Pate, et al. Acetabular alterations in untreated congenital dysplasia of the hip: computed tomography with multiplanar re-formation and three-dimensional analysis, *J. Comput. Assist. Tomogr.* 10:84–91 (1986).
128. Sutherland, C.J., S.J. Bresina, and D.E. Gayou. Use of general purpose mechanical computer assisted engineering software in orthopaedic surgical planning: advantages and limitations, *Comput. Med. Imaging Graph.* 18:435–442 (1994).

129. Rüegsegger, P., B. Münch, and M. Felder. Early detection of osteoarthritis by 3D computed tomography, *Technol. Health Care* 1:53–66 (1993).
130. Billet, F.P.J., W.G.H. Schmitt, B. Gay, and J. Lang. Conventional CT and 3D of the normal and fractured os calcis: an investigation procedure and a classification of 21 calcaneal fractures. In: Fuchs, W.A., ed. *Advances in CT* (Berlin, Germany: Springer-Verlag, 1990), pp. 154–171.
131. Allon, S.M. and D.C. Mears. Three dimensional analysis of calcaneal fractures, *Foot Ankle* 11:254–263 (1991).
132. Kirtland, S., D. Resnick, D.J. Sartoris, D. Pate, and G. Greenway. Chronic unreduced dislocations of the glenohumeral joint: imaging strategy and pathologic correlation, *J. Trauma* 28:1622–1631 (1988).
133. Müller, R., T. Hildebrand, and P. Rüegsegger. Non-invasive bone biopsy: a new method to analyse and display the three-dimensional structure of trabecular bone, *Phys. Med. Biol.* 39:145–164 (1994).
134. Niitsu, M. Three-dimensional imaging of the knee joint; diagnostic value for meniscal tears, *Nihonihoukaishi* 51:1201–1209 (1991).
135. Disler, D.G., S.V. Kattapuram, F.S. Chew, D.I. Rosenthal, and D. Patel. Meniscal tears of the knee: preliminary comparison of three-dimensional MR reconstruction with two-dimensional MR imaging and arthroscopy, *AJR* 160:343–345 (1993).
136. Pilch, L., C. Stewart, D. Gordon, R. Inman, K. Parsons, I. Pataki, et al. Assessment of cartilage volume in the femorotibial joint with magnetic resonance imaging and 3D computer reconstruction, *J. Rheumatol.* 21:2307–2319 (1994).
137. Lang, Ph., P. Steiger, H.K. Genant, N. Chafetz, T. Lindquist, S. Skinner, and S. Moore. Three-dimensional CT and MR imaging in congenital dislocation of the hip: clinical and technical considerations, *J. Comput. Assist. Tomogr.* 12:459–464 (1988).
138. Vahlensieck, M., Ph. Lang, W.P. Chan, S. Grampp, and H.K. Genant. Three-dimensional reconstruction. Part II: Optimisation of segmentation and rendering of MRI, *Eur. Radiol.* 2:508–510 (1992).
139. Bellon, R.J. and Horwitz, S.M. Three-dimensional computed tomography studies of the tendons of the foot and ankle, *J. Digital Imaging* 5:46–50 (1992).
140. Udupa, J.K., B.E. Hirsch, S. Samarasekera, and R.J. Goncalves. Joint kinematics via three-dimensional MR imaging, *SPIE Proc.* 1808:664–670 (1992).
141. Vahlensieck, M., Ph. Lang, W.P. Chan, S. Grampp, and H.K. Genant. Three-dimensional reconstruction. Part I: Applications and techniques, *Eur. Radiol.* 2:503–507 (1992).
142. Lang, Ph., H.K. Genant, P. Steiger, D.W. Stoller, and A.F. Heuck. 3-D reformatting asserts clinical potential in MRI. *Diagn. Imaging* 11(5):80–84 (1989).
143. Brody, G.A. and D.W. Stoller. The wrist and hand. In: Stoller, D.W., ed. *Magnetic resonance imaging in orthopaedics and sports medicine* (Philadelphia, PA: J.B. Lippincott, 1992) pp. 683–806.
144. Chung, H.-W., F.W. Wehrli, J.L. Williams, and S.L. Wehrli. Three-dimensional nuclear magnetic resonance microimaging of trabecular bone, *J. Bone Mineral Res.* 10:1452–1461 (1995).
145. Sohn, Ch., G.P. Lenz, and M. Ties. Die 3dimensionale Ultrashalldarstellung der Säuglingshüfte, *Ultraschall Med.* 11:302–305 (1990).
146. Böhm, K. and F.U. Niethard. Dreidimensionale Ultra-schalldarstellung der Säuglingshüfte, *Bildgebung* 61:126–129 (1994).
147. Wood, A.K.W., C.M. Sehgal, and V.B. Reef. Three-dimensional sonographic imaging of the equine superficial digital flexor tendon, *Am. J. Vet. Res.* 55:1505–1508 (1994).
148. Ali, Q.M., B. Dietrich, and H. Becker. Patterns of skull base fracture: a three-dimensional computed tomographic study, *Neuroradiology.* 36:622–624 (1994).
149. Klein, H.M., H. Bertalanffy, L. Mayfrank, A. Thron, R.W. Günther, and J.M. Gilsbach. Three-dimensional spiral CT for neurosurgical planning, *Neuroradiology* 36:435–439 (1994).
150. Takakura, K. Three-dimensional imaging diagnosis for cranial base lesions, *J. Craniofacial Surg.* 6:27–31 (1995).
151. Atzor, K.-R., H. Stoltz, H.-U. Kauczor, V. Urban, J. Tintera, A. Perneczky, et al. 3D-high resolution imaging of tumors and aneurysms at the cranial base — comparison of CT and MR, *Comput. Biol. Med.* 25:277–281 (1995).
152. Godard, J., G. Jacquet, J.F. Bonneville, Y.S. Tan, J. Guyot, and A. Czorny. Torticolis et sub-luxation rotatoire C1-C2, *J. Neuroradiol.* 21:223–227 (1994).
153. Dannenmaier, B. and W. Grodd. Anwendungsmöglichkeiten der dreidimensionalen Computertomographie an der Wirbelsäule, *Neurochirurgia* 31:58–62 (1988).

154. Salvolini, U., E.A. Cabanis, M.T. Iba-Zizen, M. De Nicola, and D.C. Hemmy. Apport diagnostique de la reconstruction tridimensionelle en scanner RX: coupes et surfaces de l'anatomie céphalique, *Ann. Chir. Plast. Esthét.* 29:339–357 (1984).
155. Vannier, M.W., M.H. Gado, and J.L. Marsh. Three-dimensional display of intracranial soft-tissue structures, *AJNR* 4:520–521 (1983).
156. Gillespie, J.E. and I. Isherwood. Three-dimensional anatomical images from computed tomographic scans, *Br. J. Radiol.* 59:289–292 (1986).
157. Gillespie, J.E., J.E. Adams, and I. Isherwood. Three-dimensional computed tomographic reformations of sellar and parasellar lesions. *Neuroradiology* 29:30–35 (1987).
158. Gholkar, A. and I. Isherwood. Three-dimensional computed tomographic reformations of intracranial vascular lesions, *Br. J. Radiol.* 61:258–261 (1988).
159. Virapongse, C., A. Gmitro, and M. Sarwar. The spine in 3D. Computed tomographic reformation from 2D axial sections, *Spine* 11:513–520 (1986).
160. Virapongse, C., M. Shapiro, A. Gmitro, and M. Sarwar. Three-dimensional computed reformation of the spine, skull, and brain from axial images, *Neurosurgery* 8:53–58 (1986).
161. Hadley, M.N., V.K.H. Sonntag, M.R. Amos, J.A. Hodak, and L.J. Lopez. Three-dimensional computed tomography in the diagnosis of vertebral column pathological conditions, *Neurosurgery* 21:186–192 (1987).
162. Naidich, T.P., B.C. Teeter, A. Nieves, C.R. Crawford, E. Prenger, and D.G. McLone. Rapid three-dimensional display of the cerebral ventricles from noncontrast CT scans, *J. Comput. Assist. Tomogr.* 13:779–788 (1989).
163. Zinreich, S.J., D.W. Kennedy, D.M. Long, B.S. Carson, and C.R. Dufresne. 3D applications in neuroradiology, *Hospimedica* 8(1):29–32 (1990).
164. Mucelli, R.P., Z. Tarjàn, and I.S. Razavi. Three-dimensional images of the brain surface from standard CT examination, *Eur. Radiol.* 5:238–243 (1995).
165. Levrier, O., P. Sabbah, N. Murayama, Ch. Brunet, J. Farisse, B.M. Mazoyer, et al. Traitement d'image morphologique et imagerie tridimentionnelle (3D) en neuroradiologie, *Radiol. J. CEPUR* 14(6):13–14 (1994).
166. Herman G.T., J.K. Udupa, D.M. Kramer, P.C. Lauterbur, A.M. Rudin, and J.S. Schneider. Three-dimensional display of nuclear magnetic resonance images, *Optical Eng.* 21:923–926 (1982).
167. Brant-Zawadzki, M.N., G.D. Gillan, D.J. Atkinson, N. Edalatpour, and M. Jensen. Three-dimensional MR imaging and display of intracranial disease: improvements with MP-RAGE sequence and gadolinium, *J. Magn. Reson. Imaging* 3:656–663 (1993).
168. Bomans, M., K.-H. Höhne, U. Tiede, and M. Riemer. 3D segmentation of MR-images of the head for 3D display, *IEEE Trans. Med. Imaging* 9:177–183 (1990).
169. Duvernoy, H. *The human brain. Surface, three-dimensional sectional anatomy and MRI* (Vienna, Austria: Springer-Verlag, 1991), pp. 1–354.
170. Hu, X., K.K. Tan, D.N. Levin, S. Galhotra, J.F. Mullan, J. Hekmatpanah, et al. Three-dimensional magnetic resonance images of the brain: application to neurosurgical planning, *J. Neurosurg.* 72:433–440 (1990).
171. Toda, T., T. Watanabe, K. Matsumura, Y. Sunada, H. Yamada, I. Nakano, et al. Three-dimensional MR imaging of brain surface anomalies in Fukuyama-type congenital muscular dystrophy, *Muscle Nerve* 18:508–517 (1995).
172. Ter Haar Romeny, B.M., ed. *Geometry-driven diffusion in computer vision* (Dordrecht, the Netherlands: Kluwer Academic Publishers, 1994,) pp. 1–439.
173. Bullmore, E., M. Brammer, I. Harvey, R. Persaud, R. Murray, and M. Ron. Fractal analysis of the boundary between white matter and cerebral cortex in magnetic resonance images: a controlled study of schizophrenic and manic-depressive patients, *Psychol. Med.* 24:771–781 (1994).
174. Phillips, W.E. II, S. Phuphanich, R.P. Velthuizen, and M.L. Silbiger. Automatic magnetic resonance tissue characterization for three-dimensional magnetic resonance imaging of the brain, *J. Neuroimaging* 5:171–177 (1995).
175. Vannier, M.W., R.L. Butterfield, D. Jordan, W.A. Murphy, R.G. Levitt, and M. Gado. Multispectral analysis of magnetic resonance images, *Radiology* 154:221–224 (1985).
176. Delibasis, K. and P.E. Undrill. Anatomical object recognition using deformable geometric models. *Image Vision Comput.* 12:423–433 (1994).

177. Haller, J.W., G.E. Christensen, S. Joshi, M.I. Miller, and M.W. Vannier. Digital atlas-based segmentation of the hippocampus. In: *Proc. CAR'95* (Berlin, Germany: Springer-Verlag, 1995), pp. 152–157.
178. Links, J.M. and M.D. Devous Sr. Three-dimensional display in nuclear medicine: a more useful depiction of reality, or only a superficial rendering?, *J. Nucl. Med.* 36:703–704 (1995).
179. Wallis, J.W. and T.R. Miller. Three-dimensional display in nuclear medicine and radiology, *J. Nucl. Med.* 32:534–546 (1991).
180. Webb, S., R.J. Ott, M.A. Flower, V.R. McCready, and S. Meller. Three-dimensional display of data obtained by single photon emission computed tomography, *Br. J. Radiol.* 60:557–562 (1987).
181. Tachibana, H., K. Kawabata, Y. Tomino, M. Sugita, and M. Fukuchi. Three-dimensional surface display of brain perfusion with ^{123}I-IMP in Parkinson's disease, *Neuroradiology* 36:276–280 (1994).
182. Tachibana, H., K. Kawabata, Y. Tomino, M. Sugita, and M. Fukuchi. Brain perfusion imaging in Parkinson's disease and Alzheimer's disease demonstrated by three-dimensional surface display with ^{123}I-Iodoamphetamine, *Dementia* 4:334–341 (1993).
183. Ishimura, J. and M. Fukuchi. Clinical application of three-dimensional surface display in brain imaging with Tc-99m HMPAO, *Clin. Nucl. Med.* 16:343–351 (1991).
184. Hashikawa, K., M. Matsumoto, H. Moriwaki, N. Oku, Y. Okazaki, Y. Seike, et al. Three-dimensional display of surface cortical perfusion by SPECT, *J. Nucl. Med.* 36:690–696 (1995).
185. Trobaugh, J.W., D.J. Trobaugh, and W.D. Richard. Three-dimensional imaging with stereotactic ultrasonography, *Comput. Med. Imaging Graph.* 18:315–323 (1994).
186. Blaas, H.-G., S.H. Eik-Nes, T. Kiserud, S. Berg, B. Angelsen, and B. Olstad. Three-dimensional imaging of the brain cavities in human embryos, *Ultrasound Obstet. Gynecol.* 5:228–232 (1995).
187. Tjan, T.G. and H.W.G. Kleine Schaars. Three-dimensional CT angiography, *Medicamundi* 34:8–15 (1989).
188. Aoki, S., Y. Sasaki, T. Machida, T. Ohkubo, M. Minami, and Y. Sasaki. Cerebral aneurysms: detection and elineation using 3-D-CT angiography, *AJNR* 13:1115–1120 (1992).
189. Rigauts, H., G. Marchal, A.L. Baert, and R. Hupke. Initial experience with volume CT scanning, *J. Comput. Assist. Tomogr.* 14:675–682 (1990).
190. Kalender, W.A., K. Wedding, A. Polacin, M. Prokop, C. Schaefer-Prokop, and M. Galanski. Grundlagen der Gefäßdarstellung mit Spiral-CT, *Akt. Radiol.* 4:287–297 (1994).
191. Dillon, E.H., M.S. Van Leeuwen, M.A. Fernández, and W.P.Th.M. Mali. Spiral CT angiography, *AJR* 160:1273–1278 (1993).
192. Schwartz, R.B. Neuroradiological applications of spiral CT, *Seminars in Ultrasound, CT, and MRI* 15:139–147 (1994).
193. Kato, Y., H. Sano, J. Zhou, N. Kanaoka, and T. Kanno. Clinical usefulness of 3D CT endoscopic imaging of cerebral aneurysms (*in japanese*), *No Shinkei Geka* 23:685–691 (1995).
194. Velthuis, B.K., M.S. Van Leeuwen, G.J. Rinkel, T.D. Witkamp, S. Boomstra, L.M. Ramos, et al. CT angiography for intracranial aneurysms: practical approach to optimization of acquisition and display techniques (abstr.), *Radiology* 197(P):482 (1995).
195. Dillon, E.H., M.S. Van Leeuwen, M.A. Fernández, B. Eikelboom, and W.Th. Mali. Computed tomographic angiography for carotid imaging, *Lancet* 340:286 (1992).
196. Schwartz, R.B., K.M. Jones, D.M. Chernoff, S.K. Mukherji, R. Khorasani, H.M. Tice, et al. Common carotid artery bifurcation: evaluation with spiral CT, *Radiology* 185:513–519 (1992).
197. Zöllner, G., M. Sadki, A. Klinkert, J.-L. Dietemann, and R. Beaujeux. Evaluation of the carotid bifurcation by CT angiography. In: *Proc. CAR'95* (Berlin, Germany: Springer-Verlag, 1995), pp. 60–66.
198. Rubin, G.D., M.D. Dake, and C.P. Semba. Current status of three-dimensional spiral CT scanning for imaging the vasculature, *Radiol. Clin. N. Am.* 33:51–70 (1995).
199. Naidich, D.P. Volumetric scans change perceptions in thoracic CT, *Diagn. Imaging* 15(4):70–74 (Apr. 1993).
200. Itoh, T. Clinical experience with Xpress helical scan in thoracic examinations, *Toshiba Med. Rev.* 44:38–41 (1993).
201. White, R.A., M. Scoccianti, M. Back, G. Kopchok, and C. Donayre. Innovations in vascular imaging: arteriography, three-dimensional CT scans, and two- and three-dimensional intravascular ultrasound evaluation of an abdominal aortic aneurysm, *Ann. Vasc. Surg.* 8:285–289 (1994).

202. Parodi, J.C., J.C. Palmaz, and H.D. Barone. Trans femoral intraluminal graft implantation for abdominal aortic aneurysms, *Ann. Vasc. Surg.* 5:491–499 (1991).
203. Rubin, G.D. CT angiography earns role in thoracic aorta, *Diagn. Imaging* 17(suppl.):CT10–CT13 (Nov. 1995).
204. Sembe, C.P., G.D. Rubin, and M.D. Dake. Three-dimensional spiral CT angiography of the abdomen, *Seminars in Ultrasound, CT, and MRI* 15:133–138 (1994).
205. Zeman, R.K., P.M. Berman, P.M. Silverman, W.J. Davros, C. Cooper, A.O. Kladakis, et al. Diagnosis of aortic dissection: value of helical CT with multiplanar reformation and three-dimensional rendering, *AJR* 164:1375–1380 (1995).
206. Lu, D.S.K., H. Lee, and R.M. Krasny. Dual-phase scan enhances hepatic imaging, *Diagn. Imaging* 17(suppl.):CT20p–CT23 (Nov. 1995).
207. Wood, E.H. New vistas for the study of structural and functional dynamics of the heart, lungs and circulation by noninvasive numerical topographic vivisection, *Circulation* 56:506–520 (1977).
208. Sinak, L.J., E.A. Hoffman, P.R. Julsrud, D.D. Mair, J.B. Seward, D.J. Hagler, et al. The Dynamic Spatial Reconstructor: investigating congenital heart disease in four dimensions, *Cardiovasc. Intervent. Radiol.* 7:124–137 (1984).
209. Boyd, D.P. and M.J. Lipton. Cardiac computed tomography, *Proc. IEEE* 71:298–307 (1983).
210. Kutoloski, K., W.J. Eldredge, R. Cha, S.D. Cha, K. Carr, and C. Dennis. Anomalous origin of coronary arteries from the aorta: evaluation of their course using ultrafast computed tomography and 3 dimensional reconstruction (abstr.), *Circulation* 86(4)(suppl. I):I-477 (1992).
211. Napel, S., B.K. Rutt, and P. Plugfelder. Three-dimensional images of the coronary arteries from ultrafast computed tomography: method and comparison with two-dimensional arteriography, *Am. J. Cardiac Imaging* 3:237–243 (1989).
212. Moshage, W.E.L., S. Achenbach, B. Seese, K. Bachmann, and M. Kirchgeorg. Coronary artery stenoses: three-dimensional imaging with electrocardiographically triggered, contrast agent-enhanced, electron-beam CT, *Radiology* 196:707–714 (1995).
213. Dove, E.L., K.P. Philip, D.D. McPherson, W. Stanford, and K.B. Chandran. Quantitative analysis of three-dimensional reconstruction of canine heart using cine-CT, *Am. J. Cardiac Imaging* 5:180–187 (1991).
214. Lessick, J., H. Sideman, H. Azhari, M. Marcus, E. Grenadier, and R. Beyar. Regional three-dimensional geometry and function of left ventricles with fibrous aneurysms. A cine-computed tomography study, *Circulation* 84:1072–1086 (1991).
215. Westra, S.J. Fast scanning permits imaging of heart defects, *Diagn. Imaging* 17(suppl.):CT28–CT31 (Nov. 1995).
216. Gehl, H.-B., K. Bohndorf, U. Gladziwa, S. Handt, and R.W. Günther. Imaging of hemodialysis fistulas: limitations of MR angiography, *J. Comput. Assist. Tomogr.* 15:271–275 (1991).
217. Valk, P.E., J.D. Hale, L. Kaufman, L.E. Crooks, and C.B. Higgins. MR imaging of the aorta with three-dimensional vessel reconstruction: validation by angiography, *Radiology* 157:721–725 (1985).
218. Hale, J.D., P.E. Valk, J.C. Watts, L. Kaufman, L.E. Crooks, C.B. Higgins, and F. Deconinck. MR imaging of blood vessels using three-dimensional reconstruction: methodology, *Radiology* 157:727–733 (1985).
219. Sebok, N.R., D.A. Sebok, D. Wilkerson, R.S. Mezrich, and M. Zatina. In-vitro assessment of the behavior of magnetic resonance angiography in the presence of constrictions, *Invest. Radiol.* 28:604–610 (1993).
220. Wilcock, D.J., T. Jaspan, and B.S. Worthington. Problems and pitfalls of 3-D TOF magnetic resonance angiography of the intracranial circulation, *Clin. Radiol.* 50:526–532 (1995).
221. Pommert, A., M. Bomans, and K.-H. Höhne. Volume visualization in magnetic resonance angiography, *IEEE Comput. Graph. Appl.* 12(5):12–13 (1992).
222. Gerig, G., R. Kikinis, and F.A. Jolesz. Image processing of routine spin-echo MR images to enhance vascular structures: comparison with MR angiography. In: Höhne, K.-H., H. Fuchs, and S.M. Pizer, eds. *3D imaging in medicine* (Berlin, Germany: Springer-Verlag, 1990), pp. 121–132.
223. Murakami, T., T. Kashiwagi, H. Nakamura, K. Tsuda, M. Azuma, K. Tomoda, et al. Display of MR angiograms: maximum intensity projection versus three-dimensional rendering, *Eur. J. Radiol.* 17:95–100 (1993).

224. Zuiderveld, K.J., A.H.J. Koning, and M.A. Viergever. Techniques for speeding up high-quality perspective maximum intensity projection, *Pattern Recognition Lett.* 15:507–517 (1994).
225. Wielopolski, P.A., E.M. Haacke, and L.P. Adler. Three-dimensional MR imaging of the pulmonary vasculature: preliminary experience, *Radiology* 183:465–472 (1992).
226. Bontozoglou, N.P., H. Spanos, P. Lasjaunias, and G. Zarifis. Intracranial aneurysms: endovascular evaluation with three-dimensional-display MR angiography, *Radiology* 197:876–879 (1995).
227. Koller, Th., G. Gerig, and G. Székely. Object-centered description for analysis and display of the cerebral vascularity. In: *Proc. CAR'95* (Berlin, Germany: Springer-Verlag, 1995), pp. 183–188.
228. Reuzé, P., J.L. Coatrieux, L.M. Luo, and J.L. Dillenseger. 3D vessel tracking and quantitation in angio MRI, *Proc. 19th Annu. IEEE Northeast Bioeng. Conf.* (New York, NY: IEEE, 1993), pp. 43–44.
229. Sun, Y., I. Liu, and J.K. Grady. Reconstruction of 3-D binary tree-like structures from mutually orthogonal projections, *IEEE Trans. Pattern Anal. Machine Intelligence* 16:241–248 (1994).
230. Meyers, S.P., S.L. Talagala, S. Totterman, M.V.U. Azodo, E. Kwok, L. Shapiro, et al. Evaluation of the renal arteries in kidney donors: value of three-dimensional phase-contrast MR angiography with maximum-intensity-projection or surface rendering, *AJR* 164:117–121 (1995).
231. Laschinger, J.C., M.W. Vannier, S. Gronemeyer, F. Gutierrez, M. Rosenbloom, and J.L. Cox. Noninvasive three-dimensional reconstruction of the heart and great vessels by ECG-gated magnetic resonance imaging: a new diagnostic modality, *Ann. Thorac. Surg.* 45:505–514 (1988).
232. Kuwahara, M. and S. Eiho. 3-D heart image reconstructed from MRI data, *Comput. Med. Imaging Graph.* 15:241–246 (1991).
233. Vannier, M.W., S. Gronemeyer, F. Gutierrez, C.E. Canter, J.C. Laschinger, and R.H. Knapp. Three-dimensional magnetic resonance imaging of congenital heart disease, *RadioGraphics* 8:857–872 (1988).
234. Vannier, M.W., F.R. Gutierrez, C.E. Canter, C.F. Hildebolt, T.K. Pilgram, R.C. McKnight, et al. Evaluation of congenital heart disease by three-dimensional magnetic resonance imaging, *J. Digital Imaging* 4:153–158 (1991).
235. Fellows, K.E. and P.M. Weinberg. Three-dimensional reconstruction of MR images in congenital heart disease, *Acta Paediatr.* 410(suppl.):60–62 (1995).
236. Yoffie, R.L., M.W. Vannier, F. Gutierrez, R.H. Knapp, and C.E. Canter. Three-dimensional magnetic resonance imaging of the heart, *Radiol. Technol.* 60:305–310 (1989).
237. Friboulet, D., I.E. Magnin, and D. Revel. Assessment of a model for overall left ventricular three-dimensional motion from MRI data, *Int. J. Cardiac Imaging* 8:175–190 (1992).
238. Haacke, E.M., D. Li, and S. Kaushikkar. Cardiac MR imaging: principles and techniques, *Top. Magn. Resonance Imaging* 7:200–217 (1995).
239. Klein, J.L., J.W. Peifer, E.V. Garcia, C.D. Cooke, R. Folks, N. Ezquerra, and S.B. King III. Three-dimensional coronary angiography, *Am. J. Cardiac Imaging* 7:187–194 (1993).
240. Fessler, J.A. and A. Macovski. 3-D reconstruction of vessels with stenoses and aneurysms from dual bi-plane angiograms, *SPIE Proc.* 1092:22–32 (1989).
241. Hulzebosch, A.A., C.H. Slump, and M.A. Viergever. Three-dimensional reconstruction of stenosed coronary artery segments with assessment of flow impedance, *Int. J. Cardiac Imaging* 5:135–143 (1990).
242. Wahle, A., E. Wellnhofer, I. Mugaragu, A. Trebeljahr, H. Oswald, and E. Fleck. Application of accurate 3D reconstruction from biplane angiograms in morphometric analyses and in assessment of diffuse coronary artery disease. In: *Proc. CAR'95* (Berlin, Germany: Springer-Verlag, 1995), pp. 208–215.
243. Scott, D., A.G. Davies, A.R. Cowen, and A. Workman. A technique for 3D reconstruction of arteries from angiographic projections. In: *Proc. CAR'93* (Berlin, Germany: Springer-Verlag, 1993), pp. 541–546.
244. Saint-Félix, D., Y. Trousset, C. Picard, and A. Rougée. 3D reconstruction of high contrast objects using a multi-scale detection/estimation scheme. In: Höhne, K.-H., H. Fuchs, and S.M. Pizer, eds. *3D imaging in medicine* (Berlin, Germany: Springer-Verlag, 1990), pp. 147–158.
245. Hildebrand, A. and S. Großkopf. 3D reconstruction of coronary arteries from x-ray projections. In: *Proc. CAR'95* (Berlin, Germany: Springer-Verlag, 1995), pp. 201–207.
246. Kawata, Y., N. Niki, and T. Kumazaki. Three-dimensional imaging of blood vessels using cone-beam CT. In: *Proc. ICIP-94* (Los Alamitos, CA: IEEE Comput. Soc. Press, 1994), vol. 2, pp. 140–144.

247. Trousset, Y., C. Picard, D. Saint-Félix, and A. Rougée. Three-dimensional computerized angiography. In: *Proc. CAR'91* (Berlin, Germany: Springer-Verlag, 1991), pp. 68–72.
248. Niki, N., Y. Kawata, H. Satoh, and T. Kumazaki. 3D imaging of blood vessels using x-ray rotational angiographic system. In: *IEEE Conf. Record Nucl. Sci. Symp. Med. Imaging Conf.* (New York, NY: IEEE, 1993), vol. 3, pp. 1873–1877.
249. Saint-Félix, D., R. Campagnolo, S. Crocci, P. le Masson, C. Picard, C. Ponchut, et al. Three-dimensional x-ray computerized angiography (abstr.), *Eur. Radiol.* 3(suppl. ECR'93):159 (1993).
250. Koppe, R., E. Klotz, J. Op de Beek, and H. Aerts. 3D vessel reconstruction based on rotational angiography. In: *Proc. CAR'95* (Berlin, Germany: Springer-Verlag, 1995), pp. 101–107.
251. Eiho, S., M. Kuwahara, and N. Asada. Left ventricular image processing, *Med. Prog. Technol.* 12:101–115 (1987).
252. Gerber, T.C., M. Belohlavek, J.F. Greenleaf, D.A. Foley, and J.B. Seward. Dynamic spatial reconstruction of cardiovascular ultrasound images: four-dimensional ultrasound imaging, *Am. J. Cardiac Imaging* 8:199–205 (1994).
253. Marx, G.R. Advances in cardiac imaging in congenital heart disease, *Curr. Opinion Pediatr.* 7:580–586 (1995).
254. Roelandt, J., A. Salustri, B. Mumm, and W. Vletter. Precordial three-dimensional echocardiography with a rotational imaging probe: methods and initial clinical experience, *Echocardiography* 12:243–252 (1995).
255. Seward, J.B., M. Belohlavek, P.W. O'Leary, D.A. Foley, and J.F. Greenleaf. Congenital heart disease: wide-field, three-dimensional, and four-dimensional ultrasound imaging, *Am. J. Cardiac Imaging* 9:38–43 (1995).
256. Binder, Th., S. Globits, H. Gabriel, W. Rothy, G. Porenta, M. Zangeneh, and D. Glogar. Three-dimensional imaging of the heart using transesophageal echocardiography. In: *Proc. Comput. Cardiol. Conf.* (Los Alamitos, CA: IEEE Comput. Soc., 1993), pp. 21–24.
257. Fulton, D.R., G.R. Marx, N.G. Pandian, B.A. Romero, B. Mumm, M. Krauss, et al. Dynamic three-dimensional echocardiographic imaging of congenital heart defects in infants and children by computer-controlled tomographic parallel slicing using a single integrated ultrasound instrument, *Echocardiography* 11:155–164 (1994).
258. Borges, A.C., T. Bartel, S. Müller, and G. Baumann. Dynamic three-dimensional transesophageal echocardiography using a computed tomographic imaging probe — clinical potential and limitation, *Int. J. Cardiac Imaging* 11:247–254 (1995).
259. Kupferwasser, I., S. Mohr-Kahaly, R. Erbel, T. Makowski, N. Wittlich, P. Kearney, et al. Three-dimensional imaging of cardiac mass lesions by transesophageal echocardiographic computed tomography, *J. Am. Soc. Echocardiogr.* 7:561–570 (1994).
260. Rosenfield, K., P. Boffetti, J. Kaufman, R. Weinstein, S. Razvi, and J.M. Isner. Three-dimensional reconstruction of human carotid arteries from images obtained during noninvasive B-mode ultrasound examination, *Am. J. Cardiol.* 70:379–384 (1992).
261. Claudon, M. CVI challenges Doppler in vascular pathology, *Diagn. Imaging Int.* 7:61–76 (Sept/Oct 1991).
262. Pretorius, D.H., T.R. Nelson, and J.S. Jaffe. 3-Dimensional sonographic based on color flow Doppler and gray scale image data: a preliminary report, *J. Ultrasound Med.* 11:225–232 (1992).
263. Carson, P.L., D.D. Adler, J.B. Fowlkes, K. Harnist, and J. Rubin. Enhanced color flow imaging of breast cancer vasculature: continuous wave Doppler and three-dimensional display, *J. Ultrasound Med.* 11:377–385 (1992).
264. Downey, D.B. and A. Fenster. Vascular imaging with a three-dimensional Power Doppler system, *AJR* 165:665–668 (1995).
265. Burns, P.N. Harmonic imaging adds to ultrasound capabilities, *Diagn. Imaging* 17(suppl.):AU7–AU10 (May 1995).
266. Hashimoto, H., Y. Shen, T. Ohashi, Y. Takeuchi, and E. Yoshitome. Ultrasound three-dimensional imaging using Power-Doppler images (*in Japanese*), *Jpn. J. Med. Ultrasonics* 22:741–744 (1995).
267. Linker, D.T., O.D. Sæther, H.O. Myhre, B.A.J. Angelsen, and P.G. Yock. Intra-arterial ultrasound: a potential tool for the vascular surgeon, *Eur. J. Surg.* 157:373–377 (1991).

268. Pasterkamp, G., C. Borst, A.-F.S.R. Moulaert, C.J. Bouma, D. van Dijk, M. Kluytmans, and B.M. ter Haar Romeny. Intravascular ultrasound image subtraction: a contrast enhancing technique to facilitate automatic three-dimensional visualization of the arterial lumen, *Ultrasound Med. Biol.* 21:913–918 (1995).
269. Lengyel, J., D.P. Greenberg, A. Yeung, E. Alderman, and R. Popp. In: Ayache, N., ed. *Computer vision, virtual reality and robotics in medicine* (Berlin, Germany: Springer-Verlag, 1995), pp. 399–405.
270. Aretz, H.T., M.A. Martinelli, and E.G. LeDet. Intra-luminal ultrasound guidance of transverse laser coronary atherectomy, *Int. J. Cardiac Imaging* 4:153–157 (1989).
271. Kluytmans, M., C.J. Bouma, B.M. ter Haar Romeny, G. Pasterkamp, and M.A. Viergever. In: Ayache, N., ed. *Computer vision, virtual reality and robotics in medicine* (Berlin, Germany: Springer-Verlag, 1995), pp. 406–412.
272. Gibson, C.J. Real time 3D display of gated blood pool tomograms, *Phys. Med. Biol.* 33:569–581 (1988).
273. Honda, N., K. Machida, T. Takishima, T. Mamiya, T. Takahashi, T. Kamano, et al. Cinematic three-dimensional surface display of cardiac blood pool tomography, *Clin. Nucl. Med.* 16:87–91 (1991).
274. DePuey, E.G., E.V. Garcia, and N.F. Ezquerra. Three-dimensional techniques and artificial intelligence in Thallium-201 cardiac imaging, *AJR* 152:1161–1168 (1989).
275. Howarth, D.M., A.E. Southee, L.W. Allen, and P.S.K. Tan. $^{99}Tc^{m}$-pyrophosphate myocardial scintigraphy: the role of volume-rendered three-dimensional imaging in the diagnosis of acute myocardial infarction, *Nucl. Med. Commun.* 16:558–565 (1995).
276. Faber, T.L., C.D. Cooke, J.W. Peifer, R.I. Pettigrew, J.P. Vansant, J.R. Leyendecker, and E.V. Garcia. Three-dimensional displays of left ventricular epicardial surface from standard cardiac SPECT perfusion quantification techniques, *J. Nucl. Med.* 36:697–703 (1995).
277. Dilhuydy, H.P., D. McNamara, R.J. Lemieux, Y. Martel, and J.A. de Guise. Three dimensional imaging of dual isotope data-sets in a case of acute myocardial infarction, *Br. J. Radiol.* 65:273–278 (1992).
278. Erratum of previous reference, *Br. J. Radiol.* 66:386 (1993).
279. Ferretti, P.P., G. Borasi, D. Salvo, D. Serafini, and A. Versari. Three-dimensional display of myocardial perfusion: detection of ischemic lesions using a new image subtraction method, *Eur. J. Nucl. Med.* 17:55–60 (1990).
280. Metcalfe, M.J., S. Cross, M.Y. Norton, A. Lomax, K. Jennings, and S. Walton. Polar map or novel three-dimensional display technique for the improved detection of inferior wall myocardial infarction using tomographic radionuclide ventriculography, *Nucl. Med. Commun.* 15:330–340 (1994).
281. Fram, E.K., J.D. Godwing, and C.E. Putman. Three-dimensional display of the heart, aorta, lungs and airway using CT., *AJR* 139:1171–1176 (1982).
282. Hoffman, E.A., L.J. Sinak, R.A. Robb, and E.L. Ritman. Noninvasive quantitative imaging of shape and volume of lungs, *J. Appl. Physiol.* 54:1414–1421 (1983).
283. Stern, R.L., H.E. Cline, G.A. Johnson, and C.E. Ravin. Three-dimensional imaging of the thoracic cavity, *Invest. Radiol.* 24:282–288 (1989).
284. Schwierz, G. and M. Kirchgeorg. The continuous evolution of medical x-ray imaging, *Electromedica* 63:2–7 (1995).
285. Kuhlman, J.E., D.R. Ney, and E.K. Fishman. Two-dimensional and three-dimensional imaging of the in vivo lung: combining spiral computed tomography with multi-planar and volumetric rendering techniques, *J. Digital Imaging* 7:42–47 (1994).
286. Silverman, P.M., A.S. Zeiberg, R.B. Sessions, T.R. Troost, and R.K. Zeman. Three-dimensional imaging of the hypopharynx and larynx by means of helical (spiral) computed tomography, *Ann. Otol. Rhinol. Laryngol.* 104:425–431 (1995).
287. Kawana, S., K. Nakabayashi, F. Kawashima, H. Watanabe, A. Namiki, and T. Hirano. Difficult intubation assisted by three-dimensional computed tomography imaging of the pharynx and the larynx, *Anesthesiology* 83:416–419 (1995).
288. Manson, D., P. Babyn, R. Filler, and S. Holowka. Three-dimensional imaging of the pediatric trachea in congenital tracheal stenosis, *Pediatr. Radiol.* 24:175–179 (1994).
289. Sokiranski, R., K. Elsner, and T. Fleiter. Double-helix scans aid diagnosis in infants. *Diagn. Imaging* 17(suppl.):CT14–CT17 (Nov. 1995).

290. Costello, P. Spiral CT of the thorax, *Semin. Ultrasound, CT and MRI* 15:90–106 (1994).
291. Rémy, J., M. Rémy-Jardin, G. Giraud, and J. Wannebroucq. Le balayage spiralé volumique et ses applications en pathologie thoracique, *Rev. Mal. Respir.* 11:13–27 (1994).
292. Shimizu, T., I. Narabayashi, Y. Uesugi, R. Namba, Y. Ogura, K. Tabushi, et al. Three-dimensional CT imaging of pulmonary nodules using helical scan CT, *(in Japanese) Nippon Acta Radiol.* 54:583–591 (1994).
293. Kuriyama, K., N. Mihara, N. Hosomi, Y. Sawai, E. Inoue, T. Kadota, et al. Three-dimensional imaging of focal lung diseases, *(in japanese) Jpn. J. Clin. Radiol.* 40:795–802 (1995).
294. Quint, L.E., D.L. McShan, G.M. Glazer, M.B. Orringer, I.R. Francis, and B.R. Gross. Three dimensional CT of central lung tumors, *Clin. Imaging* 14:323–329 (1990).
295. Kalender, W.A., H. Fichte, W. Bautz, and M. Skalej. Semiautomatic evaluation procedures for quantitative CT of the lung, *J. Comput. Assist. Tomogr.* 15:248–255 (1991).
296. Kavuru, M., D.R. Ney, E.K. Fishman, J.E. Kuhlman, R.H. Hruban, and G.M. Hutchins. Three-dimensional imaging of the lung in vivo: work in progress, *J. Digital Imaging* 4:137–142 (1991).
297. Suzuki, K., E. Kohda, M. Izutsu, N. Shiraga, and K. Hiramatsu. 3D image, MIP and MPR for pulmonary nodule. In: *Proc. CAR'95* (Berlin, Germany: Springer-Verlag, 1995), pp. 1250–1251.
298. Schaefer-Prokop, C., M. Prokop, and M. Galanski. Minimum and maximum intensity projections for evaluation of spiral CT data of the chest. In: Pokieser, H. and G. Lechner, eds. *Advances in CT III* (Berlin, Germany: Springer-Verlag, 1994), pp. 269–275.
299. Donnelly, K.J., E.R. Bank, W.J. Parks, G.S. Gussack, P. Davenport, N.W. Todd, and S. Shepherd. Three-dimensional magnetic resonance imaging evaluation of pediatric tracheobronchial tree, *Laryngoscope* 104:1425–1430 (1994).
300. Beyer-Enke, S.A., L.G. Strauss, M. Müller, J. Görich, K. Kayser, and G. Van Kaick. Spect-3-D-Rekonstruktionen der Lungen-Perfusion bei Patienten mit thorakalen Raum-forderungen, *Fortschr. Röntgenstr.* 150:211–215 (1989).
301. Conway, J.H., P. Halson, E. Moore, A. Hashish, A.G. Bailey, M. Nassim, et al. Multi-modality imaging: the use of single photon emission computed tomography and magnetic resonance imaging to assess regional intra-pulmonary deposition of nebulised aerosols, *J. Aerosol Med.* 8:293–295 (1995).
302. Gonda, I. Diagnostic aerosols: current status and future prospects, *Aerosol Sci. Technol. (USA)* 18:250–256 (1993).
303. Ros, P.R., M.M. ElRahman, R. Barreda, G.M. Torres, J.C. Honeyman, S.B. Vogel, and K.I. Bland. Three-dimensional imaging of liver masses: preliminary experience, *Appl. Radiol.* 19(7):28–32 (1990).
304. Kashiwagi, T., N. Mitsutani, T. Koizumi, and K. Kimura. Three-dimensional demonstration of liver and spleen by a computer graphics technique, *Acta Radiol.* 29:27–31 (1988).
305. Yang, N.-C., P.K. Leichner, E.K. Fishman, S.S. Siegelman, T.L. Frenkel, J.R. Wallace, et al. CT volumetrics of primary liver cancers, *J. Comput. Assist. Tomogr.* 10:621–628 (1986).
306. Soyer, P. and A. Roche. Three-dimensional imaging of the liver, *Acta Radiol.* 32:432–435 (1991).
307. Bae, K.T., M.L. Giger, C.-T. Chen, and C.E. Kahn Jr. Automatic segmentation of liver structure in CT images, *Med. Phys.* 20:71–78 (1993).
308. Woodhouse, C.E., D.R. Ney, J.V. Sitzmann, and E.K. Fishman. Spiral computed tomography arterial portography with three-dimensional volumetric rendering for oncologic surgery planning. A retrospective analysis, *Invest. Radiol.* 29:1031–1037 (1994).
309. Leppek, R. and K.J. Klose. 3D-Darstellung der Leber, *Radiologe* 35:769–777 (1995).
310. Van Leeuwen, M.S., H. Obertop, A.H. Hennipman, and M.A. Fernández. 3-D reconstruction of hepatic neoplasms: a preoperative planning procedure, *Clin. Gastroenterol.* 9:121–133 (1995).
311. Soyer, P., A. Roche, M. Gad, L. Shapeero, F. Breitt-Mayer, D. Elias, et al. Preoperative segmental localization of hepatic metastases: utility of three-dimensional CT during arterial portography, *Radiology* 180:653–658 (1991).
312. Gmeinwieser, J., A.P. Wunderlich, P. Gerhardt, and M. Strotzer. Dreidimensionale Rekonsruktion von atemver-schieblichen Organen und Gefäßstrukturen aus Spiral-CT-Datensätzen, *Röntgenpraxis* 44:2–8 (1991).
313. Van Leeuwen, M.S., J. Noordzij, A. Hennipman, and M.A.M. Feldberg. Planning of liver surgery using three dimensional imaging techniques, *Eur. J. Cancer* 31A:1212–1215 (1995).

314. Van Leeuwen, M.S., J. Noordzij, M.A. Fernández, A. Hennipman, M.A.M. Feldberg, and E.H. Dillon. Portal venous and segmental anatomy of the right hemiliver: observations based on three-dimensional spiral CT renderings, *AJR* 163:1395–1404 (1994).
315. Takahashi, S., A. Hattori, F. Machida, A. Uchiyama, and N. Suzuki. Simulation of liver tissue reproduction after hepatic lobectomy, *Comput. Aided Surg.* 1:66–67 (1994).
316. Sugioka, A., M. Shimazu, K. Katada, H. Anno, H. Sugenoya, A. Hasumi, et al. Three dimensional cholangiography of hilar cholangiocarcinoma using helical scan CT, *Comput. Aided Surg.* 1:65–66 (1994).
317. Wunderlich, A.P., M. Lenz, P. Gerhardt, H. Helmberger, and M. Groß. 3D-Rekonstruktionen aus CT-Datensätzen, *Röntgenpraxis* 46:57–65 (1992).
318. McNeal, G.R., W.H. Maynard, R.A. Branch, T.A. Powers, P.A. Arns, K. Gunter, et al. Liver volume measurements and three-dimensional display from MR images, *Radiology* 169:851–854 (1988).
319. Van Leeuwen, M.S., M.A. Fernández, H.W. Van Es, R. Stokking, E.H. Dillon, and M.A.M. Feldberg. Variations in venous and segmental anatomy of the liver, *AJR* 162:1337–1345 (1994).
320. Bennett, W.F., J.G. Bova, L. Petty, and E.W. Martin Jr. Preoperative 3D rendering of MR imaging in liver metastases, *J. Comput. Assist. Tomogr.* 15:979–984 (1991).
321. Waggenspack, G.A., D.R. Tabb, V. Tiruchelvam, L. Ziegler, and K. Waltersdorff. Three-dimensional localization of hepatic neoplasms with computer-generated scissurae recreated from axial CT and MR images, *AJR* 160:307–309 (1993).
322. Morimoto, K., M. Shimoi, T. Shirakawa, Y. Aoki, S. Choi, Y. Miyata, and K. Hara. Biliary obstruction: evaluation with three-dimensional MR cholangiography, *Radiology* 183:578–580 (1992).
323. Zoller, W.G., H. Liess, C.M. Roth, and A. Umgelter. Clinical application of three-dimensional sonography in internal medicine, *Clin. Invest.* 71:226–232 (1993).
324. Chernoff, D.M., S.E. Seltzer, S.G. Silverman, J.P. Richie, R. Kikinis, K.R. Loughlin, and D.E. Adams. Three-dimensional imaging and display of renal tumors using spiral CT: a potential aid to partial nephrectomy, *Urology* 43:125–129 (1994).
325. Leißner, J., M. Stöckle, and R. Hohenfellner. Dreidi-mensionale Rekonstruktion zur Operationsplanung bei Tumoren in Einzelnieren, *Urologe* 34:466–469 (1995).
326. Gilja, O.H., A.I. Smievoll, N. Thune, K. Matre, T. Hausken, S. ϕdegaard, and A. Berstad. *In vivo* comparison of 3D ultrasonography and magnetic resonance imaging in volume estimation of human kidneys, *Ultrasound Med. Biol.* 21:25–32 (1995).
327. Khullar, V., S. Salvatore, L.D. Cardozo, S. Hill, and C.J. Kelleher. Three dimensional ultrasound of the urethra and urethral sphincter: a new diagnostic technique, *Neurourol. Urodyn.* 13:352–353 (1994).
328. Ng, K.J., J.E. Gardener, D. Rickards, W.R. Lees, and E.J.G. Milroy. Three-dimensional imaging of the prostatic urethra — an exciting new tool, *Br. J. Urol.* 74:604–608 (1994).
329. Kelly, I.M.G., J.E. Gardener, and W.R. Lees. Three-dimensional fetal ultrasound, *Lancet* 339:1062–1064 (1992).
330. Lees, W.A. 3D ultrasound images optimize fetal review, *Diagn. Imaging* 14(3):69–73 (1992).
331. Feichtinger, W. Transvaginal three-dimensional imaging, *Ultrasound Obstet. Gynecol.* 3:375–378 (1993).
332. Sakas, G., S. Walter, W. Hiltmann, and A. Wischnik. Foctal visualization using 3D ultrasonic data. In: *Proc. CAR'95* (Berlin, Germany: Springer-Verlag, 1995), pp. 241–247.
333. Devonald, K.J., D.A. Ellwood, K.A. Griffiths, G. Kossoff, R.W. Gill, A.P. Kadi, et al. Volume imaging: three-dimensional appreciation of the fetal head and face, *J. Ultrasound Med.* 14:919–925 (1995).
334. Gombergh, R., M. Laval-Jeantet, A. Castro, and P. Bourrier. Echographie 3D en gunécologie obstétrique: etat de l'art, *Contracept. Fertil. Sex.* 22:685–693 (1994).
335. Nelson, T.R. and D.H. Pretorius. Visualization of the fetal thoracic skeleton with three-dimensional sonography: a preliminary report, *AJR* 164:1485–1488 (1995).
336. Nagata, S., T. Koyanagi, S. Fukushima, K. Akazawa, and H. Nakano. Change in the three-dimensional shape of the stomach in the developing human fetus, *Early Hum. Dev.* 37:27–38 (1994).
337. Sickler, G.K., T.J. Dubinsky, and N.F. Maklad. Enthusiasm grows for obstetrical ultrasound, *Diagn. Imaging* 17(suppl.):AU17–AU21 (May 1995).

338. Buscombe, J.R., A.J.W. Hilson, M.L. Hall, C.E. Townsend, G. Clarke, and P.J. Ell. Does three-dimensional display of SPECT data improve the accuracy of Technetium-99m DMSA imaging of the kidneys?, *J. Nucl. Med. Technol.* 23:12–17 (1995).
339. Goitein, M., J. Wittenberg, M. Mendiondo, J. Doucette, C. Friedberg, J. Ferrucci, et al. *Int. J. Radiat. Oncol. Biol. Phys.* 5:1787–1798 (1979).
340. Lee, K.R., C.M. Mansfield, S.J. Dwyer III, H.L. Cox, E. Levine, and A.W. Templeton. CT for intracavitary radiotherapy planning, *AJR* 135:809–813 (1980).
341. Mohan, R., G. Barest, L.J. Brewster, C. Chui, G. Kutcher, J. Laughlin, and Z. Fuks. A comprehensive three-dimensional radiation treatment planning system, *Int. J. Radiat. Oncol. Biol. Phys.* 15:481–495 (1988).
342. Chaney, E.L. Introduction, *Semin. Radiat. Oncol.* 2:213–214 (1992).
343. Nilles, A., C. Ehritt-Braun, G. Bruggmoser, N. Hodapp, and H. Frommhold. Spiral CT in treatment planning of intraoperative radiotherapy. In: Pokieser, H. and G. Lechner, eds. *Advances in CT III* (Berlin, Germany: Springer-Verlag, 1994), pp. 124–128.
344. Purdy, J.A. Evolution of three-dimensional radiation therapy treatment planning. In: Purdy, J.A. and B.A. Fraass, eds. *Syllabus: a cathegorical course in physics. Three-dimensional radiation therapy planning* (Oak Brook, IL: RSNA, 1994), pp. 9–15.
345. Meyer, J.L. and J.A. Purdy, eds. *3-D conformal radiotherapy: a new era in the irradiation of cancer* (Basel, Switserland: S. Karger AG, 1996), pp. 1–278.
346. Tepper, J.E. and B. Shank (Photon treatment planning collaborative working group). Three-dimensional display in planning radiation therapy: a clinical perspective, *Int. J. Radiat. Oncol. Biol. Phys.* 21:79–89 (1991).
347. Reynolds, R.A., Sontag, M.R., and Chen, L.S. An algorithm for three-dimensional visualization of radiation therapy beams, *Med. Phys.* 15:24–28 (1988).
348. Kooy, H.M., L.A. Nedzi, J.S. Loeffler, E. Alexander III, C.-W. Cheng, E.G. Mannarino, et al. Treatment planning for stereotactic radiosurgery of intra-cranial lesions, *Int. J. Radiat. Oncol. Biol. Phys.* 21:683–693 (1991).
349. Mohan, R., L.J. Brewster, G. Barest, and C.S. Chui. Computer graphics tools for radiation treatment planning, *Comput. Methods Progr. Biomed.* 28:157–170 (1989).
350. Rosenman, J., G.W. Sherouse, H. Fuchs, S.M. Pizer, A.L. Skinner, C. Mosher, et al. Three-dimensional display techniques in radiation therapy treatment planning, *Int. J. Radiat. Oncol. Biol. Phys.* 16:263–269 (1989).
351. Bloch, P. and J.K. Udupa. Application of computerized tomography to radiation therapy and surgical planning, *Proc. IEEE* 71:351–355 (1983).
352. Wernik, B. Investigating 3D radiation therapy. An interview with James A. Purdy, PhD, *Appl. Radiol.* 17(3):39–42 (1988).
353. Lichter, A.S., H.M. Sandler, J.M. Robertson, T.S. Lawrence, R.K. Ten Haken, D.L. McShan, and B.A. Fraass. Clinical experience with three-dimensional treatment planning, *Semin. Radiat. Oncol.* 2:257–266 (1992).
354. Gehring, M.A., T.R. Mackie, S.S. Kubsad, B.R. Paliwal, M.P. Mehta, and T.J. Kinsella. A three-dimensional volume visualization package applied to stereotactic radiosurgery treatment planning. *Int. J. Radiat. Oncol. Biol. Phys.* 21:491–500 (1991).
355. Kessler, M.L., R.K. Ten Haken, B.A. Fraass, and D.L. McShan. Expanding the use and effectiveness of dose-volume histograms for 3-D treatment planning I: integration of 3-D dose-display, *Int. J. Radiat. Oncol. Biol. Phys.* 29:1125–1131 (1994).
356. Sherouse, G.W., C.E. Mosher Jr., K. Novins, J. Rosenman, and E.L. Chaney. Virtual simulation: concept and implementation. In: Bruinvis, I.A.D., P.H. Van der Giessen, H.J. Van Kleffens, and F.W. Wittkämper, eds. *The use of computers in radiation therapy* (New York, NY: Elsevier, 1987), pp. 433–436.
357. Rosenman, J.G., E.L. Chaney, T.J. Cullip, J.R. Symon, V.L. Chi, H. Fuchs, and D.S. Stevenson. Vistanet: interactive real-time calculation and display of 3-dimensional radiation dose: an application of gigabit networking, *Int. J. Radiat. Oncol. Biol. Phys.* 25:123–129 (1993).
358. Purdy, J.A., W.B. Harms, J.W. Matthews, R. Drzymala, B. Emami, J.R. Simpson, et al. Advances in 3-dimensional radiation treatment planning systems: room-view display with real time interactivity, *Int. J. Radiat. Oncol. Biol. Phys.* 27:933–944 (1993).

359. Cullip, T.J., J.R. Symon, J.G. Rosenman, and E.L. Chaney. Digitally reconstructed fluoroscopy and other interactive volume visualizations in 3-D treatment planning, *Int. J. Radiat. Oncol. Biol. Phys.* 27:145–151 (1993).
360. Bendl, R., A. Hoess, and W. Schlegel. Advanced tools for 3D radiotherapy planning. In: *Proc. CAR'95* (Berlin, Germany: Springer-Verlag, 1995), pp. 1094–1099.
361. Rosenman, J. Future directions in 3-dimensional radiation treatment planning, *Oncology* 7:97–104 (1993).
362. Nagata, Y., K. Okajima, R. Murata, M. Mitsumori, T. Mizowaki, K. Tsutsui, et al. Three-dimensional treatment planning for maxillary cancer using a CT simulator, *Int. J. Radiat. Oncol. Biol. Phys.* 30:979–983 (1994).
363. Perez, C.A., J.A. Purdy, W. Harms, R. Gerber, J. Matthews, P.W. Grigsby, et al. Design of a fully integrated three-dimensional computed tomography simulator and preliminary clinical evaluation, *Int. J. Radiat. Oncol. Biol. Phys.* 30:887–897 (1994).
364. Kennedy, I., E. Thomson, M. Atherton, and K. Rotter. On the use of 3D scanning and surface matching to locate patients undergoing radiotherapy planning and treatment. In: *Proc. IEE Colloquium on "3D Imaging and Analysis of Depth/Range Images" Digest No. 1994/054* (London: Institution of Electrical Engineers, 1994), pp. 11/1–11/8.
365. Stalling, D., H.C. Hege, and T. Höllerer. Visualization and 3D interaction for hyperthermia treatment planning. In: *Proc. CAR'95* (Berlin, Germany: Springer-Verlag, 1995), pp. 1216–1222.
366. Fellingham, L.L., A. Gamboa-Aldeco, P. Dev, and G.T.Y. Chen. Three-dimensional imaging: applications to pre-operative and radiation therapy planning, *SPIE Proc.* 602:320–325 (1986).
367. Fraass, B.A., D.L. McShan, R.F. Diaz, R.K. Ten Haken, A. Aisen, S. Gebarski, et al. Integration of magnetic resonance imaging into radiation therapy treatment planning: I. Technical considerations, *Int. J. Radiat. Oncol. Biol. Phys.* 13:1897–1908 (1987).
368. Chan, M.F. and K.M. Ayyangar. Confirmation of target localization and dosimetry for 3D conformal radiotherapy treatment planning by MR imaging of a ferrous sulfate gel head phantom, *Med. Phys.* 22:1171–1175 (1995).
369. Bookstein, F.L. *Morphometric tools for landmark data: geometry and biology* (Cambridge, U.K.: Cambridge University Press, 1991), pp. 1–435.
370. Hildebolt, C.F., M.W. Vannier, and R.H. Knapp. Validation study of skull three-dimensional computerized tomography measurements. *Am. J. Phys. Anthropol.* 82:283–294 (1990).
371. Balm, R., R. Kaatee, J.D. Blankensteijn, W.P.T.M. Mali, and B.C. Eikelboom. CT-angiography of abdominal aortic aneurysms after transfemoral endovascular aneurysm management. *Eur. J. Vasc. Endovasc. Surg.* 12:182–188 (1996).
372. Hamano, K., N. Iwasaki, T. Takeya, and H. Takita. A comparative study of linear measurement of the brain and three-dimensional measurement of brain volume using CT scans, *Pediatr. Radiol.* 23:165–168 (1993).
373. Lösch, A., F. Eckstein, K.-H. Englmeier, M. Haubner, and H. Sittek. Immersive interaction techniques for the visualization of 3D image data of the knee joint articular cartilage. In: *Proc. CAR'95* (Berlin, Germany: Springer-Verlag, 1995), pp. 41–46.
374. Zuiderveld, K.J., R. Stokking, and M.A. Viergever. Integrated visualization of quantitative information with anatomical surfaces. In: *Proc. CAR'95* (Berlin, Germany: Springer-Verlag, 1995), pp. 195–200.
375. Soyama, Y., T. Yasuda, S. Yokoi, J. Toriwaki, and M. Fujioka. A hip joint surgical planning system using 3-D images (*in japanese*), *JJME* 27:70–78 (1989).
376. Vannier, M.W., B.S. Brundsen, C.F. Hildebolt, D. Falk, J.M. Cheverud, G.S. Figiel, et al. Brain surface cortical sulcal lengths: quantification with three-dimensional MR imaging, *Radiology* 180:479–484 (1991).
377. Denis, D., L. Genitori, J. Bardot, J.B. Saracco, M. Choux, and I.H. Maumenee, *Graefe's Arch. Clin. Exp. Ophthalmol.* 232:728–733 (1994).
378. Genitori, L., N. Zanon, D. Denis, P. Erdincler, M. Achouri, G. Lena, and M. Choux. The skull base in plagiocephaly, *Child's Nerv. Syst.* 10:217–223 (1994).
379. Kulynych, J.J., K. Vladar, D.W. Jones, and D.R. Weinberger. Three-dimensional surface rendering in MRI morphometry: a study of the planum temporale, *J. Comput. Assist. Tomogr.* 17:529–535 (1993).
380. Bite, U., I.T. Jackson, G.S. Forbes, and D.G. Gehring. Orbital volume measurements in enophthalmos using three-dimensional CT imaging, *Plast. Reconstr. Surg.* 75:502–507 (1985).

381. Gault, D., F. Brunell, D. Renier, and D. Marchac. The calculation of intracranial volume using CT scans, *Child's Nerv. Syst.* 4:271–273 (1988).
382. Dufresne, C.R., J.G. McCarthy, C.B. Cutting, F.J. Epstein, and W.Y. Hoffman. Volumetric quantification of intracranial and ventricular volume following cranial vault remodeling: a preliminary report, *Plast. Reconstr. Surg.* 79:24–32 (1987).
383. Lin, K.Y., S.P. Bartlett, M.J. Yaremchuk, R.F. Grossman, J.K. Udupa, and L.A. Whitaker. An experimental study on the effect of rigid fixation on the developing craniofacial skeleton, *Plast. Reconstr. Surg.* 87:229–235 (1991).
384. Dulce, M.C., G.H. Mostbeck, K.K. Friese, G.R. Caputo, and C.B. Higgins. Quantification of the left ventricular volumes and function with cine MR imaging: comparison of geometric models with three-dimensional data, *Radiology* 188:371–376 (1993).
385. Zonneveld, F.W., L. Koornneef, and D. Wittebol-Post. Quantitative volumetric assessment of orbital soft tissue. In: *Proc. CAR'91* (Berlin, Germany: Springer-Verlag, 1991), pp. 181–186.
386. Harvey, I., R. Persaud, M.A. Ron, G. Baker, and R.M. Murray. Volumetric MRI measurements in bipolars compared with schizophrenics and healthy controls, *Psychol. Med.* 24:689–699 (1994).
387. Wible, C.G., M.E. Shenton, H. Hokama, R. Kikinis, F.A. Jolesz, D. Metcalf, and R.W. McCarley. Prefrontal cortex and schizophrenia: a quantitative magnetic resonance imaging study, *Arch. Gen. Psychiatry* 52:279–288 (1995).
388. Waitzman, A.A., J.C. Poznick, D.C. Armstrong, and G.E. Pron. Craniofacial skeletal measurements based on computed tomography. Part I. Accuracy and reproducibility, *Cleft Palate Craniofacial J.* 29:112–117 (1992).
389. Ono, I., T. Ohura, E. Narumi, K. Kawashima, I. Matsuno, S. Nakamura, et al. Three-dimensional analysis of craniofacial bones using three-dimensional computer tomography, *J. Cranio-Maxillo-Facial Surg.* 20:49–60 (1992).
390. Matteson, S.R., W. Bechtold, C. Phillips, and E.V. Staab. A method for three-dimensional image reformation for quantitative cephalometric analysis. *J. Oral Maxillofacial Surg.* 47:1053–1061 (1989).
391. Vannier, M.W., T. Pilgram, G. Bhatia, B. Brundsen, and P. Commean. Facial surface scanner, *IEEE Comput. Graph. Appl.* 11(11):72–80 (1991).
392. Abbott, A.H., D.J. Netherway, D.J. David, and T. Brown. Craniofacial osseous landmark determination from stereo computer tomography reconstructions, *Ann. Acad. Med. Singapore* 19:595–604 (1990).
393. Abbott, A.H., D.J. Netherway, D.J. David, and T.A.D. Brown. Application and comparison of techniques for three-dimensional analysis of craniofacial anomalies, *J. Craniofacial Surg.* 1:119–134 (1990).
394. Cutting, C., F.L. Bookstein, B. Grayson, L. Fellingham, and J.G. McCarthy. Three-dimensional computer-assisted design of craniofacial surgical procedures: optimization and interaction with cephalometric and CT-based models, *Plast. Reconstr. Surg.* 77:877–885 (1986).
395. Matsuno, I., M. Kawakami, M. Yamamura, H. Ishikawa, A. Kudou, S. Nakamura, et al. Three-dimensional morphological analysis for craniofacial deformity (*in japanese*), *J. Jpn. Orthodont. Soc.* 49:291–301 (1990).
396. Richtsmeier, J.T. Craniofacial growth in Apert syndrome as measured by finite-element scaling analysis, *Acta Anat.* 133:50–56 (1988).
397. Lele, S. and J.T. Richtsmeier. On comparing biological shapes: detection of influential landmarks, *Am. J. Phys. Anthropol.* 87:49–65 (1992).
398. Zonneveld, F.W. Three-dimensional imaging in craniofacial surgery: a review of the role of mirror image production, *Eur. J. Plast. Surg.* 14:49–51 (1991).
399. Ayache, N. Medical computer vision, virtual reality and robotics, *Image Vision Comput.* 13:295–313 (1995).
400. Andreasen, N.C., G. Harris, T. Cizadlo, S. Arndt, D.S. O'Leary, V. Swayze, and M. Flaum. Techniques for measuring sulcal/gyral patterns in the brain as visualized through magnetic resonance scanning: BRAINPLOT and BRAINMAP, *Proc. Natl. Acad. Sci. USA* 90:93–97 (1994).
401. Kawata, Y., N. Niki, and T. Kumazaki. Quantitative analysis of blood vessels using cone-beam CT images. In: *Proc. CAR'95* (Berlin, Germany: Springer-Verlag, 1995), pp. 222–227.
402. Robb, R.A., P.B. Hefferman, J.J. Camp, and D.P. Hanson. A workstation for multi-dimensional display and analysis of biomedical images, *Comput. Methods Prog. Biomed.* 25:169–184 (1987).

403. Robb, R.A. Interactive and quantitative analysis of biomedical images, In: Kelly, P.J. and B.A. Kall, eds. *Computers in stereotactic neurosurgery* (Boston, MA: Blackwell 1992) pp. 17–32.
404. Robb, R.A. *Three-dimensional biomedical imaging: principles and practice* (New York, NY: VCH Publishers Inc., 1995), pp. 1–287.
405. Udupa, J.K., D. Odhner, S. Samarasekera, R.J. Goncalves, K. Iyer, K. Venugopal, and S. Furuie. 3DVIEWNIX: an open, transportable, multidimensional, multimodality, multiparametric imaging software system, *SPIE Proc.* 2164:58–73 (1994).
406. Hoffman, E.A., D. Gnanaprakasam, K.B. Gupta, J.D. Hoford, S.D. Kugelmass, and R.S. Kulawiec. VIDA: an environment for multidimensional image display and analysis, *SPIE Proc.* 1660:1–18 (1992).
407. Ligier, Y., O. Ratib, M. Logean, C. Girard, R. Perrier, and J.R. Scherrer. Object-oriented design of medical imaging software, *Comput. Med. Imag. Graph.* 18:125–135 (1994).
408. Höhne, K.-H., M. Bomans, A. Pommert, M. Riemer, and U. Tiede. 3D-visualization of human anatomy from tomograms. In: Barber, B., D. Cao, D. Qin, and G. Wagner, eds. *Proc. 6th Conf. Med. Informatics (MEDINFO'89)* (Amsterdam, the Netherlands: North-Holland, 1989), pp. 417–421.
409. Zuiderveld, K.J., A.H.J. Koning, R. Stokking, J.B.A. Maintz, F.J.R. Appelman, and M.A. Viergever. Multimodality visualization of medical volume data. *Comput. Graph.* 20:775–791 (1996).
410. Vannier, M.W. State of the art: imaging for simulation surgery, craniofacial surgical planning, and evaluation with computers, *Comput. Aided Surg.* 1:16–17 (1994).
411. Jackson, I.T. and U. Bite. Three-dimensional computed tomographic scanning and major surgical reconstruction of the head and neck, *Mayo Clin. Proc.* 61:546–555 (1986).
412. Fukuta, K., I.T. Jackson, C.N. McEwan, and N.B. Meland. Three-dimensional imaging in craniofacial surgery: a review of the role of mirror image production, *Eur. J. Plast. Surg.* 13:209–217 (1990).
413. Fujioka, M., H. Nakajima, S. Yokoi, T. Yasuda, and J. Toriwaki. Computer graphic simulation of craniofacial surgery in children (abstr.), *Radiology* 161(P):406 (1986).
414. Yokoi, S., T. Yasuda, Y. Hashimoto, and J. Toriwaki. A craniofacial surgical planning system. In: *Proc. Natl. Comput. Graph. Assoc. "Computer Graphics'87" 8th Annu. Conf. Expo.* (Fairfax, VA: NCGA, 1987), pp. 152–161.
415. Fujioka, M., S. Yokoi, T. Yasuda, Y. Hashimoto, J. Toriwaki, and H. Nakajima. Computer-aided interactive surgical simulation for craniofacial anomalies based on 3-D surface reconstruction CT images, *Radiat. Med.* 6:204–212 (1988).
416. Fujioka, M., S. Yokoi, T. Yasuda, and J. Toriwaki. Computer-aided interactive surgical simulation system — its clinical application. In: *Proc. CAR'89* (Berlin, Germany: Springer-Verlag, 1989), pp. 409–412.
417. Bak, D.J. and A.L. Baker. "Electronic scalpel" aids cranial surgery, *Design News* 48:89–91 (1992).
418. Yasuda, T., Y. Hashimoto, S. Yokoi, and J.-I. Toriwaki. Computer system for craniofacial surgical planning based on CT images, *IEEE Trans. Med. Imaging* 9:270–280 (1990).
419. Suto, Y. Three-dimensional surgical simulation system using X-ray CT and MR images, *Toshiba Med. Rev.* 35:32–42 (1991).
420. Marsh, J.L., M.W. Vannier, S. Bresina, and K.M. Hemmer. Applications of computer graphics in craniofacial surgery, *Clin. Plast. Surg.* 13(3):441–448 (1986).
421. Tan, A.C., S.R. Richards, and A.D. Linney. The MGI workstation: an interactive system for 3D medical graphics applications. In: *Proc. CAR'91* (Berlin, Germany: Springer-Verlag, 1991), pp. 705–710.
422. Tronnier, U., K.D. Wolff, and S. Trittmacher. A 3-D surgical planning system and its clinical applications. In: *Proc. CAR'89* (Berlin, Germany: Springer-Verlag, 1989), pp. 403–408.
423. Fujioka, M. Computer assisted radiology for infants and children. In: *Proc. CAR'91* (Berlin, Germany: Springer-Verlag, 1991), pp. 763–770.
424. Moriya, Y. and H. Aramata. Surgical planning system for osteotomy using 3-dimensional images, *Comput. Aided Surg.* 1:23–25 (1994).
425. Udupa, J.K. and D. Odhner. Fast visualization, manipulation, and analysis of binary volumetric objects, *IEEE Comput. Graph. Appl.* 11(6):53–62 (1991).
426. Odhner, D. and J.K. Udupa. Shell manipulation: interactive alteration of multiple-material fuzzy structures, *SPIE Proc.* 2431:35–42 (1995).
427. Fukuta, K. and I.T. Jackson. New developments in three-dimensional imaging: clinical application of interactive surgical planning for craniofacial disorders, *Perspect. Plast. Surg.* 6:155–177 (1992).

428. Rovetta, A., K.L. Cavalca, and W. Xia. CAD/CAM and robotics: bioengineering application in bone prosthesis (abstr.), *Comput. Aided Surg.* 1:27 (1994).
429. Esselman, G.H., J.M. Coticchia, F.J. Wippold II, J.M. Fredrickson, M.W. Vannier, and J.G. Neely. Computer-simulated test fitting of an implantable hearing aid using three-dimensional CT scans of the temporal bone: preliminary study, *Am. J. Otol.* 15:702–709 (1994).
430. Kojima, T. and T. Kurokawa. 3-D simulation and practice of corrective spinal osteotomy for scoliosis, *Comput. Aided Surg.* 1:73–76 (1994).
431. Tomihra, M., I. Miyake, K. Fukuta, and S. Tanaka. Simulation for rotation osteotomy of avascular necrosis of femoral head (abstr.), *Comput. Aided Surg.* 1:70 (1994).
432. Robertson, D.D., J.R. Essinger, J.M. Aubaniac, J.N. Argenson, and A.J. Zarnowski. Individualized femoral total hip components designed using computer generated 3-D bone models and surgical simulation of bone preparation and insertion, *Comput. Aided Surg.* 1:71–73 (1994).
433. Bo, A., S. Imura, Y. Okumura, H. Oomori, M. Ando, and H. Baba. The femoral component for secondary osteoarthritis of the hip joints in Japan. In: *Proc. CAR'95* (Berlin, Germany: Springer-Verlag, 1995), pp. 927–932.
434. Linney, A.D., S.R. Grinrod, S.R. Arridge, and J.P. Moss. Three dimensional visualization of computerized tomography and laser scan data for the simulation of maxillo-facial surgery, *Med. Inform.* 14:109–121 (1989).
435. Katoh, K., T. Yasuda, S. Yokoi, J. Toriwaki, and M. Fujioka. Improved interface functions in a computer-aided surgical planning system; manipulation on three-view images and recording of history of operations (*in japanese), Trans. Inst. Electr. Infom. Commun. Eng. D-II PRU89* 112:1897–1905 (1990).
436. Patel, V.V., M.W. Vannier, J.L. Marsh, and L.-J. Lo. Evaluation of digital surgical simulation. In: *Proc. CAR'95* (Berlin, Germany: Springer-Verlag, 1995), pp. 783–788.
437. Lo, L.-J., J.L. Marsh, V.V. Patel, and M.W. Vannier. Craniofacial surgical simulation and outcome validation. In: *Proc. CAR'95* (Berlin, Germany: Springer-Verlag, 1995), pp. 789–794.
438. Lo, L.-J., J.L. Marsh, M.W. Vannier, and V.V. Patel. Craniofacial computer-assisted surgical planning and simulation, *Clin. Plast. Surg.* 21:501–516 (1994).
439. Patel, V.V., M.V. Vannier, J.L. Marsh, and L.-J. Lo. Assessing craniofacial surgical simulation, *IEEE Comput. Graph. Appl.* 16(1):46–54 (1996).
440. Xiao, H. and I.T. Jackson. Surface matching: application in post-surgical/post-treatment evaluation. In: *Proc. CAR'95* (Berlin, Germany: Springer-Verlag, 1995), pp. 804–811.
441. Frey, P., B. Sarter, and M. Gautherie. Fully automated mesh generation for 3-D domains based upon voxel sets, *Int. J. Numerical Methods Eng.* 37:2735–2753 (1994).
442. Shibata, N., T. Ide, E.Y.S. Caho, and A. Inoue. Simplified 2-D interface stress analysis for a femoral stem: a comparative study of the finite element method, *Comput. Aided Surg.* 1:68–69 (1994).
443. Bandak, F.A., M.J. Vander Vorst, L.M. Stuhmiller, P.F. Mlakar, W.E. Chilton, and J.H. Stuhmiller. An imaging-based computational and experimental study of skull fracture: finite element model development, *J. Neurotrauma* 12:679–688 (1995).
444. Edinger, D., K. Rall, P. V. Schroeter, and S. Ehrenreich. Computer-aided single tooth restoration. In: *Proc. CAR'95* (Berlin, Germany: Springer-Verlag, 1995), pp. 964–968.
445. Earnshaw, E.A., M.A. Gigante, and H. Jones, eds. *Virtual reality systems* (London: Academic Press, 1993) pp. 1–327.
446. Faulkner, G. and M. Krauss. Evaluation of 3D input and output devices for the suitability for medical applications. In: *Proc. CAR'95* (Berlin, Germany: Springer-Verlag, 1995), pp. 1069–1074.
447. Fisher, S.S., M. McGreevy, J. Humphries, and W. Robinett. Virtual environment display system. In: Crow, F. and S. Pizer, eds. *Proc. 1986 Workshop on 3D Graphics in Chapel Hill, NC, Oct. 23–24, 1986* (New York, NY: Assoc. for Computing Machinery, 1987), pp. 77–87.
448. Graham, J.A. Virtual reality in medicine, *Austr. J. Otolaryngol.* 1:409–414 (1994).
449. Kobayashi, M., T. Fujino, T. Kaneko, H. Chiyokura, K. Enomoto, K. Shiohata, et al. The virtual reality technique in simulation surgery — mandibular fracture model, *Comput. Aided Surg.* 1:iv–viii (1994).
450. Sukthankar, S.M. and N.P. Reddy. Force feedback issues in minimally invasive surgery. In: Satava, R.M., K. Morgan, H.B. Sieburg, R. Mattheus, and J.P. Christensen, eds. *Interactive technology and the new paradigm for healthcare* (Amsterdam, the Netherlands: IOS Press, 1995), pp. 375–379.

451. Satava, R.M. Medical applications of virtual reality, *J. Med. Syst.* 19:275–280 (1995).
452. Sims, D. The point where lines converge, *IEEE Comput. Graph. Appl.* 13(7):7–9 (1993).
453. Merril, J.R., G.L. Merril, R. Raju, A. Millman, D. Meglan, G.M. Preminger, et al. Photorealistic interactive three-dimensional graphics in surgical simulation. In: Satava, R.M., K. Morgan, H.B. Sieburg, R. Mattheus, and J.P. Christensen, eds. *Interactive technology and the new paradigm for healthcare* (Amsterdam, the Netherlands: IOS Press, 1995), pp. 244–252.
454. Spitzer, V.M., M.J. Ackerman, A.L. Scherzinger, and D. Whitlock. The visible human male: a technical report, *J. Am. Med. Informatics Assoc.* 3(2):118–130 (Mar 1996).
455. Kerr, J., P. Ratiu, and M. Sellberg. Volume rendering of visible human data for an anatomical virtual environment. In: Weghorst, S.J., H.B. Sieburg, and K.S. Morgan, eds. *Health care in the information age* (Amsterdam, the Netherlands: IOS Press, 1996), pp. 352–370.
456. Sellberg, M., D. Murray, D. Knapp, T. Teske, K. Lattie, and M. Vanderploeg. Virtual Human™: an automated virtual environment for computer-aided instruction and biomechanical analysis. In: Satava, R.M., K. Morgan, H.B. Sieburg, R. Mattheus, and J.P. Christensen, eds. *Interactive technology and the new paradigm for healthcare* (Amsterdam, the Netherlands: IOS Press, 1995), pp. 340–348.
457. Cameron, B.M., A. Manduca, and R.A. Robb. Patient-specific anatomic models: geometric surface generation from three-dimensional medical images using a specified polygonal budget. In: Weghorst, S.J., H.B. Sieburg, and K.S. Morgan, eds. *Health care in the information age* (Amsterdam, the Netherlands: IOS Press, 1996), pp. 447–460.
458. Satava, R.M. Virtual reality, telesurgery, and the new world order of medicine, *J. Image Guided Surg.* 1:12–16 (1995).
459. Voelter, S. and K.-L. Kraemer. Virtual reality in medicine: a functional classification. In: *Proc. CAR'95* (Berlin, Germany: Springer-Verlag, 1995), pp. 1297–1298.
460. Alberti, C. Three-dimensional CT and structure models, *Br. J. Radiol.* 53:261–262 (1979).
461. Altschuler, B.R. and G.T. Herman. Head and neck 3-D mapping derived from computed tomographic serial scans. In: *Proc. 6th Conf. on Computer Applications in Radiology and Computer-Aided Analysis of Radiological Images* (Newport Beach, CA: IEEE Computer Soc., 1979), pp. 81–85.
462. Tonner, H.-D. and H. Engelbrecht. Ein neues Verfahren zur Herstellung alloplastischer Spezialimplantate für den Becken-Teilersatz, *Fortschr. Med.* 97:781–783 (1979).
463. Vannier, M.W., J.L. Marsh, M.H. Gado, W.G. Totty, L.A. Gilula, and R.G. Evens. Clinical applications of three-dimensional surface reconstructions from CT scans: experience with 250 patient studies, *Electromedica* 51:121–131 (1983).
464. Schmidt, G.G. Verarbeitung von Bilddaten und Modell bauprozeß, *Biomed. Technik.* 40(suppl. 3):7–11 (1995).
465. Kliegis, U.G., R. Ascherl, and H. Kärcher. Anatomical models in surgery planning — applications and manufacturing techniques. In: *Proc. CAR'95* (Berlin, Germany: Springer-Verlag, 1995), pp. 885–892.
466. White, D.N. Method of forming implantable prostheses for reconstructive surgery, *U.S. Patent 4436683* (U.S. Patent Office. 3 June 1982).
467. White, D.N. Multidimensional surgical imaging: changing the link between radiologist and surgeon, *Admin. Radiol.* 5:51–54 (1986).
468. Woolson, S.T., P. Dev, L.L. Fellingham, and A. Vassiliadis. Three-dimensional imaging of the ankle joint from computerized tomography, *Foot Ankle* 6:2–6 (1985).
469. Woolson, S.T., P. Dev, L.L. Fellingham, and A. Vassiliadis. Three-dimensional imaging of bone from computerized tomography, *Clin. Orthoped.* 202:239–248 (1986).
470. Woolson, S.T. Three-dimensional bone imaging and preoperative planning of reconstructive hip surgery, *Contemp. Orthoped.* 12(5):13–22 (1986).
471. Southard, T.E., J.H. Morris, K.A. Southard, and D.L. Zeitler. A three-dimensional system for planning orthognathic surgery, *J. Am. Dent. Assoc.* 125:452–459 (1994).
472. Donlon, W.C., P. Young, and A. Vassiliadis. Three-dimensional computed tomography for maxillofacial surgery: report of cases, *J. Oral Maxillofacial Surg.* 46:142–146 (1988).
473. Kaplan, E.N. 3D CT images for facial implant design and manufacture, *Clin. Plast. Surg.* 14:663–676 (1987).
474. Lambrecht, J.T. *3-D modeling technology in oral and maxillofacial surgery* (Carol Stream, IL: Quintessence, 1995), pp. 5–145.

475. Brix, F. Vorstellung eines Styrodyrschneide- und fräsgerätes für die Strahlentherapie, *Strahlentherapie* 157:260–263 (1981).
476. Fleiner, B., B. Hoffmeister, T. Kreusch, and T. Lambrecht. Dreidimensionale Operationsplanung am Modell — eine kritische Bestandsaufnahme, *Fortschr. Kiefer-Gesichts-Chir.* 39:13–16 (1994).
477. Zonneveld, F.W. and M.F. Noorman van der Dussen. Three-dimensional imaging and model fabrication in oral and maxillofacial surgery, *Oral Maxillofacial Surg. Clin. N. Am.* 4:19–33 (1992).
478. Brix, F. and J.T. Lambrecht. Individuelle Schädelmodellherstellung auf der Grundlage computertomographischer Informationen, *Fortschr. Kiefer-Gesichts-Chir.* 32:74–78 (1987).
479. Lambrecht, J.T. Planning orthognathic surgery with three-dimensional models, *Int. J. Adult Orthognath. Surg.* 4:141–144 (1989).
480. Maejima, S., S. Tajima, Y. Tanaka, K. Imai, and K. Yab. Use of 3-D solid model complete with study model in maxillofacial surgery, *Comput. Aided Surg.* 1:41–43 (1994).
481. Kärcher, H. and W. Kopp. Dreidimensionale CT- und Modellplanung kraniofazialer Operationen, *Z. Stomatol.* 88:183–204 (1991).
482. Matsuno, T., K. Kaneda, K. Shimakage, and S. Matsuno. Three dimensional image reconstruction of dysplastic hip using 3-D milling system, *Comput. Aided Surg.* 1:69–70 (1994).
483. Lambrecht, J.T. Clinical utility of simulation surgery models: state of the art, *Comput. Aided Surg.* 1:18–20 (1994).
484. Imai, K., S. Tajima, Y. Tanaka, S. Maejima, and K. Yab. Use of 3-D solid models in craniofacial synostosis surgery, *Comput. Aided Surg.* 1:34–35 (1994).
485. Zonneveld, F.W., M.F. Noorman van der Dussen, U. Kliegis, and P.F.G.M. Van Waes. Volumetric CT-based model milling in rehearsing surgery. In: *Proc. CAR'91* (Berlin, Germany: Springer-Verlag, 1991), pp. 347–353.
486. Schmitz, H.-J., T. Tolxdorff, J. Honsbrok, A. Harders, G. LaBorde, and J. Gilsbach. Computer-assisted 3-D reconstruction and interactive manufacturing of alloplastic cranial and maxillofacial implants. In: *Proc. SCAR'90* (Symposia Foundation, 1990), pp. 479–485.
487. Kärcher, H. Three-dimensional cranifacial surgery: transfer from a three-dimensional model (Endoplan) to clinical surgery: a new technique (Graz), *J. Cranio-Maxillo-Facial Surg.* 20:125–131 (1992).
488. Solar, P., C. Ulm, H. Imhof, G. Watzek, R. Blahout, H. Gruber, and M. Matejka. Precision of three-dimensional CT-assisted model production in the maxillofacial area, *Eur. Radiol.* 2:473–477 (1992).
489. Santler, G., H. Kärcher, C. Ruda, and R. Kern. The accuracy of three-dimensional models: analysis and correction of possible errors, *Comput. Aided Surg.* 2:3–11 (1992).
490. Zonneveld, F.W. Seeing is believing, *Medicamundi* 38:5–15 (1993).
491. Kobayashi, M., T. Fujino, T. Kaneko, I. Tanaka, H. Chiyokura, T. Kurihara, et al. Computer-aided surgery in plastic and reconstructive surgery using laser lithography models and virtual reality technique. In: *Proc. CAR'95* (Berlin, Germany: Springer-Verlag, 1995), pp. 1061–1065.
492. Ono, I., H. Gunji, F. Kaneko, S. Numazawa, and N. Kodama. Treatment of extensive cranial bone defects using computer-designed hydroxiapatite ceramics (abstr.), *Comput. Aided Surg.* 1:35 (1994).
493. Yoshimura, Y., T. Nakajima, Y. Nakanishi, K. Onishi, T. Nishiyama, K. Katada, and S. Koga. Preoperative shaping of high-strength apatite ceramics using 3D modelling method: application to craniomaxillofacial surgery, *Comput. Aided Surg.* 1:35–36 (1994).
494. Bill, J.S., J.F. Reuther, W. Dittmann, N. Kübler, J.F. Meier, H. Pistner, and G. Wittenberg. Stereolithography in oral and maxillofacial operation planning, *Int. J. Oral Maxillofacial Surg.* 24:98–103 (1995).
495. Bill, J.S., J.F. Reuther, W. Dittmann, H. Collmann, and H. Pistner. Der klinische Einsatz von Planungsmodellen in der Rekonstruktion von Schädeldefekten und Fehlbildungen, *Biomed. Technik.* 40(suppl. 3):41–46 (1995).
496. Pistner, H., J. Reuther, N. Kübler, and J. Bill. Perspektiven biodegradierbarer Materialien, *Biomed. Technik.* 40(suppl. 3):24–27 (1995).
497. Kübler, N. Defektrekonstruktion des Schädels mit osteoinduktiven Implantaten, *Biomed. Technik.* 40(suppl. 3):28–35 (1995).
498. Yabu, K., S. Tajima, and K. Imai. Evaluation and treatment of enophthalmos using solid modelling, *Comput. Aided Surg.* 1:37 (1994).

499. Fleiter, T., R. Niemeier, J. Bauer, and J.M. Brown. Preoperative planning and surgical tools with spiral CT and rapid prototyping. In: *Proc. CAR'95* (Berlin, Germany: Springer-Verlag, 1995), pp. 909–912.
500. Wehmöller, M., H. Eufinger, D. Kruse, and W. Maßberg. CAD by processing of computed tomography data and CAM of individually designed prostheses, *Int. J. Oral Maxillofacial Surg.* 24:90–97 (1995).
501. Eufinger, H., M. Wehmöller, M. Schoz, and E. Machtens. Die Rekonstruktion kraniofazialer Knochendefekte mit präoperativ gefertigten individuellen Titanimplantaten, *Biomed. Technik.* 40(suppl. 3):36–40 (1995).
502. Eufinger, H., M. Wehmöller, A. Harders, and L. Heuser. Prefabricated prostheses for the reconstruction of skull defects, *Int. J. Oral Maxillofacial Surg.* 24:104–110 (1995).
503. Neugebauer, P.J. Interactive segmentation of dentistry range images in CIM systems for the construction of ceramic inlays using edge tracing. In: *Proc. CAR'95* (Berlin, Germany: Springer-Verlag, 1995), pp. 969–974.
504. Toennies, K.D., J.K. Udupa, G.T. Herman, I.L. Wornom, and S.R. Buchman. Registration of 3D objects and surfaces. *IEEE Comput. Graph. Appl.* 10(3):52–62 (1990).
505. Hull, C.W. Apparatus for production of three-dimensional objects by stereolithography, *U.S. Patent 4575330* (U.S. Patent Office, 11 March 1986).
506. Mancovich, N.J., A.M. Cheeseman, and N.G. Stoker. The display of three-dimensional anatomy with stereolithographic models, *J. Digital Imaging* 3:200–203 (1990).
507. Herbert, A.J. Solid object generation, *J. Appl. Photogr. Eng.* 8:185–188 (1982).
508. Brennan, P., H. Stucki, A. Ghezal, P. Stucki, and W.A. Fuchs. Three-dimensional printing from Somatom Plus CT data. In: Felix, R. and M. Langer, eds. *Advances in CT II* (Berlin, Germany: Springer-Verlag, 1992), pp. 207–210.
509. Klein, H.M., W. Schneider, J. Nawrath, T. Gernot, E.D. Voy, and R. Krasny. Stereolithographische Modellfertigung auf der Basis dreidimensional rekonstruierter CT-schnittbildfolgen, *Fortschr. Röntgenstr.* 156:429–432 (1992).
510. Pomerantz, I., J. Cohen-Sabban, A. Blieber, J. Kamir, M. Katz, and M. Nagler. Three dimensional modelling apparatus, *U.S. Patent 4961154* (U.S. Patent Office, 2 Oct. 1990).
511. Pomerantz, I., S. Gilad, Y. Dollberg, B. Ben-Ezra, Y. Sheinman, G. Barequet, et al. Three dimensional modelling apparatus, *U.S. Patent 5031120* (U.S. Patent Office, 9 July 1991).
512. Ono, I., H. Gunji, K. Suda, and F. Kaneko. Method for preparing an exact-size model using helical volume scan computed tomography, *Plast. Reconstr. Surg.* 93:1363–1371 (1994).
513. Sichting, A., V,. Hietschold, and K. Köhler. Stereo-lithography of the skull: effect of CT filter kernel selection on bone segmentation. In: *Proc. CAR'95* (Berlin, Germany: Springer-Verlag, 1995), pp. 900–902.
514. Komori, T., T. Takato, and T. Akagawa. Use of a laser-hardened three-dimensional replica for simulated surgery, *J. Oral Maxillofacial Surg.* 52:516–521 (1994).
515. Wolf, H.P., A. Lindner, W. Millesi, and M. Rasse. High precision 3-D model design using CT and stereolithography, *Comput. Aided Surg.* 1:46–48 (1994).
516. Ono, I., H. Gunji, T. Tateshita, and F. Kaneko. Method for preparing an exact-size model using helical volume scan CT data and its clinical significance. In: *Proc. CAR'95* (Berlin, Germany: Springer-Verlag, 1995), pp. 903–908.
517. Yau, Y.Y., J.F. Arvier, and T.M. Barker. Technical note: maxillofacial biomodelling — preliminary result, *Br. J. Radiol.* 69:519–523 (1995).
518. Anderl, H., D. Zur Nedden, W. Mühlbauer, K. Twerdy, E. Zanon, K. Wicke, and R. Knapp. CT-guided stereolithography as a new tool in craniofacial surgery, *Br. J. Plast. Surg.* 47:60–64 (1994).
519. Tanino, R., G. Takayama, T. Sakakibara, T. Kihara, N. Shigemura, and K. Furuhata. Simulated surgery using a facial bone replica: a case study of hemifacial microsomia, *Comput. Aided Surg.* 1:43–44 (1994).
520. Millesi, W., M. Rasse, R. Eglmeier, A. Lindner, G.A. Schobel, and I. Friede. Preoperative 3D model planning for reconstruction of the maxilla and the mandible. In: *Proc. CAR'95* (Berlin, Germany: Springer-Verlag, 1995), pp. 939–944.
521. Lindner, A., M. Rasse, H.P. Wolf, W. Millesi, R. Eglmeier, and I. Friede. Stereolithographic skull reconstructions for preoperative planning in cranio-maxillofacial surgery. In: *Proc. CAR'95* (Berlin, Germany: Springer-Verlag, 1995), pp. 1223–1228.

522. Takato, T., K. Harii, S. Hirabayashi, T. Kihara, N. Shigemura, and K. Furuhata. Accurate skull replicas for simulation surgery, *Comput. Aided Surg.* 1:45–46 (1994).
523. Matsuzaki, K., I. Kasem, H. Nishitani, F. Shichijo, K. Matsumoto, Y. Fukumori, et al. 3-D solid model reconstruction for surgical approach, *Comput. Aided Surg.* 1:40–41 (1994).
524. Brown, D.R. A study of the behaviour of a thin sheet of moving liquid, *J. Fluid Mech.* 10:297–307 (1960).
525. Vancraen, W. and K. Renap. *Curtain recoating* (Heverlee, Belgium: Materialise NV, 9 Feb. 1996). Patent application (Patent bureau M.F.J. Bockstael).
526. McAloon, K., M.R. Edwards, and A.H. Popat. Selectively-coloured stereolithography models, *EARP-News.* 7:1,8–9 (Dec. 1995).
527. Vancraen, W. and B. Swaelens. Rapid prototyping techniques for medical modelling (abstr.). In: *Rapid prototyping in medicine & computer-assisted surgery, program & abstracts* (Erlangen, 19–21 Oct. 1995), p. 19.
528. Gebhardt, A., J. Bier, and B. Hell. Anatomic facsimile models: procedure, examples, trends. In: *Proc. CAR'95* (Berlin, Germany: Springer-Verlag, 1995), pp. 893–899.
529. Netherway, D.J., A.H. Abbott, J.R. Abbott, and D.J. David. Craniofacial landmarks, models and prostheses. In: *Proc. CAR'95* (Berlin, Germany: Springer-Verlag, 1995), pp. 921–926.
530. DelBalso, A.M., F.G. Greiner, and M. Licata. Role of diagnostic imaging in evaluation of the dental implant patient, *RadioGraphics* 14:699–719 (1994).
531. Bauer, J., T. Kaus, T. Grunert, T. Fleiter, R. Niemeier, and M. Schaich. CT-data-based construction of a dental drilling device. In: *Proc. CAR'95* (Berlin, Germany: Springer-Verlag, 1995), pp. 958–963.
532. Hemmy, D.C. Internal fixation of the lumbar spine: further clinical experience using computer assisted design and manufacture of a precise system (abstr.), *Comput. Aided Surg.* 1:76 (1994).
533. Radermacher, K., H.-W. Staudte, and G. Rau. Technique for better execution of CT scan planned orthopedic surgery on bone structures. In: *Proc. CAR'95* (Berlin, Germany: Springer-Verlag, 1995), pp. 933–938.
534. Rose, E.H., M.S. Norris, and J.M. Rosen. Application of high-tech three-dimensional imaging and computer-generated models in complex facial reconstructions with vascularized bone grafts, *Plast. Reconstr. Surg.* 91:252–264 (1992).
535. Englmeier, K.-H., M. Haubner, U. Fink, and B. Fink. Image analysis and synthesis of multimodal images in medicine, *Comput. Methods. Prog. Biomed.* 43:193–206 (1994).
536. Peters, T.M., C.J. Henri, P. Munger, A.M. Takahashi, A.C. Evans, B. Davey, and A. Olivier. Integration of stereoscopic DSA and 3D MRI for image-guided neurosurgery, *Comput. Med. Imaging Graph.* 18:289–299 (1994).
537. Pietrzyk, U., K. Herholz, A. Schuster, H.-M. von Stockhausen, H. Lucht, and W.-D. Heiss. Clinical applications of registration and fusion of multimodality brain images from PET, SPECT, CT, and MRI, *Eur. J. Radiol.* 21:174–182 (1996).
538. Trobaugh, J.W., W.D. Richard, K.R. Smith, and R.D. Bucholz. Frameless stereotactic ultrasonography: method and applications, *Comput. Med. Imaging Graph.* 18:235–246 (1994).
539. Barfuss, H., R. Graumann, and D. Petersen. A multimodality workstation for use in neurosurgery and neuroradiology. In: *Proc. CAR'95* (Berlin, Germany: Springer-Verlag, 1995), pp. 853–858.
540. Hemler, P.F., T.S. Sumanaweera, P.A. Van den Elsen, S. Napel, and J. Adler. A versatile system for multimodality image fusion, *J. Image Guided Surg.* 1:35–45 (1995).
541. Schad, L.R., S. Blüml, J. Debus, J. Scharf, and W.J. Lorenz. Improved target volume definition for precision radiotherapy planning of meningiomas by correlation of CT and dynamic, Gd-DTPA-enhanced FLASH MR imaging, *Radiother. Oncol.* 33:73–79 (1994).
542. Rubin, J.M. and R.E. Sayre. A computer-aided technique for overlaying cerebral angiograms onto computed tomograms, *Invest. Radiol.* 13:362–367 (1978).
543. Kikuchi, K., M. Kowada, H. Ogayama, J. Sasanuma, and K. Watanabe. Automated image processing by PACS as a simple tool for designing craniotomy: synthesis of sagittal reconstructed CT images and cerebral angiogram, *Comput. Aided Surg.* 1:56–58 (1994).
544. Gallen, C.C., R. Bucholz, and D.F. Sobel. Intracranial neurosurgery guided by functional imaging, *Surg. Neurol.* 42:523–530 (1994).

545. Ten Haken, R.K., A.F. Thornton Jr., H.M. Sandler, M.L. LaVigne, D.J. Quint, B.A. Fraass, et al. A quantitative assessment of the addition of MRI to CT-based, 3-D treatment planning of brain tumors, *Radiother. Oncol.* 25:121–133 (1992).
546. Hawkes, D.J., C.F. Ruff, D.L.G. Hill, C. Studholme, P.J. Edwards, W.L. Wong, and A. Padhani. Three-dimensional multimodal imaging in image-guided interventions, *Semin. Interv. Radiol.* 12:63–74 (1995).
547. Gandhe, A.J., D.L.G. Hill, C. Studholme, D.J. Hawkes, C.F. Ruff, T.C.S. Cox, et al. Combined and three-dimensional rendered multimodal data for planning cranial base surgery: a prospective evaluation, *Neurosurgery* 35:463–470 (1994).
548. Gamboa-Aldeco, A., L.L. Fellingham, and G.T.Y. Chen. Correlation of 3D surfaces from multiple modalities in medical imaging, *SPIE Proc.* 626:467–473 (1986).
549. Hoh, C.K., M. Dahlbom, G. Harris, Y. Choi, R.A. Hawkins, M.E. Phelps, and J. Maddahi. Automated iterative three-dimensional registration of positron emission tomography images, *J. Nucl. Med.* 34:2009–2018 (1993).
550. Shepard, S. MRI volume rendering in paediatric neuro oncology, *Medicamundi* 40:27–31 (1995).
551. Henri, C.J., G.B. Pike, D.L. Collins, and T.M. Peters. Three-dimensional display of cortical anatomy and vasculature: magnetic resonance angiography versus multimodality integration, *J. Digital Imaging* 4:21–27 (1991).
552. Peters, T.M., C.J. Henri, D.L. Collins, L. Lemieux, G.B. Pike, and A. Olivier. Stereotactic neurosurgery planning using integrated three-dimensional stereoscopic images. In: Kelly, P.J. and B.A. Kall, eds. *Computers in stereotactic neurosurgery* (Boston, MA: Blackwell, 1992), pp. 259–270.
553. Zeilhofer, H.-F., R. Sader, R. Kirsten, and M. Lenz. Computer-aided individual transplant design for reconstruction of the mandible. In: *Proc. CAR'95* (Berlin, Germany: Springer-Verlag, 1995), pp. 1353–1358.
554. Van den Elsen, P.A., M.A. Viergever, A.C. Van Huffelen, W. Van der Meij, and G.H. Wieneke. Accurate matching of electromagnetic dipole data with CT and MR images, *Brain Topogr.* 3:425–432 (1991).
555. Girod, S., E. Keeve, and B. Girod. Advances in interactive craniofacial surgery planning by 3D simulation and visualization, *Int. J. Oral Maxillofacial Surg.* 24:120–125 (1995).
556. Levin, D.N., C.A. Pelizzari, G.T.Y. Chen, C.-T. Chen, and M.D. Cooper. Retrospective geometric correlation of MR, CT, and PET images, *Radiology* 169:817–823 (1988).
557. Levin, D.N., X. Hu, K.K. Tan, S. Galhotra, C.A. Pelizzari, G.T.Y. Chen, et al. The brain: integrated three-dimensional display of MR and PET images, *Radiology* 172:783–789 (1989).
558. Kullmann, W.H. and M. Fuchs. Integrated imaging of neuromagnetic reconstructions and morphological magnetic resonance data, *Clin. Phys. Physiol. Meas.* 12(suppl. A):37–41 (1991).
559. Watanabe, E., S. Ishii, T. Watanabe, and S. Manaka. Three-dimensional reconstruction of CT and angiogram (*in japanese*), *Igakunoayumi* 135:206–210 (1985).
560. Peters, T.M., J.A. Clark, A. Olivier, E.P. Marchand, G. Mawko, M. Dieumegarde, et al. Integrated stereotactic imaging with CT, MR imaging, and digital subtraction angiography, *Radiology* 161:821–826 (1986).
561. Kall, B.A. The impact of computer and imaging technology on stereotactic surgery, *Appl. Neurophysiol.* 50:9–22 (1987).
562. Zamorano, L., Z. Jiang, and A.M. Kadi. Computer-assisted neurosurgery system: Wayne State University hardware and software configuration, *Comput. Med. Imaging Graph.* 18:257–271 (1994).
563. Kall, B.A. Comprehensive multimodality surgical planning and interactive neurosurgery. In: Kelly, P.J. and B.A. Kall, eds. *Computers in stereotactic neurosurgery* (Boston, MA: Blackwell, 1992), pp. 209–229.
564. Peifer, J.W., E.V. Garcia, C.D. Cooke, J.L. Klein, R. Folks, and N.F. Ezquerra. 3-D registration and visualization of reconstructed coronary arterial trees on myocardial perfusion distributions, *SPIE Proc.* 1808:225–234 (1992).
565. Barillot, C., B. Gibaud, J.-M. Scarabin, and J.-L. Coatrieux. 3D reconstruction of cerebral blood vessels, *IEEE Comput. Graph. Appl.* 5(12):13–19 (1985).
566. Chen, G.T.Y., M. Kessler, and S. Pitluck. Structure transfer between sets of three dimensional medical imaging data. In: *Proc. Natl. Comput. Assoc. Computer Graphics '85 Sixth Annu. Conf. Expo.* (Fairfax, VA: NCGA, 1985), pp. 171–177.

567. Pelizzari, C.A., G.T.Y. Chen, D.R. Spelbring, R.R. Weichselbaum, and C.-T. Chen. Accurate three-dimensional registration of CT, PET, and/or MR images of the brain, *J. Comput. Assist. Tomogr.* 13:20–26 (1989).
568. Van den Elsen, P.A., E.J.-D. Pol, and M.A. Viergever. Medical image matching — a review with classification, *IEEE Eng. Med. Biol.* 12:26–39 (1993).
569. Guo, J.-F., Y.-L. Cai, and Y.-P. Wang. Morphology-based interpolation for 3D medical image reconstruction, *Comput. Med. Imaging Graph.* 19:267–279 (1995).
570. Landau, P. and E. Schwartz. Subset warping: rubber sheeting with cuts, *CVGIP: Graph. Models Image Process.* 56:247–266 (1994).
571. Benson, P.J. Morph transformation of the facial image, *Image Vision Comput.* 12:691–696 (1994).
572. Boes, J.L., P.H. Bland, T.E. Weymouth, L.E. Quint, F.L. Bookstein, and C.R. Meyer. Generating a normalized geometric liver model using warping, *Invest. Radiol.* 29:281–286 (1994).
573. Christensen, G.E., M.I. Miller, J.L. Marsh, and M.W. Vannier. Automatic analysis of medical images using a deformable textbook. In: *Proc. CAR'95* (Berlin, Germany: Springer-Verlag, 1995), pp. 146–151.
574. Mac Nicol, G. 3D animation inexpensive and effective. *Comput. Graph. World* 16(4):37–44 (1993).
575. Rohlf, F.J. and F.L. Bookstein, eds. *Proceedings of the Michigan Morphometrics Workshop* (Ann Arbor, MI: The University of Michigan Museum of Zoology, 1990), pp. 1–380.
576. Ehricke, H.-H., G. Daiber, R. Sonntag, W. Straßer, M. Lochner, L.R. Schad, and W.J. Lorenz. Interactive 3D-graphics workstations in stereotaxy: clinical requirements, algorithms and solutions, *SPIE Proc.* 1808:548–558 (1992).
577. Kikuchi, K., M. Kowada, H. Ogayama, J. Sasanuma, and K. Watanabe. Sythesized image processing in clinical neurosurgery, *Eur. J. Radiol.* 10:74–83 (1990).
578. Talairach, J. and P. Tournoux. *Co-planar stereotactic atlas of the human brain: 3-dimensional proportional system — an approach to cerebral imaging* (Stuttgart, Germany: Thieme Verlag, 1988).
579. Evans, A.C., S. Marrett, P. Neelin, L. Collins, K. Worsley, W. Dai, et al. Anatomical mapping of functional activation in stereotactic coordinate space, *Neuroimage* 1:43–53 (1992).
580. Bajcsy, R., R. Lieberson, and M. Reivich. A computerized system for the elastic matching of deformed radiographic images to idealized atlas images, *J. Comput. Assist. Tomogr.* 7:618–625 (1983).
581. Tiede, U., M. Bomans, K.-H. Höhne, A. Pommert, Th. Schiemann, and W. Lierse. A computerized three-dimensional atlas of the human skull and brain, *Am. J. Neuroradiol.* 14:551–561 (1993).
582. Vannier, M.W. and D.E. Gayou. Automated registration of multimodality images, *Radiology* 169:860–861 (1988).
583. Van den Elsen, P.A., J.B.A. Maintz, and M.A. Viergever. Geometry driven multimodality matching of brain images. *Brain Topogr.* 5:153–157 (1992).
584. Schouten, J.F. The visual world of the radiologist, *Inst. Perception Res. Annu. Prog. Rep.* 4:129–130 (1969).
585. Burder, D.G. Stereoscopic imaging and its role in medical illustration, *J. Audiovisual Media Med.* 16:66–70 (1993).
586. Yanai, A., H. Segawa, S. Nagata, and H. Asato. Stereoscopy without instruments: a training device, *Radiology* 155:826 (1985).
587. Herman, G.T., W.F. Vose, J.M. Gomori, and W.B. Gefter. Stereoscopic computed three-dimensional surface displays, *RadioGraphics* 5:825–852 (1985).
588. Hildebrand, Scholtz, and Wieting-Pascha. *Das Arteriensystem des Menschen im stereoskopischen Röntgenbild* (4th ed.) (Wiesbaden, Germany: Verlag von J.F. Bergmann, 1917).
589. Bassett, D.L. *A stereoscopic atlas of human anatomy* (Portland, OR: Sawyer's Inc., 1952), reel 34.
590. Hötte, H.H. *Orbital fractures.* (Assen, the Netherlands: Van Gorkum & Co., 1970), pp. 370–383 and separate Polaroid Vectographs.
591. Caulfield, H.J. and C. O'Rear. The wonder of holography, *Natl. Geographic* 165:364–377 (1984).
592. Ogle, P. Hologram on the cover is more than a gimmick, *Diagn. Imaging* 9(11):5 (1987).
593. Hart, S.J. and M.N. Dalton. Display holography for medical tomography. *SPIE Proc.* 1212:116–135 (1990).
594. Skolnick, A.A. New holographic process provides noninvasive, 3-D anatomic views, *JAMA* 271:5–6,8 (1994).
595. Meyers, S., D.J. Sandin, W.T. Cunnally, E. Sandor, and T.A. DeFanti. New advances in computer-generated barrier-strip autostereography, *SPIE Proc.* 1256:312–321 (1990).

596. Hess, W. Lenticular screen, *U.S. Patent 1128979* (U.S. Patent Office, 16 Feb. 1915).
597. Zonneveld, F.W., A.G.M. Huitema, A.H. Joel, M.A. Fernández, P.F.G.M. Van Waes, and B. Ter Haar Romeny. Lenticular system: full-color, limited-angle, autostereoscopic alternative to holography, *RadioGraphics* 16:393–400A (1996).
598. Lam, N.L. A single-stage 3D photographic printer with a key-subject alignment method, World Patent application WO 94/28462 (1994).
599. Gautsch, T.L, E.E. Johnson, and L.L. Seeger. True three dimensional stereographic display of 3D reconstructed CT scans of the pelvis and acetabulum, *Clin. Orthoped.* 305:138–151 (1994).
600. Wentz, K.U., H.P. Mattle, R.R. Edelman, J. Kleefield, G.V. O'Reilly, C. Liu, and B. Zhao. Stereoscopic display of MR angiograms, *Neuroradiology* 33:123–125 (1991).
601. Herman, G.T., W.F. Vose, J.M. Gomori, and W.B. Gefter. Computed stereo motion of three-dimensional surfaces: a video demonstration (abstr.), *Radiology* 157(P):396 (1985).
602. Darvann, T., P. Larsen, S. Kreiborg, S.-E. Madsen, and S. Brockmann. An affordable system for 3D stereo-visualization of tomographic data (abstr.) . In: *Proc. CAR'95* (Berlin, Germany: Springer-Verlag, 1995), p. 1311.
603. Hodges, L.F. and D.F. McAllister. Stereo and alternating-pair techniques for display of computer-generated images, *IEEE Comput. Graph. Appl.* 5(9):38–45 (1985).
604. Lipton, L. and L. Meyer. A flicker-free field-sequential stereoscopic video system, *SMPTE J.* 93:1047–1051 (1984).
605. Hübner, M. and U.G. Kühnapfel. Realtime volume visualization of 3D MRI data for applications in diagnostics and computer-aided surgery (abstr.). In: *Proc. CAR'95* (Berlin, Germany: Springer-Verlag, 1995), p. 1312.
606. Von Pichler, C., K. Rademacher, W. Boeckmann, G. Rau, G. Jakse, and V. Schumpelick. In: Weghorst, S.J., H.B. Sieburg, and K.S. Morgan, eds. *Health care in the information age* (Amsterdam, the Netherlands: IOS Press, 1996), pp. 523–531.
607. Dodgson, N.A., N.E. Wiseman, S.R. Lang, D.C. Dunn, and A.R.L. Travis. Autostereoscopic 3D display in laparoscopic surgery, *Proc. CAR'95* (Berlin, Germany: Springer-Verlag, 1995), pp. 1139–1144.
608. Butterfield, J.F. Autostereoscopy delivers what holography promised, *SPIE Proc.* 199:42–46 (1979).
609. Butterfield, J.F. Autostereoscopic film display, *SPIE Proc.* 271:36–41 (1981).
610. Traub, A.C. Stereoscopic display using rapid varifocal mirror oscillations, *Appl. Optics* 6:152–159 (1967).
611. Soltan, P., J. Trias, W. Dahlke, M. Lasher, and M. McDonald. Laser-based 3D volumetric display system. In: Morgan, K., R.M. Satava, H.B. Sieburg, R. Mattheus, and J.P. Christensen, eds. *Interactive technology and the new paradigm for healthcare* (Amsterdam, the Netherlands: IOS Press, 1995), pp. 349–358.
612. Clifton III, T.E. and F.L. Wefer. Direct volume display devices, *IEEE Comput. Graph. Appl.* 13(7):57–65 (1993).
613. Lucente, M. and T.A. Galyean. Rendering interactive holographic images. In: *Comput. Graph. Proc. SIGGRAPH 95* (New York, NY: ACM Press, 1995), pp. 387–394.
614. Desbat, L. and P. Cinquin. A 3D energy distributor for 3D visualization. In: *Proc. CAR'95* (Berlin, Germany: Springer-Verlag, 1995), pp. 1174–1179.
615. Vannier, M.W. Despite its limitations, 3-D imaging here to stay, *Diagn. Imaging* 9(11):206–210 (1987).
616. Hemmy, D.C. Future directions in three-dimensional imaging. In: Udupa, J.K. and G.T. Herman, eds. *3D imaging in medicine* (Boca Raton, FL: CRC Press, 1991), pp. 331–339.
617. National Electrical Manufacturers Association (NEMA). *Digital imaging and communications in medicine (DICOM)* (Washington, DC: NEMA, 1993), Parts 1–9.
618. Udupa, J.K., D. Odhner, S. Samarasekera, and R. Goncalves. The 3D Viewnix software system data format specification: a generalization of the ACR-NEMA standards to multidimensional data (Philadelphia, PA: Medical Imaging Processing Group, Univ. of Pennsylvania, Sept. 1993) *Techn. Rep. No. MIPG202,* pp. 1–66.
619. Shellabear, M. and W. Kalender, eds. Common Layer Interface (CLI) Version 2.0 (Brite EuRam/EARP), http://www.cs.hut.fiado/rp/rp (1995).
620. Hemmy, D.C. and P.M. Brigman. A comparison of modalities. In: Udupa, J.K. and G.T. Herman, eds. *3D imaging in medicine*, 2nd ed. (Boca Raton, FL: CRC Press, 2000).
621. Satava, R.M., K. Morgan, H.B. Sieburg, R. Mattheus, and J.P. Christensen, eds. *Interactive technology and the new paradigm for healthcare* (Amsterdam, the Netherlands: IOS Press, 1995), pp. 1–459.

622. Weghorst, S.J., H.B. Sieburg, and K.S. Morgan, eds. *Health care in the information age: future tools for transforming medicine* (Amsterdam, the Netherlands: IOS Press, 1996), pp. 1–734.
623. Suzuki, H. and J. Toriwaki. Automatic segmentation of head MRI images by knowledge guided thresholding, *Comput. Med. Imaging Graph.* 15:233–240 (1991).
624. Benn, D.K., J.C. Pettigrew, M. Shim, A.F. Laine, A.A. Mancuso, C.D. De Bose, and H.E. Stambuk. In: *Proc. CAR'95* (Berlin, Germany: Springer-Verlag, 1995), pp. 1021–1027.
625. Flynn, J. Next generation computer architectures for radiology (abstr.). In: *Proc. CAR'95* (Berlin, Germany: Springer-Verlag, 1995), p. 1209.
626. Ayache, N., ed. *Computer vision, virtual reality and robotics in medicine* (Berlin, Germany: Springer-Verlag, 1995), pp. 1–567.
627. Sundaramoorthy, G., J.D. Hoford, E.A. Hoffman, and W.E. Higgins. IMPROMPTU: a system for automatic 3D medical image analysis, *Comput. Med. Imaging Graph.* 19:131–143 (1995).
628. Udupa, J.K. Three-dimensional imaging techniques: a current perspective, *Acad. Radiol.* 2:335–340 (1995).
629. Pun, T., G. Gerig, and O. Ratib. Image analysis and computer vision in medicine, *Comput. Med. Imaging Graph.* 18:85–96 (1994).
630. Polley, J.W. Three-dimensional imaging and computer-generated models in complex facial reconstructions, *Plast. Reconstr. Surg.* 92:1204–1205 (1993).
631. Zador, I.E., V. Salari, and R.J. Sokol. Computer applications in ultrasound imaging, *Ultrasound Q.* 12:205–215 (1994).
632. Akimoto, M., J. Tamai, H. Hyakosoku, and M. Fumiiri. Three-dimensional CT system using a personal computer, *Aesthet. Plast. Surg.* 15:181–185 (1991).
633. Forcade, T. Evaluating 3D on the high end. Part 1. *Comput. Graph. World* 16(10):44–56 (1993).
634. Robertson, B. Toy Story: a triumph of animation, *Comput. Graph. World* 18(8):28–38 (1995).

3 Quantification Using 3D Imaging

Gabor T. Herman

CONTENTS

3.1 INTRODUCTION

Medical three-dimensional (3D) imaging produces "pretty pictures" which, as discussed in the other chapters, can be clinically useful. However, in addition to improved qualitative assessment, 3D imaging provides us with the potential of more accurate quantification than can be done using the original slice images. In this chapter we discuss some methodologies for quantification using the 3D surface imaging approach. Specifically, we describe (1) how the location in the original slices of a point on the displayed 3D surface is identified, (2) how the (3D) distance between two such points is measured, and (3) how a volume enclosed by such a surface is calculated. We follow this by a report on some results that have been obtained regarding the reproducibility and accuracy of these methods, especially in the areas of CT-based osseous landmark identification and MRI-based volumetric analysis of the brain. We then briefly review the literature regarding the application of quantification using 3D imaging to other medical problems. We complete the chapter with a concise discussion of our conclusions.

This is not a survey article; there is a heavy concentration on the approaches taken by the author and his closest colleagues. We do not mean to imply that these are superior to other approaches; they are simply the ones with which we are the most familiar.

0-8493-3179-X/00/$0.00+$.50

3.2 METHODS

3.2.1 3D Surface Image Generation

Although this topic is treated in other chapters, to make the rest of this chapter easily understandable, we give here a brief description of a particular aspect of the MIPG perspective of 3D surface image generation.[1]

The input to a 3D surface image-generating program is a set of slice images. These provide us with one or more values associated with a large number of volume elements (voxels) of known size and location. (For example, it is quite common in MRI to assign more than one value to each voxel by the use of multiple imaging sequences.) The collection of voxels together with their values is referred to as a scene.

These scenes are often preprocessed before going on to the next stage of the program. Typical preprocessing steps are the following:

1. *Subregioning*: This is used to reduce the size of the data set by indicating which region of the original data space contains the object of interest. It can also be used to cut things open, by indicating a subregion which cuts right through the object.
2. *Interpolation*: One often uses the original data to estimate what the data would look like if voxels were smaller and/or more densely spaced. Such a preprocessing step is often performed to estimate data for cube-shaped voxels from the typically not cube-shaped voxels of a CT or MRI scanner.
3. *Derived-scene formation*: Here one assigns to each voxel one or more new values based on the previous values. In MRI, the new values may be pure T1, T2, and proton density values calculated from the values obtained by the imaging technique. A generally useful preprocessing step of this kind assigns to each voxel a gradient (a measure of the rate of change of the value in the neighborhood of the voxel) based on the prior values of that voxel and its neighbors. Often, the derived scene is binary (0–1 valued), obtained, for example, by thresholding the prior values of the voxels. However, it is important to emphasize that there are many other ways of deriving a binary scene from the original scene and these are often superior in their performance to thresholding. One particularly attractive alternative is the so-called fuzzy segmentation.[2,3]

We illustrate these ideas by an example which is quite relevant to the accuracy of volume quantification. Suppose we have CT slices in which voxels are $1 \times 1 \times 2$ mm. Suppose that a CT value of 200 and above is considered indicative of bone. So if a voxel has a CT value of 200 or more assigned to it, one can say that it is at least partially occupied by bone. Now suppose that we wish to estimate the total bone volume in the CT slices. One method is to threshold the values at 200, producing a binary scene in which we count the number n of 1-valued voxels, thus estimating the bone volume to be $2n$ mm^3 (since each voxel is 2 mm^3). Another method is to estimate what a CT scanner would do when the voxel size is $1 \times 1 \times 1$ mm. We can use linear interpolation to estimate CT values for new slices (lying halfway between the old slices) by assigning to each new voxel the average of the two voxel values above and below it. We can then threshold this interpolated scene to obtain a binary scene (of cube-shaped voxels) and count the number of 1-valued voxels as the estimate of bone volume in cubic millimeters. That this sort of approach may indeed improve accuracy has been dramatically visually illustrated by the side-by-side display of binary scenes, one derived from the uninterpolated scene and the other derived from the interpolated scene.[4] A third approach is the so-called shape-based interpolation.[5,6] Here we threshold the voxels just as was done in the first approach. Then we perform an interesting derived-scene formation. We assign a new value 0.5 to every voxel that is 1-valued and shares a face in the slice with a voxel that is 0-valued, and we assign –0.5 to every voxel that is 0-valued and shares a face in the slice with a voxel that is 1-valued. Then we assign (iteratively) values to voxels which have not been previously assigned a value: if they share a face in the slice with a voxel of positive value, they are given a value 1 greater; if they share a face in the slice with a voxel of negative value, they are given a value 1 less. We repeat this process until every voxel has been assigned a new value. The new values indicate distances from the nearest edge (positive for "inside," negative for "outside"). Now we linearly interpolate this derived scene, just as in the second method, to produce a scene with cube-shaped voxels. Finally, we threshold this interpolated scene at value 0 and count the number of 1-valued voxels to estimate bone volume in cubic millimeters. It has been demonstrated that for complex biological objects this approach is even more accurate than the second approach.[5] A comparative study of a number of interpolation methods has been recently published by Grevera and Udupa.[7]

In the MIPG perspective, it is assumed that at the end of the preprocessing stage, the region of the scene is box-shaped (i.e., it is a rectangular parallelepiped) and it is subdivided into equal-sized abutting box-shaped voxels, each with the same number of values assigned to it. The next stage in this approach is surface formation.

We think of a surface as a collection of voxel faces which unambiguously divides the region of the scene into two parts (an inside and an outside) such that one cannot get from one part to the other without crossing the surface. In the terminology of geometry, a surface has to be closed and non-self-intersecting (i.e., for each edge of each voxel face in the surface there is a unique adjacent face in the surface sharing that edge).

Surface formation is particularly simple if the scene is binary. In such a case, a surface element would be defined as a face which separates a 1-valued voxel from a 0-valued voxel. It has been mathematically proven that for any binary scene and for any such surface element, there is a unique surface (consisting of surface elements) containing the given surface element.[8,9] Furthermore, very efficient computer algorithms have been designed to find such surfaces.[10]

However, it is important to realize that computerized surface formation may be performed on scenes which are not binary. For example, Liu[11] devised a method which operates on the original, or linearly interpolated, scene. The final surface produced by Liu's method is determined globally (rather than locally); that is, for any voxel face it is impossible to tell until the computer program completes its work whether or not that face will be part of the surface. This is because Liu's program can "change its mind": if it finds that its current guess at a partial surface cannot be completed in a geometrically consistent manner (so that it becomes closed and non-self-intersecting), then it backtracks and tries again.

However, whichever approach is used, at the end of the surface-formation phase we have at hand one or more surfaces, each described as a set of voxel faces.

The final stage of 3D surface image generation in the MIPG perspective is the display of the surface(s). While our programs are general enough to display surfaces at arbitrary orientations with respect to the display screen, in this discussion we restrict our attention to a special approach.

Consider Figure 3.1. The display screen is assumed to be parallel to the xy plane. We think of the object as lying "behind" the display screen (i.e., in the positive z direction). We express the permissible orientations of the surface (relative to the screen) by a tilt followed by a rotation. As indicated in Figure 3.1, a tilt is a turning of the scene around the x axis, and a rotation is a turning of the resulting tilted scene around the y axis.

In displaying a surface on the display screen, we use the so-called orthographic projection. This can be thought of as follows: for each point d on the display screen, cast a line in the positive z direction (i.e., perpendicular to the screen). The first point s on the surface that is met by this line is going to be the one displayed on the screen at point d.

The details of how such a display can be created are discussed in Chapter 1. Here we restrict ourselves to one observation which will be important later on. For any fixed point s on the surface and for any fixed tilt of the object, the y coordinate of the projection d of s on the screen is the

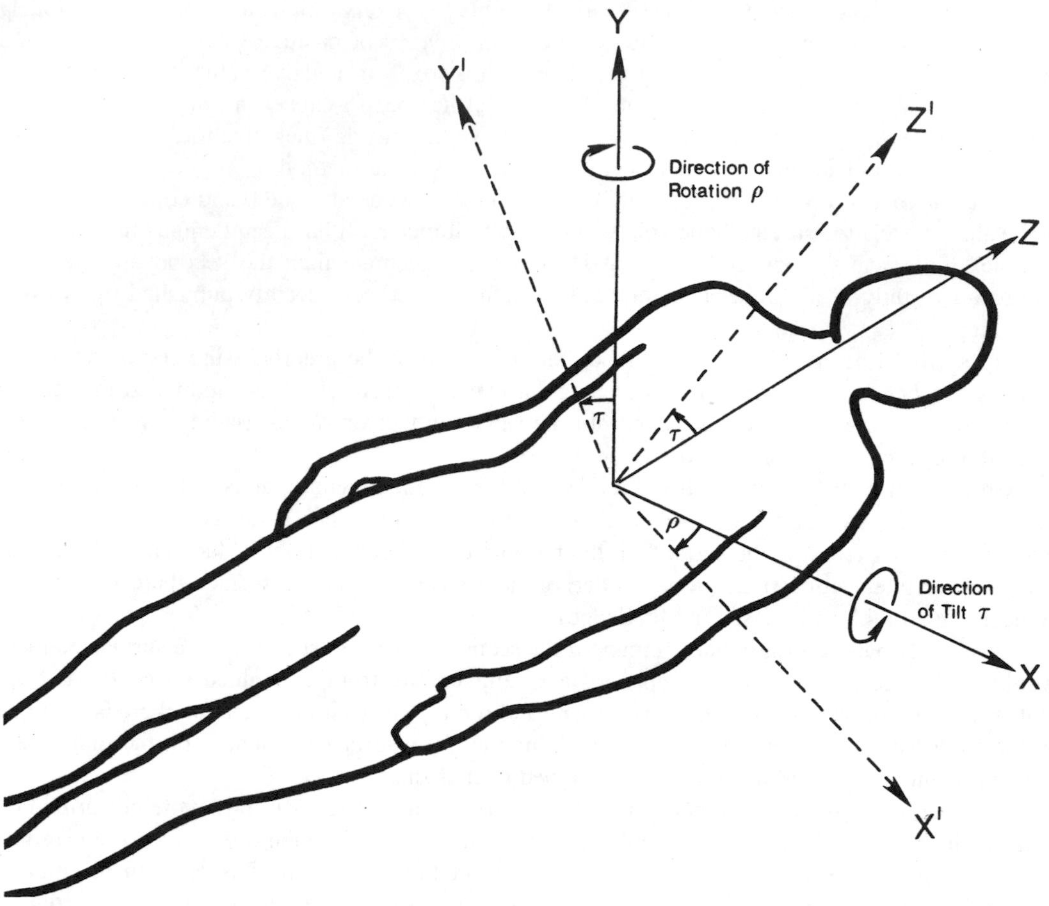

FIGURE 3.1 The definition of "tilt" and "rotation."

same for all rotations. This observation has been successfully used for rapidly obtaining a sequence of displays of a surface as it is rotating (after a single tilt). In what follows we refer to such a sequence of images as a movie.

3.2.2 Point Location

In the first half of this subsection we discuss an approach taken by a specific software package for 3D display and analysis, namely the package 3D98 which was designed to run on the GE 9800 CT scanners.[12] However, the principles that are described are easily transportable.

When 3D98 generates a movie, it stores the images in that movie in the same way the original CT slices are stored. Hence these images can be retrieved and displayed by the standard software of the CT scanner. In particular, one can superimpose a cursor on the image of the surface. A natural question is: Where in the original slices is the point s on the surface which is displayed at the position d where the cursor is on the screen? For example, if a bone surface is being displayed, we might wish to investigate the appearance of soft tissue in the neighborhood of specific points on the surface. Such information is indeed provided by 3D98; for any image in the movie and for any cursor location d on the screen, the user may request the slice location and the pixel location within the slice of the point s in the surface which projects onto d. Furthermore, the information is delivered practically instantaneously. We now explain how this is done.

The essence of the idea is to make the problem manageable by subdividing the display screen into horizontal strips.[13] Since the tilt in a movie is fixed, we can associate with each strip *D* a subset *S* of faces in the surface(s) in such a way that we know that, for any rotation, the surface point *s* displayed at a point *d* in the strip *D* must be on a face which belongs to *S*. If the strips are narrow, then the subsets associated with the strips will contain a small number of faces (relative to the total number of faces in the surface), due to the property of displayed rotations explained in the last subsection. These subsets are worked out once (at the time of the movie generation) and are stored in the computer of the scanner together with the movie. When the user puts a cursor over an image from the movie and requests the location in the original slices of the corresponding surface point, the computer first identifies the strip *D* to which the cursor location *d* belongs and then searches through the associated set of faces *S* to find the scan coordinates of the face which is visible at *d* for the given rotation. Since *S* is relatively small, this is practically instantaneous.

Clearly, such computerized determination of point locations is quite convenient to use. However, even if one has just photographic images from a movie, it is still possible to determine the scan coordinates of surface points. For example, Abbott[14,15] created movies with 9° incremental rotations (using the software system 3D83[16]) and then used consecutive images in these movies as stereo pairs to determine the 3D locations of landmarks.

3.2.3 Distance Calculation

Once the 3D locations of each of a pair of surface points have been identified, the calculation of the (3D) distance between them is quite trivial. Such a capability is provided by many 3D display packages, including 3D83,[16] 3D98,[12] ANALYZE,[17] and 3DVIEWNIX.[18] It is even possible to calculate a curvilinear distance; that is, the distance along that path on the 3D surface which corresponds to a curve drawn on the screen displaying the surface.[13]

3.2.4 Volume Calculation

A very desirable by-product of the surface-display approach to 3D imaging is that the volumes enclosed by the surfaces are obtained essentially free as a result of surface detection.[19] The reason for this is as follows.

The total volume in an object is the sum of the volumes which the object occupies in individual vertical columns of voxels. Now consider a single column of voxels. The intersection of the object with that column can be partitioned into separate segments of contiguous voxels occupied by the object. The volume which the object occupies in the column is the sum of the volumes of these segments. Each segment is bordered by two faces in the surface of the object, with one face pointing up and the other pointing down. Assuming a coordinate system in which up is positive, the volume of the segment is the product of the cross-sectional area of the column (pixel size) and the difference in the coordinate locations of the up-pointing face and the down-pointing face at the two ends of the segment. Hence, to calculate the complete volume enclosed by a surface while detecting the surface we can do the following. We set an accumulator to be initially 0-valued. During surface detection, every time a new up-pointing face is added to the surface, we add its coordinate location to the accumulator and every time a new down-pointing face is added to the surface we subtract its coordinate location from the accumulator. When surface detection is completed, we multiply the value of the accumulator with the pixel size to get the total volume enclosed by the surface.

An alternative to volume calculation via surface detection is to identify all the voxels which are contained in the object of interest and then multiply the number of such voxels with the voxel volume. Increased accuracy can be achieved by using smaller voxels (recall the discussion on bone volume determination in Section 3.2.1) or by estimating partial occupancy of voxels by the object.

3.3 RESULTS

To give a flavor of applicability, reproducibility, and accuracy of those quantitative approaches, we now discuss two different areas with which we have had personal experience: CT-based osseous landmark identification and MRI-based 3D volumetric analysis of the brain. We follow this with a review of the literature on the applicability, reproducibility, and accuracy in other areas of medicine of quantification using 3D imaging.

3.3.1 Osseous Landmark Identification Based on CT

There are a number of reasons why it is desirable to identify the 3D location of osseous landmarks; here we give two of them.

First, the use of standard sets of landmarks opens up the possibility of a mathematical study of craniofacial shape, shape deformity, and shape comparison. Having a normative data set of such landmarks allows one to quantitatively analyze deformity. The same approach can be used for growth evaluation[20] and comparison of anthropological specimens.[14] For these application areas, it is important that researchers use the same set of landmarks.

The second reason is based on the desire to register images of the same patient obtained at different times. For example, it is often useful to register images of the same patient obtained using different modalities, such as MR and PET.[21] Our involvement in this area has a different motivation; we wish to carry out a longitudinal study of the post-operative volume changes of craniofacial onlay bone grafts. Due to fusion of the bone graft to the native bone, it is not possible to accurately identify in a follow-up CT study where the native bone ends and the bone graft starts. However, assuming that the native bone is stable, taking a difference of the bony structures based on CT studies made at different times should provide us with an estimate of volume change due to bone grafts. In order to do this we need to register the two CT studies. We do this by the use of landmarks on the 3D displays of the two bone surfaces obtained from them.[22] In this application the landmarks need not be standard. The user displays the movies made from the two CT studies side by side and can thus discern any landmarks which are clearly identifiable in both 3D images.

In the rest of this subsection we discuss experiments that have been carried out to see how well we can identify osseous landmarks based on 3D surface images.

Abbott[14,15] carried out a comprehensive evaluation for her stereo method of landmark identification (discussed in the last section). Five skulls were scanned on the GE 8800 CT scanner, with a pixel size 0.8×0.8 mm, slice thickness 5 mm, and slice spacing (table shift) 3 mm. The package 3D83[16] was used to produce the surface images. In particular, this package performs an interpolation (prior to thresholding for bone) producing estimated values for abutting cubic voxels of size $0.8 \times 0.8 \times 0.8$ mm. For each of the five skulls, Abbott determined the location of 76 standard landmarks, using her stereo method twice with at least a month in-between. To measure the reproducibility of her method she used the "figure-of-merit"[23]

$$S = \left(\frac{1}{2n} \sum_{i=1}^{n} |X_i|^2 \right)^{1/2}$$

where n is the number of specimens (in this case five) and $|X_i|$ is the 3D distance between the two estimated locations of a particular landmark on the i'th skull. She found that, for the 76 landmarks, S varied between 0.4 and 5.2 mm, with a median of 1.7 mm, which is quite impressive considering the 5-mm slice thickness and 3-mm slice spacing. (Another study, involving three patients, yielded similar results.) A study of the accuracy of these landmark identifications was carried out by comparing, for 31 pairs of landmarks, the distances estimated using the 3D approach with those obtained by craniometric measurements using a caliper. The mean difference ranged from 0.2 mm (with a standard deviation of 0.2 mm) to 9.3 mm (with a standard deviation of 1.5 mm). It was observed that while some of the differences were due to inherent limitations of the CT-based approach (e.g., thin bone projections are unlikely to fully image with 5-mm-thick slices), all the significant differences were due to changes in the perceived definition of the landmarks during the two measurement processes ("the same landmarks were not being measured although referred to by the same name"). Eliminating such non-inherent differences, Abbott found that for the remaining 20 pairs of distances, the mean difference between the two measurement processes was always less than 2.7 mm with a median value of 0.8 mm. She concluded that "three dimensional CT landmark coordinates derived using the multiple stereo imaging technique are consistent with craniometric measurement, provided that the same landmark definitions can be followed for the two measurement techniques."

In order to eliminate the difficulty in landmark definition and to make the use of landmarks identification easier for the non-specialist (such as an X-ray technician), we have attempted to define a number of landmarks (24 to be precise) by unambiguous operational directives.[24] By this we mean the following. First of all, a strict protocol is given which describes precisely the head stabilization and positioning, the scanning technique, and the 3D imaging technique including the subregionings to be used and the number of images in the movies.[25] The following are the directives for the identification of 3 of the 24 landmarks.

1. To identify the left condylion, use the fourth image of the movie of the inferior–anterior subregion of the skull. Find the brightest local point on the lateral part of the condylion head (see Figure 3.2).
2. To identify the nasale, use the first image of the movie of the inferior–anterior subregion of the skull. Find the brightest point in the middle of the nose at its bottom (see Figure 3.3).
3. To identify the opisthocranion, use the seventh image in the movie of the superior–posterior subregion of the skull. Narrow the display window to produce an elliptical region on the back of the skull, and find its center (see Figure 3.4).

To validate the approach, the same skull was scanned twice (with 3 months in-between) on a GE 8800 according to the protocol mentioned in the previous paragraph. (In particular, pixel size was 0.75 mm and slice thickness and slice spacing were both 1.5 mm.) The movies of 3D surface images were generated according to the protocol (using 3D83[16]) and were provided to each of two observers. Each observer had two sessions with each CT study (with at least 2 weeks in between) in which all of the 24 landmarks had to be identified according to the operational directives. Table 3.1 shows the intra-observer and inter-observer reproducibility for the three landmarks of Figures 3.2 to 3.4.

These results are quite typical. The median of the intra-observer differences in the whole study was 0.75 mm, which is the size of one pixel side and half the size of the slice thickness and slice spacing. This is very good. However, the approach clearly fails to overcome inter-observer variability; apparently the directives are not as unambiguous as we thought.

Our experiment also allows us to comment on the inter-study variability of our approach. This is because we can calculate distances between pairs of landmarks; these distances should be the same for the two CT studies. We have found examples in which even though inter-observer variability of the estimated distances was negligible, inter-study variability was much more serious. Our worst example is the distance between the right condylion and the right gonion, which, based on Study 1, was measured to be 34.1 mm by both observers and, based on Study 2, was measured to be 36.9 mm by one and 37.4 mm by the other observer. Such a 3-mm difference between studies may not be acceptable for the applications we have in mind.

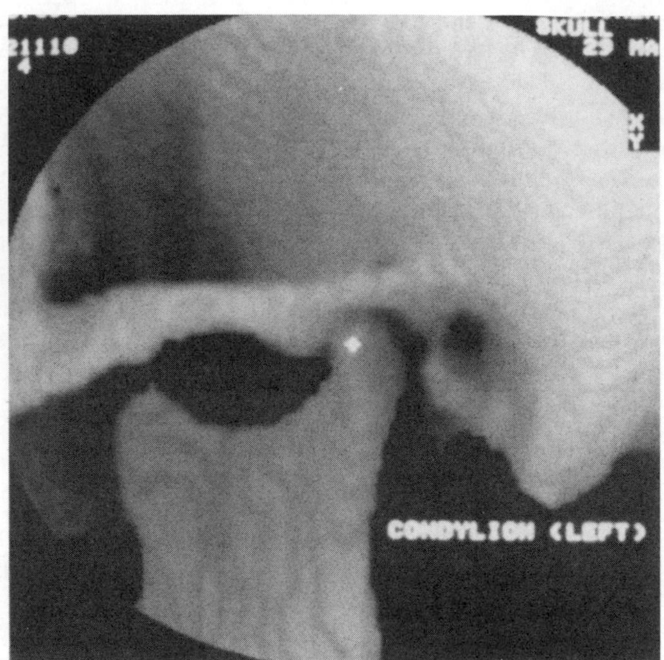

FIGURE 3.2 The location of the left condylion.

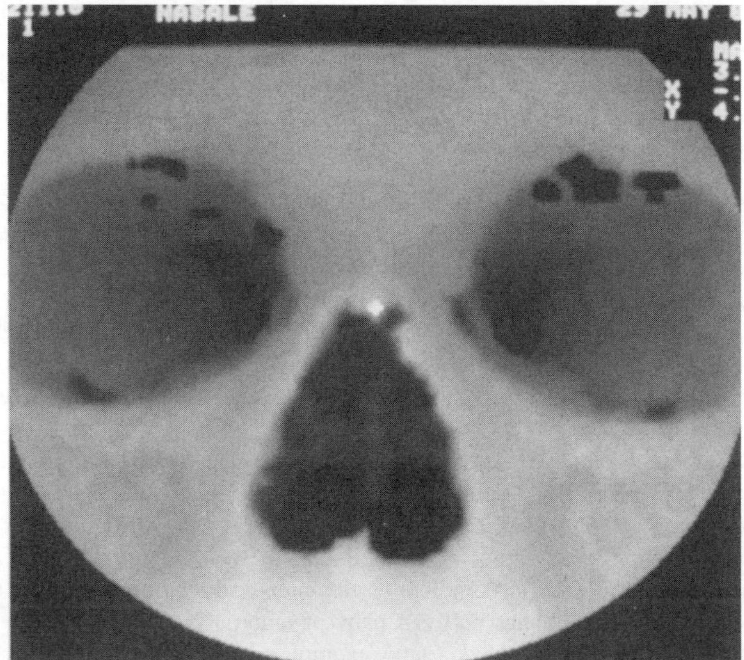

FIGURE 3.3 The location of the nasale.

In fact, the mean of the differences between the distances we calculated based on the two studies was 1.6 mm. To put this into context, we used the methodology described near the beginning of this subsection of displaying the movies made from the two CT studies side by side and

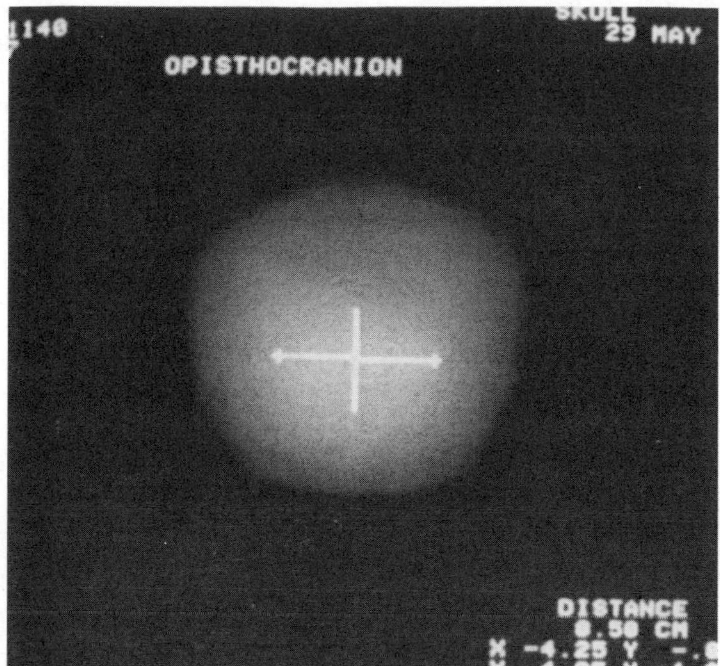

FIGURE 3.4 The location of the opisthocranion.

TABLE 3.1
Intra-Observer and Inter-Observer Variability of Landmarks Defined by Operational Directives

	Study 1			Study 2		
	O1[a]	O2[b]	IO[c]	O1[a]	O2[b]	IO[d]
Left condylion	0.0	0.0	0.8	0.8	2.4	1.1
Nasale	0.0	0.0	2.4	1.1	0.0	4.1
Opisthocranion	0.0	0.8	4.2	1.7	0.8	2.0

Note: Entries are in millimeters. Under O1 (resp. O2) we record the distance between the locations identified as the landmarks in two readings by Observer 1 (resp. 2). Under IO we record the distance between the averages of the two locations identified by each of the observers.

[a] Observer 1.
[b] Observer 2.
[c] Intra-observer.
[d] Inter-observer.

determining landmarks in an ad-hoc way, just because they appear to match. The mean of the differences of distances between these landmarks based on the two studies was less than 0.8 mm. That is about the size of a pixel side and is twice as good as what we obtained based on our operational directives.

It does appear, therefore, that our operational-directive approach, while resulting in excellent intra-observer reproducibility (the size of a pixel side on average), still allows unacceptably large variations between observers (sometimes as much as 4 mm or more). Furthermore, its inter-study reproducibility is not as good as what can be achieved by quite ad-hoc methods. It seems that the very restrictive image-oriented nature of our directives ("find the brightest point" on a certain image) makes them sensitive to minor variations in head positioning and the conciseness of the directives makes them not as unambiguous as is desirable.

We judge the results reported here to be rather encouraging. It appears that even if slice thickness and spacing is twice (or more) the size of a pixel side, variations in estimated landmark locations and inter-landmark distances can be kept down to the size of a pixel side on average and that the same is true regarding accuracy of the distances. However, in order to achieve this level of reproducibility and accuracy for a standard set of landmarks, they and the procedures for identifying them will have to be carefully defined and validated. Studies in this direction have been published by Matteson et al.,[26] Abbott et al.,[27] Hildebolt et al.,[28] and Patel et al.,[29] with the last of these publications assessing the capability not only for landmark identification but also for other quantifications used in craniofacial surgical simulation.

3.3.2 3D Volume Analysis of the Brain Based on MRI

Our research group got involved in MRI-based regional brain volume analysis as a result of our collaboration with researchers in neuropsychiatry. To indicate one motivation in this area, we quote from Herman et al.[30]

> More specifically, we conjecture the following. (i) Specific patterns of atrophy, cerebral blood flow and metabolism can help to distinguish the various sub-types of dementia as well as predict the clinical course and prognosis. (ii) Anatomic differences exist between rapid and slow declining Alzheimer's patients. (iii) Three-dimensional analysis can help to identify the earliest changes of Alzheimer's disease in the temporal lobes. (iv) Detection of subtle regional volume alternations of the temporal lobe can help the diagnosis and therapy of unremitting temporal lobe seizures. (v) Subclassifying clinical variants of schizophrenia requires identification of regional dysfunction. (vi) Clinically valid regional analysis of positron emission tomography images requires correction for spaces occupied by cerebrospinal fluid, and such correction can be achieved based on appropriately registered and segmented magnetic resonance images.

More recently we have been looking into additional hypotheses regarding various diseases of the brain. We list three examples: (1) In babies with cerebral nervous system injury there will be an increase with age in the ratio of unmyelinated to myelinated white matter, with regions of greatest damage showing the greatest increase. (2) The ratio of tumor volume which enhances as a result of intravenous Magnevist to the total tumor volume is directly correlated with survival in gliomas. (3) The ratio of brain volume in multiple sclerosis (MS) to the total brain volume corresponds to clinically defined subgroups of MS.

In order to be able to investigate such hypotheses, in the late 1980s we developed two computer packages for volumetric measurement of brain tissue based on MRI. One package, developed by Kohn,[30,31] requires a certain amount of human decision making. It is an interactive tool which utilizes the window and graphics techniques available on Sun workstations. It has been popular with our colleagues in psychiatry, nuclear medicine, and neuroradiology.[32–34] The other package uses a rule-based approach and is intended to be totally automatic.[35] Since only the first of these packages is available for routine clinical use, we restrict our attention to roughly describing it, as it can be applied to the last of the hypotheses listed above. (More recently we have been using the 3DVIEWNIX[18] package and fuzzy-connectedness principles[36] for this purpose.)

What we need is an estimate of the total brain volume and the volume involved in MS. In our approach we attempt to obtain this information from the MRI study which for each voxel provides us with two values, commonly referred to as PD (for proton density) and T2W (for T2-weighted).[31] As a first step we perform a subregioning to restrict our attention to the intracranial

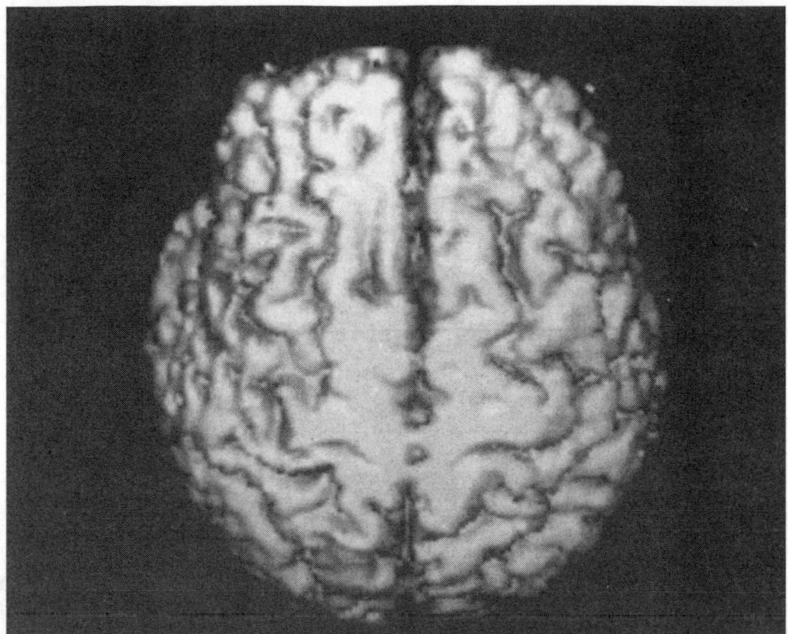

FIGURE 3.5 3D display of surface enclosing brain voxels, based on MRI.

content. This we do based on the observation that the gradient (rate of change) in T2W is particularly large at the interior surface of the skull and hence we can apply a gradient-based surface detector.[11] From this point on we deal only with voxels inside this surface. The total volume inside the surface is occupied by three types of tissue: normal brain (NB), multiple sclerotic lesion (MS), and cerebrospinal fluid (CSF). We attempt to classify each voxel as being associated with one of these categories. (Partial occupancy is taken care of later on by the use of shape-based interpolation.)

The classification is based on a two-feature scatter plot.[37] This is a function defined over a two-dimensional space whose coordinates correspond to the (PD, T2W) values. The idea is that every voxel has a PD and a T2W value and so corresponds to a unique point in the (PD, T2W) plane. The underlying assumption is that the values associated with each of the classes NB, MS, and CSF cluster together and are separable from each other. To find these clusters, one uses Kohn's software package as follows. One draws over the magnetic resonance slice images little regions which contain voxels all of which are unambiguously in the same one of the three classes, and one indicates which class that is. Based on this information, the package automatically subdivides the (PD, T2W) plane into three regions, associated with NB, MS, and CSF, respectively. We have found that this process classifies some voxels as MS, even though they are clearly not, and a further subregioning (for MS only) is a desirable adjunct. This consists of free-hand tracing boundaries enclosing the lesions in each slice. Voxels within these boundaries will be classified into NB, MS, and CSF; voxels outside them will be classified into NB and CSF only.

We can now think of the result obtained so far as three binary scenes, one associated with each of the classes. For the binary scenes associated with NB and MS, we perform shape-based interpolation[5] (described in the last section) to obtain a binary scene with small cubic voxels. The total volumes occupied by these voxels provide us with our desired estimates. In Figure 3.5, we show the 3D display of the surface enclosing the brain voxels in one such binary scene.

The total study described above takes less than half an hour for an experienced user. We have carried out a series of experiments to evaluate the reproducibility and accuracy of such approaches. We now describe one of them.

This experiment was designed to check intra-observer, inter-observer, and inter-study reproducibility. Three volunteers with MS lesions were scanned repeatedly (two of them three times and the other one twice). In each study, approximately 30 slices of 5-mm thickness were obtained, both for PD and for T2W. Three readers were used: (1) a radiology resident, (2) a radiology fellow, and (3) a medical student. Each was asked to estimate total brain and MS lesion volumes. Each reader had four reading sessions arranged such that, by the end, each reader read two studies of each patient and each study was read by at least two readers who read both studies twice. In each session three studies were read, one of each patient, in a randomized order. The readers had no way of identifying (other than by the images) the patients from session to session. Table 3.2 summarizes the experiment and its results.

To analyze these results we define the variability between two estimates α and β of a volume by

$$v = \frac{|\alpha - \beta|}{|\alpha + \beta|} \times 100$$

and say that the variability is $v\%$.

Since every study was read twice by each of at least two readers, we can measure intra-observer variability (see Tables 3.3 and 3.4). The entries are the values of v, when α and β are the estimates given by the same reader for the same study at different times. Brain volume variability was below 6.5% in all cases and averaged 1.7% overall; a very respectable result. On the other hand, the results for MS were much less uniform. The variability of the radiology fellow (Reader 2) was always below 10% and averaged below 5%, but the variability of the medical student (Reader 3) averaged over 25% and got up to 81% in one case. Clearly, careful training is necessary if the system is to be used for MS volume determination.

Inter-observer variability is reported in Table 3.5. Here the entries are the values of v, when α and β are defined as the averages of the estimates by the two observers who are being compared. Pairwise comparisons are given for Patient II, whose scans have been read by all three observers. For brain, the results are again very good; inter-observer variability is always less than 4% and averages 1.6%. In view of the unreliability (as indicated by the large intra-observer variability) of two of the readers for estimating MS volumes, the bad result for inter-observer variability for MS volume estimation is not surprising.

Inter-study variability is reported in Tables 3.6 and 3.7. Here the entries are the value of v, when α and β are defined as the averages of the estimates given at the two readings of the two studies that are being compared. Again, the results for brain are excellent; inter-study variability is always less than 3%, with the overall average less than 1%. On the other hand, the inter-study variability of the MS volume estimates is disappointing. Even for the best reader, all we can say is that the average is under 7%. There is the possibility that this is due to our 5-mm slice thickness (too thick for such small lesions); however, a phantom experiment by Kohn et al.[38] did not yield a significant effect of section thickness.

Accuracy studies for such applications are much more difficult, since there is no reliable gold standard with which we can compare our brain-volume and MS-volume estimates. Our accuracy studies[38] therefore involved scanning bottles containing mainly one type of agarose gel into which we inserted a known volume of another type of agarose gel. A sample result from one such study is shown in Figure 3.6.

To summarize, we found the reproducibility of total brain-volume measurements to be excellent. Other experiments, not reported here, showed similar results for regional brain volumes (such as that of the temporal lobes) and CSF volumes. Our experiments with lesion volumes indicate that to obtain good results we have to improve the training of our users and adjust the imaging method used to obtain data; the accuracy studies with phantoms show that such improvements are likely to be achievable.

TABLE 3.2
Summary of the Reproducibility Experiment

		Patient I			Patient II		Patient III		
Reader	**Session**	**Study I**	**Study II**	**Study III**	**Study I**	**Study II**	**Study I**	**Study II**	**Study III**
1	1		1.1.2 1079 11.5			1.1.1 1037 18.0	1.1.3 1316.5 28.0		
	2			1.2.3 1109 17.3	1.2.1 1093 11.6			1.2.2 1378 17.0	
	3		1.3.1 1095 16.5			1.3.3 1069 15.4	1.3.2 1333 30.2		
	4			1.4.3 1067 20.9	1.4.1 1126 13.1			1.4.2 1326 34.2	
2	1	2.1.1 1070 12.9			2.1.3 1082 10.7				2.1.2 1316 6.2
	2		2.2.1 1077 11.7			2.2.3 1005 12.3		2.2.2 1308 5.4	
	3	2.3.3 1051 15.7			2.3.1 1011 11.0				2.3.2 1335 5.9
	4		2.4.1 1051 14.0			2.4.2 970 14.0		2.4.3 1316 5.4	
3	1			3.1.2 1066 16.6		3.1.1 1067 23.3	3.1.3 1279 77.3		
	2	3.2.3 1086 12.4			3.2.1 1083 12.2				3.2.2 1399 5.5
	3			3.3.1 1091 19.6		3.3.3 1068 19.5	3.3.2 1456 8.1		
	4	3.4.1 1034 11.2			3.4.3 1057 18.7				3.4.2 1319 10.2

Note: The first line of each entry indicates reader number, session number, and the order in which the study was read. The second line is the estimated total brain volume in cubic centimeters. The third line is the estimated MS lesion volume in cubic centimeters.

Validation of brain tissue classification based on MRI is also discussed by Vannier et al.[40] Three-dimensional MRI-based volume analysis of the brain has many uses. We used the software package of Kohn to study gender differences in the age effect on brain atrophy[32] and schizophrenia.[33,34] Recent publications include studies by Robb et al.,[41] which illustrates the use of the ANALYZE[17]

TABLE 3.3
Intra-Observer Variability for Brain

	Patient I			Patient II		Patient III			
Reader	**Study I**	**Study II**	**Study III**	**Study I**	**Study II**	**Study I**	**Study II**	**Study III**	**Average**
1		0.7	1.9	1.5	1.5	0.6	1.9		1.4
2	0.9	1.2		3.4	1.8		0.3	0.7	1.4
3	2.4		1.2	1.2	0.1	6.5		2.9	2.4
Average	1.7	1.0	1.5	2.0	1.1	3.5	1.1	1.6	1.7

TABLE 3.4
Intra-Observer Variability for MS

	Patient I			Patient II		Patient III			
Reader	**Study I**	**Study II**	**Study III**	**Study I**	**Study II**	**Study I**	**Study II**	**Study III**	**Average**
1		17.9	9.4	6.1	7.8	3.8	33.6		13.1
2	9.8	8.9		1.4	6.5		0.0	2.5	4.8
3	5.1		8.3	21.0	8.9	81.0		29.9	25.7
Average	7.4	13.4	8.9	9.5	7.7	42.5	16.8	16.2	14.5

TABLE 3.5
Inter-Observer Variability

	Patient I			Patient II		Patient III			
	Study I	**Study II**	**Study III**	**Study I**	**Study II**	**Study I**	**Study II**	**Study III**	**Average**
Brain	0.0	1.1	0.4	2.9	3.2	1.6	1.5	1.2	1.6
				1.8	0.7				
				1.1	3.9				
MS	9.6	4.3	2.7	6.5	11.9	18.9	65.2	12.9	16.4
				11.1	12.3				
				17.5	23.9				

software system for analyzing brain tumors, and Haller et al.,[42] on the measurement of the human hippocampus based on magnetic resonance images. The quantification of MS based on MRI remains a hotly pursued topic.[43–47] Three-dimensional images of the brain from MR are also used for measuring distances, such as the cortical sulcal lengths.[48]

3.3.3 Other Medical Applications

As stated in the introduction, this is not a survey article. In this subsection we note some of the developments that have taken place in the last decade in the area of quantification using 3D imaging.

Higgins et al.[49] reported on the measurement of the left ventricular chamber volume from 3D CT images, while Boxerman et al.[50] used MRI to evaluate the heart and the great vessels. Studies of lung volumes based on CT were reported by Holbert et al.[51] and Hartman et al.[52] Quantification

TABLE 3.6
Inter-Study Variability for Brain

Reader	Patient I	Patient II	Patient III	Average
1	0.0	2.6	1.0	1.2
2	0.2	2.9	0.5	1.2
3	0.9	0.1	0.3	0.4
Average	0.3	1.9	0.6	0.9

TABLE 3.7
Inter-Study Variability for MS

Reader	Patient I	Patient II	Patient III	Average
1	15.4	15.0	6.4	12.3
2	5.3	9.6	5.7	6.9
3	21.1	16.1	68.9	35.4
Average	13.9	13.6	27.0	18.2

of the airways using "virtual bronchoscopy" was discussed by Summers et al.[53] and McAdams et al.[54] An evaluation of the virtual bronchoscopy methodology was provided by Higgins et al.[55]

Another organ for which volumetric quantification is useful is the liver. McNeal et al.[56] reported on liver volume measurements and 3D display from MRI. Soyer et al.[57] used hepatic volumetric analysis based on CT for surgical decision making.

Finally, we turn to the skeletal system. Vannier et al.[58] carefully compared the diagnostic performance in determining the presence, type, and extent of calcaneal and pelvic fractures using various 3D and 2D imaging modes. A most interesting and edifying part of their conclusion was the following:

> 3D shaded was the most useful of the 3D reconstruction techniques, but only slightly superior to 3D volume. The objective results for the 3D modalities were opposite to the subjective rankings of volumetric and shaded 3D images based on perceived diagnostic value. For subjective rankings, observers expressed a marked preference for volumetric images.

Laine et al.[59] reported on a study for making measurements on the femur which is very similar in nature to the studies for the skull discussed in Section 3.3.1. 3D imaging is also used while doing bone densitometry.[60,61] The ultimate quantification moves to the fourth dimension: temporal sequences of 3D images can be used to quantify the internal kinematics of joints.[62]

3.4 CONCLUSIONS

On the promising side, there have already been a number of good results obtained, and there is every hope that reproducibility and accuracy of quantification based on 3D imaging will continue to improve. For example, both of the studies on osseous landmark identification that we have discussed in Section 3.3.1[14,24] used the old software package 3D83[16] to produce the images. The quality of these images (Figures 3.2 to 3.4) is nowhere near that which can be obtained by the surface-imaging techniques of today (see the illustrations in the other chapters). There is every

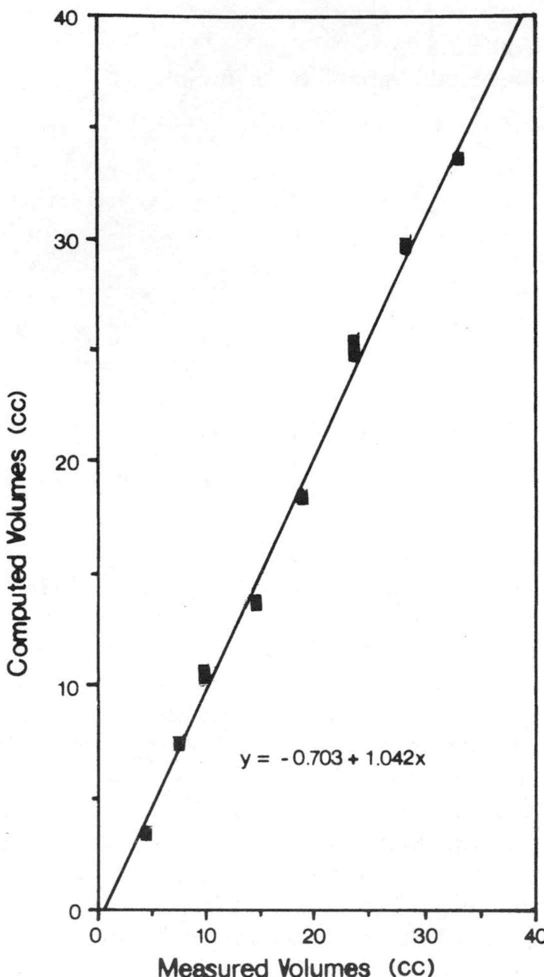

FIGURE 3.6 Plot of computed volumes (superposition of three readings) versus measured volumes for an agarose gel phantom.[38]

reason to believe that improved image quality will result in better performance in landmark identification. Similarly, more work can be done to optimize magnetic resonance image acquisition for the purpose of volumetric analysis of various structures inside the brain. It is hard to imagine that a judicious effort in that direction will not result in significant improvements over the results reported in Section 3.3.2. (An example of what can be done along such lines is provided by the so-called magnetization transfer imaging for the quantification of MS.[46,47]) As we acquire experience, we can improve on rule-based approaches[35] and fuzzy segmentation[2,3,36] resulting in programs which automatically (and hence reproducibly) deliver clinically relevant numbers based on 3D imaging techniques.

It is worth pointing out that the word "accuracy" was not used in the last sentence. It is indeed important not to get hung-up on accuracy; that may unnecessarily impede useful progress. In an area such as MS lesion volume estimation, method accuracy is just about impossible to test. The important question is not whether the number produced is indeed the "volume," but rather whether it is a reliable indicator of the clinical state of the patient. A number which strongly correlates with the volume would serve just as well as the volume itself.[34]

A word of caution: we must point out that there is a danger in computerized quantification: programs provide us with numbers without giving us a feel for their reproducibility and accuracy. To use these numbers without having performed careful validation studies, along the lines of those described in Section 3.3, is foolhardy. Alas, such studies are time consuming and, frankly, boring. It is tempting to simply accept the output of the computer; this temptation must be resisted.

In conclusion, quantification using 3D imaging can, after proper validation, be a useful tool in various areas of medicine. This has been demonstrated in some cases already and the potential for future applications is wide ranging.

ACKNOWLEDGMENT

The research of the author is currently supported by NIH Grant HL28438.

REFERENCES

1. G.T. Herman. Three-dimensional computer graphic display in medicine: The MIPG perspective. In K.H. Höhne, editor, *Pictorial Information Systems in Medicine*, pages 181–210. Springer-Verlag, Berlin, 1986.
2. J.K. Udupa and S. Samarasekera. Fuzzy connectedness and object definition: Theory, algorithms and applications in image segmentation. *Graph. Models Image Process.*, 58:246–261, 1996.
3. B.M. Carvalho, C.J. Gau, G.T. Herman and T.Y. Kong. Algorithms for fuzzy segmentation. In S. Singh, editor, *International Conference on Advances in Pattern Recognition*, pages 154–163. Springer, London, 1998.
4. S.S. Trivedi. Interactive manipulation of three-dimensional binary scenes. *Visual Comp.*, 2:209–218, 1986.
5. S.P. Raya and J.K. Udupa. Shape-based interpolation of multidimensional objects. *IEEE Trans. Med. Imaging*, 9:32–42, 1990.
6. G.T. Herman, J. Zheng and C.A. Bucholtz. Shape-based interpolation. *IEEE Comput. Graph. Appl.*, 12(3):69–79, 1992.
7. G.J. Grevera and J.K. Udupa. An objective comparison of 3-D image interpolation methods. *IEEE Trans. Med. Imaging*, 17:642–652, 1998.
8. G.T. Herman and D. Webster. A topological proof of a surface tracking algorithm. *Comput. Vision Graph. Image Process.*, 23:162–177, 1983.
9. G.T. Herman. *Geometry of Digital Spaces*. Birkhäuser, Boston, MA, 1998.
10. D. Gordon and J.K. Udupa. Fast surface tracking in three-dimensional binary images. *Comput. Vision Graph. Image Process.*, 45:196–241, 1989.
11. H.K. Liu. Two- and three-dimensional boundary detection. *Comput. Vision Graph. Image Process.*, 6:123–134, 1977.
12. J.K. Udupa, G.T. Herman, L.S. Chen, P.S. Margasahayam and C.R. Meyer. 3D98: A turnkey system for the 3D display and analysis of medical objects in CT data. *Proc. SPIE*, 671:154–168, 1986.
13. S.S. Trivedi, G.T. Herman, J.K. Udupa, L.S. Chen and P. Margasahayam. Measurement on 3-D displays in the clinical environment. In *Proceedings of the 7th Annual Conference and Exposition of the National Computer Graphics Association*, volume III, pages 93–100. National Computer Graphics Association, Fairfax, VA, 1986.
14. A.H. Abbott. *The Acquisition and Analysis of Craniofacial Data in Three Dimensions*. Ph.D. thesis, University of Adelaide, Adelaide, South Australia, 1988.
15. A.H. Abbott, D.J. Netherway, D.J. David and T. Brown. Craniofacial osseous landmark determination from stereo computer tomography reconstructions. *Ann. Acad. Med.*, 19:595–604, 1990.
16. L.S. Chen, G.T. Herman, C.R. Meyer, R.A. Reynolds and J.K. Udupa. 3D83 — An easy to use software package for three-dimensional display from computed tomograms. *Proc. SPIE*, 515:309–316, 1984.
17. R.A. Robb and D.P. Hanson. ANALYZE: A software system for biomedical image analysis. In *First Conf. Visualization Biomed. Comput.*, pages 507–518. IEEE, Atlanta, GA, 1990.

18. J.K. Udupa, D. Odhner, S. Samarasekera, R. Goncalves, K. Iyer, K. Venugopal and S. Furuie. 3DVIEWNIX: An open, transportable, multidimensional, multimodality, multiparametric imaging software system. *Proc. SPIE*, 2164:58–73, 1994.
19. J.K. Udupa. Determination of 3D shape parameters from boundary information. *Comput. Graph. Image Process.*, 17:52–59, 1981.
20. J.T. Richtsmeyer, C. Hildebodt and M.W. Vannier. Data collection from C-T images. In *Proceedings of the 10th Annual Conference and Exposition of the National Computer Graphics Association*, volume I, pages 199–206. National Computer Graphics Association, Fairfax, VA, 1989.
21. D.N. Levin, X. Hu, K.K. Tan, S. Galhotra, C.A. Pelizzari, G.T.Y. Chen, R.N. Beck, C.-T. Chen, M.D. Cooper, J.F. Mullan, J. Hekmatpanah and J.-P. Spire. The brain: Integrated three-dimensional display of MR and PET images. *Radiology*, 172:783–789, 1989.
22. K.D. Toennies, J.K. Udupa, G.T. Herman, I.L. Wornom and S.R. Buchman. Registration of three-dimensional objects and surfaces. *IEEE Comput. Graph. Appl.*, 10(3):52–62, 1990.
23. G. Dahlberg. *Statistical Methods for Medical and Biological Students*. George Allen and Unwin, London, 1940.
24. G.T. Herman and A.H. Abbott. Reproducibility of landmark locations on CT-based three-dimensional images. In *Proceedings of the 10th Annual Conference and Exposition of the National Computer Graphics Association*, volume I, pages 144–148. National Computer Graphics Association, Fairfax, VA, 1989.
25. G.T. Herman. Three-dimensional imaging on a CT or MR scanner. *J. Comput. Assist. Tomogr.*, 12:450–458, 1988.
26. S.R. Matteson, W. Bechtold, C. Phillips and E.V. Staab. A method for three-dimensional image reformation for quantitative cephalometric analysis. *J. Oral Maxillofacial Surg.*, 47:1053–1061, 1989.
27. A.H. Abbott, D.J. Netherway, D.J. David and T. Brown. Application and comparison of techniques for three-dimensional analysis of craniofacial anomalies. *J. Craniofacial Surg.*, 1:119–134, 1990.
28. C.F. Hildebolt, M.W. Vannier and R.H. Knapp. Validation study of skull three-dimensional computerized tomography measurements. *Am. J. Phys. Anthropol.*, 82:283–294, 1990.
29. V.V. Patel, M.W. Vannier, J.L. Marsh and L.-J. Lo. Assessing craniofacial surgical simulation. *IEEE Comput. Graph. Appl.*, 16(1):46–54, 1996.
30. G.T. Herman, M.I. Kohn and R.E. Gur. Computerized three-dimensional volume analysis from magnetic resonance images for characterization of brain disorders. In J.B. Myklebust and G.F. Harris, editors, *Proceedings of a Special Symposium on Maturing Technologies and Emerging Horizons in Biomedical Engineering*, pages 65–67. IEEE, Piscataway, NJ, 1988.
31. M.I. Kohn. Segmentation of magnetic resonance brain images. In *Proceedings of the 10th Annual Conference and Exposition of the National Computer Graphics Association*, volume I, pages 168–171. National Computer Graphics Association, Fairfax, VA, 1989.
32. R.C. Gur, P.D. Mozley, S.M. Resnick, G.L. Gottlieb, M. Kohn, R. Zimmerman, G. Herman, S. Atlas, R. Grossman, D. Berretta, R. Erwin and R.E. Gur. Gender differences in age effect on brain atrophy measured by magnetic resonance imaging. *Proc. Natl. Acad. Sci. USA*, 88:2845–2849, 1991.
33. R.E. Gur, P.D. Mozley, S.M. Resnick, D. Shtasel, M. Kohn, R. Zimmerman, G. Herman, S. Atlas, R. Grossman, R. Erwin and R.C. Gur. Magnetic resonance imaging in schizophrenia: I. Volumetric analysis of brain and cerebrospinal fluid. *Arch. Gen. Psychiatr.*, 48:407–412, 1991.
34. P.D. Mozley, R.E. Gur, S.M. Resnick, D.L. Shtasel, J. Richards, M. Kohn, R. Grossman, G. Herman and R.C. Gur. Magnetic-resonance-imaging in schizophrenia — relationship with clinical measures. *Schizophrenia Res.*, 12:195–203, 1994.
35. S.P. Raya. Low-level segmentation of 3-D magnetic resonance brain images — a rule based system. *IEEE Trans. Med. Imaging*, 9:327–337, 1990.
36. J.K. Udupa, L. Wei, S. Samarasekera, Y. Miki, M.A. van Buchem and R.I. Grossman. Multiple sclerosis lesion quantification using fuzzy-connectedness principles. *IEEE Trans. Med. Imaging*, 16:598–609, 1997.
37. K. Fukunaga. *Introduction to Statistical Pattern Recognition*. Academic Press, New York, 1972.
38. M.I. Kohn, N.K. Tanna, G.T. Herman, S.M. Resnick, P.D. Mozley, R.E. Gur, A. Alavi, R.A. Zimmerman and R.C. Gur. Analysis of brain and cerebrospinal fluid volumes with MR imaging. Part I: Methods, reliability, and validation. *Radiology*, 178:115–122, 1991.
39. M.D. Mitchel, H.L. Kundel, L. Axel and P.M. Joseph. Agarose as a tissue equivalent phantom material for NMR imaging. *Magn. Resonance Imaging*, 4:263–266, 1986.

40. M.W. Vannier, C.M. Speidel, D.L. Rickman, L.D. Schertz, L.R. Baker, C.F. Hildebolt, C.J. Offutt, J.A. Balko, R.L. Butterfield and M.H. Gado. Validation of magnetic resonance imaging (MRI) multispectral tissue classification. In *Proceedings of the 9th International Conference on Pattern Recognition*, pages 1182–1186. IEEE Computer Society Press, Washington, D.C., 1988.
41. R.A. Robb, J.J. Camp, J.D. Bourland, C.R. Jack, Jr. and B.P. O'Neill. Tumor volume analysis using 3-D image registration and segmentation by feature analysis. *J. Biomed. Eng. Soc. India*, 14:106–115, 1997.
42. J.W. Haller, A. Banerjee, G.E. Christensen, M. Gado, S. Joshi, M.I. Miller, Y. Sheline, M.W. Vannier and J.G. Csernansky. Three-dimensional hippocampal MR morphometry with high-dimensional transformation of a neuroanatomic atlas. *Radiology*, 202:504–510, 1997.
43. J.P. Broderick, S. Narayan, M. Gaskill, A.P. Dhawan and J. Khoury. Volumetric measurement of multifocal brain lesions: Implications for treatment of trials of vascular dementia and multiple sclerosis. *J. Neuroimaging*, 6:36–43, 1996.
44. J.R. Mitchel, S.J. Karlik, D.H. Lee, M. Eliasziw, G.P. Rice and A. Fenster. The variability of manual and computer assisted quantification of multiple sclerosis lesion volumes. *Med. Phys.*, 23:85–97, 1996.
45. B. Johnson, M.S. Atkins, B. Mackiewich and M. Anderson. Segmentation of multiple sclerosis lesions in intensity corrected multispectral MRI. *IEEE Trans. Med. Imaging*, 15:154–169, 1996.
46. M.A. van Buchem, R.I. Grossman, C. Armstrong, M. Polansky, Y. Miki, F.H. Heyning, M.P. Boncoeur-Martel, L. Wei, J.K. Udupa, M. Grossman, D.L. Kolson and J.C. McGowan. Correlation of volumetric magnetization transfer imaging with clinical data in MS. *Neurology*, 50:1609–1617, 1998.
47. M.D. Phillips, R.I. Grossman, Y. Miki, L. Wei, D.L. Kolson, M.A. van Buchem, M. Polansky, J.C. McGowan and J.K. Udupa. Comparison of T2 lesion volume and magnetization transfer ratio histogram analysis and of atrophy and measures of lesion burden in patients with multiple sclerosis. *Am. J. Neuroradiol.*, 19:1055–1060, 1998.
48. M.W. Vannier, B.S. Brusden, C.F. Hildebolt, D. Falk, J.M. Cheverud, G.S. Figiel, W.H. Perman, L.A. Kohn, R.A. Robb, R.L. Yoffie and S.J. Bresina. Brain surface cortical sulal lengths: Quantification with three-dimensional MR imaging. *Radiology*, 180:479–484, 1991.
49. W.E. Higgins, N. Chung and E.L. Ritman. LV chamber extraction from 3-D CT images – accuracy and precision. *Comput. Med. Imaging Graph.*, 16:17–26, 1992.
50. J.L. Boxerman, T.J. Mosher, E.R. McVeigh, E. Atalar, J.A.C. Lima and D.A. Bluemke. Advanced MR imaging techniques for the evaluation of the heart and great vessels. *RadioGraphics*, 18:543–564, 1998.
51. J.M. Holbert, M.L. Brown, F.C. Sciurba, R.J. Keenan, R.J. Landreneau and A.D. Holzer. Changes in lung volume and volume of emphysema after unilateral lung reduction surgery: Analysis with CT lung densitometry. *Radiology*, 201:793–797, 1996.
52. T.S. Hartman, H.D. Tazelaar, S.J. Swensen and N.l. Müller. Cigarette smoking: CT and pathologic findings associated with pulmonary diseases. *RadioGraphics*, 17:377–390, 1997.
53. R.M. Summers, W.S. Selbie, J.D. Malley, L.M. Pusanik, A.J. Dwyer, N.A. Courcoutsakis, D.J. Shaw, D.E. Kleiner, M.C. Sneller, C.A. Langford, S.M. Holland and J.H. Shelhamer. Polypoid lesions of airways: Early experience with computer-assisted detection by using virtual bronchoscopy and surface curvature. *Radiology*, 208:331–337, 1998.
54. H.P. McAdams, S.C. Palmer, J.J. Erasmus, E.F. Patz, J.E. Connolly, P.C. Goodman, D.M. Delong and V.F. Tapson. Bronchial anastomotic complications in lung transplant recipients: Virtual bronchoscopy and noninvasive assessment. *Radiology*, 209:689–695, 1998.
55. W.E. Higgins, K. Ramaswamy, R.D. Swift, G. McLennan and E.A. Hoffman. Virtual bronchoscopy for three-dimensional pulmonary image assessment: State of the art and future needs. *RadioGraphics*, 18:761–778, 1998.
56. G.R. McNeal, W.H. Maynard, R.A. Branc, T.A. Powers, P.A. Arns, K. Gunter, J.M. Fitzpatrick and G.L. Partain. Liver volume measurements and three-dimensional display from MR images. *Radiology*, 169:851–854, 1988.
57. P. Soyer, A. Roche, D. Elias and M. Levesque. Hepatic metastasis from colorectal cancer: Influence of hepatic volumetric analysis on surgical decision making. *Radiology*, 184:695–697, 1992.
58. M.W. Vannier, C.F. Hildebolt, L.A. Gilula, T.K. Pilgram, F. Mann, B.S. Monses, W.A. Murphy, W.G. Totty and C.J. Offutt. Calcaneal and pelvic fractures: Diagnostic evaluation by three-dimensional computed tomography scans. *J. Digital Imaging*, 4:143–152, 1991.

59. H.-J. Laine, K. Kontola, M.U.K. Lehto, M. Pitkänen, P. Jarske and T.S. Lindholm. Image processing for femoral endosteal anatomy detection: Description and testing of a computed tomography based program. *Phys. Med. Biol.*, 42:673–689, 1997.
60. H.K. Genant. Current state of bone densitometry for osteoporosis. *RadioGraphics*, 18:913–918, 1998.
61. T.F. Lang, P. Augat, N.E. Lane and H.K. Genant. Trochanteric hip fracture: Strong association with spinal trabecular bone mineral density measured with quantitative CT. *Radiology*, 209:525–530, 1998.
62. J.K. Udupa, B.E. Hirsch, H.J. Hillstrom, G.R. Bauer and J.B. Kneeland. Analysis of *in vivo* 3-D internal kinematics of the joints of the foot. *IEEE Trans. Biomed. Eng.*, 45:1387–1396, 1998.

4 Evaluation of 3D Imaging

Michael W. Vannier

CONTENTS

0-8493-3179-X/00/$0.00+$.50

4.1 INTRODUCTION

3D medical imaging and measurement systems are used for non-destructive inspection of the body and its component regions *in vivo* and *in vitro*. These systems provide 3D data as discrete points, surfaces, or volumes. 3D medical imaging is used for diagnosis, treatment planning, execution and monitoring of interventions, to extract quantitative measurements, to determine if an abnormality is present by comparison with normal controls, to assess change over time, or all of these. Once acquired, 3D digital image data is visualized, measured, and compared to perform these tasks. The evaluation of 3D imaging system performance depends on the specific application, body region, modality used, observers involved, and subject being studied. This chapter deals with the subjective and objective evaluation of 3D imaging as it is used in diagnostic radiology, anthropometry, radiotherapy, and surgery. Basic principles and evaluation of 3D anthropometry for measurement of body shape and size are reviewed. Rigorous methods for subjective and objective evaluation of 3D images are described with examples from craniofacial surgery and 3D anthropometry.

4.1.1 EVALUATION OF 3D IMAGING

Evaluation of 3D medical imaging serves two main purposes: (1) to objectively assess anatomical regions and features using 3D images, and (2) to determine the performance of 3D imaging systems in visualization and measurement of biological structures. 3D medical imaging systems are used to inspect and measure anatomic points (e.g., landmarks), surfaces, slices, or volumes that comprise organs and body regions. Medical imaging modalities that provide 3D data include computed tomography and magnetic resonance imaging, as well as ultrasound, surface scanners, point digitizers and many others. Potentially any imaging modality can provide 3D data using principles of geometry and tomography. 3D medical imaging systems are used to evaluate biological structure by acquiring and processing digital data for static or interactive visualization, measurement, and comparison — processes that usually involve a human operator or interpreter. The evaluation of 3D imaging system performance therefore depends on the specific application, body region, modality used, observers involved, and subject being studied to estimate relative diagnostic performance, measurement error, image artifacts, and user preference.

Evaluation of imaging systems and procedures is done to assess their quality using subjective or preferably objective methods. The principal applications of 3D imaging are visualization and intervention. Process or outcome evaluation of 3D medical imaging systems begins with images and measurements. For example, the distance between homologous landmarks calculated for each pair of images taken at a single measurement session, averaged over measurement sessions and individuals, provides a measure of error due to the imaging device. Each measurement requires judgment by an operator, also known as an observer, at every point selected. Since intra- and inter-observer judgments are known to vary, evaluation of test–retest repeatability and operator error is essential for objective assessment of measurements. Assessment of user preference using side-by-side comparison of 3D and alternative imaging methods, for example, is used for subjective evaluation.

Computed tomography (CT) is a 3D imaging modality that allows more accurate diagnosis than plain radiography in some diagnostic applications, while three-dimensional (3D) CT reconstruction has been shown to facilitate other more complex or demanding diagnostic tasks. It is generally agreed that 3D CT is the most useful imaging modality for planning surgical management in craniofacial imaging, having supplemented and replaced cephalometry in many instances. Similar observations have been made to support the use of 3D imaging in certain orthopedic, neurosurgical, radiotherapy, and otolaryngological applications.

Anthropometry is the study of human body measurement, especially to characterize groups rather than individuals and subpopulations according to age, gender, demographics, or other criteria. Medical diagnosis and treatment is often based on precise image-based measurements obtained in individuals using 3D anthropometric methods. Examples include radiotherapy treatment planning and intra-operative surgical navigation. Data collection and format standards are required for transfer and subsequent postprocessing of raw image data obtained from projection, surface, or volumetric scanner systems. These standards, such as DICOM for medical imaging data, have stimulated the development of many add-on systems to plan, administer, and assess physical and surgical interventions.

Disciplines that use human body surface dimensions require accurate, repeatable measurements. The analysis of repeatability, precision, and validation of a 3D measurement device, the Cencit Imaging System (CIS) (an optical surface scanner), is presented as an example. A pair of 3D images was scanned during each of two sessions, and each image was digitized twice by two operators to estimate repeatability. Surface scanners such as the CIS have been found useful in a variety of anthropometric applications.

Three factors influence the validation and testing of an imaging system for anthropometric measurement: (1) the digital images produced must be as clear and accurate as possible, allowing visual identification of contrasting intensities or colors and depths by an observer or by electronic means (i.e., error in detecting visible landmarks in digitized images should be evaluated); (2) repeated images of the same individual should be nearly identical (i.e., error in producing a digital image from a living subject should be evaluated more than once); and (3) the locations of the anatomical structures chosen for data collection must be reliably identifiable by a trained observer (i.e., error in locating and marking landmarks by human operators should be evaluated).

An image comparison methodology has been defined and applied to clinical studies where 3D images are used as the basis for synthesis of surgical plans. Validated image comparison methods allow evaluation of 3D image-based surgical planning by measuring the discrepancy between surgical outcome observed on post-operative scans and a surgical plan based on pre-operative scans. These methods are applied to 3D imaging systems and the results show that errors due to operator variability predominate in most practical applications.

In summary, this chapter introduces subjective and objective methods for evaluation of 3D imaging systems, gives examples of their use, and explains the principal sources of error in anthropometric measurement. The multiplicity of modalities used for 3D imaging and the diversity of present and future applications are described. Visualization and measurement of 3D images for diagnosis, planning, execution of interventions, and comparison are evaluated by formal methods, to determine their relative diagnostic performance, measurement repeatability, and validity.

4.2 3D IMAGING SYSTEMS

3D medical imaging systems measure points, surfaces, slices, or volumes in digital data sets. By convention, 3D refers to three spatial dimensions rather than a single plane observed at several temporal increments. Medical imaging modalities that provide 3D data include computed tomography and magnetic resonance imaging, as well as ultrasound and others. Serial 3D examinations or multimodality examinations may be combined and analyzed as four- or higher dimensional data sets. Real-time 3D imaging (e.g., 4D imaging) has been implemented for experimental purposes, such as the Mayo Dynamic Spatial Reconstructor (DSR), a 3D CT scanner built to image the moving heart. Higher dimensions are possible, but their use in medical imaging is infrequent.

Individual points in three dimensions are localized by interactive digitizers that employ manual optical, mechanical, electrostatic, or electromagnetic styli. These instruments locate and record individual points on the body surface or interactively report the location of hand-held instruments relative to organs and body regions. Point digitization is the basis of landmark analysis, such as that used in craniometry, skull measurement, and orthognathic surgical planning.

4.2.1 Point Digitizers

Instruments that report 3D coordinate locations of a stylus tip, typically held in the operator's hand, have been developed using ultrasonic arrays, articulated arms with potentiometer or graycode angle encoders, or electromagnetic and optical elements. The purpose of these instruments is to report the 3D coordinates of specific surface points designated by the operator. A list of points may be collected in an attached computer for subsequent use in object modeling and computation of measurements.

4.2.1.1 Polhemus 3Space™ Digitizer

A common instrument used in 3D point digitization is based on electromagnetic measurements of spatial location with a hand-held stylus. The operator moves the stylus to each desired point and the digitizer reports three corresponding spatial coordinates (x,y,z). The Polhemus 3Space™ digitizer has been validated.[26,51] The unit consists of a tablet containing the computer, a hand-held stylus, a keypad, and a footpad. The hand-held stylus contacts each landmark, and an electromagnetic field generated within the unit determines the location of the stylus. There are many other designs of stylus digitizers that have been built and commercially distributed employing ultrasonic, mechanical, and optical technology. These devices are integrated into interactive surgical navigation systems.

Point digitizers are important in 3D medical imaging, since several points on the body surface have special anatomic significance. These points, known as landmarks, include the nasion, gonion, and many others. These points are tabulated in the anatomy and physical anthropology literature, and they form a common basis for comparison of instruments, studies of skull growth and development, as well as planning and prediction of outcomes from various surgical procedures.

4.2.2 Surface Scanner/Digitizers

Three-dimensional surface coordinates may be obtained by active optical scanning where a light source illuminates the surface and image sensors at known locations are used to triangulate the object's location at every visible point on the surface. There are many practical examples of such scanners in use today, and we introduce two examples here — the Cencit and the Cyberware scanners.

4.2.2.1 Cencit and Cyberware Facial Surface Scanners

The Cencit Imaging System is a non-contact, stationary three-dimensional active optical imaging system employing structured light and multiple sensors which are enclosed in a stand-alone unit. Individual subjects are digitized (scanned) and the data processed and displayed on a graphics workstation (Silicon Graphics Indigo 2). This system has been described in detail in a series of publications on its design, application to biomedicine, and assessment of its performance in anthopometry.

Cyberware, Inc. manufactures a popular commercially available facial surface digitizer. This scanner obtains millimeter resolution data sets from 360° coverage of the head, neck, and upper

TABLE 4.1
Average Precision (in cm) of Landmark Locations Measured from the Cencit Facial Scanner and the Polhemus 3Space Digitizer

	Average Minimum		Average Maximum	
Method	**Men**	**Women**	**Men**	**Women**
Cencit				
Marking	0.11	0.13	0.64	0.56
Scan	0.04	0.14	0.46	0.32
Digitize	0.02	0.02	0.41	0.32
3Space				
Marking	0.13	0.18	0.64	0.61
Scan	0.03	0.10	0.26	0.31

Note: The average minimum and maximum distances between homologous landmarks resulting from differences in digitizing landmarks, scanning the image, marking the landmarks, and differences between individuals are presented. Note that the dots used to mark the landmarks are 0.64 cm in diameter.

torso. It has been applied to portrait sculpture, orthotics and prosthetics, synthetic actors, medical diagnosis, and communications research.

Many other designs of optical surface scanners based on active sensors with fixed geometry and structured sources have been built and tested in a variety of applications. Several newer 3D optical surface scanner instruments have been developed, as these devices are essential components of systems for intra-operative use, to enable 3D ultrasound image acquisition, for 3D whole-body anthropometry, and many others.

4.2.2.2 Facial Scanner Validation Analysis

The use of the Polhemus 3Space digitizer and Cencit scanner to study skull and facial surface structure serves as an example of how these systems are evaluated. The principal issues for evaluation include the quantitative accuracy, precision, and especially repeatability of measurements.

Human volunteers were examined after placing markers on the facial surface at anatomically significant points. Quantitative evaluation of the Cencit scanner and Polhemus digitizer measurement precision indicated that the minimum and maximum distances between homologous landmarks at the level of digitizing, scanning, and landmark marking were all less than or equal to the diameter of black dots used to mark the landmarks (0.64 cm) (Table 4.1). Homologous landmarks measured by the Polhemus 3Space digitizer have comparable minimum and maximum distances. The precision of the Cencit facial scanner was comparable to that of the Polhemus 3Space digitizer. The greatest amount of error was in the marking of the landmarks. However, the magnitude of the imprecision was smaller than or equal to the diameter of the black dots (0.64 cm) used to mark the landmarks. The size of the black dots used was determined by current constraints of the Cencit facial scanner. Greater precision can be expected if smaller markers could be used to identify landmarks.

The average proportions of the total variance explained by digitizing, scanning, landmark location and individual differences (repeatability) are comparable (Table 4.2). In the location of the x, y, and z coordinates from the Cencit facial scanner, an average of 2% (males) to 6% (females) of the total variation is due to differences in digitizing, 2% (males) to 4% (females) of the total variation is due to differences in scanning, 18% (males) to 34% (females) of the variation is due

TABLE 4.2
Average Percentage of Total Variation in Location of *x, y,* and *z* Coordinates and Bilateral Distances Explained by Digitizing, Scanning, Marking Landmarks, and Individual (Repeatability) for the Cencit Facial Scanner and the Polhemus 3Space Digitizer

	x, y, z Axis Location		Bilateral Distances	
Method	**Men**	**Women**	**Men**	**Women**
Cencit				
ID	79	56	83	69
Marking	18	34	13	115
Scan	2	4	2	12
Digitize	2	6	2	4
3Space				
ID	89	67	80	83
Marking	9	24	14	5
Scan	2	9	7	11

Note: The averages were calculated within each level of analysis (e.g., average for ID, average for marking). Therefore, the portion of the variation explained by all levels of the analysis may not total 100% for males or females measured by either the Cencit facial scanner or the 3Space digitizer.

to differences between locating the landmarks in the two measurement sessions. The repeatability of the *x, y,* and *z* landmark coordinates measured with the Cencit facial scanner averages 56% (females) to 79% (males). For *x, y,* and *z* landmark coordinates measured with the Polhemus 3Space digitizer, an average of 2% (males) to 9% (females) of the variation is due to differences in scanning, and 9% (males) to 24% (females) of the variation is due to differences in landmark location between the two measurement sessions. The repeatability of the *x, y,* and *z* landmark coordinates measured with the Polhemus 3Space digitizer averages 67% (females) to 89% (males). Measurements of bilateral distances (e.g., bi-zygomatic breadth, bi-ectocanthus) are more highly repeatable, with 69% (females) to 83% (males) repeatability using the Cencit facial scanner and 80% (males) to 83% (females) repeatability using the Polhemus 3Space digitizer. The proportions of variance explained by digitizing, scanning, and landmark location are roughly comparable between the two systems.

The precision and repeatability of the Cencit facial scanner and the Polhemus 3Space digitizer are similar. The proportion of the variance due to digitizing and scanning is low. A large proportion of the variance within individuals is due to error in landmark location. This human error can be reduced by training of the anthropometrist, thus increasing repeatability. The repeatability of bilateral distances is greater than repeatability of the *x, y,* and *z* landmark coordinate locations. The imprecision of locating the landmarks is generally much less than 0.64 cm (the diameter of a marking black dot), and we are therefore explaining the repeatability of finding a landmark within a very small region. Small measurements can be expected to be less repeatable than large measurements. Large measurements are expected to be measured with greater repeatability because the errors are distributed across a greater distance.

4.2.2.3 Evaluation of the Cencit Facial Scanner

The Cencit facial scanner was shown to perform comparably to the Polhemus 3Space digitizer. The Cencit facial scanner accurately images facial landmarks. A large amount of data can be collected from electronically stored facial images. Images can be collected and processed at a researcher's convenience, and stored images may be useful. Such a system is used in studies of landmarks, surfaces, and volumes and in comparisons within or between populations. The majority of the error was found to be in the location of the landmarks (i.e., human error). This source of error is common to all measurement devices and can be reduced by training and judicious choice of landmarks.

4.2.3 Volume Imaging Systems

Volume imaging is achieved clinically by computed tomography (CT) and magnetic resonance imaging (MRI). Spiral or helical computed tomography has been developed to acquire body region volume images in less than 1 min. Similarly, MRI scanners can acquire a volumetric head scan with approximately 256 × 256 × 128 or 256 voxels at 1 mm resolution in less than 10 min.

4.2.3.1 3D CT Images

3D craniofacial imaging was introduced in the early 1980s and has become routine in many centers. Typical CT scans are obtained at 512 × 512 resolution at 1 or 2 mm intervals throughout the skull in children and adults with congenital and acquired deformities of the head.

CT scans for 3D visualization and analysis are routinely performed in patients with craniosynostosis, a group of disorders that deform the skull during growth due to abnormalities of the sutures between cranial bones. The results of a 3D imaging study can help distinguish between normal and synostosed (or "closed") sutures. This question was evaluated using three kinds of evidence: the incorrect diagnoses of the least experienced reader, the confidence levels of diagnosis in the most experienced readers, and examination of the images ourselves in an unblinded fashion.

Craniosynostosis has historically been treated as an inherently binary abnormality. Sutures have been diagnosed as either normal or abnormal, based on skull morphology with confirmation by imaging procedures. Our detailed comparison of surgical results, histological examination of excised sutures, and results from inspection of 3D CT images suggests that this historical approach is correct. In our sample, although suture histopathology varied about normal and abnormal values, the distinction between normal and abnormal sutures was clear both histologically and clinically. Our results indicate that the appropriate model for craniosynostosis is binary with variation, rather than a gradient of abnormality with an arbitrary decision threshold.

For purposes of evaluation, the results suggest the addition of a third gold standard. Surgeon's opinion based on intra-operative findings and histological analysis of excised sutures have been used separately as gold standards. They are combined in this study, and they agreed perfectly. The diagnoses made by the most experienced readers from 3D images agreed nearly perfectly with the combined gold standard. The results from all three kinds of information are therefore interchangeable, and it appears reasonable to use diagnoses made by experienced readers from good quality images as an additional gold standard.

4.3 MEASUREMENTS

3D imaging systems are used to quantify and model the geometry of biological structures. Measurements of points, surfaces, and volumes are obtained by manual interaction with the digital data sets or by automated processes.

4.3.1 Spatial — Point, Displacement, Area

The simplest and most common types of measurements extracted from 3D medical image data sets include spatial coordinates of individual points, the distance between points representing displacements or offsets between identifiable landmarks, and surface area.

4.3.2 Mass Properties

Mass properties of scanned or imaged objects include volume, centroid, and moments of inertia. Using material properties estimated from the literature, several authors have computed mass properties in scanned volumes with satisfactory results.

4.3.3 Target Definition

Target definition is an essential step in the planning of radiation therapy. 3D conformal radiotherapy is an emerging technology for precision delivery based on volumetric imaging with target definition on 3D CT scans of the body region. The tumor itself, its margins, and critical normal structures in the treatment fields are identified, segmented, and labeled before the dosimetry and evaluation of plans can be done.

4.3.4 Anatomic Fidelity

3D imaging systems have varying degrees of temporal, contrast, and spatial resolution that determine their relative ability to delineate anatomic structure. The anatomic fidelity of renderings is judged subjectively in most cases, where comparison is made by experts between known or expected levels of quality in medical images and those synthesized from scan data sets. The acceptance and use of visualization results is highly dependent on the perceived level of anatomic fidelity in images.

4.4 EVALUATION

Evaluation of imaging systems and procedures is a means of assessing their quality. Evaluation is a collection of methods and processes that measure the quality of an entity, such as usability, validity, repeatability, effectiveness, or other aspect. In three-dimensional imaging, the principal applications involve visualization and interventional tasks. Diagnosis and therapy planning, delivery, and assessment necessitate medical tests, of which clinical three-dimensional imaging is but a part. Three-dimensional medical imaging is among the group of medical tests that receives special scrutiny by many observers concerned with cost, due to several factors: (1) the high costs associated with medical testing; (2) the fact that many tests, even the most familiar and common ones, are often inaccurate, misused, and misleading; (3) such tests are sometimes administered unnecessarily; and (4) they can be dangerous to patients on whom they are used, either because of inherent risks in high-technology tests or because of the consequences of their inaccuracies.[73]

Evaluations are undertaken for a variety of reasons: to judge the worth of ongoing applications, and to estimate the usefulness of attempts to improve them; to assess the utility of new applications and initiatives; to increase the effectiveness of management and administration; and to satisfy the accountability requirements of sponsors.[121] Only rarely are evaluation studies conducted for the primary purpose of contributing new knowledge. Instead, they are done to measure the contribution of a system and thereby determine its quality. An evaluation must ask specific questions or test hypotheses about a program or technology that are useful for future decision making. The results of an evaluation study are quality measures used for future decisions regarding system applications in the same or other settings.

Evaluation of medical imaging systems can be done on the basis of outcome or process criteria. Outcomes of medical procedures are evaluated by survival, morbidity, or morbidity criteria. Since diagnostic imaging is performed most often as a component of a more extensive episode of care, separating the contribution of the imaging is often difficult, requiring very large sample sizes and lengthy studies. As a general rule, every evaluation should ask questions about outcome.

The significance of three-dimensional imaging can be defined as an outcome that makes a meaningful difference in meeting the goals that 3D systems are intended to meet. This difference should be a non-trivial amount that impacts an important place or aspect at a reasonable cost. The basis for operational or programmatic significance can be viewed as a matter of judgment through expert review, past experience, statistical rules of evidence, or theory.

Alternatively, evaluation may be done according to statistical significance. Statistical findings are valid only when viewed along with program standards. By rule of thumb, we may ascribe meaning to an increase from pre- to post-intervention if it exceeds the criterion of half a standard deviation gain. If the intervention under evaluation is 3D imaging, we seek to detect improvements in diagnostic performance or other metric by half a standard deviation or more. Numerous statistical experimental designs are employed in evaluatory testing, including case, time-series, or comparison group studies.

Evaluation can be performed according to process descriptors such as cost, timeliness, safety, user preference, reliability, or many other criteria. The specific criteria applied to perform an evaluation assess aspects of quality that measure how well an intervention, such as three-dimensional imaging, satisfies specific needs.

Three-dimensional imaging systems produce images and measurements. The images are visualized and manipulated for diagnosis and planning of surgical or radiotherapy procedures. Image-based navigation is the basis of percutaneous non-palpable lesion biopsy or minimally invasive therapy.

The quality of 3D images can be assessed by ROC analysis, a well-established set of methods for measuring relative diagnostic performance in a rated response experiment (Figure 4.1). ROC (receiver operating characteristic) analysis has been widely used to quantify a subjective process — the observation of images by experts for detection and localization of specific features in images, especially for diagnosis of abnormalities.

There are no widely accepted evaluation standards and guidelines that pertain directly to three-dimensional imaging. Ad hoc comparisons of images generated with simulations, phantom test devices, cadaver parts, and *in vivo* have been reported. Anatomic–pathologic correlation is often used to verify image-guided interventions, including specimen radiography or direct histopathological comparison.

Evaluation is concerned with internal and external validity. To possess internal validity, it must be possible to distinguish changes caused by the program being evaluated from other causes, whereas external validity determines whether the evaluation's findings will hold at another place.

Current methods of morphometry do not effectively capture information about the shape of structures. Although the volumes of brain structures and substructures may be related to some aspects of normal brain morphology, critical aspects of disease may not be reflected in such simple measures. Preliminary attempts have been made to quantify the qualitative features of morphometric shape measures, such as the patterning of sulci and gyri on the cortical surface,[154] but under only the most limited circumstances (i.e., a method for quantifying the similarity of sulcal patterns between individuals cannot similarly quantify shapes of subcortical 3D structures). The precise and quantitative assessment of shape characteristics of volumes and surfaces may offer entirely new insights into a multitude of critical questions.

It is necessary to evaluate the precision and repeatability of new neuromorphometric methods and to compare these methods to simpler and previously validated methods for collecting morphological data. Models have been introduced and used to evaluate repeatability and precision in surface anthropometry.[69] Further, it is necessary to determine the repeatability and precision of the methods used in all aspects of data collection. To interpret our analysis, we must be able to evaluate whether the data have been collected in a consistent manner. If data collection consists of more than one step, the overall repeatability of the data collection process will reflect error in data collection at each step. A method for the evaluation of repeatability, precision, and validation is described here, with application to 3D anthropometry:

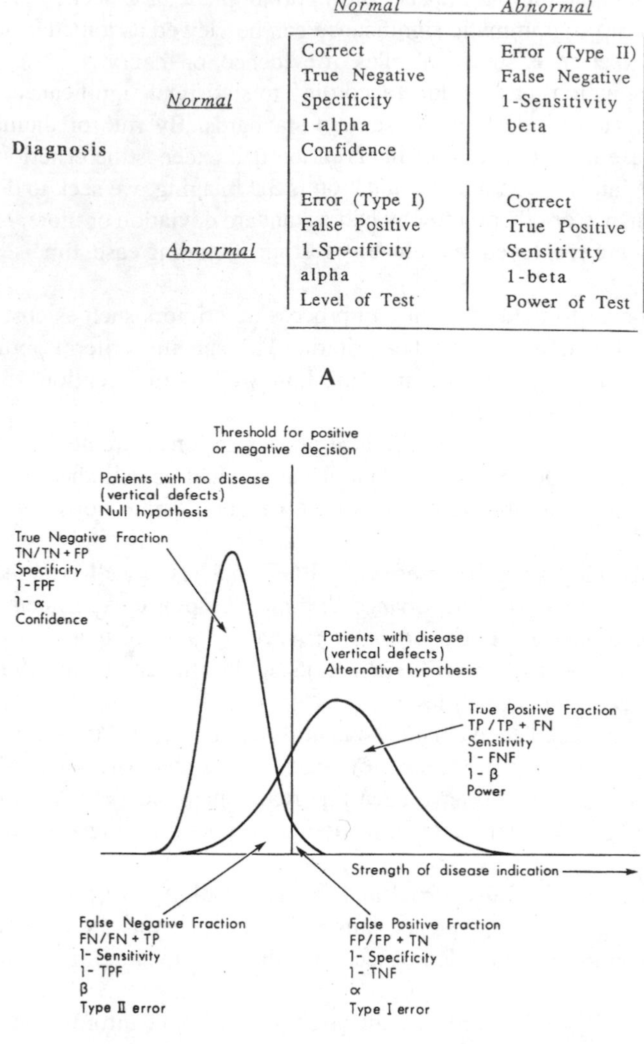

		Normal	*Abnormal*
Diagnosis	*Normal*	Correct True Negative Specificity 1-alpha Confidence	Error (Type II) False Negative 1-Sensitivity beta
	Abnormal	Error (Type I) False Positive 1-Specificity alpha Level of Test	Correct True Positive Sensitivity 1-beta Power of Test

A

B

FIGURE 4.1 (A) Two × two (2 × 2) contingency table of relationships and statistical terms associated with ROC analysis. (B) Two overlapping distributions of subjects with and without disease (vertical bony defects). The strength of the indicators of disease increases from left to right. TN = true negative; FN = false negative; FP = false positive; TP = true positive; β = Type II error = false rejection of alternative hypothesis: α = Type I error = false rejection of null hypothesis. (From Hildebolt CF, Vannier MW, Shrout MK, Pilgram TK. ROC analysis of observer-response subjective rating data — application to periodontal radiograph assessment. *Am J Phys Anthropol.* 84:351–361, 1991. With permission.)

1. The digital volumetric images available for study should be as clear and accurate as possible, allowing visual identification of object features by an observer or by automatic means (i.e., error in detecting visible landmarks and image features should be evaluated).
2. Repeated images of the same individual should be nearly identical (i.e., error in producing a digital image from a living subject should be evaluated).
3. The locations of the anatomic structures chosen for data collection must be reliably identifiable by a trained observer (i.e., error in locating and marking landmarks or delineating volumes by experts [radiologist and/or pathologist] should be evaluated).

Tests of new imaging methods need to deal with these three issues in terms of precision and repeatability. Precision is the average absolute difference between repeated measures of the same individual. Repeatability is the precision of the measurement relative to the differences among individuals contrasted in any given study. It is measured as the proportion of total variance resulting from differences between individuals using a repeated-measures analysis-of-variance (ANOVA) design. One minus the repeatability is the proportional error resulting from measurement inaccuracy. The level of repeatability and the imprecision that can be tolerated in any particular study will vary with the size of the contrast being made. For example, measurements that are precise enough for a comparison of infants with adolescents may not be precise enough for studying variation among adolescents. Usually, repeatability is judged within a single homogeneous population because this places the most stringent constraint on error levels.

Although we can use precision and repeatability assessments to determine the replicability of measurements, these measurements may still be inaccurate or biased. The potential bias of the measurement system can be judged by validation studies in which measurements taken from some simpler, already validated system are compared with those obtained by the new method. If measurements taken by the new device are consistently larger or smaller than those taken by the already validated system, the device is said to be biased.

Three-dimensional imaging provides measurements and visualizations. The measurements are typically made as landmarks, displacements, or volumes. Mass properties such as the volume, centroid, and moments of inertia can be measured and evaluated for repeatability, precision, and validity using these methods.

4.4.1 Precision, Repeatability, and Validity

The statistical analysis of the repeated measures allows estimation of the precision and repeatability of the measurement device. Precision of three-dimensional coordinates can be measured by superimposing repeated images in such a way that the squared distance between homologous landmarks is minimized. This registration procedure is called Procrustean rotation.

- First, the two separate digitizations of a single image are compared by deriving the distance between homologous landmark positions after Procrustean rotation. These differences are averaged over images, measurement sessions, and individuals to provide a measure of error due to the digitizing process. Error at this level is the result of interaction between the device and the operator.
- Second, the two digitizations of each image are averaged (after Procrustean rotation). These averages represent each of the two images obtained at each measurement session. The image averages are then compared to one another after Procrustean rotation. The distance between homologous landmarks is calculated for each pair of images taken at a single measurement session and then averaged over measurement sessions and individuals to provide a measure of error due to the imaging device.
- Third, the two image averages obtained at each measurement session are averaged (after Procrustean rotation). These new averages represent the separate landmark markings done at each measurement session. The marking averages are then compared to one another after Procrustean rotation. The distance between homologous landmarks is calculated for each pair of coordinates from a single individual and then averaged over individuals to provide a measure of error due to marking by the anthropometrist.

With these three sets of comparisons we can measure imprecision due to digitizing from the images, making the images, and marking the landmarks on a living subject (Figure 4.2).

Analysis of Variance for Analysis Outlined in Figure 4.2

Source	df^a	Expected M^2
ID	a – 1	Var (error) + 2 var (scan [ID marking]) + 4 var (marking [ID]) + 8 var (ID)
Marking (ID)	a (b – 1)	Var (error) + 2 var (scan [ID marking]) + 4 var (marking [ID])
Scan (ID marking)	ab (c – 1)	Var (error) + 2 var (scan [ID marking])
Error	abc (d – 1)	Var (error)
Corrected total	abcd – 1	

[a] The degrees of freedom are determined by the number of individuals (a), the number of measurement or marking sessions (b), the number of scans (c), and the number of measurements of each scan (d).

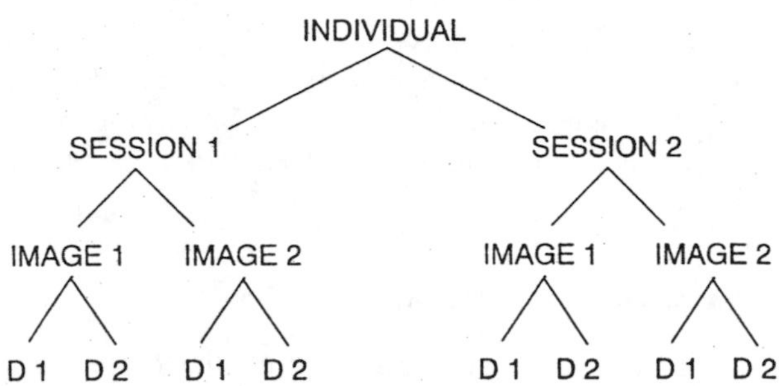

FIGURE 4.2 Scheme for validation study of Cencit three-dimensional facial scanner. For each individual, identification of landmarks (SESSION), facial surface images (IMAGE), and digitizing (D) of identified landmarks are each repeated twice to estimate the amount of variance resulting from measurement error compared with a variance caused by individual differences. The measurement error can then be divided into error in identifying landmarks, error in producing an image from a living subject, and error in digitally recording landmark locations.

Repeatability can also be measured with this design. First, a Procrustean rotation is performed using all coordinate sets (eight per individual) in a single analysis. The *x, y,* or *z* coordinates are then used as the dependent variables in a nested ANOVA with three factors: (1) individual, (2) measurement session nested within individual, and (3) image (scan) nested within measurement session and individual. The separate digitizations of each image serve as the residual or error term. This can be expressed by the equation

$$\text{dependent variable} = \text{ID} + \text{SESSION (ID)} + \text{SCAN (ID SESSION)} + \text{ERROR}$$

The variance due to each of these random effects is derived from the ANOVA procedure. The proportion of the total variance due to individual differences is the repeatability [Var(ID)/Var(total)]. The proportion of the total variance due to measurement session represents error due to marking [Var(marking)/Var(total)]. The proportion of the total variance due to image represents error due to the imaging device [Var(scan)/Var(total)]. Finally, the proportion of the total variance due to the residual represents the error due to digitization of the images [Var(error)/Var(total)].

Validation consists of comparing the results from the new imaging device to results obtained from other, previously validated, techniques. These comparisons were done using Procrustean techniques, as described above. The Procrustean-derived average coordinate locations for each individual obtained with the new device are compared, using Procrustean rotation, to the locations derived for that same individual using the previously validated Polhemus 3Space digitizer. Homologous landmarks digitized by the two devices are to be superimposed after Procrustean rotation. Distances between homologous landmarks indicate error in the new device. If the images from the new device are consistently larger (or smaller) than images from the other device, then the new device is said to be biased.

The procedures described above for three-dimensional coordinate data can be applied to other kinds of data derived from anthropometric images. Linear distances and angles can be derived either directly from the subjects or from the digitized images. Alternatively, surfaces can be compared after registration using some measure of difference between the repeated surfaces, such as the volume separating the surfaces. This volume would be treated in the same way as the distance between repeated landmarks in the discussion above.

4.4.1.1 Validation of the Cencit 3D Facial Surface Scanner

A validation study of the Cencit 3D optical digitizing system (CIS), a facial surface scanner, was conducted. The objective was to test the suitability of Cencit system for applications in anthropometry and medical imaging of the human face. The study was designed to test whether the Cencit system could produce repeatable facial images and whether landmarks could be accurately located on the images produced by the Cencit facial scanner.

Recruited for the study were 10 normal adult men and 10 normal adult women. Twenty-seven facial landmarks were identified on each individual, and the landmark locations were marked with a ¼-in. non-reflective black adhesive dot (Figure 4.3). The landmarks chosen were used in a previous anthropometric study of facial morphology and their locations had been found to be highly reproducible. The measurement scheme outlined above was followed. On each of two measurement sessions, landmarks were marked on each participant and two Cencit facial scanner images were recorded. Each Cencit facial scanner image was digitized twice, yielding eight sets of three-dimensional coordinates for each individual. All landmark location and digitizing was performed by one observer to eliminate inter-observer error. The procedure was repeated with the Polhemus 3Space electromagnetic digitizer.

4.4.2 Subjective Assessment of Diagnostic Performance with 3D Visualization

To measure diagnostic performance and subjective preference between two 3D CT reconstruction modalities (voxel gradient and surface projection) displayed two ways (conventional and unwrapped). The diagnostic task was craniosynostosis, confirmed by surgical inspection and histology of resected sutures. High-resolution 2-mm contiguous CT scan slices were obtained and 3D reconstruction images generated for 25 infants and children with skull deformities prior to surgical management of craniosynostosis. Two pediatric radiologists and two neuroradiologists first ranked images by subjective preference for diagnostic use. Then they diagnosed the presence or absence of craniosynostosis from images presented in random order and blinded fashion. The gold standard was inspection during surgery and histologic evaluation of excised sutures. Finally, reviewers repeated their subjective preference test. The least experienced radiologist had 100% specificity for all imaging modalities and specificities ranging from 43 to 83%. The two most experienced radiologists performed nearly identically, with sensitivities of 96% and specificities of 100%. After performing diagnostic tasks using all image types, all radiologists preferred conventional surface projections. Experienced readers can achieve nearly perfect diagnostic performance using the latest 3D CT reconstruction images, making it a contribution to the diagnostic process. Although performance is nearly identical for all modalities, readers strongly prefer conventionally presented surface projection images.

Landmarks Included in Anthropometric Analysis

1. Alare (right): the lateral point on the flare or wing of the nose
2. Alare (left)
3. Cheilion (right): the lateral point of the juncture of the fleshy tissue of the lips with the facial skin at the corner of the mouth
4. Cheilion (left)
5. Ear top (right): the highest point of the ear on its long axis
6. Ear top (left)
7. Ectocanthus (right): the outside corner of the eye formed by the meeting of the upper and lower eyelids
8. Ectocanthus (left)
9. Frontotemporale (right): the point of the deepest indentation of the temporal crest of the frontal bone above the browridges
10. Frontotemporale (left)
11. Gonion (right): the lateral point on the posterior angle of the mandible
12. Gonion (left)
13. Infraorbitale (right): the lowest point on the anterior border of the boney eye socket
14. Infraorbitale (left)
15. Otobasion superior (right): the superior point of juncture between the ear and the head
16. Otobasion superior (left)
17. Tragion (right): the superior point of juncture of the cartilaginous flap (tragus) of the ear with the head
18. Tragion (left)
19. Zygion (right): the lateral point of the zygomatic arch
20. Zygion (left)
21. Zygofrontale (right): the lateral point of the frontal bone on its zygomatic process
22. Zygofrontale (left)
23. Chin: the most protruding point on the bottom edge of the chin along the jawline
24. Crinion: the lowest point of the hairline on the forehead in the midsagittal plane
25. Promenton: the anterior projection of the soft tissue of the chin
26. Pronasale: the point of the anterior projection of the tip of the nose
27. Sellion: the point of the deepest depression of the nasal bones at the top of the nose

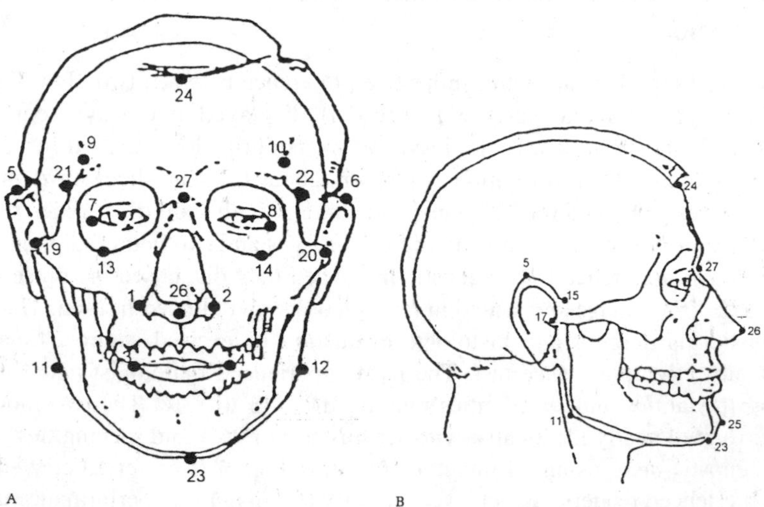

FIGURE 4.3 Landmarks used in the validation study of the Cencit three-dimensional facial scanner. Landmark descriptions are listed in the table. (A) Anterior view. (B) Lateral view.

4.4.3 Diagnostic Testing

Readers were presented with the images one set at a time, so the diagnosis was made using one rendering/presentation combination at a time for each patient. Images were identified only with random numbers, and these numbers determined the presentation order of the images. Therefore, the images were randomly ordered with regard to both image type and patient.

For each image set, the readers were asked to diagnose craniosynostosis for six sutures: metopic, sagittal, right and left coronal, and right and left lambdoidal. Diagnosis was made in the form of a six-point scale (definitely or almost definitely abnormal, probably abnormal, possibly abnormal, possibly normal, probably normal, definitely or almost definitely normal).

This study was designed from the outset for ROC analysis. However, the level of observer performance was so high that the results were degenerate in all but 2 of the 16 cases, and in these two A_z was greater than 0.99. Because ROC analysis did not provide enough results to make comparisons feasible, sensitivity and specifity were calculated. Sensitivity and specificity make fewer assumptions about the data, but are based on the same principles: normal and abnormal cases share characteristics and are divided on the basis of a decision threshold which results in inevitable errors (Figure 4.4A).

The four readers in this study[107] were all board-certified radiologists, with a minimum of 15 years experience. Two were pediatric radiologists, who were experienced in the evaluation and diagnosis of craniosynostosis and had both participated in a previous study which used 3D CT reconstructions in the diagnosis of craniosynostosis. Two readers were neuroradiologists who had less familiarity with craniosysnostosis and no experience making this diagnosis from 3D CT reconstruction images.

4.5 3D ANTHROPOMETRY

Anthropometry is the study of human body measurement. Surface points (e.g., landmarks) and simple scalar measures (e.g., circumferences, breadths, and heights), from individuals and populations have traditionally been used for anthropometry. 3D anthropometry extends body measurements to 3D surface geometry and morphology of both external and internal human body regions. Modern 3D anthropometry includes the acquisition, storage, and analysis of body surface measurements throughout growth and development to adulthood.

3D anthropometry is defined as the quantitative study of human body region and organ surface, volume, and shape characteristics using non-invasive methods. This information is essential to design and manufacture human environments, personal items, protective gear, clothing, and health aids such as orthotics and prosthetics. Medical diagnosis and treatment is often based on precise image-based measurements obtained using 3D anthropometric methods. Volumetric and surface 3D data are gathered, analyzed, and interpreted using computer graphics visualization tools on networked interactive workstations.

3D anthropometry is an emerging discipline that improves productivity of design and manufacturing operations by assuring the quality of fit before the final item is acceptable. Accommodation for variability in groups as well as tailoring products to individual characteristics in human size and shape are supported. Visualization of human models is an essential element in contemporary design of manufactured environments, protective gear, medical treatment, and personal items.

3D anthropometry defines population norms and evaluates individual subjects or groups for the design and fabrication of tailored products. Software tools and normative databases are used in prosthetics and orthotics, human factors studies, electronic atlases, anatomic replicas, surgical and radiation therapy planning, clothing and protective gear design, and others. Optical surface scanning systems have been integrated with spatial databases, CAD/CAM, and rapid prototype

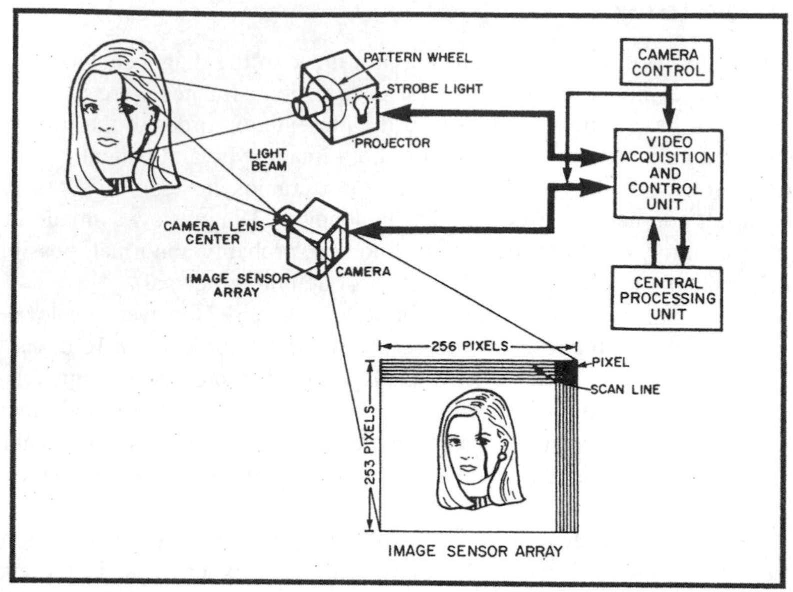

A

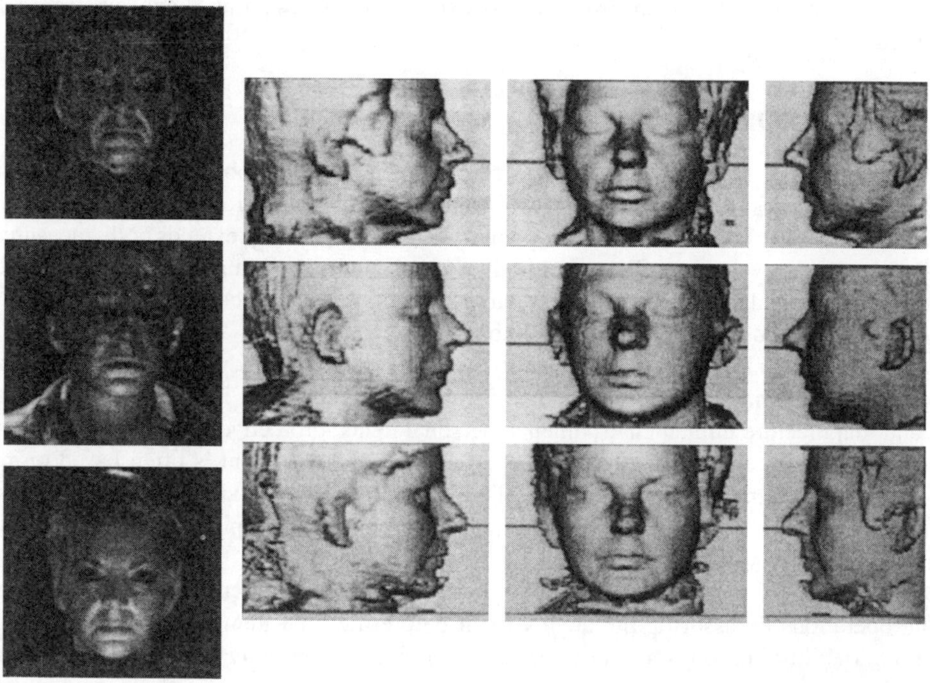

B

FIGURE 4.4 (A) Projection of a single pattern on a subject to form a profile that is captured by the camera image sensor array. (B) Facial surface scanner.

manufacturing technologies to serve these needs. Traditionally, users of anthropometric information have been the military and aircraft manufacturers, with recent expansion of services to aid in the design of personal products, clothing, health services, and rehabilitation aids.

While 3D surface anthropometry methods are relatively new, traditional surveys using simple tools such as calipers and tape measures are well established. Recorded studies of the human form date back to at least the 17th century.[155] Since then, many investigators have measured physical properties of the human body such as weight, size, and center of mass. Martin[156] documented "standard" body measurement methods in a handbook.

In the early 1970s the U.S. Air Force began assembling an anthropometric data repository of worldwide military and civilian surveys. Originally called the AMRL (Aerospace Medical Research Laboratory) Anthropometric Data Bank, it was a collection of magnetic tapes in a "standardized" format. These data were utilized as a source for military standards and handbooks, for ergonomics texts, and by NASA to create a source book containing lists of selected summary statistics and measurement descriptions.

3D anthropometry data has been collected since the 1970s as (1) a finite set of "homologous" points either static or during motion, and (2) an exhaustive sampling of surface point loci on static objects. The first type requires precise definition of specific points, also known as landmarks, prior to measurement. On static objects these points have been measured mechanically by moving a stylus to each of the predefined (and often manually premarked) points while recording stylus position. For example, Snyder et al.[157] used moveable scales and plumb bobs to record points on cadavers. Reynolds and Leung[158] implanted targets in unembalmed cadavers which were then captured with X-rays in stereo pairs. Gordon et al.[159] used a mechanical stylus with a computerized 3D locator for head measurement of living U.S. Army personnel. A box with a special clamp was used to steady the head as the stylus was moved from point to point.

For traditional motion studies, a small number of landmarks are recorded at multiple points in time as the subject changes position. The points are marked prior to data collection with special reflective markers for photographic or video tracking systems[100,160] or with sound emitters for sonic tracking. These are then located in 3D using camera pairs for the visual methods or microphone arrays for the sonic methods.

Stereophotography[23,46,50] and especially stereophotogrammetry, which captures an exterior surface with linked pairs of photographs, are examples of projection image methods. Images for stereophotogrammetry can be acquired rapidly, but the subsequent manual digitization of the desired points in images is extremely slow, tedious, and error prone. As a result, the number of subjects digitized in any one study is small; one set of studies which used stereophotogrammetry for estimating mass distribution properties of body segments measured just 31 men[96] and 46 women.[161]

Designers of aircraft cockpits and aircrew equipment have long recognized the importance of accurate measurements of the flying population. In fact, one of the first symposia of the new Advisory Group for Aeronautical (now Aerospace) Research and Development (AGARD) was devoted to anthropometry and human engineering.[162,163] For example, if an aircraft seat does not provide sufficient height adjustment, a pilot with short stature cannot see over the instrument panel. Likewise, a poorly fit flight helmet may slip on the wearer's head and lead to injury in an aircraft accident.[164] All components of an aircraft system, including control layout, visual displays, crash-worthy or ejection seats, flight clothing, and protective equipment make use of anthropometric data to "fit" the aircraft and life support equipment to the aviator.

The success of 3D anthropometry and its usability for design and fitting are largely dependent on the adoption of standards for display, storage, and communication. Standards are required for raw image data obtained from surface or volumetric scanner systems, as well as reduced and analyzed data.

Multidimensional anthropometric data, including demographic, spatial, temporal, mechanical, and other properties, comprise the anthropometry database. Rigid or deformable and static or dynamic structures are modeled. Range data, CAD geometry,[166] and biomedical image standards have been adopted for acquiring, transforming, storing, and communicating anthropometry data, augmented by information on the method and body position or pose used for image acquisition.

4.5.1 Human Factors Engineering

Body size and shape must be specified for the design of protective clothing used in hostile environments, such as special "G" suits for military aircraft pilots and for protective clothing for chemical warfare and many hazardous industrial environments. Realistic body shapes are required for architectural models and ergonomics and in the evaluation of escape envelopes. Interference checks, fit and integration, assessment of equipment interfaces, and mannequins for crash research require body shape data.

Crew Chief[31] is an interactive computer design 3D modeling system. Because it creates a digital human model that has the correct body size and proportions, it is of particular use in the design of clothing and personal protective equipment. It has 35 segments, which correspond functionally to the human skeletal system and is able to represent the limits of mobility and the physical capacities of the human body.

Another CAD system has been developed by Thalmann and Yang.[165] Here the skeleton or a simple representation is used to convey size information to the designer to convert the two dimensions to three. This is important for seeing the lay of a fabric envelope over the 3D shape.

COMputerized BIomechanical MAN-model, COMBIMAN,[9] is an interactive computer graphics human factor evaluation system. It is used to assess the capabilities and the accommodation of the human operator. It represents the geometric and physical properties of an operator, which is useful for the design of car or aircraft control seats.

Paquette[166] reviewed six computerized analog models including Crew Chief and COMBIMAN. One of these models, JACK,[7] has been designed for the evaluation of the space shuttle and the space station. Programs for animation and visual fields analysis are written in C under UNIX. A second, SAFEWORK, is designed for evaluation of human–machine incompatibilities including safety and health concerns. Positioning of the model and its segments is interactive and a zoom is available for precise positioning. The model is a 35-link skeleton and enfleshment is realized using Bezier curves. Indeed, the U.S. Navy has abandoned man-models for digitized images of living human subjects, but such images are static and require prior knowledge of the design.

Traditional anthropometry does not record the relationship between measurements, so 3D variations in body shape are not detected and a given set of measurements does not uniquely define any individual.

Research has also been done to establish a relationship between readily measured body dimensions and mass distribution.[96,161] Stereophotogrammetry was used for volume measurements and regression equations on anthropometric data for predicting mass distribution characteristics of the total body and its segments. These studies included 31 male and 46 female subjects. The photogrammetric system consisted of stereopair cameras integrated in a single coordinate system using control stands as reference planes, for front and back views.

Greiner and Gordon[167] assessed long-term changes of the human body shape. This secular trend study was based on 22 variables taken from the 1966 and 1988 U.S. Army surveys. Individuals were grouped by birth year into 12 five-year cohorts that span the years 1911 to 1970. It was observed that, with few exceptions, the greatest relative rates of change were found in dimensions related to soft-tissue development rather than skeletal dimensions.

Finally, Roebuck[120] predicted future developments in the fields of anthropometry, computer modeling of the human form, and electronic imaging of the human body. He stressed the importance of measuring the location of joint centers of rotation and development of standards for dividing body parts for determining mass properties of moving segments. He suggests a very interesting strategy for compact mathematical data description and storage of electronic images, based on a skeleton reference axis and a cylindrical coordinate system for compact surface data representation.

4.5.2 Anthropometry

Disciplines using human body surface dimensions require accurate, repeatable measurements. The study by Kohn et al.[69] presents a design for the analysis of repeatability, precision, and validation of a new anthropometric device. This model enables estimation of the proportion of the total variation attributable to each level of data collection. This model is applied to an analysis of repeatability, precision, and validation of the CIS, an optical surface scanner. Twenty-seven facial landmarks were marked on 10 adult males and 10 adult females at two measurement sessions. Two images were scanned during each session, and each image was digitized twice. The CIS results were compared to a previously validated digitizer. The CIS was found to produce accurate, highly repeatable images. Most of the error in this study was found attributable to human error in marking landmarks on the subjects. The CIS was found useful in a variety of anthropometric applications.

Human body surface dimensions are useful to researchers in many disciplines, including anthropometrists who characterize the morphology of a population, developers of clothing or protective devices, plastic and reconstructive surgeons who diagnose and treat abnormal morphology, and forensic scientists who attempt to reconstruct facial dimensions from cranial material.

These disciplines share the requirement for accurate, highly repeatable measurements of homologous anatomical structures, either landmarks or surfaces. Traditional anthropometric studies are based on anatomical locations (or landmarks) and dimensions defined by Hrdlicka,[56] for example. Anthropometers, calipers, and tape measures have traditionally been used to collect these dimensions. The traditional measures have been used to characterize and compare a variety of human populations. The standard list of measurements has also been augmented for use in medicine and human engineering. Traditional anthropometric techniques have been limited to linear distances of unknown configuration in three-dimensional space.

Several recent studies have introduced new methods for the measurement of three-dimensional surface landmark coordinates and the use of these coordinates to reconstruct surfaces and volumes. Burke and co-workers[168–169] used stereophotogrammetry to collect three-dimensional locations on the human face. Cheverud et al.[20] and Donelson and Gordon[171] report variation and covariation among measurements based on three-dimensional coordinates of head landmarks obtained from over 9000 U.S. Army personnel with an automated measurement device. These methods are accurate in the collection of three-dimensional data. Laser scanners are being developed for surface scanning. Systems for use in sensing complex three-dimensional surfaces are being developed by several groups, including Cencit, Inc., St. Louis, MO; Cyberware, Inc., Pacific Grove, CA; Robotic Vision Systems, Inc., Hauppague, NY; and Laser Design Inc., MI. Several of these three-dimensional optical active ranging systems have been reviewed by Besl.[12]

It is necessary to evaluate the precision and repeatability of all new surface imaging devices, and to compare the new device to a simpler and previously validated device for collecting morphological data. Models have been introduced and used to evaluate repeatability and precision. Further, it is necessary to determine the repeatability and precision of the methods used in all aspects of data collection. To interpret analyses, we must be able to evaluate whether the data have been collected in a repeatable manner. If data collection is comprised of more than one step, the overall repeatability of the data collection will reflect error in data collection at each of the composite steps. A method for the evaluation of repeatability, precision, and validation is outlined, and an example of its use in the evaluation of a new three-dimensional facial surface scanner is given below.

4.5.3 Optical Surface Scanners

Optical surface scanners for head and skull measurement include the Cencit and Cyberware devices described above. Active optical scanning methods have been applied to the construction of instruments for whole-body surface measurement used in 3D anthropometry. These recently developed systems are intended for use in surveying populations to characterize the size and shape distributions of various groups, especially for the military and the clothing industry and in some biomedical applications.

4.5.4 Body Imaging System: Requirements and Validation

Several factors must be considered in the validation and testing of an imaging system for anthropometric measurement:

1. The digital images produced must be as clear and accurate as possible, allowing visual identification of contrasting colors and depths by an observer or by electronic means (i.e., error in detecting visible landmarks in digitized images should be evaluated).
2. Repeated images of the same individual should be nearly identical (i.e., error in producing a digital image from a living subject should be evaluated).
3. The locations of the anatomic structures chosen for data collection must be reliably identifiable by a trained observer (i.e., error in locating and marking landmarks by the anthropometrist should be evaluated).

Tests of new imaging devices need to deal with these three issues in terms of precision and repeatability. Precision is the average absolute difference between repeated measures of the same individual. Repeatability is the precision of the measurement relative to the differences among individuals contrasted in any given study. It is measured as the proportion of total variance due to differences between individuals using a repeated-measures ANOVA design. One minus the repeatability is the proportional error due to measurement inaccuracy. The level of repeatability and the imprecision that can be tolerated in any particular study will vary with the size of the contrast being made. For example, measurements that are precise enough for a comparison of infants with adolescents may not be precise enough for studying variation among adolescents. Usually, repeatability is judged within a single homogeneous population since this places the most stringent constraint on error levels.

Although the concepts described above determine the replicability of measurements taken using a device, these measurements may still be inaccurate or biased. The potential bias of the measurement system can be judged by validation studies in which measurements taken from some simpler, already validated system are compared to those obtained by the new device. If measurements taken by the new device are consistently larger or smaller than measurements taken by the already validated system, the device is said to be biased.

A method for testing and validating electronic imaging systems allows a researcher to test whether structures can be reliably located on the images produced by the imaging system, whether an imaging system can produce repeatable images, and whether structures can be reliably located on individuals. Structures located by the new imaging device are compared to a previously validated measurement system. The structures to be tested can be anatomic landmarks, surfaces, or linear dimensions; however, for ease of reference this discussion will focus on the analysis of anatomic landmarks.

4.5.4.1 Data Collection

Prior to recruitment of volunteers, landmarks or surfaces are identified for study. For example, if the imaging device is to be used in plastic surgery applications, facial contours or landmarks may be identified which are commonly used in characterizing normal and abnormal facial morphology. This would include bony landmarks or surfaces which would be changed by plastic surgery (e.g., regions around the eyes, cheeks, or nose) and those which may be expected to remain unchanged by surgical intervention (e.g., the ears).

The number of volunteers necessary for a validation study is dependent on whether the imaging device will be used to characterize a single population (within population) or differences between two or more populations (between populations). For example, approximately 10 volunteers should be recruited for the repeatability study within a single population. This sample size is sufficient to provide a general level of precision and repeatability. It allows us to identify which component, or components, of the measurement process is the major source of error so that this component can be targeted for further development and improvement.

Following this scheme, each volunteer is scheduled for two separate measurement sessions. At each measurement session, landmarks are first identified and marked. Differences in measurements taken on these two occasions are due to error in landmark localization and marking. Two images of each marked individual are collected at each measurement session. Differences between these two images are due to error in digital recording by the device being tested. Finally, the three-dimensional landmark coordinates are recorded twice from each digital image. Differences in measurements taken at separate times on the same image are due to recording error. Thus we can separate error due to (1) locating landmarks on subjects, (2) the imaging device itself, and (3) the digitizing of landmarks from the images. With this design, the data for each individual in the repeatability study consists of eight sets of landmark locations.

4.5.5 Whole-Body Surface Scanning

Recently, several designs for whole-body scanners have been proposed and prototype instruments are undergoing testing for field use.[142,172] Among these are the NKK mobile unit used for population studies in Japan, the Canadian NRC scanner,[111,112] and a new Cyberware instrument. Bhatia et al.[14] simulated a whole-body scanner based on structured light. Many other scanners have been proposed and some built and tested. In an AGARD report,[116,117] a section on data collection reviews these instruments and the principles that underlie their operation. Early attempts to define an "average man"[173] using univariate methods[174] have been superseded by multivariate statistics.[175]

4.5.6 Optical Facial Surface Morphometry

Optical surface scanning systems capture 3D facial surface geometry using on- or off-axis methods. Laser[6] or structured light sources have been used in systems such as Cyberware[3] and Cencit.[25,42,140] The precision, accuracy, and repeatability of landmark localization using an optical scanner was investigated,[69] and the technology was applied to the quantitative assessment of facelift procedures.[143] Facial surface changes in plastic surgery have been objectively evaluated and quantified using optical surface scanning.[13] Facial surface models were synthesized using SDRC I-Deas on a workstation (SGI 4D/340) from optical surface coordinates acquired using the Cencit scanner. Mass properties of the head have been derived from image data sets.[126] Methods for quantitative morphometric analyses were pioneered by Bookstein[18] and other investigators.[20,80]

4.5.6.1 Helmets and Face Masks

Helmets are by far the most common form of personal protection. Types include construction worker safety, motorcycle, football, baseball, diving, welding, bicycle, fire fighter, protective crash, wrestling, explosive ordinance disposal, and flight (pilots). Similarly, facemasks are used for cold protection, surgical and medical procedures, and anesthesia. They are used by physicians, dentists, sculptors, scuba divers, welders, fire fighters, and others.

In the case of an aircraft pilot, the helmet is used not only for personal protection but also for interfacing with the aircraft controls and instruments. Hall and Campbell[45] describe the helmet of the future, showing the complexity of the design task and the importance of integration for lightweight design and comfort.

A pilot's head was digitized (using a Cyberware scanner) with and without the helmet to study stability and fit.[176] Anthropometric methods must accurately represent the shape of the head, especially local surface curvature, for proper helmet design. This laser scanning system has been used to digitize over 1000 U.S. Air Force subjects. Scanning time is 12 s for 130,000 surface points with a resolution of about 1 mm. The main advantage of the method is that a helmet axis system is defined that can be used to standardize the alignment and assess population variability.

Case et al.[177] reported on face mask fitting tests to determine the facial characteristics associated with seal breakage. They found significant differences between races and sexes and noted the lack of anthropometric data available for studying the effects of secular and demographic changes. It is suspected that substantial overlap exists in the current sizing interval for face masks and a better fit test could result in the reduction of the total number of sizes.

Oestenstad et al.[178] used fluorescent tracer aerosol at the leaking sites of respirators to study their distributions. Seventy-three subjects were used to link anthropometric data with leaks. Their findings were as follows: (1) 79% of the leaks occurred at the nose, (2) 73% of leaks approximated the shape of a slit, (3) there is a difference between the sexes, (4) there is a significant association between facial dimensions and leak sites, and (5) the amount of leakage is highest through the chin area. Facial dimensions and fit factor for three facial dimensions were correlated, but this is not currently used for respirator mask design.

Hidson[179] described experiments using CAD/CAM technology for the design of a respirator facepiece. The geometry was constructed using biparametric cubic patches, and a three-axis numerically controlled milling machine cut the final shape.

Rash et al.[180] described a helmet equipped with a night vision system for operation in darkness or under adverse weather conditions, considering sensor inputs, display parameters, temporal characteristics, visual acuity, field of view, environment, and the effects of internal/external sources of information. Accident experiences were carefully analyzed in the context of an improved process of helmet design.

4.6 CRANIOFACIAL DEFORMITIES

3D graphical simulation of craniofacial surgery procedures is often done prior to these operations. However, before surgical simulation can be fully accepted as a planning and educational tool, its accuracy (validity) must be proven. Objective quantitative comparison of 3D CT reconstruction images to surgical results has been done to establish the basis for use of computer graphics in this application.

To characterize the 3D CT scan-based accuracy of volumetric image measurements, we investigated the error involved in each step of the imaging and measurement process using mathematically simulated electronic test objects (exclusive of CT scanning error) and a custom-designed phantom (to test intra-scan and inter-scan image acquisition and 3D reconstruction error).

We compared image volumes based on their associated mass properties, angular orientation, and Boolean subtraction of image objects. Fresh, unpreserved cadaver heads with lead point marker skull implants served as a testing standard for the methodology by allowing both physical measurement of surgical change and comparison of simulation images with post-operative images. The same methodology was applied to actual patient simulation and post-operative images in three pediatric patients who underwent surgery for major craniofacial deformities (Figures 4.5 and 4.6).

The results showed that linear, angular, and coordinate measurement error was well within tolerable limits. Accuracy of coordinate system matching to overlay objects was also acceptable. Subtraction methods yielded the largest error (7% worst case) along the z axis. Application of image comparison methodology to cadaver and patient simulations with post-operative images yielded minimal discrepancy.

An image comparison methodology has been defined and applied to actual patient studies. Validity has been established using this methodology that shows computer graphics simulation can

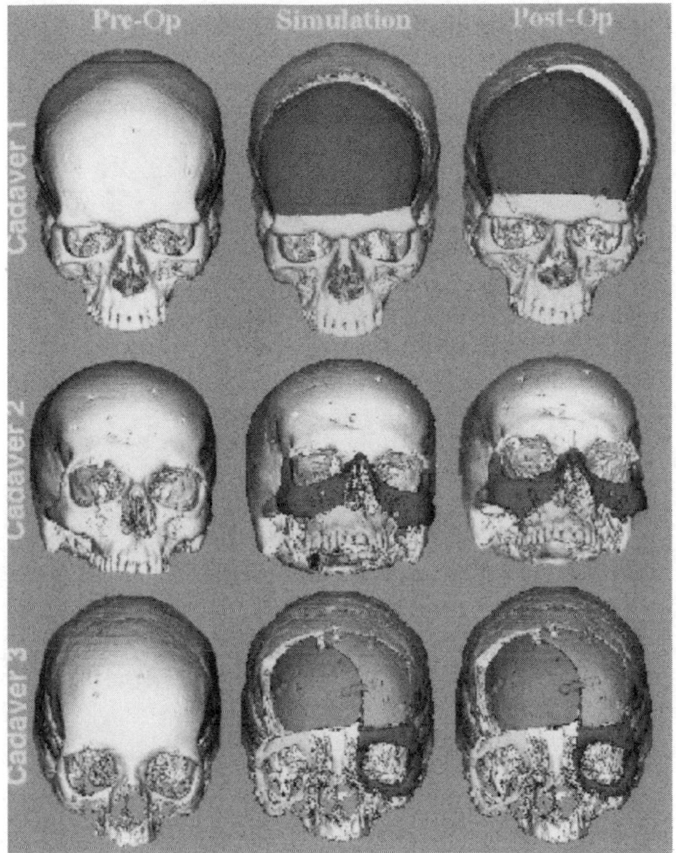

FIGURE 4.5 Cadaver study. Three cadaver skulls are shown, one in each row. The three columns depict: (1) a baseline pre-operative view, (2) a computer-generated surgical simulation which resulted from interaction with the pre-operative scan at the workstation, and (3) a post-operative view obtained upon rescanning after the surgery. The surgical procedures and methods used to assess the differences among the three volumetric data sets are explained in the text. (From Patel VV, Vannier MW, Marsh JL, Lo L-J. Assessing craniofacial surgical simulation. *IEEE Comp Graph Appl* 16(1):46, 1996. With permission.)

be used effectively for surgical planning and for post-operative description of surgical and traumatic change. Validated image comparison methods can also allow evaluation of surgical technique by showing discrepancies between the surgical outcome and surgical plan.

4.6.1 Craniofacial Imaging

Radiography plays an important role in diagnosing craniosynostosis and planning its surgical management. It is generally agreed that 3D CT is the most useful imaging modality for planning surgical management. It has been demonstrated that CT allows more accurate diagnosis than plain radiography and that 3D CT reconstructions allow more accurate diagnosis than ordinary CT. Diagnostic performance of, and subjective preference for, two greatly improved 3D CT rendering methods (voxel gradient and surface projection) and a new technique of image presentation (unwrapped) have been evaluated.[145] The diagnoses from these images are compared against a gold standard comprising both inspection during surgery and histology of resected sutures.

The gold standard in this study was derived by comparing inspection during surgery and histology of resected sutures (Table 4.3). Comparison of these independent sources of information showed that, if the division between pathology normals and abnormals was set between categories

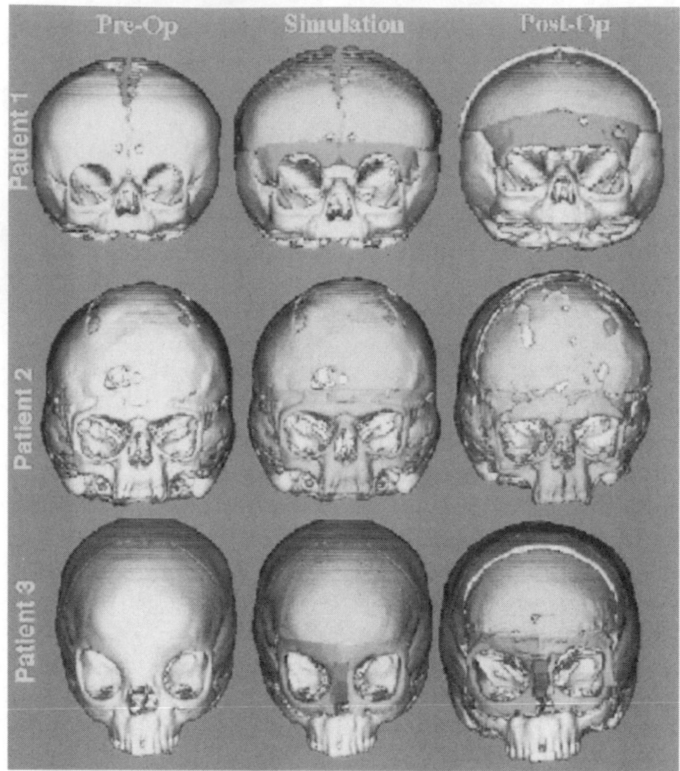

FIGURE 4.6 Patient study. Three patient skulls are shown, one in each row. These are based upon archived CT scan data sets where both pre- and post-operative scans were available *a priori*. There are three columns: (1) a baseline pre-operative view, (2) a computer-generated surgical simulation which resulted from interaction with the pre-operative scan at the workstation, and (3) a post-operative view obtained after the surgical procedure and rescanning. The surgical procedures and methods used to assess the differences among the three volumetric data sets are explained in the text. Patient 1: Female aged 4 years 1.5 months (pre-operative and simulation), with the post-operative scan at 4 years 5.8 months (7 days after surgery). Patient 2: Female aged 1.8 months (pre-operative and simulation), with the post-operative scan at 4.0 months (6 days after surgery). Patient 3: Female aged 4 years 9.7 months (pre-operative and simulation), with the post-operative scan at 4 years 10.5 months (7 days after surgery). (From Patel VV, Vannier MW, Marsh JL, Lo L-J. Assessing craniofacial surgical simulation. *IEEE Comp Graph Appl* 16(1):46, 1996. With permission.)

two and three, there were disagreements with surgical truth in only 6 of 66 sutures (Figure 4.1). Four of the disagreements resulted from the two patients with partial bilateral lambdoidal synostosis. The synostosed portions of the lambdoidal sutures were excised with the synostosed sagittal suture, while the normal portions were excised separately and correctly judged to be histologically normal. The other two disagreements were metopic sutures which had closed normally. The surgeon rated them as normal, while the histological results, which were blinded and did not consider the age of the patient, identified them as closed. In all six cases, therefore, the disagreements resulted from procedural difficulties, and the surgeon's findings were used as the gold standard.

Two types of 3D images were generated: voxel gradient rendering and surface projection rendering. Voxel gradient rendering treats the computer reconstruction as a solid object and creates the image by calculating the angle at which a ray of light originating at the observer would strike the object. The closer the surface is to a right angle relative to the light ray, the brighter that portion of the image. Therefore, flat surfaces are highlighted and angled surfaces are shaded. Although these principles are identical to those used to create the images in the most recent diagnostic test

TABLE 4.3
Pathology Categories and Description of Physical Characteristics for Cross-Sectioned Slices of Excised Sutures

Pathology Category	Description
0	Completed patent suture
1	Minimal osseus encroachment of fibrous suture; no overlapping bony trabeculae
2	Fibrous suture predominates; overlapping bony projections
3	Minimal persistence of fibrous suture; bony trabeculae
4	Fused suture

of 3D imaging of craniosynostosis, the images themselves are much improved because the algorithms which create the object surface preserve much more detail.

Projection rendering creates the image by calculating cumulative object density along a ray perpendicular to the display surface. In a situation directly analogous to X-ray films, the brightness of the image is determined by the density. If the rendering makes brightness inversely proportional to cumulative density, as ours did, the image will be very similar to an X-ray film. Our images had two important improvements over X-ray images or previously evaluated projection (then called "volumetric") images. First, images were rendered using only the half of the skull facing the viewer. This technique eliminates the possibility of confusing anatomical features from different sides of the skull. Second, we used surface projection, which calculates cumulative density only for those features a chosen distance below the object surface. Because calvarial shape and suture characteristics are both surface or near-surface features, we were able to select only the information relevant to them, and eliminate potentially confusing internal structures.

Unwrapped images have two theoretical advantages over conventional images. First, the projection rays are always orthogonal to the surface of the skull, rather than to the plane of the image, as is the case with conventional views. This eliminates the "blotting out" of the suture at the edges of projection images, where the curvature of the skull increases the quantity of bone through which the projected ray must pass. Second, the entire skull can be viewed at once, which makes it easier to examine bilateral sutures for symmetry.

Two aspects of using these images were evaluated: diagnostic performance and subjective preference. To measure subjective preference, readers were presented with all images for each patient, one patient at a time, and asked to rank the images in terms of their perceived ability to diagnose craniosynostosis using them. The random numbers assigned to the images determined the left-to-right presentation order, although readers were told they were free to change the order of the images if they thought this would aid them in making comparisons. The same images were presented in identical fashion before and after the diagnostic phase, and ranking was done the same way. Because these imaging modalities were unfamiliar to all reviewers at the beginning of the study, we were interested to see how well first impressions related to both diagnostic performance and subjective preference after diagnostic use.

For testing diagnostic performance, readers were presented with one set of images, containing one rendering/presentation combination, at a time. Presentation order of the images was determined by their randomly assigned numbers, so the images were randomly ordered with regard to both image type and patient. For each image set, readers were asked to diagnose craniosynostosis for six sutures: metopic, sagittal, right and left coronal, and right and left lambdoidal. Diagnosis was made in the form of a six-point scale (definitely or almost definitely abnormal, probably abnormal, possibly abnormal, possibly normal, probably normal, definitely or almost definitely normal).

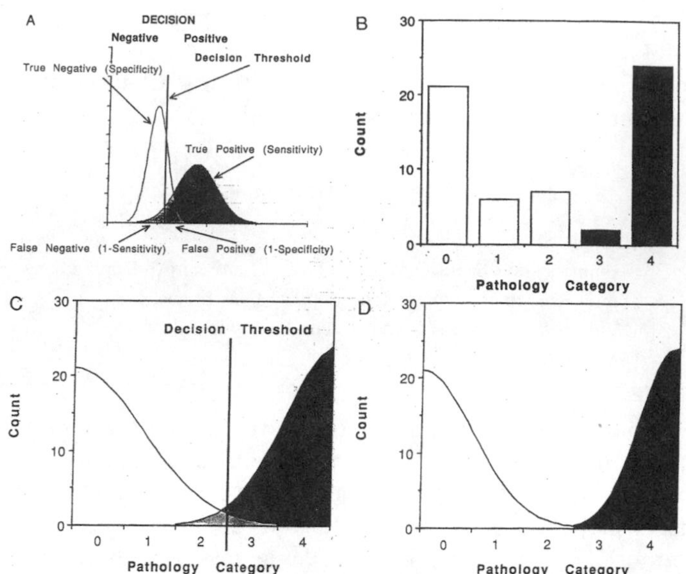

FIGURE 4.7 (A–D) Two models of craniosynostosis. (A) Decision theory principles applied to hypothetical populations with Gaussian distributions of normal and abnormal characteristics, showing overlap in characteristics and a decision threshold dividing normal and abnormal. (B) Comparison of surgical truth to pathology truth, with the apparent errors due to logistics removed. (C) A model for the data in (B), assuming an overlap in characteristics with a decision threshold. (D) A model for the data in (B), assuming no overlap in characteristics. In all graphs, the solid areas are abnormal, the open areas are normal, and the shaded areas are overlap.

In addition to making the diagnosis, readers were asked to evaluate the quality of the image set for evaluating each suture on a three-point scale (good, satisfactory, poor). Before beginning this phase of the study, each reader was presented with a set of standardized instructions.

Although this study was designed from the outset for ROC analysis, the level of performance was so high with these images that ROC analysis was impossible in almost all cases. The ROC analysis software used, ROCFIT and CORROC2, were unable to fit ROC curves to the data in all but 2 of the 16 cases. In these two cases A_z, the area under the ROC curve which equals the proportion of correct responses regardless of the decision threshold, was greater than 0.99. In place of ROC analysis, sensitivity and specifity were compared. Sensitivity and specificity were nearly perfect for most sutures, imaging modalities, and readers.

Although the radiologists who participated in the study achieved similar diagnostic performance with all imaging modalities, their level of confidence in their diagnosis, as measured by relative strength of the diagnostic category they chose, varied with the imaging modality. The differences in confidence were clearest with the normal sutures. Readers were most confident with the surface projection images, particularly when they were conventionally displayed, and least comfortable with the voxel gradient images, particularly the unwrapped versions. The differences in level of confidence were echoed in subjective evaluations of image quality. Surface projection images were given the highest quality ratings, with conventional images slightly favored over unwrapped ones. Voxel gradient images received quality ratings markedly lower than surface projection images, with no real difference between conventional and unwrapped images.

The difficulty of diagnosing craniosynostosis varies by case. In some cases, especially the simpler abnormalities, the diagnosis is clear. For more complex abnormalities the diagnosis can be more difficult. Improvements in radiologic imaging have consistently improved its accuracy in

TABLE 4.4
Physical Models Compared with Graphical Models

Physical Models	Digital Models
Physical replica	3D computer images
Fixation plate preparation facilitated	Difficult plate preparation
Implant preparation	Difficult implant preparation
High cost	Low cost
Significant operator time	Less operator time
Difficult to create	Easy to create
Destructive simulation	Unlimited simulations
Milling equipment required	Total simulation on computer

diagnosing craniosynostosis by making the more difficult cases clearer. CT allows more accurate diagnosis than plain radiography, and 3D CT reconstructions allow more accurate diagnosis than ordinary CT. This study, using the most recent 3D CT algorithms, found nearly perfect performance with experienced readers. Gellad, et al. suggested that plain radiography is adequate for the diagnosis of most craniosynostosis, but that CT could be useful in cases which are not clearly positive or negative. Our results suggest that 3D CT reconstructions may perform the same role in relation to CT.

Although all the 3D reconstruction algorithms we tested achieved similar levels of diagnostic performance, and therefore have the same clinical potential, our readers strongly preferred conventionally displayed surface projection images. The pediatric radiologists, who were most familiar with diagnosis of craniosynostosis, described their pattern of viewing images as, first, looking at calvarial shape to see if there was a reason to suspect craniosynostosis, and second, looking at the sutures to see which were open. The unwrapped images required more effort to interpret shape, and the voxel gradient images required more effort to interpret suture patency.

Craniofacial malformations and trauma can require complex procedures for treatment, especially surgical correction. Surgical planning using cephalograms (skull X-rays) with comparison to normative data has become standard, augmented by sectional imaging including CT and MRI. 3D reconstruction of CT scans was introduced in the 1980s and has increasingly been used to plan operative procedures on the skull.[3–6] Interactive computer graphics visualization allows simulation of craniofacial procedures before surgical intervention. Two simulation modes are currently available: (1) physical replicas created with CT data applied to numerically controlled milling machines or stereolithography machines and (2) 3D graphical images created from tomographic data (Table 4.4). Physical replica models make structural conflicts more apparent and enable pre-operative preparation of rigid fixation plates and implants. The disadvantages of these models include high construction cost and time and the destructive nature of simulation. Digital volume replicas allow repeated simulation trials and allow simulations to be performed with modest desktop equipment.

Simulation of surgical procedures allows selection of a best technical approach based on predictions of functional and aesthetic results. Surgical simulation can also be used as an educational tool to inform the patient and allow students to non-invasively and non-destructively practice surgical procedures. Finally, simulation can describe physical, surgical, or traumatic change based on comparison to pre- and post-operative images. Before surgical simulation becomes widely used, however, its accuracy (validity) must be established. Previous testing has been limited principally to subjective comparison of simulations with actual surgical outcomes. Objective measurements made on test objects or cadavers to quantify the accuracy and measurability of surgical simulation processes have not been reported.

TABLE 4.5
Comparison Methods Validation Summary

Measurement Method	Test	Error
Linear measurement	Electronic cube	0
Landmark coordinates	Electronic landmark	<1 voxel
Surface match	Rotated electronic cube	<1°
		<1 voxel
Mass properties	Electronic "F" object	0
Measurement of physical change	Phantom: surface match	< (3 mm),[a] 1–2°
between scans	Phantom: mass properties	<1 mm
Subtraction	Phantom	<7% in objects rotated about z axis
		<4% in all others

[a] Method not used for measurement.

4.6.2 Object Comparison

Among the procedures required for comparison of two image volumes are segmentation and registration. Segmentation is defined as the parceling of 3D image data sets into contiguous subvolumes that share a common signal or structural property. Segmentation was performed in this project to isolate bone sections that function as separate intra-operative objects. For surgical simulation, these individual bone objects are translated and rotated to alter the skull configuration and achieve a predefined goal, such as normalization. For the actual post-operative images, mobilized bones are also segmented for pairwise object comparison. To allow such comparison, registration between the pre-operative and post-operative skull volumes is necessary. This was achieved by placing the pre-operative skull images in the same orientation and position in the reference coordinate system as the post-operative images. This essentially overlays the images to allow accurate comparison of landmark coordinates, object position, mass properties, and other metrics.

4.6.3 Validation of Measurements (Table 4.5)

The error involved in each step of the surgical simulation process was quantified to characterize 3D CT-based measurement. Possible error sources considered included:

1. CT scanning
2. 3D image reconstruction and reformatting
3. Image manipulation (translation, rotation, and dissection)
4. Operator landmark identification and measurement

Since CT imaging has been validated previously as a measurement system, it is most important to concentrate on validation of the three-dimensional reconstruction images themselves. To test reconstruction and measurement capability, 3D electronic objects free of CT imaging-generated error and of known dimensions were synthesized as a series of planar images.

The results of direct comparison between simulation and post-operative image volumes have been reported as measurements taken at the skull base (surgically unaltered), for the entire skull, and for individual bone objects. For each object pair, the principal metrics used include differences between their centroids, angular orientation discrepancy in degrees, and displaced moments of inertia that describe changes in the mass distribution along each principal axis reported as percentages. Finally, discrete bony objects (such as an isolated frontal bone fragment) subjected to volume subtraction (Boolean differencing) after surface matching were used to define the maximum intersection possible. Manually aligned bony fragments result in an intersection (or Boolean difference) that is influenced by variations in their shape, position, and orientation between the simulation and post-operative images. The overall orientation error is expressed as a percentage based on the actual intersection as a fraction of the ideal given by surface matching. All three cadaver results show that the skull bases match well. Their centroids are within 1.5 mm and moments of inertia are within 3%. In patient studies, the skull base and total skull measurements correspond well, whereas individual object correspondence varies with (1) difficulty of dissection, (2) object shape, and (3) extent of movement.

4.6.4 Surgical Simulation

Surgical simulation promises to improve patient outcomes by better informing the operating surgeon of the abnormal anatomy, allowing comparison and selection of the best alternative procedure for an individual patient, and reducing procedure time so fewer complications occur and better outcomes result. The cost of such simulations is minimal and dropping as the computer graphics hardware and software needed to accomplish it become commonplace and the requisite high-speed digital networks proliferate in hospitals. The benefits are difficult to quantify, since randomized controlled trials have not been done. Because the technology is evolving so rapidly, it is not practical to conduct such evaluations on a regular basis. However, the application of computer graphics in surgery is growing and there is a great imbalance between claims made for the benefits of the technology and rigorous and systematic studies that support these assertions. We chose to study and compare the quality of the results obtained from surgical simulations against independent standards for truth, including phantom test objects and cadavers. The results are encouraging, but not sensational. The discrepancies between the simulated and actual results that we report here serve to demonstrate that the problem we are attempting to solve is complex and demanding. Real progress in this important area can best be made by such carefully designed systematic studies, since the feasibility of generating and manipulating graphical images of biological objects has already been demonstrated many times in the past decade.

4.6.5 Surgical Imaging

Imaging in surgery is used for diagnosis, planning, intra-operative navigation, and post-operative evaluation. Digital medical imaging modalities include CT, MRI, MR therapy (MRT), fluoroscopy, and ultrasound. These modalities are applied singly or jointly (multimodality). Surgical requirements differ according to the nature of intervention, and real-time guidance is sometimes needed such that a sequence of images is generated and displayed as acquired. Soft-copy display on CRT screens is satisfactory for intra-operative use, whereas hard-copy film images or physical replica modeling may be needed in other cases. Computed tomography, developed more than 20 years ago, remains important in craniofacial and orthopedic surgery. Newer imaging systems, especially ultrasound, magnetic resonance imaging, and digital fluoroscopy, are used for neurosurgery, oncology, and cardiothoracic and abdominal surgery. Each modality offers specific qualities that serve specific needs in diagnosis, planning, intra-operative navigation, and evaluation.

The principal modalities used for surgical applications include radiography, CT, MRI, ultrasound, PET/SPECT, and others. No single modality serves every need in an efficient manner, and tailoring the imaging procedure and technology to match the specific requirements is a major challenge. In some instances, combinations of multiple modalities are needed to achieve the desired results. For example, an abnormal focus of activity found in a PET scan may be insufficiently defined anatomically. By combining the PET scan with a CT or MRI scan of the same body region such that the two examinations are superimposible, the anatomic locus of the abnormal functional region can be identified. The process used to unite the PET and CT/MRI scans is frameless stereotaxy.

Recent developments in imaging methods have advanced minimally invasive medicine by allowing image guidance and introduction of new therapeutic modalities, especially focused ultrasound, cryotherapy, stereotactic radiotherapy, interstitial laser therapy, and brachytherapy. Among these developments, the fusion of multiple images without use of a stereotactic frame by frameless stereotaxy is most important. Combination of optical images derived from a video camera with previously acquired CT or MRI scans facilitates the localization of lesions and critical structures.

4.7 LOWER LIMB PROSTHETICS

Lower limb prosthesis quality of fit assessment is purely subjective in routine clinical practice, based upon patient reports of discomfort, skin redness or localized pain, and palpation. Wide variation in residual limb physical characteristics and condition preclude a rigid approach to prosthesis prescription.[181] With relatively long life expectancy for many lower limb amputees,[182] outcome is measured in return to work and quality of life, which have important social and economic consequences.

An estimated 400,000 amputees live in the United States, with approximately 60,000 lower extremity amputations performed each year.[183] Many of these amputees are classified as "hard to fit," having prostheses that are unsatisfactory in both comfort and function.[184–188] 3D anthropometry has been applied to automate the fitting of lower limb prostheses.[125,146]

4.8 ELECTRONIC ANATOMIC ATLAS

The conventional printed textbook anatomic atlas is familiar and important in medical education and practice. Electronic atlases have been constructed which contain the information found in the traditional printed versions, with some interesting and important new capabilities.

An electronic atlas consists of a volumetric data set from a body region with an integrated knowledge base that contains the anatomic nomenclature and ancillary information (such as tissue type, vascular territory, functional significance, etc.) linked to the image data. By combining the stored atlas volume with interactive computer graphics rendering tools, the user can generate unique views from any desired perspective. Hoehne and associates[55] at the University of Hamburg pioneered the development of electronic atlases in their Voxel Man project.

The Visible Human Project at the National Library of Medicine is an important source of anatomic information. Adult male and female cadavers have been imaged by tissue section, CT, and MRI at high resolution. These data are now available in the public domain and are found in many electronic atlases.

3D deformable anatomical atlas matching algorithms based on Grenander's global shape models have been developed that accommodate both global and local shape differences. Anatomical shape is modeled using a deformable atlas (template), and individual shape variation is modeled using probabilistic transformations that are applied to the atlas coordinate system. Continuum mechanical models based on elasticity and fluidity are used to constrain the transformations applied to the atlas to ensure anatomical relationships are maintained.

The deformable atlas is matched to a target volume by estimating the transformation that deforms it into the shape of a particular data set. Once deformed, the resulting individualized atlas contains information such as tissue type, structure names, landmarks, and other information keyed to the target data set. Thus, the individualized atlas provides a means of automatically labeling and quantifying the shape of a particular anatomy. Analysis of the atlas transformation also provides information for quantifying shape differences and growth trajectory.

A deformable textbook that mathematically represents the shape and variability of the developing cranium (skull vault) has been created. The textbook consists of anatomic information in the form of digitized image volumes (such as CT or MR 3D data sets) and descriptive information such as structure names, locations, and shapes. The deformable textbook is used to generate individualized ones. Each individualized textbook provides subject-specific information (such as structure location, volume, shape, etc.) normally only known for the textbook anatomy. It is generated by deforming a generalized textbook into the shape of a particular individual's anatomy.

4.8.1 Surgical Simulation

Computer-based imaging for simulation surgery implies graphical display and manipulation of anatomy, typically derived from volumetric CT and MR imaging. Virtually any surgical procedure can be simulated, although this does not imply that the simulation will be accurate, complete, or useful, nor that it can be accomplished efficiently. In fact, it may be the case that simulation of a surgical procedure is more complex, awkward, and difficult to perform than the procedure itself. This is especially true when the surgeon involved has relatively little computing experience. Improvements in interactive computer graphics and the availability of networked low-cost desktop graphical workstations allow the pre-operative visualization of complex anatomic abnormalities, surgical planning, and post-operative evaluation.

4.8.1.1 Subjective Evaluation — Craniofacial 3D Imaging

Improvements in radiologic imaging have consistently resulted in improved accuracy in diagnosing craniosynostosis. Computed tomography allows more accurate diagnosis than plain radiography, and 3D CT reconstructions allow more accurate diagnoses than ordinary CT. A study using the most recent 3D CT algorithms has found nearly perfect performance with experienced readers. This pattern of findings suggests that uncertainty in diagnosing craniosynostosis may be the result of ambiguous imaging rather than genuine similarities of normal and abnormal states. In this chapter, we have compared surgical reports, suture histology, and diagnoses made from 3D CT reconstructions by readers with different levels of experience, to evaluate the possibility that craniosynostosis is inherently binary in nature and therefore, in principle, capable of being diagnosed with perfect accuracy.

To this end, two independent gold standards have been compared with subjective diagnoses from 3D CT images. Surgical reports, histology of excised sutures, and 3D CT images were compared for 25 children undergoing surgical craniosynostosis management. Surgical reports identified sutures as normal or abnormal. Histology reported suture closure on a five-point scale. Four radiologists used 3D CT images to diagnose sutures on a six-point rated response scale. Sutures with histology 0, 1, or 2 were normal on surgical reports, and those with histology 3 or 4 were abnormal. Most readers achieved nearly perfect sensitivity and specificity. Reader confidence was unrelated to degree of pathology The diagnosis of craniosynostosis appears to be binary in this sample. Surgical reports, pathology results, and 3D CT images read by experienced viewers achieved nearly perfect agreement.

4.8.2 The Visible Human Project

The Visible Human Project from the National Library of Medicine has created volumetric digital image data sets of complete human male and female cadavers in MRI, CT, and cryosection blockface modes.

The male data set consists of axial MRI images of the head and neck taken at 4-mm intervals and longitudinal sections of the rest of the body also at 4-mm intervals. The MRI images are 256×256 pixel resolution. Each pixel has 12 bits of gray tone resolution.

The CT data consists of axial CT scans of the entire body taken at 1-mm intervals at a resolution of 512×512 pixels where each pixel is made up of 12 bits of gray tone. The axial anatomic images are 2048×1216 pixels where each pixel is defined by 24 bits of color, about 7.5 megabytes. The anatomic cross-sections are also at 1-mm intervals and coincide with the CT axial images. There are 1871 cross-sections for each mode, CT and anatomy, obtained from the male cadaver.

The data set from the female cadaver has the same characteristics as the male cadaver with one exception. The axial anatomic images were obtained at 0.33-mm intervals instead of 1.0-mm intervals, resulting in over 5000 anatomic images about 40 gigabytes in size. Distribution began in mid-1995, and these data have been placed in the public domain.

4.9 FUTURE DEVELOPMENTS

A number of problems arise in validation studies such as that done with the Cencit facial scanner, Polhemus 3Space electromagnetic digitizer, or surgical simulations with cadaver heads, presenting areas in which additional effort is needed to ensure that any given electronic imaging system is fully suitable for an anthropometric application.

Not all desired landmarks were easily visible on the scanned images. Landmarks which were not visible were regarded as missing, and further analysis of these landmarks was not possible. We identified landmarks on all areas of the face and ears; however, ears were rarely imaged sufficiently to identify the marked landmarks. In addition, landmarks on the margins of the face were often unobservable due to variations in lighting. Landmarks in the center of the face were the most clearly visible because the system's cameras were concentrated on this region. These shortcomings can be overcome with changes in lighting, camera location, and data processing. Future developments may also enable landmark locations and their defining surfaces to be identified electronically, perhaps by locating landmarks of a particular color density. This will reduce error and time spent in data acquisition.

Despite these limitations, there is a considerable body of evidence to show that 3D visualization and 3D anthropometry are practical and useful. As the technology on which they are based improves, re-evaluation of their relative quality must be assessed subjectively and objectively.

4.9.1 Craniofacial Surgery — Objective Assessment

Craniofacial surgery is guided by 3D images reconstructed from CT or MR scans, but the validity of these graphically rendered images has not been tested under controlled circumstances. We simulated craniofacial surgical procedures and tested each step in the process used to create and apply the images against an independent standard for truth. The ability to measure 3D bony objects in these image volumes was tested for accuracy and repeatability. Surgery was simulated and performed on cadavers and the results compared with direct measurements. Surgical correction of craniofacial abnormalities in pediatric patients was tested for the validity of the simulations.

We found that the 3D spatial measurement accuracy of 3D image volumes obtained from CT scans was high, allowing surface landmark identification within 1 voxel, physical change detection within 1 mm and 2°, and matching of surfaces within 1° and 1 voxel under ideal conditions. The error increased to 4 mm and 3° on average in cadaver and patient simulations.

3D CT reconstructions provide acceptable bony structural detail for planning and describing craniofacial surgical interventions, and surgical simulation images accurately depict post-operative outcome.

4.9.2 Summary

Interactive computer-based simulation is gaining acceptance for craniofacial surgical planning. Subjective visualization without objective measurement capability, however, severely limits the value of simulation since spatial accuracy must be maintained. This study investigated the error sources involved in one method of surgical simulation evaluation. Linear and angular measurement errors were found to be within ±1 mm and 1°. Surface match of scanned objects was slightly less accurate, with errors up to 3 voxels and 4°, and Boolean subtraction methods were 93 to 99%

accurate. Once validated, these testing methods were applied to objectively compare craniofacial surgical simulations to post-operative outcomes, and verified that the form of simulation used in this study yields accurate depictions of surgical outcome. However, to fully evaluate surgical simulation, future work is still required to test the new methods in sufficient numbers of patients to achieve statistically significant results. Once completely validated, simulation cannot only be used in pre-operative surgical planning, but also as a post-operative descriptor of surgical and traumatic physical changes. Validated image comparison methods can also show discrepancy of surgical outcome to surgical plan, thus allowing evaluation of surgical technique.

REFERENCES

1. Adams L, Gilsbach JM, Krybus, W. et al. CAS — A navigation support for surgery. In Hoehne KH, Fuchs H, Pizer SM, eds. *3D Imaging in Medicine*. NATO ASI Series F: Computer and Systems Sciences, vol 60, Springer, Berlin, 1990, 411–423.
2. Adams L, Krybus W, Meyer-Ebrecht D, et al. Computer assisted surgery. *IEEE Comp Graph Appl* 5:43–50, 1990.
3. Addleman D, Addleman L. Rapid 3D digitizing. *Comp Graph World* Nov. 42–44, 1985.
4. Altobelli DE, Kikinis R, Mulliken JB, et al. Computer-assisted three-dimensional planning in craniofacial surgery. *Plast Reconstr Surg* 92:576, 1993.
5. Apuzzo ML, Sabshin JK. Computed tomographic guidance stereotaxis in the management of intracranial mass lesions. *Neurosurgery* 12:277, 1983.
6. Arridge S, Moss JP, Linney AD, James DR. Three-dimensional digitization of the face and skull. *J Maxillofacial Surg* 13:136–143, 1985.
7. Badler NI, Phillips CB, Webber BL. *Simulating Humans. Computer Graphics Animation and Control*. Oxford University Press, New York, 1993.
8. Bailey RC, Byrnes J. A new, old method for assessing measurement error in both univariate and multivariate morphometric studies. *Syst Zool* 39:124–130, 1990.
9. Bapu P, Korna M, McDaniel J. User's Guide for Combiman Programs (COMputerized BIomechanical MAN-Model). Version 6. Report UDR-TR-83-51, AFAMRL-TR-83-097. National Technical Information Service, U.S. Dept. of Commerce, Washington, DC, 1983.
10. Barnett GH, Kormos DW, Steiner CP, et al. Use of a frameless, armless stereotactic wand for brain tumor localization with two-dimensional and three-dimensional neuroimaging. *Neurosurgery* 3:674, 1993.
11. Beddar, AS, Thomason C, Leung PM. Description and evaluation of a new 3-D computerized treatment planning dose compensator system. *Med Dosim* 19(4):227–235, 1994.
12. Besl PJ. Active optical range imaging sensors. *Mach Vision Appl* 1:127–152, 1988.
13. Bhatia GH, Vannier MW, Commean PK, Smith KE. Surface imaging of the human body. *Proc Visualization Biomed Comp SPIE* 2359:493–503, 1994.
14. Bhatia GH, Vannier MW, Smith KE, et al. Quantification of facial surface change using a structured light scanner. *Plast Reconstr Surg* 94(6):768–774, 1994.
15. Bookstein F, Green W. Edge information at landmarks in medical images. In Robb R, ed. *Visualization in Biomedical Computing. SPIE Proc* 242–258, 1992.
16. Bookstein F. *The Measurement of Biological Shape and Shape Change*. Lecture Notes in Biomathematics, Springer, New York, 1978.
17. Bookstein F. Morphometrics. In Toga AW, ed. *Three-Dimensional Neuroimaging*. Raven Press, New York, 1990, 167–188.
18. Bookstein FL. *Morphometric Tools for Landmark Data — Geometry and Biology*. Cambridge University Press, London, 1991.
19. Cheng CW, Das IJ, Stea B. The effect of the number of computed tomographic slices on dose distributions and evaluation of treatment planning systems for radiation therapy of intact breast. *Int J Radiat Oncol Biol Phys* 30(1):183–195, 1994.
20. Cheverud J, Lewis JL, Banchrach W, and Lew WE. The measurement of form and variation in form: an application of three-dimensional quantitative morphology by finite-element methods, *Am J Phys Anthrop* 62:152–165, 1983.

21. Christiansen EL, Thompson JR, Kopp S. Intra- and inter-observer variability and accuracy in the determination of linear and angular measurements in computed tomography. *Acta Odontol Scand* 44:221–229, 1986.
22. Churchill E, McConville J. Sampling and Data Gathering Strategies for Future USAF Anthropometry, AMRL-TR-74-102. Aerospace Medical Research Laboratory, Air Force Systems Command, Wright-Patterson AFB, OH, 1976.
23. Coblentz A, Ignazi G, Mollard R. Ergodata: a complete system of data and research in human biometry and biomechanics: new advances, *Am J Phys Anthtop* 69(2):188, 1986.
24. Commean P, Smith K, Bhatia G, Vannier M. Validation of spiral computed tomography and optical surface scanning for 3D limb prosthesis design. IMAGE VIII Conference, Image Society, Tucson, AZ, 1994.
25. Commean PK, Smith KE, Bhatia G, Vannier MW. Geometric design of a multisensor structured light range digitizer. *Opt Eng* 33(4):1349–1358, 1994.
26. Corner BD, Lele S, Richtsmeier JT. Measuring precision of three-dimensional landmark data. *J Quant Anthrop* 3:347–359, 1992.
27. Cutting C, Bookstein FL, Grayson B, et al. Three dimensional computer assisted design of craniofacial surgery procedures: optimizations and interaction with cephalometrics and CT based models. *Plast Reconstr Surg* 77:877–885, 1986.
28. Cutting C, McCarthy JG, Karron D. Three-dimensional input of body surface data using a laser light camera. *Ann Plast Surg* 21:38–45, 1988.
29. Demaria R, Godlewski G, De Guilhermier P, Tang J, Seguin J, Chaptal PA. Static morphometric bases for CT identification and evaluation of the outflow chamber of the left ventricle. Preliminary study in formalin-fixed heart. *Surg Radiol Anat* 15(2):145–150, 1993.
30. Dumoulin CL, Souza SP, Darrow RD. Real-time position monitoring of invasive devices using magnetic resonance. *Magn Reson Med* 29:411, 1993.
31. Easterly JA. Crew Chief: a model of a maintenance technician. NTIS AFHRL-TP-90-18, 1990.
32. Ehricke HH, Schad LR, Gademan G, et al. Use of MR angiography for stereotactic planning. *J Comp Assisted Tomogr* 16:35, 1992.
33. Ellis DS, Toth BA, Stewart WB. Three dimensional imaging and computer-designed prostheses in the evaluation and management of orbitocranial deformities. *Adv Ophthalmic Plast Reconstr Surg* 9:261–272, 1992.
34. Ende G, Treuer H, Boesecke R. Optimization and evaluation of landmark-based image correlation. *Phys Med Biol* 37(1):261–271, 1992.
35. Esselman GH, Coticchia JM, Wippold FJ, Fredrickson JM, Vannier MW, Neely JG. Computer-stimulated test fitting of an implantable hearing aid using three-dimensional CT scans of the temporal bone: preliminary study. *Am J Otol* 15(6):702–709, 1994.
36. Evans JL, Ng KH, Wiet WG, Vonesh MJ, Burns WB, Radvany MG, Kane BJ, Davidson CJ, Roth SI, Kramer BL, Meyers SN, McPherson DD. Accurate three-dimensional reconstruction of intravascular ultrasound data. Spatially correct three-dimensional reconstructions. *Circulation* 93:567–576, 1996.
37. Farkas LG. *Anthropometry of the Head and Face in Medicine*. Elsevier, New York, 1981.
38. Fujino T, ed. *Simulation and Computer-Aided Surgery.* John Wiley & Sons, New York, 1994.
39. Galvin JM, Sims C, Dominiak G, Cooper JS. The use of digitally reconstructed radiographs for three-dimensional treatment planning and CT-simulation. *Int J Radiat Oncol Biol Phys* 31(4):935–942, 1995.
40. Gandhe AJ, Hill DL, Studholme C, Hawkes DJ, Ruff CF, Cox TC, Gleeson MJ, Strong AJ. Combined and three-dimensional rendered multimodal data for planning cranial base surgery: a prospective evaluation. *Neurosurgery* 35(3):463–470, discussion 471, 1994.
41. Gleason PL, Kikinis R, Altobelli D, et al. Video registration virtual reality for frameless stereotactic surgery. *Stereotact Funct Neurosurg* 62/63 (in press).
42. Godhwani A, Bhatia G, Vannier MW. Calibration considerations in a multisensor 3D scanner. *Opt Eng* 33(4):1359–1367, 1994.
43. Goodall C, Bose A. Models and Procrustes methods. 19th Symposium of the Interface Between Computer Science and Statistics, 1987, 86–92.
44. Guthrie BL, Adler JR Jr. Computer-assisted preoperative planning, interactive surgery, and frameless stereotaxy. *Clin Neurosurg* 38:112–131, 1992.

45. Hall PS, Campbell BL. Helmet-mounted systems technology planning for the future. *SPIE Proc* 1695:2–8, 1992.
46. Herron RE. Biostereometric measurement of body forms. *Yearbook Phys Anthrop* 16:80–121, 1972.
47. Heilbrun MP, Roberts TS, Apuzzo ML, et al. Preliminary experience with Brown-Roberts-Wells (BRW) computerized stereotaxic guidance system. *J Neurosurg* 59:217, 1983.
48. Heilbrun MP, McDonald P, Wilker C, et al. Stereotactic localization and guidance using a machine vision technique. *Stereotact Funct Neurosurg* 58:94, 1992.
49. Heilbrun MP, Koehler S, McDonald P, et al. Implementation of a machine vision method for stereotactic localization and guidance. In Maciunas RJ, ed. *Interactive Image-Guided Neurosurgery.* American Association of Neurological Surgeons, Boston, 1993, 169–177.
50. Hertzberg HT, Dupertuis CW, Emanual I. Sterophotogrammetry as an anthropometric tool. *Photogrammetric Eng* 23:942–947, 1957.
51. Hildebolt CF, Vannier MW. Three-dimensional measurement accuracy of skull surface landmarks. *Am J Phys Anthrop* 76:497–503, 1988.
52. Hildebolt CF, Vannier MW, Knapp RH. Validation study of skull three-dimensional computerized tomography measurements. *Am J Phys Anthrop* 82:283–294, 1990.
53. Hildebolt CF, Vannier MW, Shrout MK, Pilgram TK. ROC analysis of observer-response subjective rating data — application to periodontal radiograph assessment. *Am J Phys Anthrop* 84:351–361, 1991.
54. Himes JJ. Repeatability of anthropometric methods and replicate measurements. *Am J Phys Anthrop* 79:77–80, 1989.
55. Hoehne KH, Fuchs H, Pizer SM, eds. *3D Imaging in Medicine.* NATO ASI Series F: Computer and Systems Sciences, vol 60, Springer-Verlag, Berlin, 1990.
56. Hrdlicka A. *Anthropometry.* Wistar Institute, Philadelphia, 1920.
57. Hu X, Tan KK, Levin DN, et al. Three-dimensional magnetic resonance images of the brain: application to neurosurgical planning. *J Neurosurg* 72:433, 1990.
58. Huijsmans DP, Lamers WH, Los JA, Strackee J. Toward computerized morphometric facilities: a review of 58 software packages for computer-aided three-dimensional reconstruction, quantification, and picture generation from parallel serial sections. *Anat Rec* 216:449–470, 1986.
59. Jamison PL, Ward RE. Brief communication: measurement size, precision and reliability in craniofacial anthropometry: bigger is better. *Am J Phys Anthrop* 90:495–500, 1993.
60. Jamison PL, Zegura SL. A univariate and multivariate examination of measurement error in anthropometry. *Am J Phys Anthrop* 40:197–204, 1974.
61. Kato A, Yoshimine T, Hayakawa T, et al. A frameless, armless navigational system for computer assisted neurosurgery. *J Neurosurg* 74:845, 1991.
62. Kaufman A. *Volume Visualization.* IEEE Computer Society Press, New York, 1991.
63. Kelly PK, Kall BA, Goerss S, et al. Computer-assisted stereotaxic laser resection of intra-axial brain neoplasms. *J Neurosurg* 64:427, 1986.
64. Kelly PK, Kall BA, Goerss S, et al. Results of computer-assisted stereotactic laser resection of deep-seated intracranial lesions. *Mayo Clin Proc* 61:20, 1986.
65. Kelly PK. *Tumor Stereotaxis.* W.B. Saunders, Philadelphia, 1991.
66. Kikinis R, Jolesz FA, Gerig G, et al. 3D morphometric and morphologic information derived from clinical brain MR images. In Hoehne KH, Fuchs H, Pizer SM, eds. *3D Imaging in Medicine.* NATO ASI Series F: Computer and Systems Sciences, vol 60, Springer-Verlag, Berlin, 1990, 441–454.
67. Klein HM, Bohndorf K, Hermes H, Schutz WF, Gunther RW, Schlondorff G. Computed tomography and magnetic resonance imaging in the preoperative work-up for cochlear implantation. *Eur J Radiol* 15(1):89–92, 1992.
68. Knapp RH, Vannier MW, Marsh JL. Generation of three dimensional images from CT scans: technological perspective. *Radiol Technol* 56(6):391–398, 1985.
69. Kohn LAP, Cheverud JM, Bhatia G, Commean P, Smith K, Vannier MW. Anthropometric optical surface imaging system repeatability, precision, and validation. *Ann Plast Surg* 34:362–371, 1995.
70. Kooy HM, van Herk M, Barnes PD, et al. Image fusion for stereotactic radiotherapy and radiosurgery treatment planning. *Int J Radiat Oncol Biol Phys* 28:1229, 1994.
71. Kosecoff J, Fink A. *Evaluation Basics — A Practitioner's Manual.* Sage, Newbury Park, CA, 1982.
72. Kosugi Y, Watanabe E, Goto J, et al. An articulated neurosurgical navigation system using MRI and CT images. *IEEE Trans Biomed Eng* 35:147, 1988.

73. Kraemer HC. *Evaluating Medical Tests — Objective and Quantitative Guidelines*. Sage, Newbury Park, CA, 1992.
74. Kragskov J, Sindet-Pedersen S, Gyldensted C, Jensen KL. A comparison of three-dimensional computed tomography scans and stereolithographic models for evaluation of craniofacial anomalies. *J Oral Maxillofacial Surg* 54(4):402–411; discussion 411–412, 1996.
75. Kreiborg S, Marsh JL, Cohen Jr. MM, Liversage M, Pedersen H, Skovby F, Borgesen SE, Vannier MW. Comparative three-dimensional analysis of CT-scans of the calvaria and cranial base in Apert and Crouzon syndromes. *J Craniomaxillofacial Surg* 21(5):181–188, 1993.
76. Kuszyk BS, Ney DR, Fishman EK. The current state of the art in three dimensional oncologic imaging: an overview. *Int J Radiat Oncol Biol Phys* 33(5):1029–1039, 1995.
77. Lambrecht JT. *3-D Modeling Technology in Oral and Maxillofacial Surgery.* Quintessence, Chicago, 1995.
78. Lavallee S, Cinquin P. Computer assisted medical interventions. In: Hoehne KH, Fuchs H, Pizer SM, eds. *3D Imaging in Medicine.* NATO ASI Series F: Computer and Systems Sciences, vol 60, Springer-Verlag, Berlin, 1990, 301–312.
79. Lavallee S, Taylor R. *Computer Aided Surgery.* MIT Press, Cambridge, MA, 1995.
80. Lele S, Richtsmeier JT. Euclidian distance matrix analysis: a coordinate free approach for comparing biological shapes using landmark data. *Am J Phys Anthrop* 86:415–427, 1991.
81. Lemke HU, Inamura K, Jaffe CC, Vannier MW, eds. *Computer Assisted Radiology — CAR'95.* Springer-Verlag, Berlin, 1995.
82. Lemke HU, Vannier MW, Inamura K, Farman A, eds. *Computer Assisted Radiology — CAR'96.* Elsevier, Amsterdam, 1996.
83. Lemke HU, Vannier MW, Inamura K, eds. *Computer Assisted Radiology — CAR'97.* Elsevier, Amsterdam, 1997.
84. Levin DN, Pelizzari CA, Chen GTY, et al. Retrospective geometric correlation of MR, CT, and PET images. *Radiology* 169:817, 1988.
85. Levin DN, Hu X, Tan KK, et al. Surface of the brain: three-dimensional MR images created with volume rendering. *Radiology* 171:277, 1989.
86. Levin DN, Hu X, Tan KK, et al. The brain: integrated three-dimensional display of MR and PET images. *Radiology* 172:783, 1989.
87. Lo LJ, Marsh JL, Vannier MW, Patel VV. Craniofacial computer-assisted surgical planning and simulation. *Clin Plast Surg* 21(4):501–516, 1994.
88. Lo LJ, Marsh JL, Pilgram TK, Vannier MW. Plagiocephaly: differential diagnosis based on endocranial morphology. *Plast Reconstr Surg* 97(2):282–291, 1996.
89. Lohrum R, Becker G, Boesecke R, Werner T, Schlegel W, Lorenz WJ. A medical workstation for the evaluation of alternative 3D radiotherapy treatment plans. *Comput Med Imaging Graph* 16(5):301–309, 1992.
90. Maciunas RJ, ed. *Interactive Image-Guided Neurosurgery.* American Association of Neurological Surgeons, Boston, 1993.
91. Maciunas RJ, Galloway Jr. RL, Latimer J, et al. An independent application accuracy evaluation of stereotactic frame systems. *Stereotact Funct Neurosurg* 58:103, 1992.
92. Marks GC, Habicht J-P, Mueller WH. Reliability, dependability, and precision of anthropometric measurements. *Am J Epidemiol* 130:578–587, 1989.
93. Marsh JL, Vannier MW, Stevens WG. Computerized imaging for soft tissue and osseous reconstruction in the head and neck. *Plast Surg Clin N Am* 12:279–291, 1985.
94. Marsh JL, Vannier MW. Cartographic mapping of the skull from computed tomography scans. *J Craniofacial Surg* 5(3):188–194, 1994.
95. Marsh LH, Robertson JM, McShan DL. Simplified method for three-dimensional evaluation of interstitial brachytherapy applications. *Med Dosim* 19(4):203–210, 1994.
96. McConville JT, Clauser CE, Churchill TD, Cuzzi J, Kaleps I. *Anthropometric Relationships of Body and Body Segment Moments of Inertia.* Air Force Aerospace Medical Research Laboratory, Air Force Systems Command, Wright-Patterson AFB, OH, 1980.
97. Miller MI, Christensen GE, Amit Y, Grenander U. A mathematical textbook of deformable neuroanatomies. *Proc Natl Acad Sci USA* 90:11944–11948, 1993.

98. National Library of Medicine (U.S.) Board of Regents. *Electronic Imaging: Report of the Board of Regents.* U.S. Dept of Health and Human Services, Public Health Service, National Institute of Health, NIH Publication 90-2197, 1990.
99. Nielson GM, Shriver B, Rosenblum LJ. *Visualization in Scientific Computing.* IEEE Computer Society Press, Los Alamitos, CA, 1990.
100. Nixon JH, Cater JP. *A Functional Video-Based Anthropometric Measuring System.* Final report. National Aeronautics and Space Administration, Washington, DC, 1982.
101. Offutt CJ, Vannier MW, Gilula LA, Marsh JL, Sutherland CJ. Volumetric 3-D imaging of computerized tomography scans. *Radiol Technol* 61(3):212–219, 1990.
102. Patel VV, Vannier MW, Marsh JL, Lo L-J. Evaluation of craniofacial surgical simulation. *IEEE Comp Graph Appl* 46–54, January 1996.
103. Patel VV, Vannier MW, Marsh JL, Lo L-J. Evaluation of digital surgical simulation. In Lemke HU, Inamura K, Jaffe CC, Vannier MW, eds. *Computer Assisted Radiology — CAR'95.* Springer-Verlag, Berlin, 1995, 783–794.
104. Pelizzari CA, Chen GT, Spelbring DR, Weichselbaum RR, Chen CT. Accurate three-dimensional registration of CT, PET, and/or MR images of the brain. *J Comput Assist Tomogr* 13(1):20–26, 1989.
105. Perez CA, Purdy JA, Harms W, Gerber R, Matthews J, Grigsby PW, Graham ML, Emami B, Lee HK, Michalski JM, et al. Design of a fully integrated three-dimensional computed tomography simulator and preliminary clinical evaluation. *Int J Radiat Oncol Biol Phys* 30(4):887–897, 1994.
106. Perez CA, Purdy JA, Harms W, Gerber R, Graham MV, Matthews JW, Bosch W, Drzymala R, Emami B, Fox S, et al. Three-dimensional treatment planning and conformal radiation therapy: preliminary evaluation. *Radiother Oncol* 36(1):32–43, 1995.
107. Pilgram TK, Vannier MW, Marsh JL, Kraemer BB, Rayne SC, Gado MH, Moran CJ, McAlister WH, Shackelford GD, Hardesty RA. Binary nature and radiographic identifiability of craniosynostosis. *Invest Radiol* 29(10):890–896, 1994.
108. Polacin A, Kalender WA, Marchal G. Evaluation of section sensitivity profiles and image noise in spiral CT. *Radiology* 185(1):29–35, 1992.
109. Purdy JA, Fraass BA, eds. *Syllabus: A Categorical Course in Physics — Three-Dimensional Radiation Therapy Treatment Planning.* Radiological Society of North America, Oak Brook, IL, 1994, 167.
110. Richtsmeier JT, Paik CH, Elfert PC, III Cole TM, Dahlman HR. Precision, repeatability, and validation of the localization of cranial landmarks using computed tomography scans. *Cleft Palate Craniofacial J* 32(3):217–227, 1995.
111. Rioux M, Bechthold G, Taylor D, Duggan M. Design of a large depth of view three-dimensional camera for robot vision. *Optical Eng* 26(12):1245–1250, 1987.
112. Rioux M. Laser range finder based on synchronized scanners. *Appl Optics* 23(21):3837–3844, 1984.
113. Robb RA, Barillot C. Interactive display and analysis of 3D medical images. *IEEE Trans Med Imaging* 8(3):217–226, 1989.
114. Robb RA, Hanson DP, Karwoski RA, Larson AG, Workman EL, Stacy MC. Analyze: a comprehensive, operator-interactive software package for multidimensional medical image display and analysis. *Comput Med Imaging Graph* 13(6):433–454, 1989.
115. Robb RA. Multidimensional biomedical image display and analysis in the biotechnology computer resource at the Mayo Clinic. *Mach Vision Appl* 1:75–96, 1988.
116. Robinette KM, Vannier MW, Rioux M, Jones PRM. 3-D Surface Anthropometry: Review of Technologies. NATO Advisory Group for Aeronautical Research and Development, Aerospace Medical Panel Working Group 20 Report, 1997.
117. Robinson J, Robinette, KM, Zehner GF. *User's Guide to the Anthropometric Data Base at the Computerized Anthropometric Research and Design (CARD) Laboratory,* AL-TR-1992-0036, Crew Systems Directorate, Human Engineering Division, Armstrong Laboratory, Wright-Patterson AFB, OH, 1992.
118. Roebuck Jr. JA, Kroemer KHE, Thomson WG. *Engineering Anthropometry Methods.* John Wiley & Sons, New York, 1975.
119. Roebuck JA. Calibration, validation, and evaluation of scanning systems: anthropometric issues and recommendations for electronic imaging, in *Proceedings of the Electronic Imaging of the Human Body Workshop.* Dayton, OH, 1992, 131–146.

120. Rossi PH, Freeman HE. *Evaluation — A Systematic Approach,* 5th ed. Sage, Newbury Park, CA, 1993.
121. Sadler LL, Chen X, Figueroa A, Aduss H. Medical applications of three dimensional and four dimensional laser scanning of facial morphology. *SPIE Biostereometr Technol Appl* 1380:158–162, 1990.
122. Sandeman DR, Patel N, Chandler C, Nelson RJ, Coakham HB, Griffith HB. Advances in image-directed neurosurgery: preliminary experience with the ISG Viewing Wand compared with the Leksell G frame. *Br J Neurosurg* 8(5):529–544, 1994.
123. Schellhas KP, El Deeb M, Wilkes CH, et al. Three-dimensional computed tomography in maxillofacial surgical planning. *Arch Otolaryngol Head Neck Surg* 114:438, 1988.
124. Smith K, Commean P, Bhatia G, Vannier MW. (1995) Validation of Spiral CT and Optical Surface Scanning for Lower Limb Remnant Volumetry. Prosthetics and Orthotics International. 19, 97–107, 1995.
125. Smith KE, Bhatia G, Vannier MW. Assessment of mass properties of human head using various three-dimensional imaging modalities. *Med Biol Eng Comput* 33(3):278–284, 1995.
126. Sutherland GH, Bresina SJ, Gayou DE, Blair VP. Application of computer-assisted engineering (CAE) software to orthopedic surgical planning. *SOMA Eng Hum Body* 3(4):49–56, 1989.
127. Tiede U, Bomans M, Hohne KH, Pommert A, Riemer M, Schiemann T, Schubert R, Lierse W. A computerized three-dimensional atlas of the human skull and brain. *AJNR Am J Neuroradiol* 14(3):551–559, 1993.
128. Toga AW, Banerjee PK. Registration revisited. *J Neurosci Meth* 8(1–2):1–13, 1993.
129. Udupa JA, Herman GT, eds. *Three-Dimensional Imaging in Medicine.* CRC Press, Boca Raton, FL, 1991.
130. Udupa JK, Hung HM, Chuang KS. Surface and volume rendering in three-dimensional imaging: a comparison. *J Digital Imaging* 4:159–168, 1991a.
131. Udupa JK, Samarasekera S, Alavi A. Integrated display, manipulation and analysis of MR and PET images. *J Nucl Med* 34(5):124, 1993.
132. Vannier MW, Marsh JL, Warren JO. Three dimensional computer graphics for craniofacial surgical planning and evaluation. *Comput Graph* 17:263–273, 1983.
133. Vannier MW, Marsh JL, Warren JO. Three dimensional CT reconstruction images for craniofacial surgical planning and evaluation. *Radiology* 150:179–184, 1984.
134. Vannier MW, Conroy GC, Marsh JL, Knapp RH. Three-dimensional cranial surface reconstructions using high-resolution computed tomography. *Am J Phys Anthrop* 67:299–311, 1985.
135. Vannier MW, Pilgram TK, Bhatia G, Brunsden B, Commean P. Facial surface scanning. *IEEE Comput Graph Appl* 11:72–80, 1991.
136. Vannier MW, Brunsden BS, Hildebold CF, et al. Brain surface cortical sulcal lengths: quantification with three-dimensional MR imaging. *Radiology* 180:479–484, 1991.
137. Vannier MW, Gutierrez FR, Canter CE, Hildebolt CF, et al. Evaluation of congenital heart disease by three-dimensional magnetic resonance imaging. *J Digital Imaging* 4:153–158, 1991.
138. Vannier MW, Hildebolt CF, Gilula LA, Pilgram TK, et al. Calcaneal and pelvic fractures: diagnostic evaluation by three-dimensional computed tomography scans. *J Digital Imaging* 4:143–152, 1991.
139. Vannier MW, Pilgram T, Bhatia G, Brunsden B. Facial surface scanner. *IEEE Comput Graph Appl* 11(6):17–24, 1991.
140. Vannier MW, Yates RE, Whitestone JJ, eds. *Proceedings of the Cooperative Working Group in Electronic Imaging of the Human Body.* Crew Systems Ergonomics Information Analysis Center (CSERIAC), Wright-Patterson AFB, Dayton, OH, 1992.
141. Vannier MV, Bhatia G, Commean P. Medical facial surface scanner. *SPIE, Image Capture, Formatting and Display* 1653:177–184, 1992.
142. Vannier MW, Pilgram TK, Bhatia G, Nemecek JR, Young VL. Quantitative three-dimensional assessment of face-lift with an optical facial surface scanner. *Ann Plast Surg* 30:204–211, 1993.
143. Vannier MW, Yates RE, Whitestone J, eds. Proceedings of the USAF/MIR/NLM Workshop on Electronic Imaging of the Human Body. Harry G. Armstrong Human Factors Laboratory, Crew Systems Ergonomics Info Center, Wright-Patterson AFB, Dayton, OH, 1993.
144. Vannier MW, Pilgram TK, Marsh JL, Kraemer BB, Rayne SC, Gado MH, Moran CJ, McAlister WH, Shackelford GD, Hardesty RA. Craniosynostosis: diagnostic imaging with three-dimensional CT presentation. *AJNR Am J Neuroradiol* 15(10):1861–1869, 1994.

145. Vannier MW, Smith KE, Commean PK, Bhatia G. In situ evaluation of lower limb prosthesis fit by spiral computed tomography. *Phys Med Imaging SPIE Med Imaging* 2434:438–451, 1995.
146. Vannier MW, Marsh JL, Wang G, Christensen GE, Kane AA. Surgical imaging systems. *Surg Tech Int* 1996.
147. Vannier MW, Marsh JL. Three-dimensional imaging, surgical planning, and image-guided therapy. *Radiol Clin N Am* 34:545–563, 1996.
148. Waitzman AA, Posnick JC, Armstrong DC, Pron GE. Craniofacial skeletal measurements based on computed tomography: part I. accuracy and reproducibility. *Cleft Palate J* 29:112–117, 1992.
149. Ward RE, Jamison PL. Measurement precision and reliability in craniofacial anthropometry: implications and suggestions for clinical applications. *J Craniofacial Gen Dev Biol* 11:156–164, 1991.
150. Watanabe E, Mayanagi Y, Kosugi Y, et al. Open surgery assisted by the Neuronavigator, a stereotactic, articulated, sensitive arm. *Neurosurgery* 28:792, discussion 799, 1991.
151. Webb Associates. *Volume II: A Handbook of Anthropometric Data.* NASA Reference Publication 1024, NASA. Houston, TX, 1978.
152. Zonneveld FW, Lobregt S, van der Meulen JCH, et al. Three-dimensional imaging in craniofacial surgery. *World J. Surg* 13:328–ff, 1989.
153. Zonneveld FW, Noorman van der Dussen MF. Three-dimensional imaging and model fabrication in oral and maxillofacial surgery. *Oral Maxillofacial Surg Clin N Am* 4(1):19–33, 1992.
154. Noga JT, Bartley AJ, Jones DW, Torrey EF, Weinberger DR (1996) Cortical Gyral Anatomy and Gross Brain Dimensions in Monozygotic Twins Discordant for Schizophrenia. *Schizophr. Res.* 1996 Oct 18;22(1):27-40.
155. Borelli, G. (1608-1679). De Motu Animalium (On Animal Motion). Lugduni Batvorum. Translated and reprinted in E Balaguer Periguell, La introduccion del modelo fisico-matematico en la medicina moderna : Analisis de la obra de G.A. Borelli (1608-1679) : De motu animalium (Valencia, 1974).
156. Martin, R. *Lehrbuch der Anthropologie* (2nd edition), vol. 3. G. Fischer, Jena.
157. Snyder, R.G., Chaffin, D.B . and Schutz, R.K. Link System of the Human Torso (AMRL-TR-71-88). Aerospace Medical Research Laboratory, Air Force Systems Command, Wright-Patterson Air Force Base, OH.
158. Reynolds H.M. and S. Leung. (1983). Foundation for Systems Anthropometry-Lumbar/Pelvic Kinematics, Final Report, Air Force Aerospace Medical Research Laboratory, Air Force Systems Command, Wright-Patterson AFB, OH.
159. Gordon C. C., T. Churchill, C.C. Clauser, B. Bradtmiller, J.T. McConville, I. Tebbets and R. Walker, (1989) 1987-1988 Anthropometric Survey of U.S. Army Personnel: Summary Statistics Interim Report, Technical Report NATICK/TR-89/027 (AD A209 600), U.S. Army Natick Res, Devt and Engrg Center, Natick, MA.
160. Probe J.D. (1990). Quantitative assessment of human motion using video motion analysis. Proceedings of the 3rd Annual Workshop on Space Operations Automation and Robotics (SOAR 1989), pp. 155-157, NASA Johnson Space Ctr, Houston TX.
161. Young J.W., R.F. Chandler, C.C. Snow, K.M. Robinette, and G.F. Zehner. (1983). Anthropometric and Mass Distribution Characteristics of the Adult Female. Revised. Federal Aviation Administration, Washington DC, Office of Aviation Medicine.
162. Hertzberg H.T., Daniels, G., and E. Churchill. (1954). Anthropometry of Flying Personnel, Wright Air Development Center TR-52-321, AD 47 953, Wright Air Development Center, Wright-Patterson AFB, OH.
163. Hertzberg H.T., Churchill, E., Dupertius C., White, R., and Damon A., Anthropometric Survey of Turkey, Greece, and Italy. AGARDograph 73. Pergamon Press, Oxford. 1963.
164. Whitestone J. W, (1993), Design and evaluation of helmet systems using 3D data. Proceedings of the 37th Annual Meeting of the Human Factors and Ergonomics Society, The Human Factors and Ergonomics Society, Santa Monica CA.
165. Thalmann N.M. and Y. Yang. (1991) Techniques for Cloth Animation. In *New Trends in Animation and Visualization,* N. M. Thalmann and D. Thalmann, eds., John Wiley & Sons Ltd.: London, pp. 243-256.
166. Paquette SP. (1990). Human analogue models for computer-aided design and engineering applications. U. S. Army Natick Research, Development and Engineering Center, Natick, Massachusetts. NTIS No. NATICK-TR-90-054.

167. Greiner TM and Gordon CC. (1990). Assessment of long-term changes in anthropometric dimensional: Secular trends of US Army males. U. S. Army Natick Research, Development and Engineering Center, Natick, Massachusetts. NTIS No. NATICK-TR-91-006.
168. Burke PH, Beard L. Stereophotogrammetry of the face. *Am J Orthod* 1967;53:769-82.
169. Burke PH. Stereophotogrammetric measurement of normal facial asymmetry in children. *Human Biol* 1971;43:536-48.
170. Burke PH. Serial stereophotogrammetric measurements of the soft tissues of the face. *Br Dent J* 1983;155:373-9.
171. Donelson SM, Gordon CC. 1988 Anthropometric Survey of U. S. Army Personnel: Pilot Summary Statistics. Technical Report NATICK/TR-91/040. U. S. Army Natick Research, Development and Engineering Center, Natick, Massachusetts, 1991.
172. Whitestone J.J. and Robinette, K.M. (1992). High resolution human body surface data for the design of protective equipment. Proc 2nd Pan Pacific Conference on Occupational Ergonomics, "Ergonomics in Occupational Safety and Health", Safety and Environmental Protection Research Institute, MMI, Wuhan, China.
173. Daniels G.S. The Average Man. Report WADC-TR. Wright Air Development Center, Wright-Patterson AFB, OH.
174. Churchill E., Churchill, T., McConville, J. and White, R. (1977a). Anthropometry of Women of the U.S. Army--1977, Report No. 2-The Basic Univariate Statistics. Technical Report NATICK/TR-77/024, U.S. Army Natick Research and Development Command, Natick, MA.
175. Hendy K.C. (1990). Aircrew/Cockpit compatibility-a multivariate problem seeking a multivariate solution, in AGARD, Recruiting, Selection, Training and Military Operations of Female Aircrew. Defence and Civil Institute of Environmental Medicine, Ownsview Ontario.
176. Robinette KM. (1992). Anthropometry for HMD Design. *SPIE Proceedings* Vol 1695, Helmet Mounted Displays III, pp. 138-145.
177. Case H, Erving C, and Robinette KM. (1989). Anthropometry of a fit test sample used in evaluating the current and improved MCU-2/P. Armstrong Aerospace Medical Research Laboratory, Wright Patterson Air Force Base, NTIS No. AAMRL-TR-89-009.
178. Oestenstad RK, Dillon HK, and Perkins LL. (1990). Distribution of face seal leak sites on half-mask respirators and their association with facial dimensions. Cincinnati, Ohio: National Institute for Occupational Safety and Health.
179. Hidson DJ. (1984). Computer-aided design of a respirator facepiece model. Canadian Defense Research Establishment, NTIS No. DREO-902.
180. Rash CE, Verona RW, and Crowley JS. (1990). Human factors and safety considerations of night vision systems flight using thermal imaging systems. *SPIE Proceedings* Vol 1290, 142-164.
181. Rubin G., E. Fischer, M. Dixon: Prescription of above-knee and below-knee prostheses, *Prosth Orthot Int,* 10:117-24 (1986).
182. Jensen J.S. Life expectancy and social consequences of through-knee amputations, *Prosth Orthot Int,* 7:113-15 (1983).
183. Walsh N.E., J.L. Lancaster, V. Faulkner, W.E. Rogers: A computerized system to manufacture prostheses for amputees in developing countries, *J Prosth Orthot,* 1(3):165-181 (1989).
184. Nielsen C.C. A survey of amputees: Functional level and life satisfaction, and information needs, *J Prosth Orthot,* 3(3):125-129 (1991).
185. Nicholas J.J., L.R. Robinson, R. Schulz, C. Blair, R. Aliota, G. Hairston: Problems experienced and perceived by prosthetic patients, *J Prosth Orthot,* 5(1):36-9 (1993).
186. Millstein S., D. Bain, G.A. Hunter: A review of employee patterns of industrial amputees - factors influencing rehabilitation. *Prosth Orthot Int,* 9:69-78 (1985).
187. Chatterton H.C. Consumer concerns in prosthetics, *Prosth Orthot Int,* 7:15-16 (1983).
188. Narang I.C., B. Mathur, P. Singh, V. Jape: Functional capabilities of lower limb amputees, *Prosth Orthot Int,* 8:43-51 (1984).

5 An Overview of Computer-Integrated Surgery and Therapy

Stéphane Lavallée, Eric Bainville, and Ivan Bricault

CONTENTS

0-8493-3179-X/00/$0.00+$.50

Computer-integrated surgery and therapy (CIST): Methods and systems to help the surgeon or the physician use multimodality data (mainly medical images) in a rational and quantitative way, in order to plan but also to perform medical interventions through the use of passive, semi-active, or active guiding systems.

5.1 CLINICAL OBJECTIVES AND APPLICATIONS

5.1.1 Existing Clinical Applications

Historically, stereotactic neurosurgery has been probably the first surgical discipline to benefit from CIST technology. The fact that some accurate mechanical systems had been used for a long time (stereotactic frames) and the conjunction of the advent of CT imaging and sufficiently powerful low-cost computers may explain that phenomenon. Figure 5.1 shows an example of one of the numerous successful systems that have been developed in the 1980s for frame-based stereotactic neurosurgery.[67] Now, the situation has changed — many physicians and surgeons coming from very different specialties have realized the potential benefits of CIST technology. The literature of the domain shows an impressive collection of successful clinical applications, in various surgery and therapy disciplines. The reader may refer to the following references for an overview of the most successful systems (this is not an exhaustive list):

- Neurosurgery
  - — In stereotactic neurosurgery, pre-operative CT and MR images have been connected with articulated stereotactic frames[68,81] or positioning robots.[87,91,92,162]
  - — In open neurosurgery, passive navigation of a tool in pre-operative CT and MR images has been proposed using mechanical arms,[90,151] ultrasonic localizers,[130] or optical localizers.[141]
  - — Surgical microscopes have been interfaced with pre-operative CT or MR images using passive localizers[51,134] or robotic manipulators (MKM™ system of Zeiss, Surgiscope™ system of DeeMed-Elekta).
- Ear, nose, and throat surgery (ENT)
  - — Free navigation of a tool in CT and MR images has been developed using mechanical arms[118] or optical localizers.[2]
  - — In endonasal surgery, recent systems have proposed to overlay MR and CT segmented structures with endoscopic images.[70]
- Radiation therapy
  - — Optimal patient setup during radiation therapy can be performed in conjunction with planning of dose delivery based on CT and MR images. Different techniques have been developed for patient setup: registration using external markers for the abdomen,[17] internal markers for the prostate,[14] images of portal imaging devices (PID) for the prostate[65] or X-ray images for the brain,[32] ultrasound images for the prostate,[158] and video range images for the brain.[161]
  - — Optimal dose delivery planning delivered with a large robotics system has been reported.[4]
  - — Accurate and image-based insertion of radioactive seeds using magnetic fields has been developed and is under clinical validation.[66]

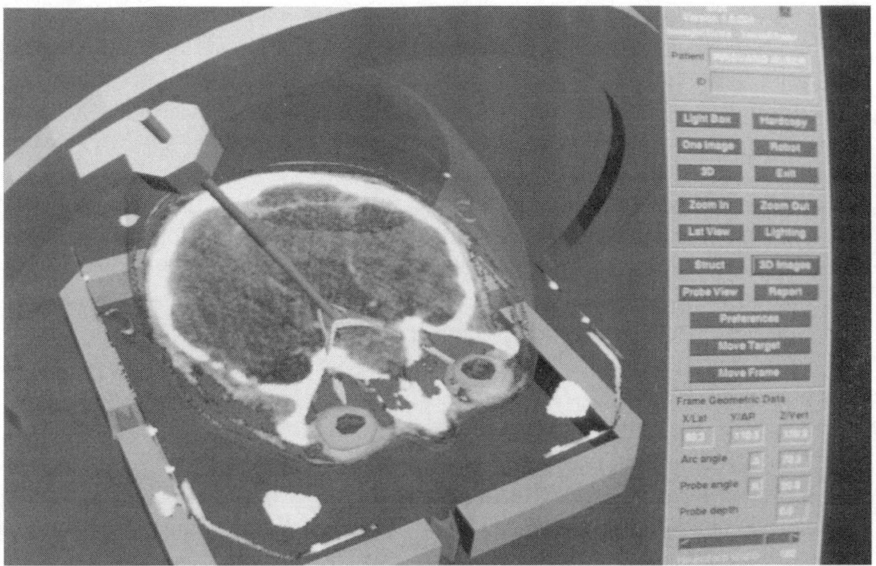

FIGURE 5.1 Interactive stereotactic neurosurgery: positioning of a probe on pre-operative CT images using an articulated stereotactic frame. (With courtesy of Dr. Cesare Giorgi, Istituto Nazionale Neurologico C. Besta, Milano, Italy.)

- Orthopedics and traumatology
  - — In spine surgery, insertion of pedicle screws based on pre-operative CT images and passive navigation help has been reported.[60,99,119]
  - — In hip surgery, insertion of prosthesis using CT-based planning and an active robot for bone machining has been widely validated clinically.[148]
  - — For total knee arthroplasty (TKA), prototypes of systems for insertion of prosthesis using CT-based planning and an active robot for bone machining has been reported,[88,109] while it is also possible to consider only intra-operative geometric data.[104]
  - — For knee optimal placement of the anterior cruciate ligament (ACL), an intra-operative passive system has been proposed.[49]
  - — An elegant solution for accurate tool positioning based on CT images using individual templates has been reported for pelvis surgery and spine surgery.[127]
  - — Simulation of arthroscopic procedures using a virtual reality system has been developed.[167]
- Craniofacial surgery
  - — Optimal bone placement based on CT images and anatomical models has been clinically validated.[43]
  - — Mandibular condyle repositioning in orthognathic surgery using a 3D localizer has been reported.[21]
- Eye surgery
  - — Different prototypes of robotics micro-manipulators including force feedback and vocal commands have been developed.[74,78,138]
  - — Simulators of surgery are also beeing developed.[113]
- Cardiac surgery
  - — A prototype of computer-assisted pericardiac surgery using ultrasound images and a 3D localizer has been validated on animals.[15]

- Minimal-access surgery
  - Interventional radiology in open MRI is one of the most important breakthroughs of the domain that has been validated in many clinical cases and still offers many possibilities.[85]
  - Laparoscopic robotic arms that hold endoscopic cameras have been extensively developed and successfully validated.[59,62,135]
  - A robot has been developed for prostatectomy based on ultrasound images.[111]
  - A prototype of passive navigation in CT and MR images for retroperitoneoscopy has been reported.[11]
  - Simulation of interventions on soft tissues using visual models and force feedback is being developed by several research groups (e.g., see Ref. 42).
  - Superimposition of real video bronchoscopic images with CT synthetic images has been reported.[28]
- Dentistry
  - Clinical validation of accurate dental implant surgery using CT has been reported.[61]
  - A system for robotic control of intra-oral radiography has been developed.[50]
  - Various configurations of CAD/CAM systems for dental implants have been proposed.[131]

5.1.2 Clinical Added Value of CIST Systems

The above list is not exhaustive and many other projects are being developed successfully in various disciplines. However, the definition of success in this domain is difficult to assess and excessive enthusiasm must be avoided. It is crucial that any CIST system bring a well-defined clinical added value, instead of producing technically impressive results with poor improvement over a standard therapy or surgical procedure. We will try to define clinical added value in a general sense.

The criteria corresponding to a given CIST system are many and dependent on the type of surgery. However, it is possible to define a list of global objectives at which any CIST system designer should aim. The following items describe the potential benefits for the patient, the medical staff, and society. They provide a basis to define precise criteria that enable us to evaluate specific systems.

- Less invasive surgery — A major goal of CIST systems is to make surgery less invasive, trying to get close to ambulatory treatment, with limited post-operative consequences. Performing small incisions in the skin, instead of large open surgery, decreases the risk of infections and the duration of post-operative stay for the patient at the hospital. However, minimally invasive surgery raises a difficulty: the human operator no longer has any direct control on the operated organs. The surgeon's eyes are assisted by various sensors (X-ray intensifiers, ultrasound probes, endoscopes); the doctor's hands may not touch the tissues directly but they must guess and predict the obstacles that exist for the therapeutic tools. CIST technology can help the surgeon in this difficult task.
- Improvement of accuracy — Improving the accuracy of an operation strongly influences its success rate. However, one must be careful with the meaning of "accuracy," which is in fact twofold. First, it is desirable to be able to define surgical planning accurately. This means that morphological and functional consequences of an operation must be taken into account quantitatively. Here, the questions are to know whether there are enough data for planning the surgery, and whether the model that is used to predict the results of the surgery is accurate. A related problem is to be able to manipulate these data without losing pertinent and relevant information. The question arises as to why submillimetric planning is done if the real surgery cannot be performed with similar precision. This leads us to the second aspect of accuracy: it is necessary to deploy the

defined surgical plan accurately. This implies that we must set up guiding systems that "know" exactly the plan defined by the therapist, and that are able to help or take over from the operator in situations where such accuracy is more important than dexterity. Conversely, in some clinical applications, dexterity is the main problem, and robotics help is intended to make the gesture more accurate for better functional results and less damage. Another factor related to accuracy is the number of iterations or multiple trials required to perform a defined action. The CIST technology should aim at reducing this number to one.

- Improvement of reliability and safety — CIST technology aims at improving the success rate of interventions. For many applications, surgeons experience a non-negligible percentage of failures. An improvement of even a few percentage points would be very valuable in many instances.
- Reduction of complication risks — Decreasing the access size of surgery and improving the accuracy of the intervention obviously tends to limit the post-operative consequences for the patient.
- Reduction of intervention length — Although the major objective of CIST is to improve the intervention quality, in some cases, an interesting clinical added value is the reduction of the operation time: less risks of contamination, reduced anesthesia, shorter tourniquet duration, possibility for the medical staff to consider more interventions per day (or to get some well-deserved rest).
- Easier for the surgeon — By using effective and reliable tools, the operator stress may be reduced. However, this is strongly dependent on the reliability and ergonomy of the system. Making surgery easier for the operator is particularly important for young surgeons, who may gain confidence and efficiency with the help of CIST systems.
- Decreased danger for the medical staff — Exposure to ionizing radiation should be reduced for the medical staff. However, requiring more patient data could lead to extra examinations (such as CT with small slice spacing), which may cause more irradiation for the patient. The use of telesurgery and the reduction of invasiveness may reduce contamination risks. However, this should not be counterbalanced by the introduction of sophisticated devices that are more difficult to sterilize properly than standard surgical material. The CIST technology may find use also in dangerous or inaccessible places.
- Possible use in a difficult intervention — In some cases, CIST systems may make possible an intervention that was not possible before, but was considered necessary.
- Accounting for clinical results accurately — Providing quantitative data for surgical planning makes it also possible to validate and optimize new surgical protocols in a rigorous manner, using for instance databases that collect and statistically analyze all post-operative clinical results with the corresponding surgical planning parameters.
- Basis for surgical simulators — Similarly, surgical planning systems linked to real surgery guiding systems provide interesting platforms for developing surgical simulators. Training therapists on virtual patients instead of cadavers (or real patients) offers obvious advantages for medical students. Surgical simulators are also useful for collecting information about difficult clinical cases and for teaching larger groups of surgeons than possible through conventional means.

Usually, a system does not meet all these objectives at once, and some objectives are very often contradictory. For instance, improving the accuracy is counterbalanced by an augmentation of X-ray dose if CT must be used, or by an augmentation of infection risks if the system is bulky and not sterilizable with autoclave. There is also the issue of cost. In general, the systems will be able to save money because they improve the success rates of interventions and reduce the complication rates, intervention lengths, and hospital stays. Nevertheless, the added clinical value that any system brings has to be demonstrated on clinical validations, and the benefits have to be compared with the global cost, in terms of money but also added problems. This comparison can be made according to the factors previously mentioned but this is not sufficient, and for each specialty some specific scores must be given and guidelines for clinical validation must be followed . This is probably the most challenging aspect of this research. For this purpose, several long-term evaluation studies have been initiated in different clinical sites all over the world (e.g., see Ref. 79).

5.2 CIST TECHNOLOGY, INTEGRATION, AND METHODOLOGY

To meet the aforesaid objectives, CIST technology has two strings to its bow:

1. Information help — It brings considerable help at the information level. Indeed, CIST technology helps to merge all the available data in a single patient model, thus allowing the operator to exploit the specificity of each item of information. It also enables the surgeon to reach targets which are not visible directly, and to use only information that has been selected for its relevance and that has been processed to reduce its complexity. Similarly, the surgical planning step, which can be iteratively defined using interactive tools or optimization methods, becomes itself a piece of information. Most important, it becomes possible to use this surgical planning information accurately during the intervention and to correlate the positions of the various tools with the global patient model that contains pre- and intra-operative information.
2. Action help — CIST technology offers some capabilities to improve the action itself through the use of semi-active guiding systems that can constrain the action to a particular task, through the use of active robots that improve dexterity or perform themselves a subtask of the whole procedure, or through teleoperation systems that can filter, reduce in size, or remotely transfer the surgical motions.

Whatever CIST capability is considered, information help or action help, it must be realized that CIST systems are not intended to replace the surgeon in all tasks. There must be a real partnership between the system and the operator.[147] CIST technology must be used when the system and the human make something better than the human can do alone. In many applications, CIST systems solve geometrical problems in three or six dimensions that are difficult for the human to solve and memorize. This is the typical case of registration between pre- and intra-operative data. But the capacity of the human to deal with unforeseen and unmodeled events cannot be replaced by the machine.

Note that in this chapter, the operator in charge of the intervention will be referred to as a surgeon, an operator, or a therapist. This abuse should not be interpreted as a limitation of CIST to surgical operations only which would exclude interventional radiology, radiation therapy, and the like.

Examining carefully the literature across medical disciplines, one can notice that many projects have similar problems, related global objectives, and common technical solutions. Just for the capability of image-guided linear introduction of a tool toward a defined target, we can find many clinical applications: insertion of a biopsy probe in stereotactic neurosurgery, screw introduction in the pedicle of a vertebra, disc puncture in nucleolysis, intramedullary nail locking in traumatology and beam positioning relative to the patient in external radiation therapy. From this observation, we can conclude that many clinical applications raise very similar problems, and therefore it is necessary to define a general CIST concept that encapsulates basic tools.

This general concept is now presented and the whole chapter will follow the outline of the defined methodology. At Grenoble Hospital in France, a team of computer scientists, mathematicians, physicians, and surgeons has been involved in a project called Computer Assisted Medical Interventions (CAMI) since 1985.[37] Using this experience, a methodology which is based on a

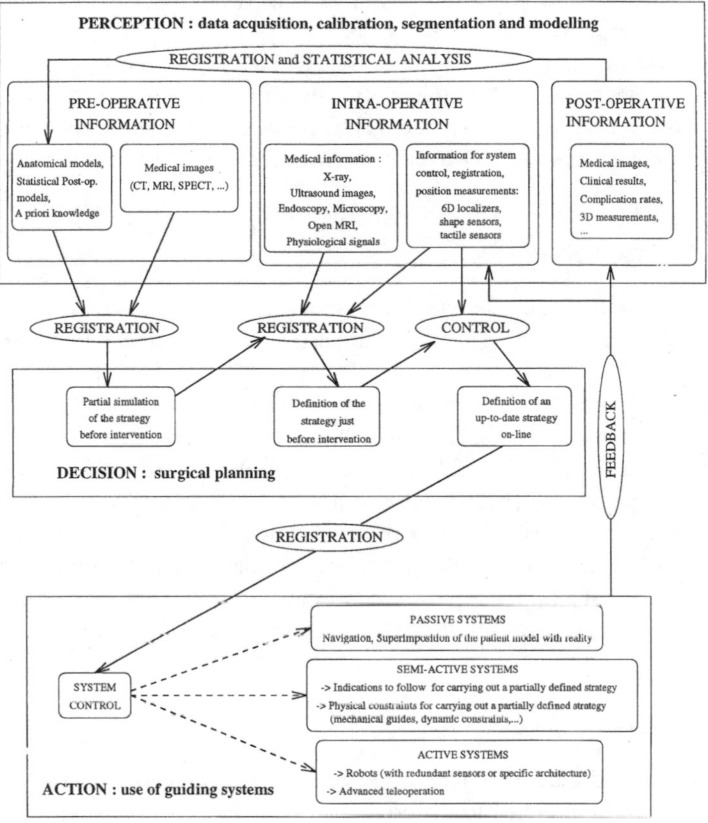

FIGURE 5.2 CIST methodology: a perception/decision/action loop.

standard loop (perception/decision/action) was defined in 1989.[93,96] Interestingly, we feel that this methodology is still valid and even reinforced by recent developments. A schematic representation of this methodology is shown in Figure 5.2; it describes the flow of information in CIST technology.

At the perception level, multimodal data are acquired (pre-operative data and models, intra-operative data, and post-operative data). At the same level, these data are intrinsically calibrated, segmented, and modeled. At the decision level, the medical strategy is defined on the basis of all the available models and data. At the action level, the strategy is carried out through the use of passive, semi-active, or active guiding systems. In the middle of these three boxes, registration acts as a glue that links all the steps together.

In the rest of this chapter, the steps of this methodology are detailed and illustrated with clinical examples.

5.3 PERCEPTION

5.3.1 Data Acquisition

At the first stage, multimodal data are acquired with standard medical imaging devices (CT, MRI, digital radiology, echography, PET, SPECT, etc.), but also with various sensors from the field of computer vision and robotics (3D localizers, shape sensors, force and tactile sensors), or devises to analyze various physiological signals (electrophysiology, pressure, Doppler, tactile feelings). Geometrical and anatomical models (such as atlases) and rules (such as empirical geometrical constraints) must be taken into account, as well as statistical data obtained by analysis of post-operative data of previous cases.

Among those data modalities, we assume that the reader is familiar with standard medical images and signals, since they are extensively described in other chapters of this book and elsewhere.[164] We now concentrate on a piece of information which is much more specific to CIST systems: optical shape sensors and 3D localizers. More details about those sensors can be found in Ref. 117.

5.3.1.1 Optical Shape Sensors

Shape sensors provide information about the surface of anatomical structures. Any 3D imaging system can be considered a shape sensor, provided that some segmentation algorithm is able to detect the surface of a structure on raw images. For instance, a 2.5D ultrasound sensor presented in the next section constitutes a shape sensor. However, when the surface of the structure is external and visible, some contactless optical sensors which are now standard in the field of computer vision give the 3D shape automatically. Optical range finders provide a set of points that belong to the surface of the studied structure. They consist of a video camera and a laser or pattern projector that make an angle of 20 to 60° between them. Triangulation techniques reconstruct the x,y,z coordinates of the surface points where the patterns are projected and that are visible to the camera. Section 5.5.4 will present the application of such range imaging sensors to registration problems for patient positioning in external radiotherapy. Figure 5.9 will show a range imaging sensor and the surface it provides.

5.3.1.2 3D Localizers

3D localizers, also called digitizers, navigation systems, and trackers, yield relative positions and orientations of rigid bodies attached to different "objects" in a sensor coordinate system $\text{Ref}_{\text{sensor}}$. In the general case, the sensor provides the 3×3 rotation matrix $\mathbf{R}$ and the three-component translation vector $\mathbf{t}$ that defines the rigid body coordinate system Ref_{body} in $\text{Ref}_{\text{sensor}}$. Different sensor technologies exist; they differ in accuracy (from 0.2 mm to 1 cm in 1 m^3), the number of rigid bodies or points that can be tracked (from 2 points to 10 complete rigid bodies), the measuring frame rate (from 0.5 to 50 Hz), and the constraints of use (see Refs. 38 and 117 for more technical details and discussions). Some of these are listed below (see also Figure 5.4):

1. Active video systems using linear CCD cameras synchronized with infrared LEDs mounted on rigid bodies (e.g., Optotrak™ from Northern Digital or Flashpoint™ 5000 from Surgical Navigation Systems) (Figure 5.3).
2. Passive video systems using pattern recognition techniques.[39]
3. Hybrid passive and active video systems using stereovision (Polaris™) from Northern Digital.
4. Passive 6 degrees of freedom mechanical arms.[90]
5. Ultrasonic systems that measure time of flight between emitters and receivers.[130]
6. Electromagnetic sensors (e.g., Flock of Bird™ from Ascencion Technology or Fast Track™ from Polhemus).

Among the above technologies, the first is currently the most efficient, robust, and accurate in clinical environments. Passive video systems still suffer from problems of robustness and speed. Passive mechanical arms are cumbersome and they can track only one rigid body. Ultrasonic systems are sensitive to air motions and temperature gradients. Electromagnetic sensors are strongly influenced by the presence of metallic objects and therefore they can be used only in restricted environments.

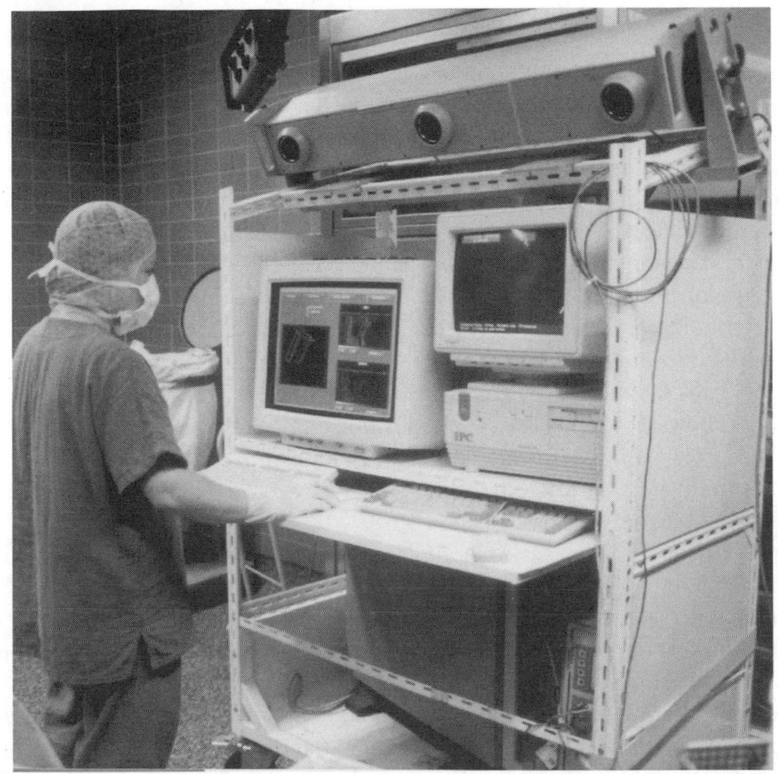
a

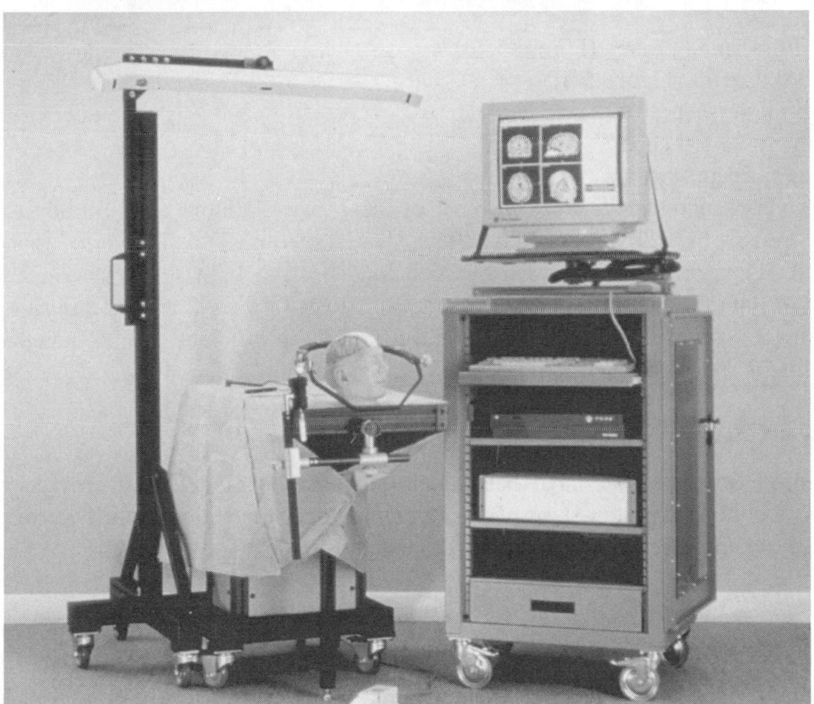
b

FIGURE 5.3 Computer-integrated surgery workstations based on 3D localizers. (a) Laboratory system including the Optotrak (Northern Digital) optical 3D localizer. (b) Commercial system of Sofamor-Danek SNT including the Flashpoint 5000 optical 3D localizer (Image Guided Technologies).

The main applications of 3D localizers are the following:

- Digitization of 3D points with a pointer — Pointers equipped with a rigid body enable digitization of points in 3D: the operator places the tip of the pointer on the anatomical point to be digitized and then presses a manual or foot switch (Figure 5.4a). Repeating the operation for points randomly taken on an anatomical surface yields a manual surface sensor (Figure 5.4b). These points can be used for registration purposes[103] or a spline surface can be fitted for further modeling.[49]
- Tracking of standard surgical tools — The 3D position of a drill, a probe, a scalpel, an aspirator, a planar cutting guide, and the like can be tracked in real time (Figure 5.4d).
- Measurement of the position and orientation of reference anatomical structures — Fixing a rigid body on a reference anatomical structure, which is usually a bone, makes it possible to track the motion of this structure in real time. This has two applications:
  First, it allows computation of all positions in a relative coordinate system and therefore compensation for any structure motions in real time. For example, this is the case in Figure 5.4a wherein the 3D points are acquired in the rigid body coordinate system fixed to the vertebra.
  Second, kinematics data corresponding to motions of articulated joints can be acquired intra-operatively. For instance, in knee surgery, for ACL reconstruction where the problem is to insert a ligament graft that replaces the normal ACL, it is useful to acquire the relative motion of the tibial bone with respect to the femoral bone during passive flexion/extension (Figure 5.4c).[49]
- Measurement of the spatial position of portable imaging sensors — Fixing a rigid body to an imaging device makes it possible to know the relative positions of the sensor in a fixed coordinate system. As examples, rigid bodies can be attached on the following devices:
  2D ultrasound probes (Figure 5.4e)[16]
  X-ray C arms (Figure 5.4f)[72]
  Rigid endoscopes[70]
  Surgical microscopes[51]
  Range image systems
  This is very important because in most of these cases, adding a rigid body to such a device transforms a 2D sensor into a 3D sensor (sometimes, this is referred to as a 2.5D sensor). 3D information provided by such low-cost and light sensors is an invaluable source of data for anatomy-based registration between pre-operative and intra-operative coordinate systems (see Section 5.5), and it is also an efficient way to navigate in the 3D surgical space (see Section 5.6.1).

5.3.2 Sensor Calibration and Data Modeling

All the multimodality data that have been acquired must be modeled to provide appropriate representations for the subsequent steps of the perception/decision/action loop. There are two main technical issues at this level: calibration and segmentation.

Calibration

Intrinsic and extrinsic calibration of the sensors and devices is essential for global CIST system accuracy. Intrinsic calibration refers to the techniques that model the basic sensor itself, thus providing a function f that transforms raw sensor data d into geometrical entities $v = f(d)$, which are expressed in a coordinate system associated with the sensor. CT, SPECT, and PET images are usually assumed to present no distortion and to be accurately calibrated. In this case the f function becomes an identity function, but this is not always the case for MR and X-ray images.

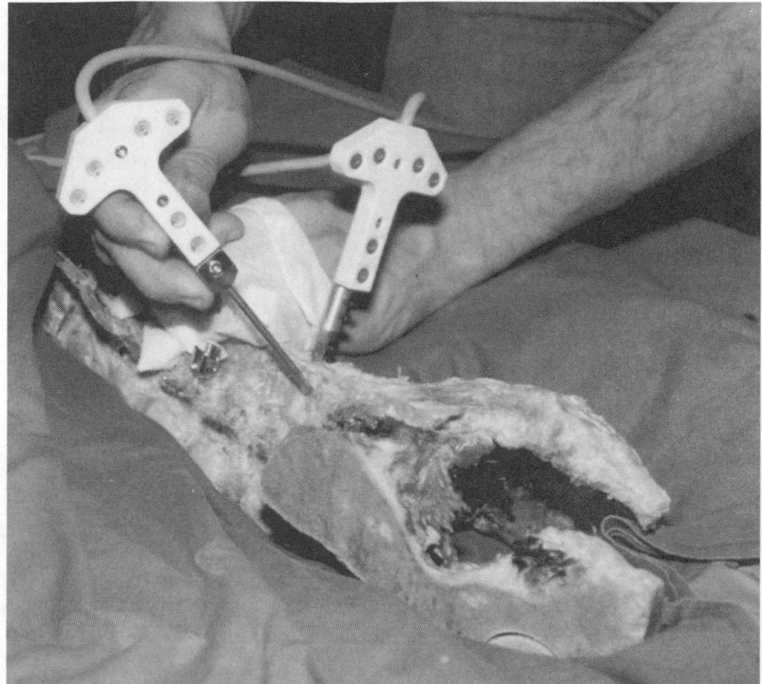

a

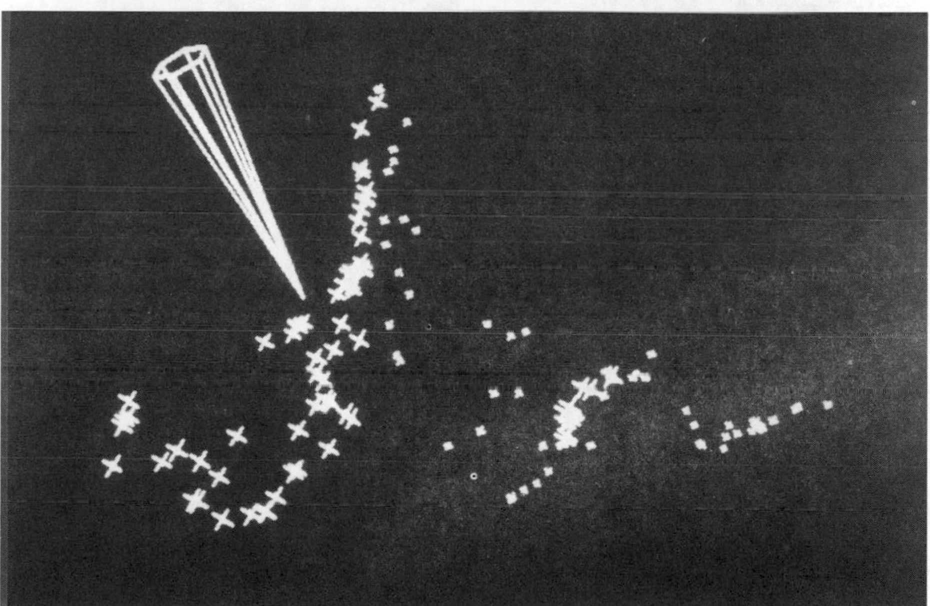

b

FIGURE 5.4 Multiple use of 3D localizers in computer-integrated surgery. (a) Digitization of 3D points with a pointer in a relative coordinate system attached to a bone (*in vitro* experiment on spine). (b) 3D view of points digitized on the vertebra surface.

In order to use MRI for accurate surgical planning, distortions could be compensated in two ways. One solution is to place a calibration cage around the patient and compute a 3D warping function from images of calibration points (see, e.g., Refs. 63 and 137 for preliminary attempts). This is quite cumbersome and does not compensate for all local distortions. Another solution would be to use CT images as reference images and perform an elastic matching between CT and MRI,

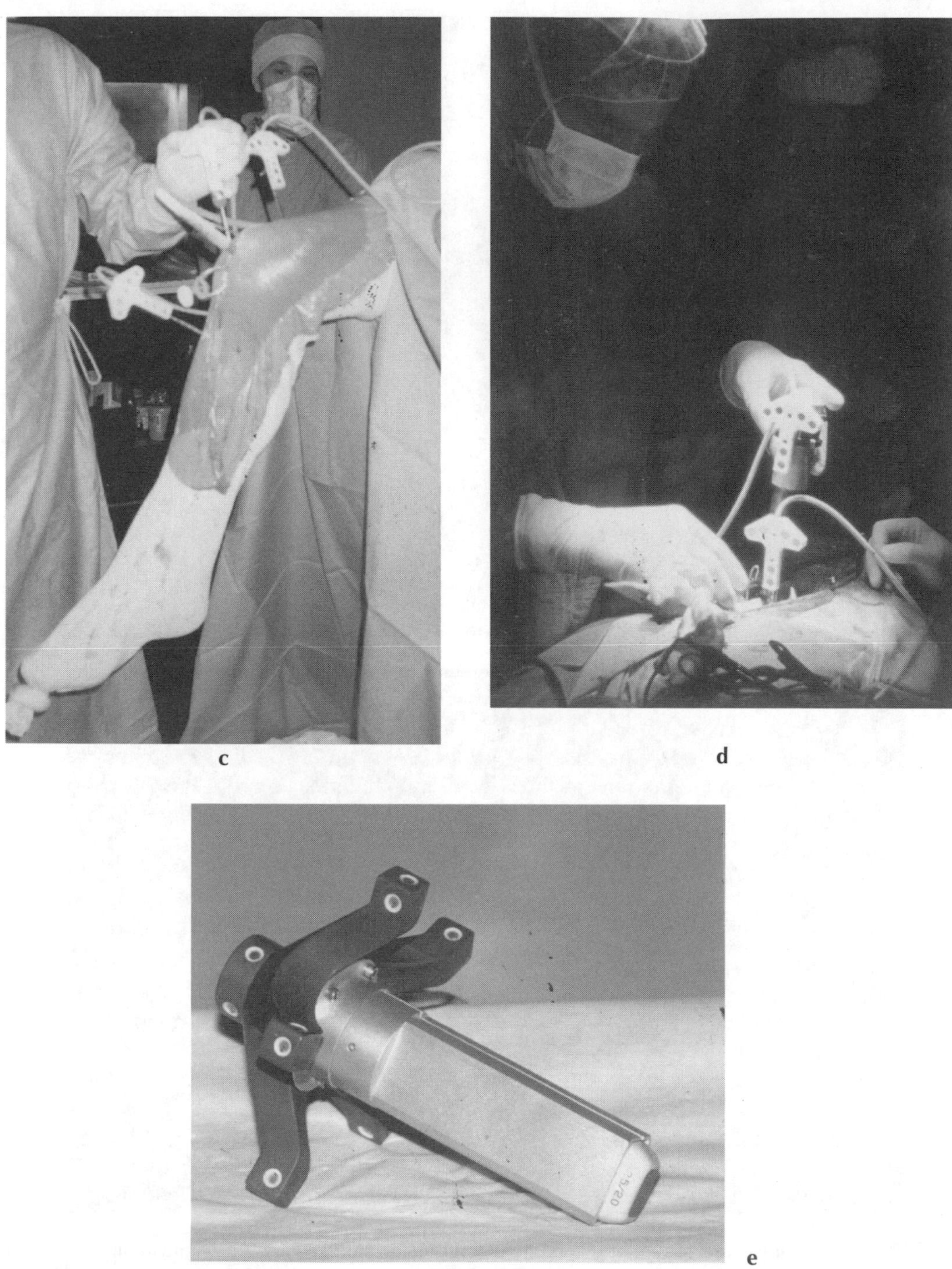

FIGURE 5.4 (c) Acquisition of bone kinematics of the knee using two rigid bodies; the flexion/extension motion of the knee is acquired during surgery. (d) 3D position of surgical instrument in real time. (e) 2D ultrasound probes.

in order to transform MR images in the non-distorted CT space.[143] Both solutions need further investigation. So far, the only requirement with MRI is to perform an accurate tuning of the magnetic gradients in order to make the images as linear as possible, which has been shown to be accurate enough in many cases (e.g., see Refs. 110 and 166).

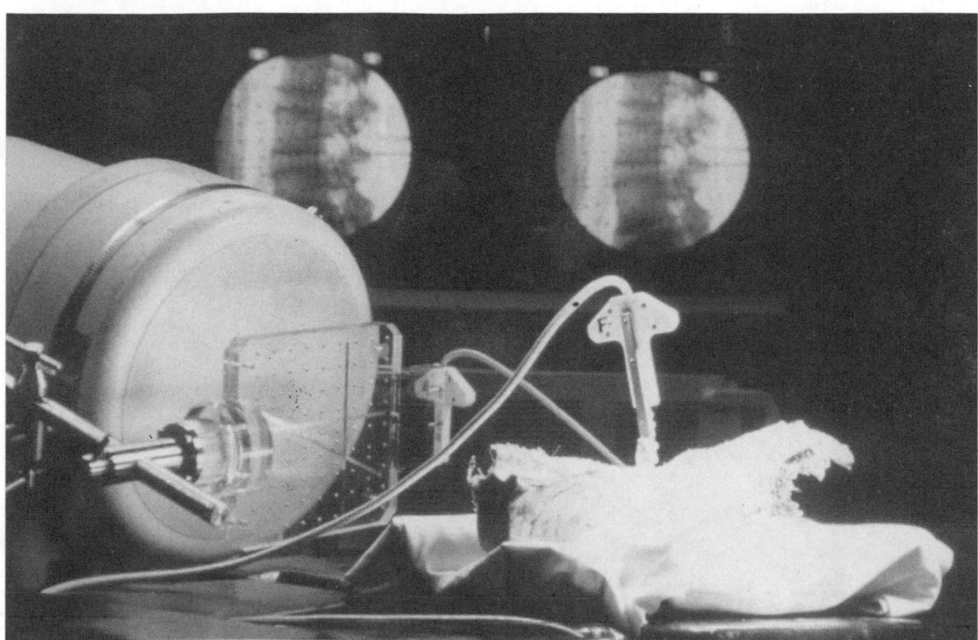

f

FIGURE 5.4(f) X-ray C arms.

In order to use X-rays for surgical planning or for registration, it is necessary to correct distortions of these images. For instance, the N-planes bicubic spline (NPBS) method uses spline approximation to correct local distortions.[34] It computes a function *f* that transforms distorted pixels of an X-ray image into a bundle of 3D X-ray projection lines in a sensor coordinate system.

Extrinsic calibration refers to the methods that can link various sensors and devices together, in a unique coordinate system. For instance, in Refs. 92 and 94, a robot was calibrated with respect to a pair of X-ray systems more or less orthogonal in a stereotactic neurosurgery room. A calibration cage made of Plexiglas plates containing radio-opaque small spheres was fixed to the robot end effector (see Figure 5.21). X-ray images of the radio-opaque spheres taken at the beginning of the operation allowed linkage of the coordinate system of the robot base with the coordinate systems associated with the images. After this calibration step, any pixel of an X-ray image corresponds a 3D projection line of which the equation is known in the robot reference system. A more flexible configuration developed in the instance of spine surgery is shown in Figure 5.4f: a calibration plate is fixed to a standard X-ray intensifier and is equipped with a rigid body localized by the Optotrak sensor. Figure 5.5 shows an image of the calibration plate that enables correction of any image distortion. The relation between image coordinates u,v and calibration plate coordinates x,y taken for two plate positions is obtained by interpolation with B-spline functions applied to the observed reference metallic balls. In this example, the result of the NPBS method which combines intrinsic and extrinsic calibration, is a function f that transforms pixels into 3D lines represented in the reference system of the vertebra.[72]

Segmentation

In many applications, using raw sensor data is usually insufficient for subsequent processing. Extraction of high-level representations such as the surface of a particular anatomical structure is very useful for registration and surgical planning steps. There are some cases where structures can be segmented automatically or at least semi-automatically (e.g., bones on CT images, skin surface on CT or MRI), but in many instances, manual adjustment is still necessary. However, current work on deformable models is very promising.[8,36,145] Segmentation is in fact a very large issue, and it is

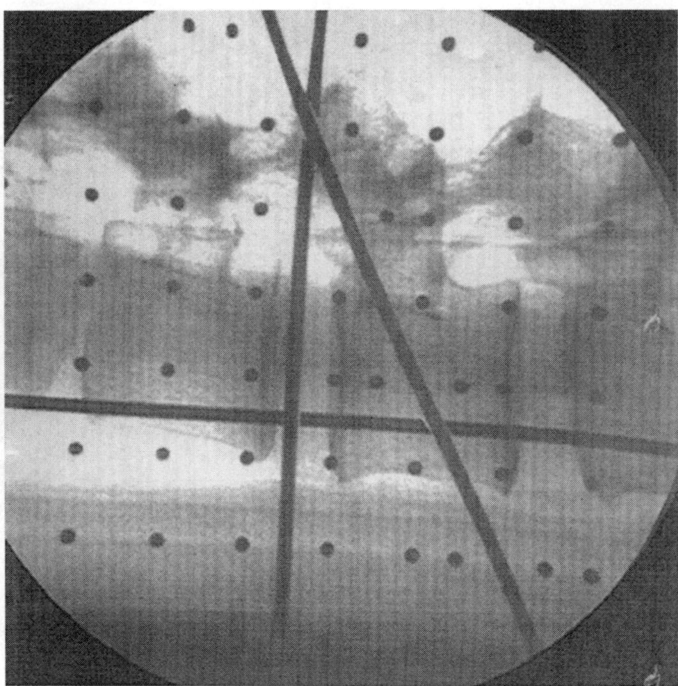

FIGURE 5.5 Digitized X-ray of a calibration plate that enables X-ray system calibration and compensation for image distortions.

very specific to CIST. Therefore, we do not address this in this chapter; the reader should refer to other chapters of this book and its first edition. The accuracy of segmentation is usually much more critical in CIST applications than in standard diagnosis problems.

5.4 DECISION (SURGICAL PLANNING)

At the decision level, the surgeon defines an optimal strategy based on the available multimodal data that constitute the patient model. However, explicit surgical planning is not necessary in instances where the surgeon just reacts directly to the information delivered by imaging sensors. Here we consider all the other cases.

5.4.1 Interactive Planning

The patient model that has been obtained using registration of multimodal images is the basis on which the user defines a surgical strategy. The intervention is simulated, taking morphological and functional consequences into account. To respect the autonomy of the physician at that level, this intervention simulation is usually interactive. Many interactive tools for 3D images handling and visualization are already available[133,159] (volume or surface rendering, reslicing, CAD models, etc.), but there remains a lot of work to integrate these tools in specific user interfaces corresponding to particular clinical applications. Figure 5.6 shows a typical interface for spine surgery that allows the surgeon to define a 3D line on CT images that goes through the pedicle of a vertebra.

5.4.2 Optimal Planning

Planning optimization is necessary when the information is too complex to be handled by just interactive planning. For instance, it may be necessary to optimize the trajectory of a needle to ensure that it keeps as distant as possible from structures such as blood vessels.

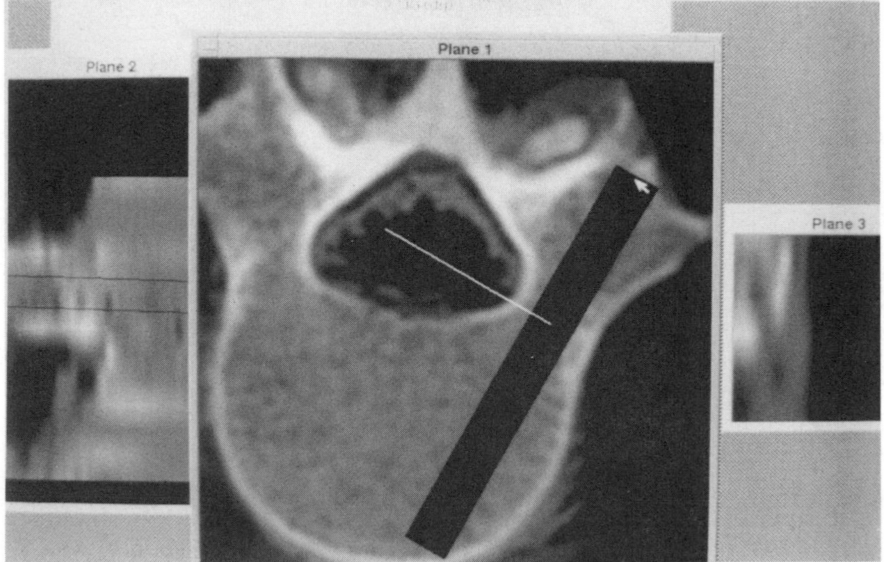

FIGURE 5.6 Interactive selection of a screw position on pre operative CT images of a vertebra. By reslicing the volume of CT images, the surgeon first selects an oblique slice and then defines a line in this plane. A second slice passing through the selected line and a third slice orthogonal to the line are also computed and displayed. The size of the screw is made to materialize by a cylinder around the selected axis.

In radiotherapy, the strategy consists of finding a radiation scheme that delivers high doses inside the tumor or the organ to irradiate (e.g., the prostate) and not in the adjacent structures that must be preserved from radiation (e.g., the bladder). Therefore, optimization tools capable of solving this difficult inverse problem are required. Some preliminary attempts to solve this problem have been presented in Refs. 4, 18, and 112.

In ACL reconstruction for the knee, functional criteria such as "minimal anisometry of the graft ligament" have to be optimized. Preliminary results are reported in Ref. 49 (see Section 5.6.1.2).

In such examples, the system helps the surgeon or the physician define the strategy. However, this optimization must always be controlled and validated by the physician.

5.4.3 Training Using Virtual Reality

The simulation of the strategy may also be useful to assist in teaching surgical techniques in realistic conditions, or to enable a well-trained surgeon to "repeat" a difficult intervention on the model of the patient. For applications on bones, CAD/CAM techniques enable production of a real replica of the patient bones based on CT images, which make it possible to rehearse an intervention on a realistic model.[89] Simulators of difficult techniques, such as retroperitoneoscopy (introduction of a rigid endoscope behind the peritoneum) are also being developed.[10,11] In the latter case, two components must be taken into account. On one hand, the difficulty is to learn where the endoscope is. This is difficult because the part of the body that may be seen through the endoscope is very limited (about 1 cm^2): the tip of the endoscope is indeed in direct contact with the tissues, which is different from classical endoscopic surgery, in which natural free space or insufflation enables the user to see the organs from some distance. The other difficulty is to learn which forces should be applied to the endoscope to make its movements possible, but without risk of hurting critical organs, such as vessels. The solution to these problems requires modeling of the 3D structures of interest, from a geometrical point of view as well as from a physical point of view (to take elasticity into account). Work in this domain of modeling is still in progress, with interesting feasibility demonstrations (see, e.g., Refs. 64, 75, 163, and 167).

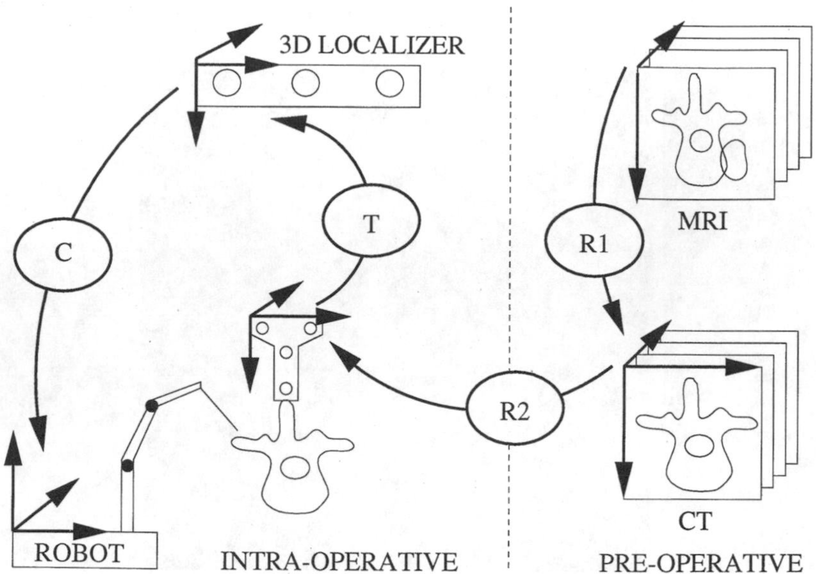

FIGURE 5.7 Registration: graph of relationships between coordinate systems. C: calibration transforms; Rl: registration transform between pre-operative data; R2: registration transform between pre-operative and intra-operative data; T: tracking transforms.

5.5 REGISTRATION

In CIST, registration of all information available for a given patient is an essential step. The purpose is to represent pre-operative images (usually CT, MR, SPECT, PET, or MEG), statistical models such as atlases, intra-operative images (X-rays, ultrasound, and endoscope or microscope images), intra-operative shape and position information (data from 3D localizers), intra-operative tools, devices, and robots, and post-operative images and data in a common coordinate system. This registered data set is called a *hybrid patient's model.*[97]

Obviously, not all applications need to register all types of information. A typical application will have to register only pre-operative CT images with a 3D passive or active manipulator during surgery. Moreover, some techniques do not rely on registration. For instance, open MRI[85] and intra-operative CT offer some obvious advantages over registration of pre-operative images with the intra-operative space, namely real-time feedback. However, these techniques are very expensive, they do not allow combining multimodality data, and they still need some CIST systems for providing passive or active manipulation aids. Similarly, specific geometric and kinematic data output from 3D localizers used intra-operatively yield efficient solutions in a few applications.[49,104] However, for all these systems, the registration of intra-operative data with models is likely to be very valuable in the future.

Figure 5.7 illustrates the concept of registration for a virtual application in spine surgery that would use pre-operative CT and MR images, a 3D localizer for tracking spine motion during surgery, and a robot that would hold a drill.

We can now make a subtle and minor distinction between registration and extrinsic calibration. First, for each modality of information (pre-, intra-, and post-operative medical imaging systems, anatomical atlas, and intra-operative devices), a coordinate system is defined. The purpose of registration and calibration is to build a graph of the relationships between all the coordinate systems involved. If two coordinate systems are in the same spatial and temporal domain (i.e., they are rigidly connected to the same object), then their relation will be estimated through *calibration* procedures. Otherwise, these coordinate systems are totally independent and they are linked through *registration* procedures. Let us consider our example illustrated in Figure 5.7. To estimate a relation C between the intra-operative 3D localizer and the intra-operative robot arm is a calibration problem, whereas to estimate a relation R2 between pre-operative CT images and the reference intra-operative coordinate system is a registration problem. Similarly, estimating the transform R1 between pre-operative MR and pre-operative CT images is a registration problem. The estimation of the relation T between the intra-operative localizer and the reference coordinate system attached to the bone is also a calibration problem, however because this transform is continuously estimated over time, it enters into the subcategory of *tracking* problems. In the rest of this chapter, we focus on techniques exclusively devoted to registration problems.

Over the past few years, many solutions have been proposed to deal with image registration problems in general, not only in the medical field but also in computer vision (see Refs. 19, 30, and 52 for surveys). In this chapter, we focus on registration methods involved in surgery and therapy, specifically addressing the problem of linking the pre-operative images with the intra-operative space (relation R2 in our example).

In Ref. 95 we have proposed a general framework for registration between two modalities A and B, in which the expression "modality" can describe any device that encompasses a sensor (imaging device, 3D localizer, shape sensor, passive or active robot). It is based on three steps as described below.

5.5.1 Step 1: Definition of a Relation Between Coordinate Systems

First, a coordinate system Ref_A and Ref_B is associated with each modality A and B, which means that each sensor is intrinsically calibrated. Then the model of a transform **T** that links coordinates of A with coordinates of B is selected. In the literature, different types of rigid or elastic transforms have been used:

- rigid body transforms parameterized by Euler angles,[102] quaternions,[77] or rotation vectors[7]
- rigid body transforms with scaling[160]
- global warping or affine transforms[82,143]
- high-order polynomial transforms[139]
- regular grids of displacement vectors[12,36]
- local transforms using thin plates[24,53]
- locally affine transforms[56]
- hierarchical adapative splines (octree-splines)[145]

5.5.2 Step 2: Segmentation of Reference Features and Definition of a Disparity (or Similarity) Function Between Extracted Features

The second step is to extract corresponding features in Ref_A and Ref_B, and at the same time, to define a disparity function (or a similarity function) between these features. Here, "feature" refers to geometrical structures such as points, curves, and surfaces as well as basic gray-level derived properties of images. However, for sake of clarity, we will distinguish feature-based methods and image-based methods.

In the literature, different types of features have been used for registration purposes in CIST. From the practical point of view, these may be further divided into material and anatomical features. Many different geometric representations have been used. The following list indicates the major classes of registration techniques available, distinguished and classified according to the type of features and disparity functions they use. There are two main groups.

5.5.2.1 Group A: Material-Based Registration

In this class of methods, material structures such as pins or balls are fixed to the patient during examinations of both modalities to be registered. Such structures are usually easy to segment on images and acquire with manual sensors. Therefore, these techniques are very suitable for accurate, robust, and semi-automatic registration. However, they can be invasive and they raise many problems for the organization of the medical staff and for the patient (e.g., pain, discomfort, additional surgery to install pins, additional image examination). They are

- Minimization of distances between matched fiducial lines (least-squares fitting) — Stereotactic frames for neurosurgery are implanted before CT and MR examination: they are made of N-shaped bars that constitute a set of 3D lines, easily segmented on images and matched with a geometric model.[87]
- Minimization of distances between matched fiducial points (least-squares fitting) — In a first instance, small markers are pasted on the skin or screwed in the skull, their center is automatically detected on CT or MR images, and they are manually digitized during surgery with a 3D localizer.[141,151] In a second instance, titanium pins are screwed into the bones; they are automatically segmented on CT images and detected during surgery using a force-controlled robot.[148]

5.5.2.2 Group B: Anatomy-Based Registration

Alternatively, it is possible to use only the information contained in the data and images of the patient for registration purposes. These methods of anatomy-based registration can be split into two groups, depending on the nature of features they use:

1. Segmented feature-based techniques — In this class of methods, anatomical features corresponding to reference structures are segmented in both modalities to be registered. Then, algorithms of point, curve, surface, or volume matching are used. These methods are very convenient for CIST because they do not require any additional preparation for the patient, they are non-invasive, and they can be percutaneous. The main issue is to segment the anatomical features in a robust and accurate manner. However, some recent approaches propose to combine segmentation and anatomy-based registration in a unique robust process,[72] which fills the gap between segmented feature-based and image-based methods.
   - Minimization of distances between interactively matched points (least-squares fitting) — A few anatomic feature points can be interactively defined in CT or MR images and manually digitized during surgery.[60,119] The same principle has been used to register multimodality images together or images with atlases.[54,155]
   - Minimization of distances between series of singular points or lines (least-squares fitting) — Singular points or crest lines can be extracted on two pairs of 3D images and then matched together and registered.[116,153] These methods are limited to intra-modality image registration.
   - Fitting of inertia axes of volumes — Volumes of anatomic structures segmented can be registered by their three inertia axes.[5] These methods are sensitive to shape symmetries. Even a non-symmetrical complex shape can have two or three of its inertia values nearly equal, which makes impossible accurate and robust registration.
   - Minimization of point-to-surface or surface-to-surface distances (least-squares fitting) — A reference surface is segmented on modalities A and B. Surface B is discretized in N 3D points and the sum of squares between those points and the surface A is minimized. Several authors have proposed to build 3D distance maps to speed

up the computation of point-to-surface distances, using octree-spline distance maps[101] or chamfer distance maps.[25,84] Distances more complex than 3D Euclidean distances (e.g., taking normals into account) can also be optimized by using Kd-trees.[56] Because they prove to be very efficient for multimodality image registration, these methods have been developed and refined by several authors.[84,102,121,122] Moreover, they have proved to be very efficient for registration between pre-operative CT or MR data and intra-operative sensor data, which can be of different types, including the following:
— a 3D digitizing pointer handled manually[99,102]
— a 2.5D ultrasound probe (percutaneously)[16,158]
— a range imaging sensor (for visible and stable surfaces)[161]
The latter methods will be illustrated in Section 5.5.4.
- Minimization of distances between anatomical surfaces segmented on CT or MR images registered with contours of X-ray projections of those surfaces[57,72,100,101] (see Section 5.5.4 for illustration).
- Minimization of distances between branching of bronchi segmented on bronchoscopy video images and pre-operative CT images.[28]

2. Image-based techniques — In this class of methods, images or sensor data are directly matched together without need for intermediary segmentation. Correlation methods usually turn out to be slow and sensitive to differences in the images. Conversely, methods that optimize mutual information (derived from entropy) seem to be more robust and faster. Extensive work is still required to validate and extend the clinical use of these methods, but there is no doubt that they offer very promising solutions for the future.
   - Gray levels of images matched together using maximization of correlation (limited to intramodality image registration).[12,33,160] — Actually, correlation can be applied directly on the images or on the images previously convolved by a filter.
   - Gray levels of images matched together using directly the difference between gray levels,[82] the difference multiplied by the gradient[29] or the difference between filtered images.[36,41]
   - Gray levels of images matched together using maximization of mutual information or entropy,[40,76,165] with possibility to match intra-operative video images with pre-operative CT or MR models[73] (see Figure 5.8).
   - Gray levels of 3D CT images registered with gray levels of X-ray projections, using correlation[105] or extreme gray level points.[65]

5.5.3 Step 3: Optimization of the Disparity (or Similarity) Function

Reference systems Ref_A and Ref_B are assumed to be registered when the defined disparity function (or similarity function) is minimal (or maximal).

Different optimization methods have been used in the literature. Usually, these methods depend directly on the choice of features; however, the association between features and optimization methods is not always obvious and one should always consider all the following classes and characteristics:

- Registration of paired 3D points by a rigid body transform — This is probably the only case where there exists a direct (non-iterative) solution. Here, the optimization can be solved by a simple least-squares system [using, e.g., singular value decomposition (SVD)[6] or unit quaternions[77]]. Otherwise, iterative algorithms are used.
- Iterative closest point (ICP) — Still in the case of rigid body transforms, authors[20] have generalized the direct 3D point-to-3D point registration to least-squares minimization of euclidean distances between any feature A represented by N 3D points and any feature

B represented by M 3D points, provided that the euclidean distance between points of A and B can be computed. The method is iterative. Starting from an initial rigid body transform (position and orientation), the ICP algorithm first searches for each data point $P_{Bj}, j = 1 \ldots M$, of feature B, the corresponding nearest point P_{Aj} on the reference feature A. Then, the rigid body transform that matches both point sets P_{Aj} and P_{Bj} is computed by a direct method using quaternions (an SVD method could have been used as well). The result is applied to data points P_{Bj} and the whole procedure is iterated. The resulting transform is given by the product of the transform matrices computed at each iteration. Although this elegant solution can be applied to many features including points and surfaces, it requires finding nearest points on the model feature very quickly, which is not always possible for complex shapes. An improved implementation of the basic algorithm has been described in Ref. 140 which makes it possible to register a few points acquired with an ultra-fast sensor on a face in real time. Another modification of this algorithm has been proposed in Ref. 22 where surface normals are used to improve the robustness of the registration.

- Non-linear minimization — More generally, standard non-linear minimization algorithms are used.[126] Best results are obtained when analytic expressions of gradients of the disparity function are known, for instance using conjugate gradients. When the disparity function is expressed as a least-squares formulation, the Levenberg-Marquardt algorithm has proved to be very efficient for registration problems (see its extended use in Refs. 101 and 106). A variation of this algorithm is the generalized Kalman filter.[22]
  Basically, non-linear minimization applied to rigid body registration problems does not raise real problems except for local minima (see next sections). But for non-rigid registration problems, several thousands of local displacement parameters need to be estimated, instead of six for rigid body transforms. Standard methods can prove to be very slow or even not practical. To solve this problem, an adaptive hierarchical basis (octree-splines)[145] has been used to speed up the iterative search, which reduces to a preconditioning of conjugate gradients algorithm that is used to solve one step of the Levenberg-Marquardt algorithm.
- Physical models (forces) — An alternative to energy minimization is using partial differential equations (PDEs) in the framework of a physical modeling. The simplest model has been to consider springs between points and surfaces. This approach is equivalent to the least-squares minimization of distances.[31] In Ref. 108, the authors take the approach of minimizing the energy with the addition of a damping factor to prevent oscillations. Actually, this intuitive physical approach is very close to standard mathematical minimization techniques, and unfortunately, local minima still exist.
  A more complex modeling has been developed for non-rigid registration between images and atlases. It consists in applying elastic models that are deformed under local forces derived from correlation measurements.[12] Each organ has its own elastic coefficients, that are set by hand. Unfortunately, these methods are very slow in convergence.
  A still more complex modeling that has been used for the image to atlas non-rigid registration problems is based on fluid modeling.[36] Instead of searching local displacements directly, these methods consider the local speed of motion of a reference fluid whose final state is given by the image. Basically, elastic equations are applied to the motion speed instead of the displacement vectors. Such methods are also very slow to converge but they give excellent results when small displacements need to be estimated.
- Local versus global optimization — The methods mentioned above use global optimization, in which a cost function such as least-squares criterion or entropy is minimized or maximized according to the parameters of the searched transform. An alternative is to consider local optimization in which different local matches create individual votes

for a transform (or for some parameters of the transform), and the winning transform is the one with the maximum number of votes. For example, with generalized Hough transforms,[13] an accumulator corresponding to a discretization of the parameter (or Hough) space is incremented in all points that are possible matching parameters for a given pair of corresponding features. This is repeated for each pair of features, and the winner is simply the point of the Hough space which has the maximum value. However, Hough transforms are difficult to implement for high-dimensional spaces, but it is also possible to use hashing tables. Registration between two volumes of CT or MR images by matching two sets of 3D crest lines have been developed with such a method.[154] Actually, local methods are not popular in the field of computer-integrated surgery. They are useful only when few parameters are searched and correspondences between a large number of features are unknown. The usual problem of local minima in global methods is simply replaced by a combinatorial pairing problem in local methods, and expensive algorithms are usually required to take into account constraints between features (e.g., relaxation methods,[129] clustering techniques,[142] dynamic programming[107]).

Optimization Issues: Local Minima, Robustness, and Uncertainties

The above optimization methods face three problems for which solutions are sometimes incompatible:

- Local minima
- Presence of outliers (false data)
- Estimation of the uncertainty of the resulting transform.

To our knowledge, there is no general method that can cope with the three problems simultaneously.

The basic method to avoid local minima is to use stochastic algorithms such as simulated annealing, but usually they turn out to be extremely slow. In Ref. 82, the authors present genetic algorithms for determining a non-rigid transform built on 24 parameters. A crude approach is to start local minimization from a few seed points randomly selected in a bounding box of the parameter space. This is sometimes efficient but does not guarantee an optimal solution. Another popular strategy is to use a multilevel search. First, the transform is estimated on low-resolution images, then the result is applied to the next level of resolution and the process is iterated until the finest resolution is reached. This method is often efficient but it makes the assumption that the result found at a low resolution is inside the real convergence domain of the function, which is never guaranteed. Moreover, the generalization of this process to irregularly distributed data is not trivial.

The second problem is the presence of outliers. For instance, when the surgeon manually digitizes 3D points that are registered with a model, there might be some points that are on a wrong part of the anatomic structures (i.e., not included in the model). Similarly, there are often some points that are acquired when a button click or a switch is activated at a wrong time. Automatic sensors or data processing techniques also provide different sources of outliers. Usually the simplest method to cope with erroneous data is to temporarily eliminate data that correspond to an error which is above an adaptive threshold.[69,84,101] For instance, one can decide that 5% of the worst data are removed at each iteration of the optimization process but re-injected in the pool of data at the next iteration. These methods are quite efficient, but they introduce local minima and the threshold is difficult to select. If not enough data are eliminated, the algorithm will converge toward an inaccurate solution, and if too many data are eliminated, the uncertainty of the result will be very high. An adaptive solution has been proposed in Ref. 23 but more work is still required in this domain.

The third problem is to obtain a solution with a low level of uncertainty. This problem is in fact divided into two subproblems. First, the function that is minimized must not have a flat profile along any direction of the parameter space. This is strongly related to the shape of the registered features. For instance, the problem would occur when 3D points are registered with a surface that is more or less spherical, cylindrical, or planar; such a problem is ill-posed and there is an infinite set of solutions for which the residual error will be very low. An estimation of the uncertainty can be easily computed by analyzing the eigenvalues of an approximation of the Hessian at the minimum of the function. For instance, a usual score is the condition number of the Hessian (smallest eigenvalue divided by the maximum eigenvalue).[140] However, this approach is not always efficient since it indicates the purely local curvature of the function, whereas we are usually interested in its shape at a given scale. Similarly, approximation errors in the Hessian can significantly influence the results. Finally, the errors of registration must be propagated to the region of interest, which is also non-trivial and requires more work.

In summary, ad-hoc recipes have to be developed for each problem, using as much as possible any available information. First, the domain of possible solutions must be accurately identified by an initial transform and by the range of parameters around this initial point. Second, there are often some constraints in the data that are not used (e.g., the normals of surface points), and image gradients must be coherent in surface-based registration techniques. Dividing the data into blocks of different anatomic regions is also very valuable. When such information cannot be obtained automatically, the operator can help, provided that the ergonomics of data acquisition and data processing is simple and efficient. Similarly, the question of whether outliers should be taken into account is still open and application dependent. Our point of view is that outliers should be admissible for only a very low percentage, such as 1%, and the system should detect the presence of more outliers and conduct a test of registration failure. Because all these problems need further investigation, it is important that the validity of a solution be assessed by the operator before use. For instance, in passive navigation systems, the surgeon has to check the coherence between the information indicated on the screen and the real pointer position, using a few checkpoints.

5.5.4 Illustration of Registration Methods

In this section, we illustrate the previously described methods by a few examples. These represent efficient and validated techniques of registration. The first example comes from the work of S. Wells et al. at Brigham and Women Hospital (Boston, MA), and the other examples come from TIMC laboratory and Grenoble Hospital.

5.5.4.1 Image-to-Image Registration Using Mutual Information

Figure 5.8 shows an instance of accurate registration between PET and MR images, and SPGR MR with T2 MR images of a same patient, using the method of Wells et al.[165] Since it is an image-based method, there is no need for segmentation of features prior to segmentation. Entropy-based methods can be formulated as follows. Consider the 2D histogram of 3D images A and B for a given transform **T** between them: if images have their discrete values m and n in $[0 \ldots M]$, the 2D histogram is a function $h(m,n)$ from $[0 \ldots M] \times [0 \ldots M]$ to IN that associates every pair of image values (m,n) with the number of occurrences where image A equals m and image B equals n at the same spatial point x in 3D (for the given transform **T** that depends on parameters p: $m = A(x)$ and $n = B(T(x))$. If we consider 3D images A and B to be from the same modality, when the images are registered, the histogram $h(m,n)$ is an array which has accumulation points on the line $m = n$. These accumulation points are therefore very concentrated. If we move image B from its registered position, the histogram h is more and more equally distributed. If we normalize the histogram h to consider it as a probability density $P(m,n)$ of the two image value variables $m = A(x)$ and

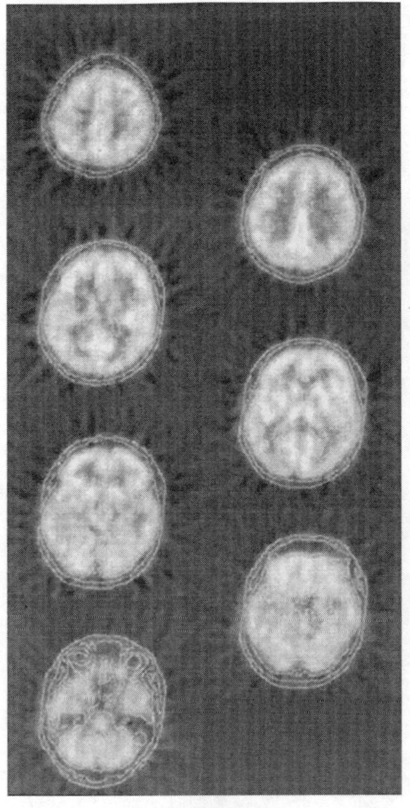

a

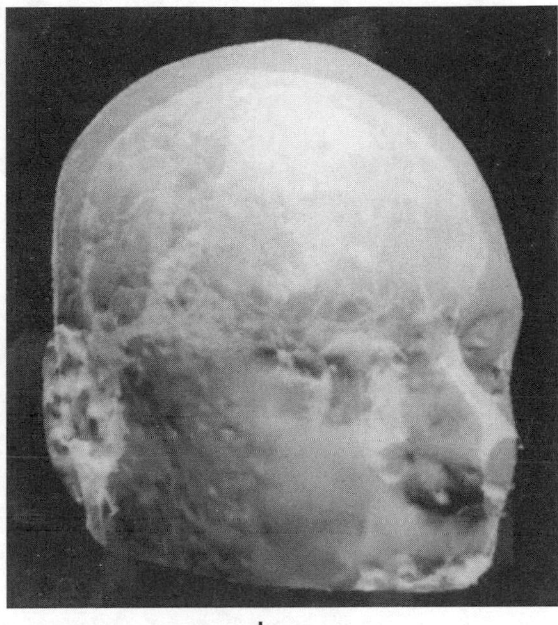

b

FIGURE 5.8 Registration of multimodality images using entropy-based methods. (With courtesy of S. Wells from Brigham and Women Hospital, Boston, MA. With permission of reprint from *MEDIA Journal*, Oxford University Press [WVA+96]. (a) The different PET slices are shown with the edges from the registered and reformatted MR data overlaid. (b) A rendering of the 3D models constructed from different MR acquisitions that were registered together: anatomic information (the skin, the brain, the vessels, the ventricles) was generated from the post-contrast gradient echo (SPGR) MR images, whereas the tumor was segmented from the registered and reformatted T2-weighted MR images.

$n = B(T(x))$, a possible way to charaterize the complexity of the 2D histogram is to consider entropy. Entropy $e(p)$ is minimum when the histogram is concentrated on very few accumulation points. It is given by the following equation:

$$e(p) = -\int P(m,n)\ln\big(P(m,n)\big)dm\,dn \tag{5.1}$$

When images are registered, the entropy will be minimized. One can say that B explains A for the exact registration transform **T**. In order to obtain a non-trivial local maximum in which images would be completely separated, it is in fact necessary to add a term that encourages the transform **T** for which the images A and B have some high complexity in their common support S. Thus, Equation 5.1 is now replaced by the expression of mutual information, which has to be maximized:

$$h(m,n) = -\int_S P(m)\ln\big(P(m)\big)dm - \int_S P(n)\ln\big(P(n)\big)dn + \int P(m,n)\ln\big(P(m,n)\big)dm\,dn \tag{5.2}$$

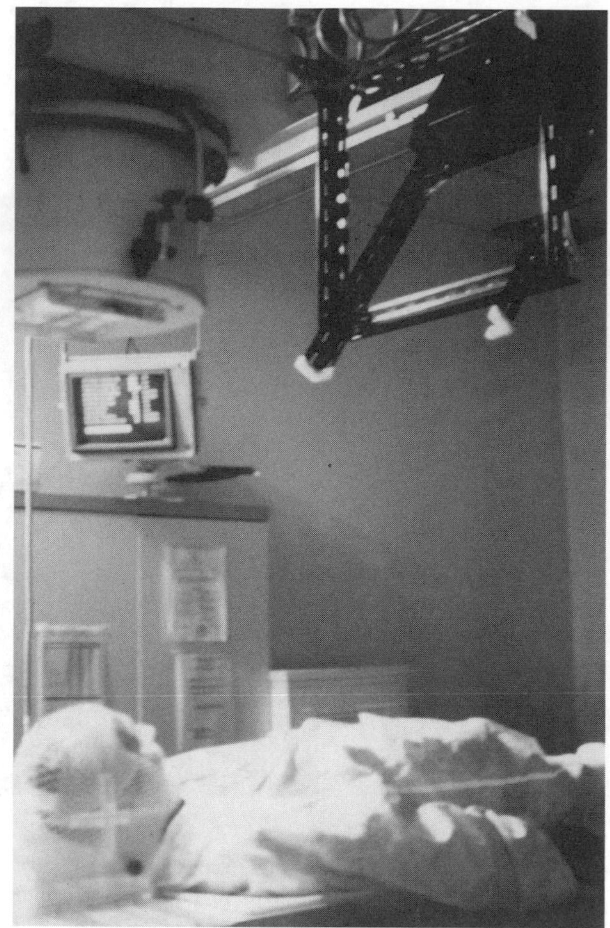

FIGURE 5.9a

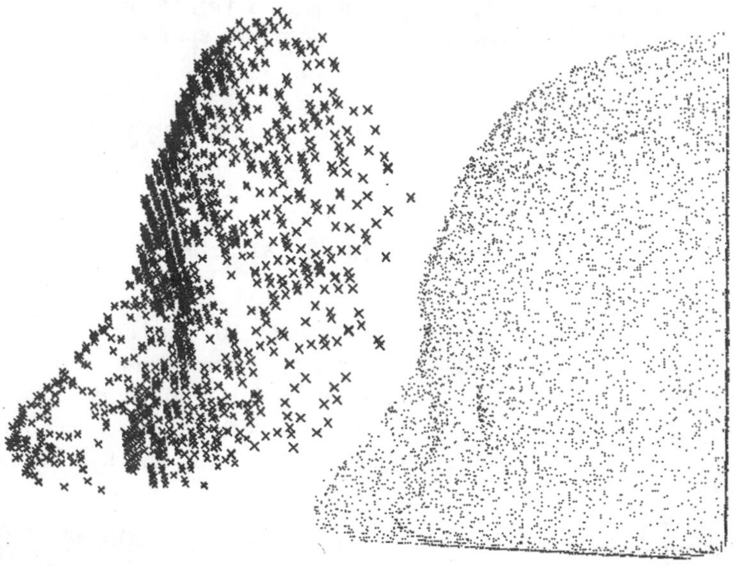

FIGURE 5.9b

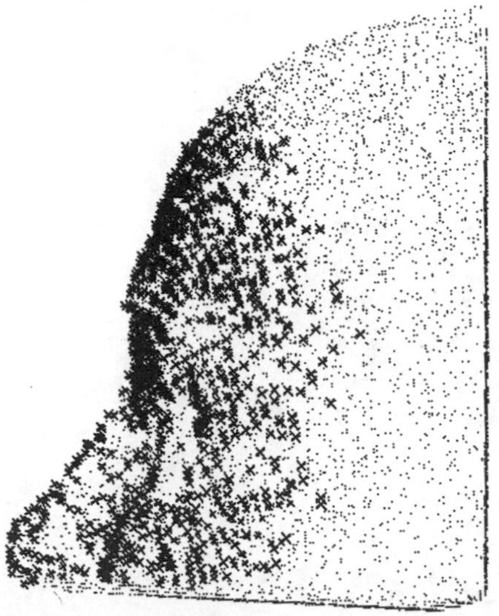

FIGURE 5.9 Frameless and accurate patient positioning in brain radiotherapy. (a) Range sensor made of a pattern projector and a video camera is fixed above the patient's head. (b) Before registration: initial transform between the data surface points (crosses in bold) acquired with the range sensor in the radiotherapy coordinate system and the skin surface points segmented on pre-operative CT images (represented by dots). Starting from such an initial transform, the registration algorithm iteratively minimizes the sum of the distances between the data surface points and the complete surface. (c) Final registration after 10 iterations of the registration algorithm: the transform between CT images and the radiotherapy coordinate system has been computed such that the data points are lying on the surface of the CT model. Using this final transform, the target defined on CT images can be positioned at the radiation isocenter. (Courtesy of Dr. M. Bolla, Radiotherapy Dept., Grenoble Hospital.)

See the method of Wells et al.[165] for a very efficient implementation of this principle. In practice, images do not need to be of the same modality; they just need to "look similar." Obviously, there are some limitations to these methods and many aspects remain to be explored, but they have shown very efficient results in various instances. In some cases where images are very different, the use of these methods might be dangerous. Then the principle of adding an intermediate sensor between images A and B is more reliable.[122]

5.5.4.2 Image-to-Physical Space Registration Using 3D Point-to-Surface Distance Minimization

For image-to-physical space registration, which is central to computer-integrated surgery, anatomy-based registration methods that register the surface of a reference anatomic structure segmented on pre-operative images with intra-operative data have shown very good results in many instances.[102]

CT/range imaging systems for brain radiotherapy

For brain radiation therapy, patient positioning in the radiotherapy system is usually done through the use of individual molded head holders or stereotactic frames. A better approach is to install a range imaging sensor above the radiotherapy system and use it as an intermediary sensor for registration (Figure 5.9). In CT or MR images, it is easy to segment the patient skin and obtain a 3D surface model S. This represents the model virtual mask. Using the range imaging sensor, we can obtain a set of N 3D points P_i that belong to the same surface in the radiotherapy coordinate system (provided this system is calibrated with respect to the sensor). This set of points represents the sensor virtual mask. Both virtual masks are registered using a 3D/3D surface registration algorithm that minimizes a least-squares criterion C with respect to the six parameters **p** of the searched rigid transform **T**(**p**):[102]

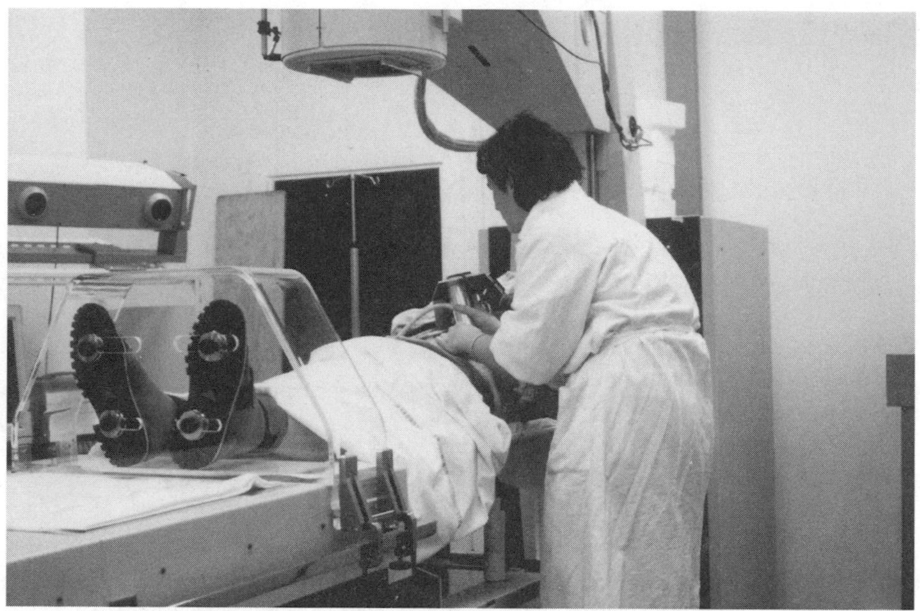

FIGURE 5.10a

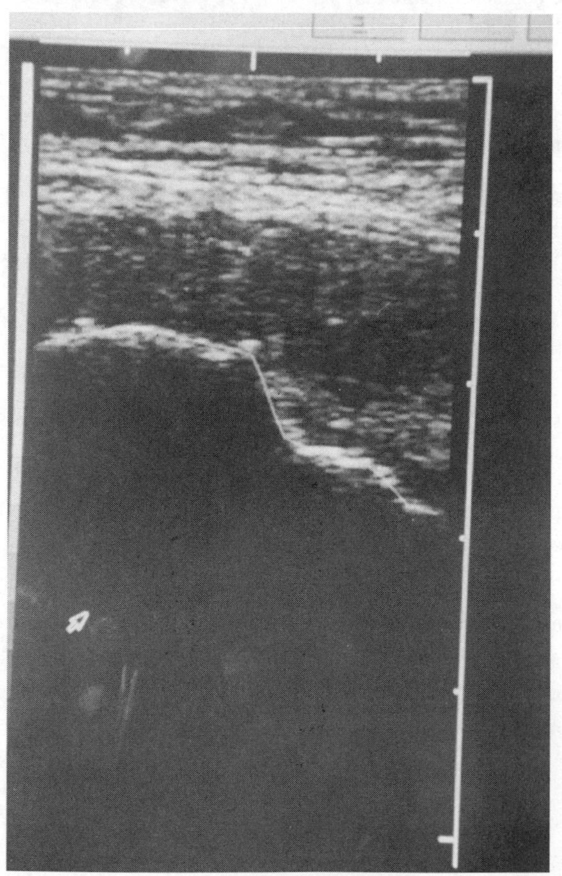

FIGURE 5.10b

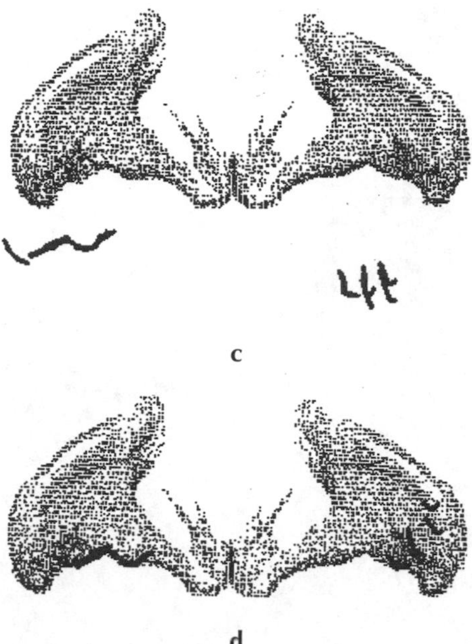

FIGURE 5.10 Patient positioning in prostate radiotherapy. (a) Acquisition of 2.5D ultrasound data on pelvic bones and prostate. (b) Segmentation of the pelvic bone edges on a typical ultrasound image. Using the measurements of the position and orientation of the ultrasound probe, such an edge is transformed in a set of coplanar 3D points in the radiation device coordinate system. About 5 to 10 slices are acquired to constitute a volumetric set of data points. (c) Before registration, an initial transform is defined using *a priori* knowledge to constitute the input for iteration 0 of the registration algorithm: it is the transform between a surface model (represented by dots) of the pelvic bones segmented on CT images and the set of 3D points (crosses in bold) obtained with the 2.5D ultrasound sensor in the radiation device coordinate system. (d) Final registration: data points fit the CT model. This view enables the operator to check that the registration is correct. Using this transform between the CT and radiation device coordinate systems, the patient table can be moved accordingly such that the tumor center defined on CT images is positioned at the radiation isocenter. (Courtesy of Dr. M. Bolla, Radiotherapy Dept., Grenoble Hospital.)

$$C(\mathbf{p}) = \sum_i \left[\tilde{d}\left(S, \mathbf{T}(\mathbf{p})P_i\right)\right]^2 / \sigma_i^2 \tag{5.3}$$

where $\tilde{d}(S,M)$ is the signed euclidean distance between a surface S and a point M, σ_i^2 is the variance of the noise for point P_i. In our current implementation, the distance $\tilde{d}$ is implemented using an octree-spline distance map,[101] and the minimization is performed using the Levenberg-Marquardt algorithm[126] (see Ref. 102 for details). Once registration has been performed, the patient table is moved until the tumor center defined on CT images is positioned at the radiation isocenter. This method is under clinical investigation at Grenoble Hospital.[161]

CT/2.5D ultrasound registration in prostate radiotherapy

The same method as in the previous case can be applied to prostate radiotherapy, provided that the range imaging sensor is replaced by a 2.5D ultrasound sensor, presented in Figure 5.4e. Figure 5.10 shows the registration process between CT images and the radiation coordinate system which is performed on the pelvic bones that are considered as a stable reference anatomic structure. Clinical validation of this method is ongoing.[157,158] Importantly, this registration method can be readily applied to orthopedics surgery on pelvic bones.

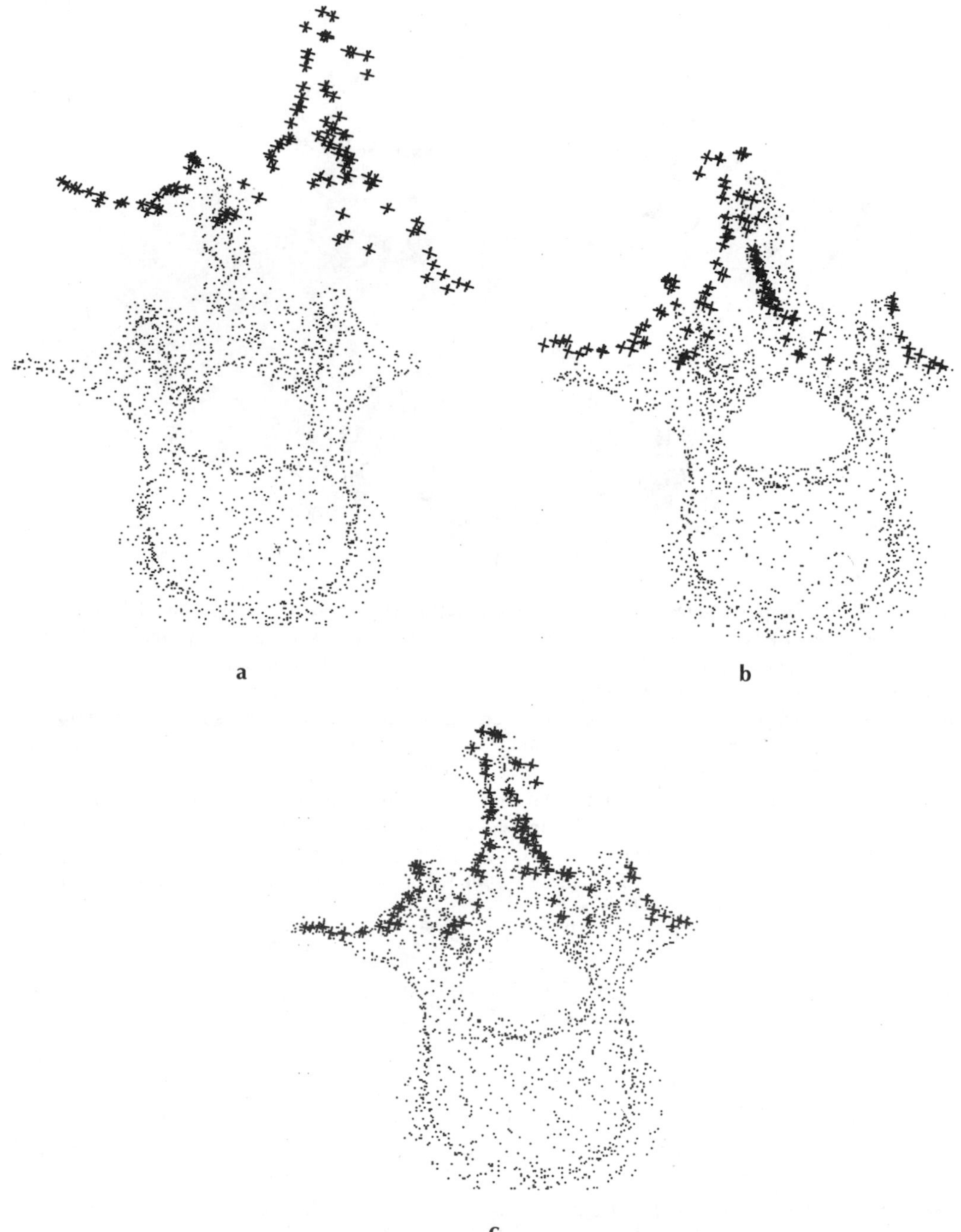

FIGURE 5.11 Convergence of 3D/3D registration algorithm. During spine surgery, a set of 50 surface points acquired manually with an optical 3D localizer (in bold) converges toward the 3D model of the vertebra segmented on pre-operative CT images (dots). Convergence is shown at iteration 0 for an *a priori* known transform (a), at iteration 3 (b), and at final iteration 7 (c). It requires about 0.1 s on a DEC-Alpha computer.

CT/3D points registration for orthopedics surgery

Figure 5.11 shows registration between 3D surface points manually digitized on a vertebra during surgery and the 3D surface model of this vertebra segmented on CT images. This technique has been validated for open spine surgery.[99]

MRI/brain atlas elastic registration

The extension of our rigid registration method to elastic registration has been reported in Refs. 144 and 145. It is illustrated in Figure 5.12, where a brain atlas is registered with a few patient MR images previously segmented. A volume deformation is computed in about 1 mn on a DEC-Alpha 5000 workstation. Instead of searching for six parameters, as in rigid registration, the algorithm searches hundreds of displacement vectors of a grid that embeds the volume of data. In order to speed up the convergence, a hierarchical and non-uniform representation of this grid is used, called an octree-spline. This is a typical ill-posed problem with an infinite set of solutions. To cope with this issue, we add a regularization term to the points-to-surface distance to be minimized. Using this regularization, we obtain a smooth and continuous deformation.

5.5.4.3 Image-to-Physical Space Registration Using 3D/2D Matching Between Surfaces and X-Ray Projections

The use of intra-operative calibrated X-ray projection enables us to register pre-operative CT images with the intra-operative space. Here, we use an extension of the 3D points-to-surface distance minimization methods presented above. A least-squares criterion $C(\mathbf{p})$ is minimized with respect to the six parameters $\mathbf{p}$ of the searched rigid transform $\mathbf{T}(\mathbf{p})$ between CT images and the intra-operative coordinate system.[71,100–102] After automated extraction of edge points on X-ray images, 3D projection lines L_i, $i = 1 \ldots N$, associated with these edge points are computed in the intra-operative coordinate system. The idea is to estimate the transform $\mathbf{T}(\mathbf{p})$ such that these 3D projection lines become tangential to the 3D surface. This is achieved by minimizing a criterion of the following form:

$$C(\mathbf{p}) = \sum_i \left[\tilde{d}_l\left(S, \mathbf{T}(\mathbf{p})L_i\right)\right]^2 / \sigma_i^2 \tag{5.4}$$

where $\tilde{d}_l\,(S,L)$ is the signed euclidean distance between a surface S and a 3D projection line L (i.e., the minimum of $\tilde{d}\,(S,P)$ for all points P on the line L), $\mathbf{T}(\mathbf{p})L_l$ is a 3D line L_l transformed by $\mathbf{T}(\mathbf{p})$, σ_i^2 is the variance of the noise of edge point segmentation that gave line L_i. In our current implementation, the distance $\tilde{d}_l$ is implemented using an adaptive distance map called octree-spline,[100] and the minimization is performed by using the Levenberg-Marquardt algorithm.[126]

Figure 5.13 shows the application of our rigid 3D/2D algorithm to skull images: a CT model of a skull is registered with two calibrated X-rays. Applications to the spine can be found in Ref. 72.

5.6 ACTION

In the final stage of computer-integrated surgery, the physician or the surgeon can be assisted by "guiding systems" to perform the intervention. Guiding systems can be divided into three classes, depending on the autonomy that is left to the physician or surgeon.

5.6.1 Passive Guiding Systems

With passive systems, the assistance consists of making possible a real-time comparison between images and tool positions. Depending on the existence of a surgical planning step, we can distinguish between two types of passive systems: free navigation systems and alignment passive systems.

5.6.1.1 Free Navigation Systems

With free navigation systems, surgical planning does not need to be defined accurately before the operation. The surgeon uses the system to know where he or she is with respect to the anatomy presented on the images. The surgeon navigates in images and in the patient simultaneously, exactly

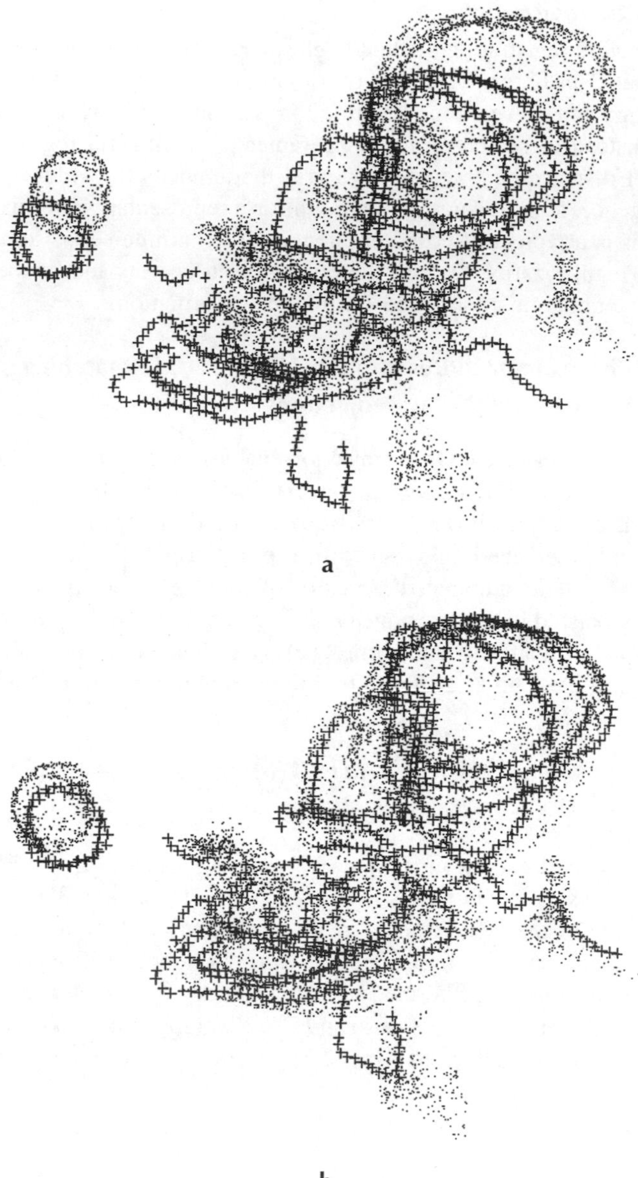

FIGURE 5.12 Elastic registration of Delmas brain atlas with patient MR images. (a) Atlas and MR data before registration. Bold crosses represent the points segmented on MR images. Thin dots represent the surfaces of the Delmas atlas. (b) After rigid registration. (Original MR images and Delmas atlas were provided by Pr. Von Keyserlinck, Aachen, Germany.)

like a satellite positioning system such as GPS, which helps one to sail and to locate oneself in marine maps.

- Tool navigation systems — With tool navigation systems, the surgeon sees the location of the tip of a tool on pre-operative images. For instance, three slices in the sagittal, frontal, and axial plane passing through the tip of a foreceps, pointer, surgical aspirator, or the like are reformatted and displayed in real time. The tool can also be displayed using a 3D rendering technique. This class of systems is probably the most widespread

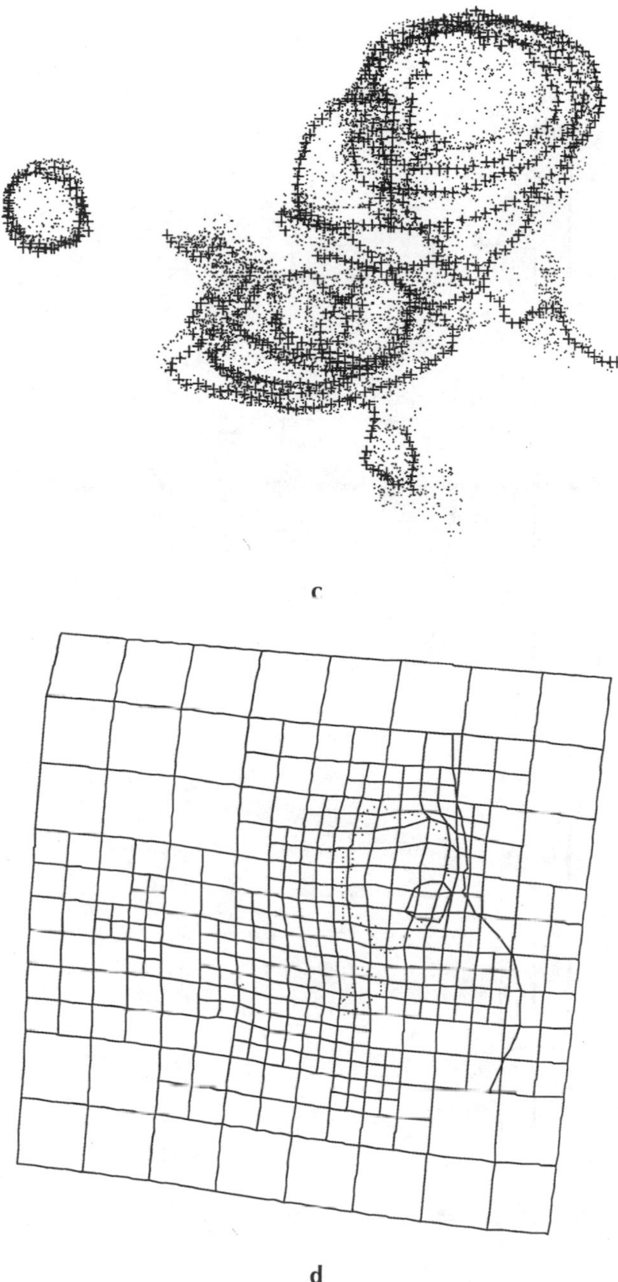

FIGURE 5.12 (c) Final result after elastic registration. (d) A 2D slice in the deformed volume mesh showing the smooth deformation of the volume that made possible the matching between MR data points and atlas surfaces.

(see the pioneering work in ENT surgery[3,118] and neurosurgery[90,130,141]). Now there exists a large variety of commercial navigation systems. Figure 5.14 shows one of the first navigation systems used in surgery.[118] These systems are also being used more and more in orthopedics surgery; for instance, in spine surgery for pedicle screw insertion[60,119] (see Figure 5.15). See also Ref. 10 for an application in the case of retroperitoneoscopy, where the tip of a rigid endoscope is tracked in real time in the

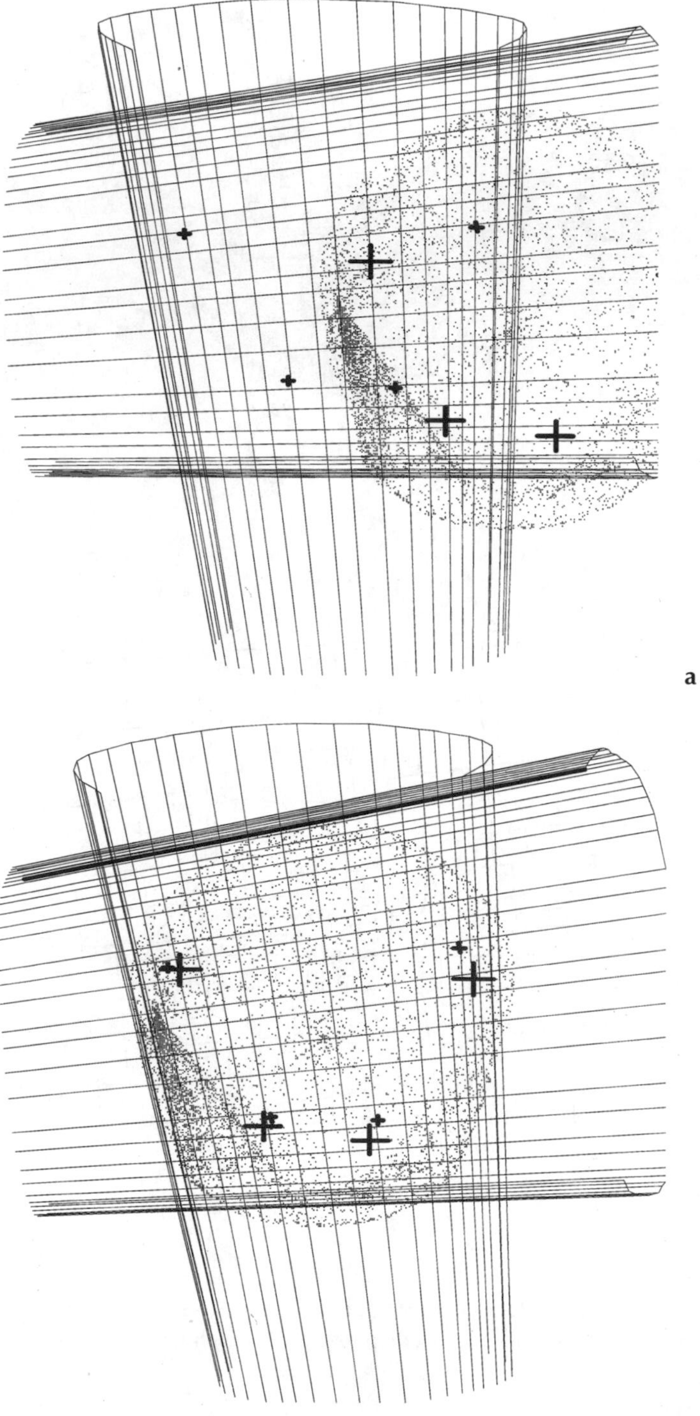

FIGURE 5.13 Convergence of 3D/2D algorithm: rigid registration between CT images and two X-ray images of a skull. On lateral and frontal X-rays, about 50 pixels are segmented on the edges of the skull. From each pixel, a 3D projection line is computed in the coordinate system of the calibrated X-rays. Starting from an initial transform between the X-ray coordinate system and the CT coordinate system, the algorithm minimizes the distances between the X-ray projection lines and the 3D surface. In the final position, all the projection lines are tangential to the skull surface. Such a convergence is obtained in 0.2 s on a DEC-Alpha workstation.

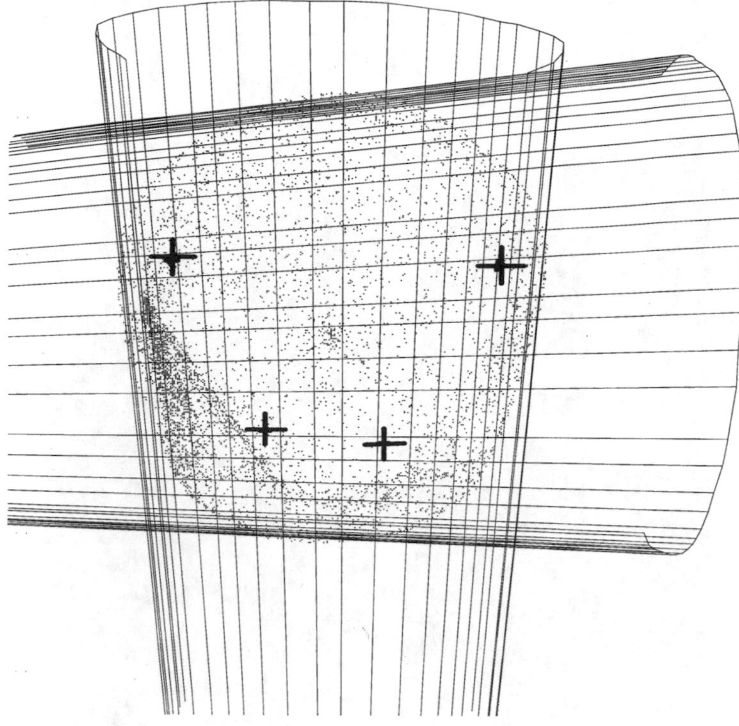

FIGURE 5.13c

abdomen: the mediastinoscope is used to explore a region located between the intestines and the spine. Visual feedback on the position of the endoscope from pre-operative CT or MR images is crucial to avoid damaging important structures such as vessels (see Figure 5.16).

- Image navigation systems — Image navigation systems constitute a different class of purely passive systems. With such devices, real images are merged with virtual images, thus constituting image-based augmented reality systems.

In Refs. 51, 87, and 134, the optical output of surgical microscopes were merged with synthetic video images computed from a registered CT or MR model, with applications in neurosurgery. Different visualization modes are possible, but the more efficient seems to inject in the image only a few structures, such as a tumor or some vessels, which have been pre-segmented and modeled by surfaces or curves. Commercial robotics surgical microscopes of Zeiss, Oberkochen, Germany (MKM™ system) and Elekta-Deemed, Grenoble, France (Surgiscope™ system) also provide a similar capability, with the difference that the microscope not only is encoded in position but also it is moved by a robot which is controlled by the user via joysticks or force sensors. The accuracy of these systems in neurosurgery is severely limited by brain shift and deformation that occurs during surgery (errors of 3 mm or more are not rare). The use of intra-operative sensors such as ultrasounds, open MR, or intra-operative CT complemented by non-rigid registration methods is necessary to obtain a better accuracy.

It is also possible to superimpose virtual images on video outputs of endoscopes. In Ref. 70, an electromagnetic localizer was used to track a rigid endoscope position in real time, which enables one to compute a virtual perspective view of the scene that corresponds to the current endoscope position. The same principle would not be possible for

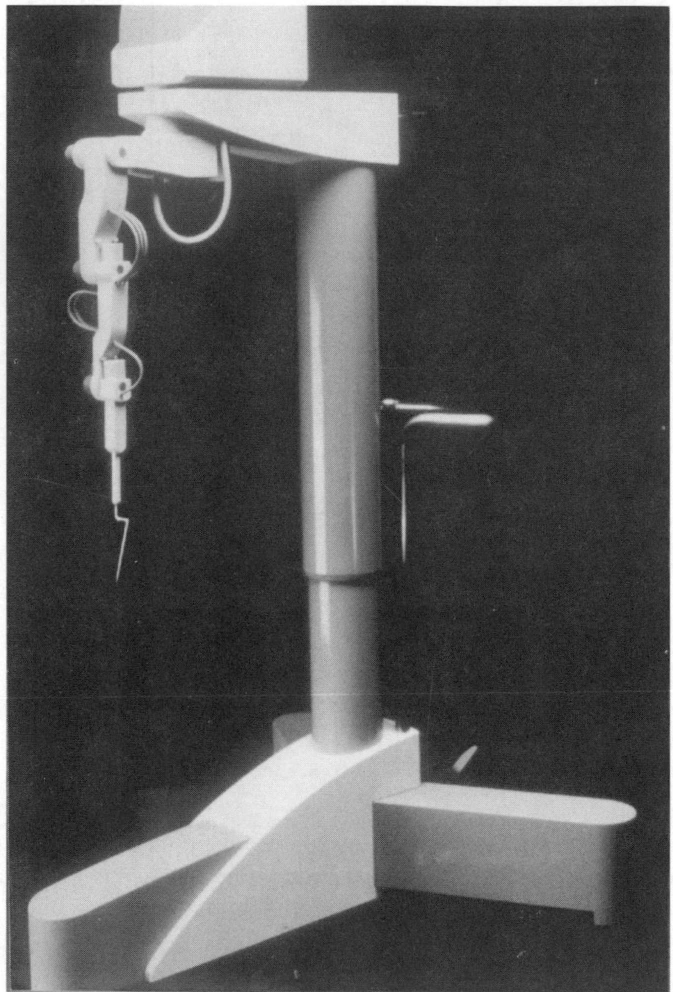

FIGURE 5.14a Navigation system for ENT surgery. (a) A 6 degrees-of-freedom mechanical arm gives the position of a tool tip in real time, using a simple forward kinematics model and encoders readings. (Courtesy of Prof. Ralph Mosges, Aachen, Germany.)

flexible endoscopes, except if micro-electromagnetic localizers could be added at the tip of a flexible endoscope (e.g., using a localization system developped by Biosense, Israel). However, an alternative to the use of localizers has been proposed recently for bronchoscopy[27,28] in using only the video image information to register the endoscope position with a patient CT model. This allows superimposing real images of the flexible endoscope and virtual images without using any additional sensor. The geometric information contained in real video images is used to register the endoscope position with pre-operative CT images. Figure 5.17 illustrates a result of this system.

Finally, head-mounted displays with semitransparent glasses offer the possibility to merge directly the visible reality with models. However, many problems of accuracy, lighting conditions, and display rates still remain to be solved. An interesting variation of head-mounted displays uses image projection on a semitransparent glass placed above the surgical field.[124]

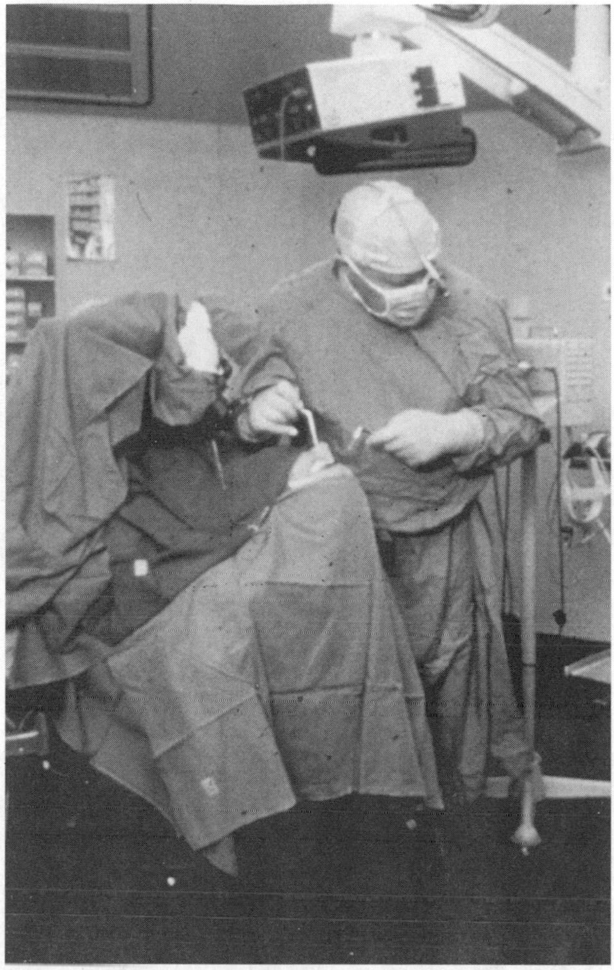

FIGURE 5.14b Clinical use of the system at Aachen Hospital: the surgeon is looking at the position of the tool tip on registered pre-operative images.

5.6.1.2 Alignment Passive Systems

For this second category of passive systems, it is necessary that a surgical planning step be performed pre-operatively or at the beginning of the operation. Then, the guiding system helps the surgeon to reproduce the planned strategy. The basic idea of alignment passive systems is to let the surgeon manipulate a tool freely, as in free navigation systems, but to provide information that allows him or her to align the current tool position with the optimal position previously defined. The system is still passive because the physical action is not constrained, but it is less free than in the previous case since the operator is not supposed to escape from the planned strategy. Different systems have been used clinically in this category:

- Aiming systems with graphics user interfaces — On these systems, the surgeon watches a computer display that represents the real-time position of a tool and tries to align the tool with respect to a position that corresponds to the defined strategy. This principle can be used to aim at a defined point, to align a linear tool with an optimal line segment,

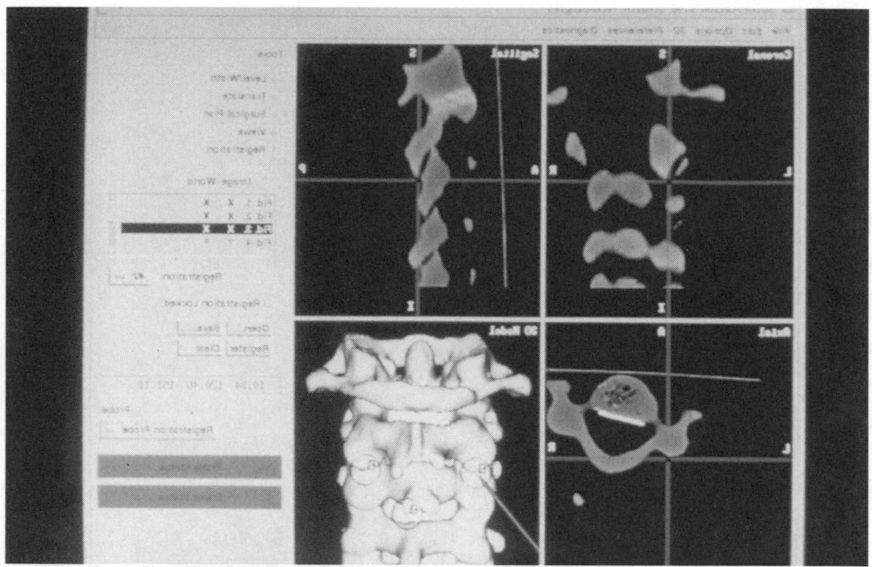

FIGURE 5.15 Standard interface for passive navigation: three reformatted slices passing through the tool tip are displayed in real time. This user interface is used for spine surgery on the Stealth workstation. (Courtesy of Sofamor-Danek.)

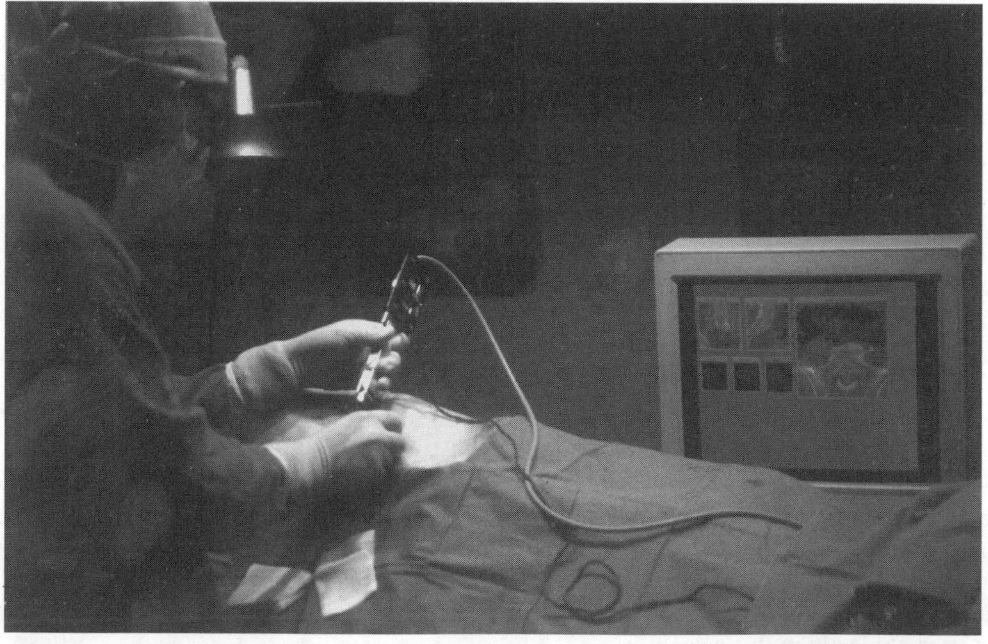

FIGURE 5.16 Computer-assisted retroperitoneoscopy. The position of a rigid endoscope is tracked in real time in pre-operative CT images. Three orthogonal CT slices passing through the tip of the endoscope are computed and displayed at a frequency of 1 Hz. It was found that using the original CT orientation (axial, sagittal, frontal) was the most acceptable for the surgeon. This method has been validated on cadavers. (Courtesy of Dr. Chaffanjon, Pr. Sarrazin, General, Thoracic and Infantile Surgery Department, Grenoble Hospital.)

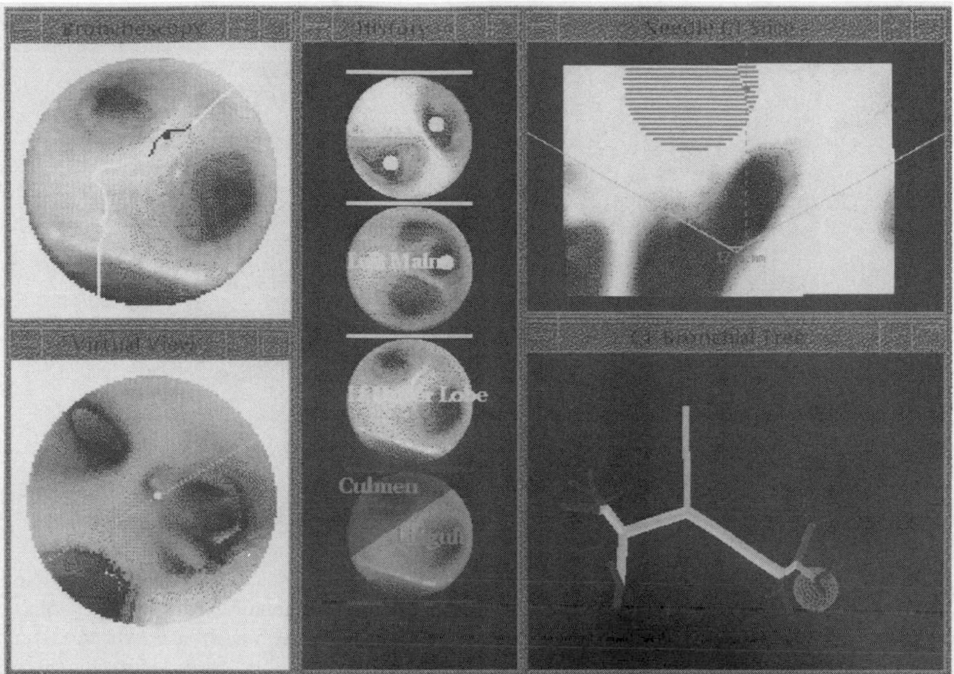

FIGURE 5.17 Computer-assisted bronchoscopy. The system achieves an automatic matching between real and virtual bronchoscopy. This permits a guidance to transbronchial needle biopsy. In the upper left window, the real bronchoscopic video sequence is analyzed in quasi real time by the computer. In the current subdivision image, we see the automatic segmentation of the wall that split both bronchi. In the middle column, the computer is able to recognize the different explored bronchi. From top to bottom, each subdivision level encountered is extracted. The bottom view identifies both current bronchi (culmen and lingula). In the bottom right window, the computer tracks the trajectory of the flexible endoscope inside a 3D geometrical model of the bronchial tree. Both current bronchi are located by specific colors. We can see a spherical target defined in the model for transbronchial needle biopsy. In the bottom left window, the system can synthesize a virtual view from CT scan data. The target appears in transparency. Using specific image processing algorithms, bronchoscopic camera position is automatically computed, so that the virtual view follows the actual camera movements and automatically matches the real view. In the upper right window, the computer shows the CT slice containing the bronchoscopic center of view and the expected biopsy needle trajectory. (Courtesy of Dr. Ferretti, Pr. Coulomb, Radiology Department, Grenoble Hospital.)

or to align two reference coordinate systems. These three cases are illustrated below by concrete clinical examples of work done at Grenoble:

1. *Point alignment for knee ACL reconstruction.* For ACL reconstruction of the knee, a system that helps to place a graft at the best points of insertion on the femur and on the tibia has been described[48,49,120] (see Figure 5.4c). The best positions are based on functional criteria that facilitate obtaining the least anisometry of the central graft fiber: the length variation of this fiber observed during passive flexion/extension of the knee is minimized. Moreover, a constraint of no collision (also called impingement) between the ligament in full extension and the femoral notch is preserved. The two optimal points on the femoral and tibial surface are proposed by the system and controlled by the surgeon. Once these points are defined, the aiming system projects in real time the position of the tip of a tool equipped with a rigid body on the tibial and femoral surfaces (Figure 5.18). A first cross-hair indicates the current position while a second cross-hair indicates the optimal position. The surgeon moves the tip

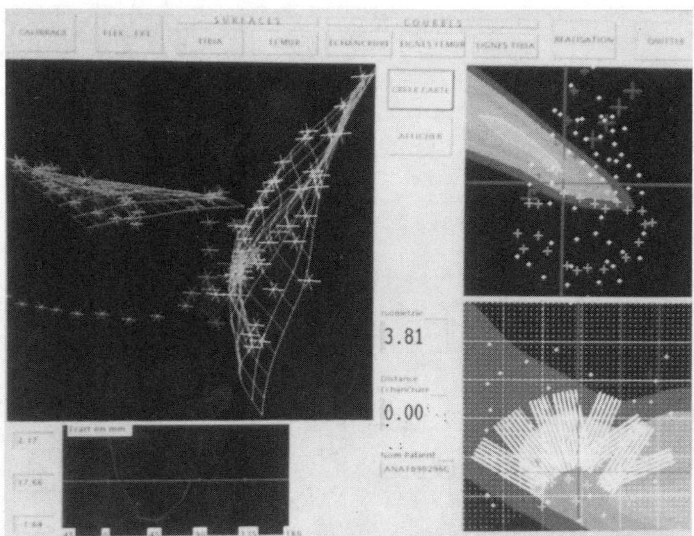

FIGURE 5.18 User interface for passive help to optimal knee ACL placement. Left part of the screen shows a 3D view of the tibial surface trajectory with respect to the femoral surface. Right part shows pseudocolor representations of the anisometry criterion on both femur and tibia surfaces, with representations of notch impingement. The surgeon locates the projection of a drilling tool tip on those images by watching the cross-hairs positions. (Courtesy of Dr. Julliard, Orthopedics Department at Cliniquie Mutualiste de Grenoble.)

on the bone surface and tries to match the two cross-hairs as accurately as possible, but he or she can also integrate some possible constraints that the system has not taken into account. This is an example of an alignment passive system, in which 2 degrees of freedom are adjusted for each point.

2. *Line alignment for spine surgery.* For transpedicular screwing in spine surgery, which is performed in cases of scoliosis or discal instability, a difficult problem is to insert the largest screw possible inside the pedicle of a vertebra without touching critical adjacent structures like vessels and the spinal cord. This is particularly difficult for thoracic and cervical vertebrae as well as for very twisted lumbar vertebrae in scoliosis cases. The optimal position of the screw can be defined interactively on pre-operative CT images (see Figure 5.6). After registration between CT images and an intra-operative 3D localizer using either a simple pointer,[98] X-ray images,[136] or 2.5D echography,[16] the optimal position is known in an intra-operative coordinate system attached to the vertebra and it is defined by an entry point Q1 and an endpoint Q2. An alignment passive guiding system is used then to align the tool position with the optimal trajectory. The surgeon's drill is equipped with a rigid body that is localized in space (see Figure 5.4d). After drill calibration, two points P_1 and P_2 on the drill axis are known in this rigid body coordinate system and therefore the coordinates of these two points are known in real time in the vertebra coordinate system, in which the optimal trajectory is also known. The graphics user interface simply compares the distances between the line segment P_1P_2 and the optimal line segment. It shows a view orthogonal to the line (Q_1Q_2), and a square or circle in the middle gives an idea of the view scale (usually, the square corresponds to 1 mm). The points P_1 and P_2 are projected on this view. First, the surgeon aligns the tool tip P_1 in the central square, then he or she aligns the tool orientation by placing the point P_2 in the central square,

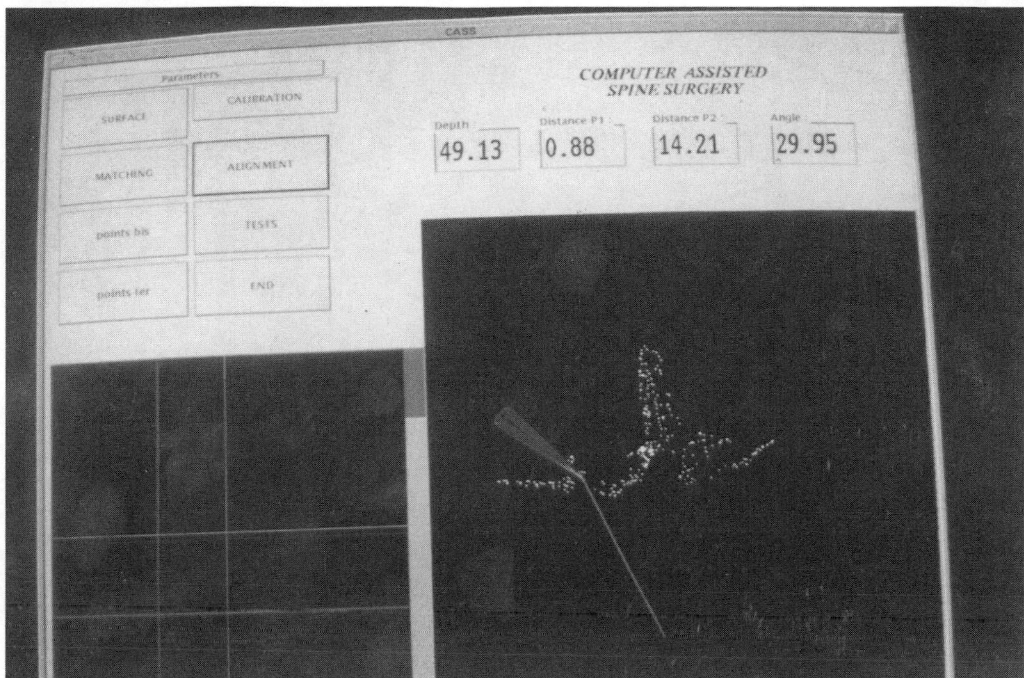

FIGURE 5.19 Passive alignment for pedicle screw insertion in spine surgery. An aiming system helps the surgeon to drill inside the vertebra pedicle according to a 3D line defined on CT images. The drill is equipped with a rigid body and its position is compared with the optimal position using cross-hairs superimposition for two points. A color bar indicates the depth of tool penetration. Graphics data are also displayed in 3D and as distances in millimeters. (Courtesy of Pr. Merloz, Orthopedics Department, Grenoble Hospital.)

and finally the penetration length is controlled by a color bar (see Figure 5.19). This simple interface was first published in Refs. 99, but it has numerous other applications (e.g., see Ref. 15). During this process, two crosses are aligned with a central cross, which corresponds to a passive alignment of 4 degrees of freedom.

3. *Alignment of coordinate systems for craniofacial surgery.* In craniofacial surgery, it may be important to place a bone in a position defined during a complex pre-operative planning phase.[149] In a simpler application described in Refs. 21 and 47, it is necessary to reposition a bone fragment of the mandible exactly as it was at the beginning of the operation. Figure 5.20 shows a graphics interface which allows the surgeon to reach this alignment of 6 degrees of freedom. The design of the user interface that must take into account the relative orientation of the surgeon with respect to the screen is essential to make such a complex alignment possible.

- Laser-guided alignment — To constrain a little more the surgeon to align a tool such as a drill with a predefined 3D line (as in the previously mentioned aiming system), it is possible to position a laser beam in space using a robot and then have the surgeon manually align the tool with the laser beam by using a sight placed at the rear part of the tool.[99,136] The action is still unconstrained but more constrained than in the previous cases, because outside of the laser alignment, no information is provided: the surgeon must not choose a slightly different trajectory because he or she would not be able to envisage the effects of a misalignment.

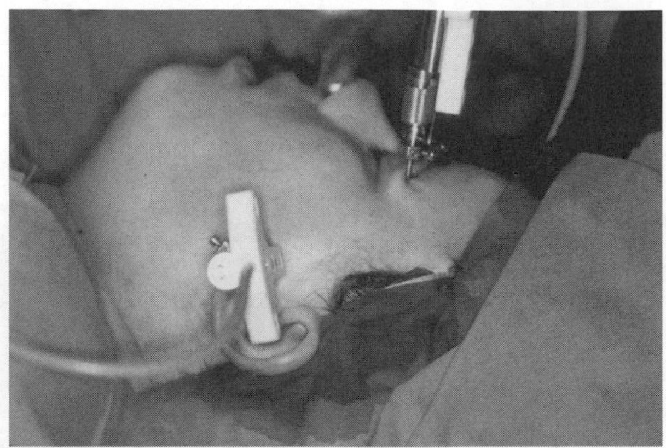

a

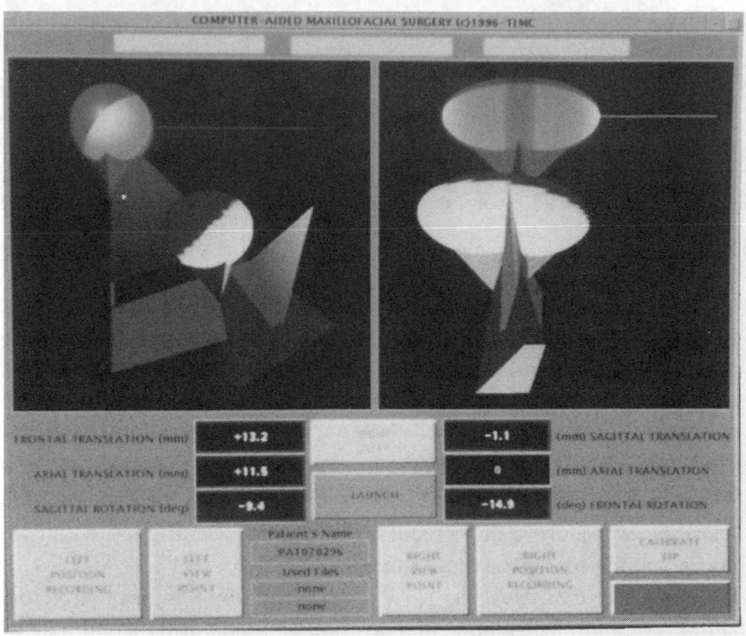

b

FIGURE 5.20 Interactive bone positioning in craniofacial surgery. (a) A rigid body is fixed to the skull, another on the condyle. (b) The surgeon manipulates the condyle fragment and looks at this screen in order to superimpose the current condyle position with the reference position obtained before mandible osteotomy. Two orthogonal 3D views are presented. (Courtesy of Dr. Bettega and Pr. Raphael, Cranio-facial Deparment, Grenoble Hospital.)

5.6.2 Semi-Active Guiding Systems

In these systems, the action is physically constrained by the system. The surgeon is responsible for the final action, while the system prevents deviation from a defined strategy. There are three classes of semi-active systems that have been reported in the literature.

5.6.2.1 Mechanical Guides

A simple semi-active guiding system is provided by the use of mechanical guides. Such semi-active systems have been developed for stereotactic neurosurgery with applications in tumor biopsy, stereo-electroencephalography, electrode implantation for Parkinson's disease, and interstitial brachytherapy. Once a linear trajectory has been defined using multimodal images, a motorized mechanical system positions a linear guide which is aligned with the selected trajectory. The motorized system is fixed in this position, the motor's power is cut off, and the surgeon introduces a drill, probe, or electrode through the mechanical guide until a predefined mechanical stop is encountered. Different systems based on this semi-active approach have been developed to position a mechanical guide at the desired location. In one study[86] a motorized frame that has the same mechanical architecture as a standard articulated stereotactic frame was used. Others have used a six-axis robot instead of a motorized stereotactic frame, which gives more flexibility[92,94] (see Figure 5.21). This system uses an intra-operative feedback through the use of X-rays with which the robot is calibrated. In the pioneering work of Kwoh et al.,[91] the authors used a standard six-axis robot but this system was installed in the CT device directly instead of in a more conventional surgical theater, which raises several problems of sterilization, organization, and cost.

The use of such semi-active systems that position a linear guide in which the surgeon introduces various tools have also been reported in orthopedics applications.[58,115]

5.6.2.2 Individual Templates

Individual templates have been recently proposed by Radermacher et al.[128] to solve the registration and guiding problems at once, for applications in orthopedics surgery. The idea is to use a CAD/CAM system to machine a template that has one surface that fits a bone surface exactly and also contains a linear or planar guide. The template is in fact a negative mold of the bone. The surface and the guide positions are defined pre-operatively using CT images. During the operation, the surgeon simply finds the best match between the template and the bone surface by a simple tactile adjustment. This manual matching step naturally places the guide at the optimal location, which enables the surgeon to introduce a drill or a saw at the planned positions. This principle has been validated successfully in different cases of orthopedics applications including spine and pelvis surgery.[128] This approach is similar to the dental application presented in Ref. 61, in which a template is placed in the patient's mouth during CT scan acquisition. The template is used as a reference system in which a linear guide can be drilled at a location defined on CT images. When it is replaced in the patient's mouth, the dentist uses the machined mechanical guide to drill in the bone and place an implant.

5.6.2.3 Passive Arm with Dynamic Constraints

To merge the flexibility and safety of passive systems with the accuracy of more active systems such as active robots, a new robot concept called passive arm with dynamic constraints (PADYC) has been designed.[46,156] To solve safety problems of active robots, some authors have proposed to impose mechanical constraints in the robot architecture so that the motions of the robot cannot physically escape from a predefined safe region (see examples in the next section). The PADYC concept is an extension of this idea. Instead of having constraints in the architecture, the physical constraints are modulated and controlled by software. For instance, from a starting position of the robot, the user is constrained to go toward a definite final position. No motors act on the system, which solves many safety issues. Robot movement is brought about by forces exerted by humans or gravity only. The arm motions can also be constrained to follow a 3D trajectory or to remain

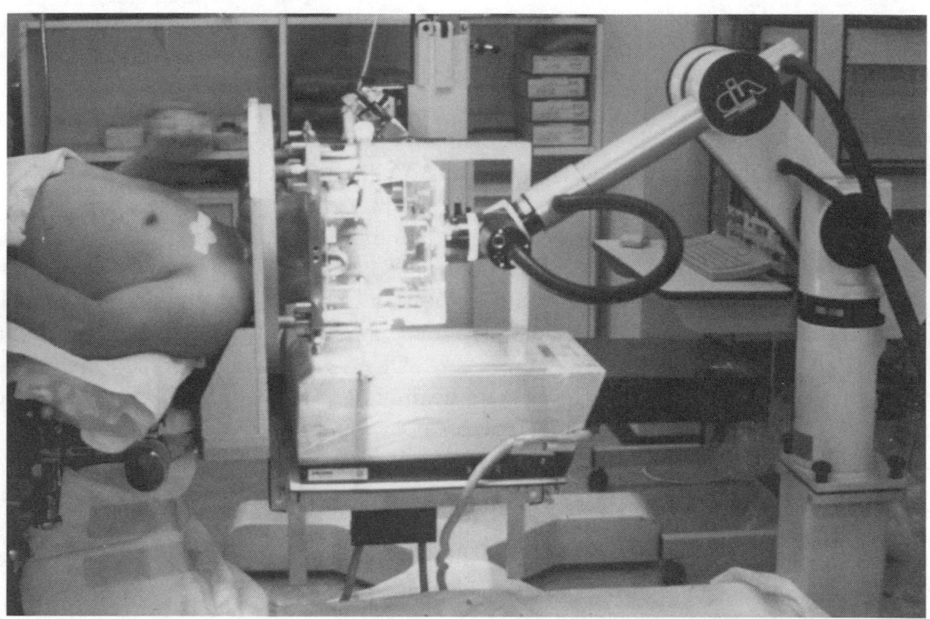

a

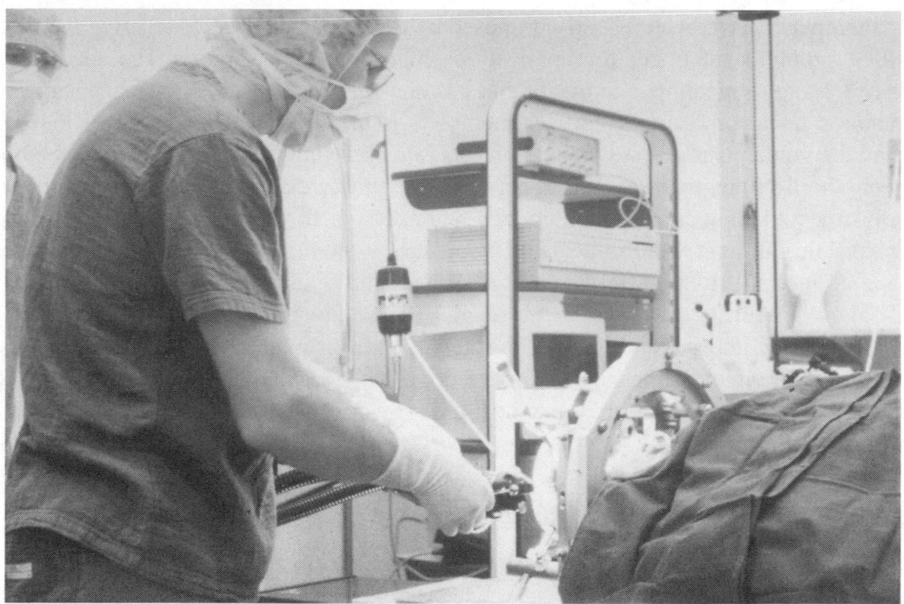

b

FIGURE 5.21 A mechanical guide for stereotactic neurosurgery. (a) A six-axis robot is calibrated with respect to intra-operative X-rays through the use of a calibration cage. (b) The robot positions a linear guide according to an optimal linear trajectory defined by the surgeon on images, and the surgeon controls the final action by inserting tools through this guide. This system has been used on more than 2000 patients since 1989. (Courtesy of Pr. Benabid, Neurosurgery Department, Grenoble Hospital.)

within a safe region. Dangerous regions to avoid, such as a nerve or a vessel, can be defined and the PADYC will leave the surgeon to operate freely outside of this area. The surgeon is entirely in charge of the action. The system only constrains the action to meet an objective previously defined

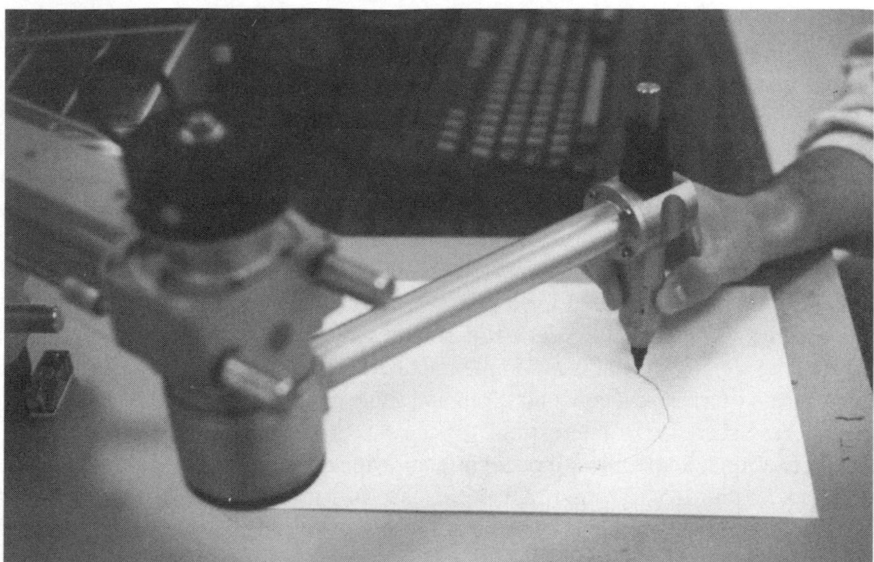

FIGURE 5.22 Two degrees of freedom prototype of a passive arm with dynamic constraint (PADYC). On each axis of the PADYC arm, two free wheels are mounted in opposite directions with clutching systems. By switching the clutching systems at a high rate, the instantaneous direction of motion is controlled on each axis. In the example shown, the system is programmed to make possible only a circular trajectory. The arm cannot move by itself but is constrained to stay in a definite area or trajectory. For example, the surgeon will be able to work freely in a safe region but will not be allowed to touch some planned obstacles such as vessels or nerves.

by the surgeon. This concept is interesting in all cases where passive systems using purely manual skills are not accurate enough. Technical details of the PADYC systems are found in Refs. 46 and 156. The basic principle is to use two free wheels mounted in opposite directions on each axis. By clutching and declutching these free wheels at a high rate, one can control the instantaneous direction and speed of motion (Figure 5.22). A similar semi-active principle can be developed using gear reduction ratio control,[123] which is more accurate than PADYC for trajectory constraints and less accurate for region constraints. One can also use brake control[146] but it is then necessary to add force control, which becomes inaccurate if the reaction of the environment is large. Standard active robots with force control can also be considered semi-active.[45] This, however, raises safety issues, because robot motions are due to motors and they are delicate to control when the interaction with the environment creates high forces or when fine movements have to be controlled freely by the surgeon in six dimensions.

5.6.3 Active Guiding Systems

With active systems, some subtasks of a predefined strategy are performed with the help of an autonomous robotic system, supervised by the surgeon and controlled by redundant sensors. This is the case where difficult actions are performed according to a complex strategy, which is interactively defined on the basis of multimodal data. This is also the case when dexterity is to be enhanced through the use of advanced teleoperation technology. Such devices are increasingly becoming available but most of them are still in development. There are two categories of active systems depending on the type of mechanical architecture: constrained and non-constrained active systems.

5.6.3.1 Constrained Active Guiding Systems

Some authors have proposed to impose mechanical constraints in the robot architecture so that the motions of the robot cannot physically escape from a predefined safe region. In other terms, the degrees of freedom are decoupled such that only a few of them are active while the others are used to position the active part.

In the simplest systems of this class, a six-axis robot positions a linear guide at a given position, the robot is fixed, and a tool is automatically inserted in the guide using force-feedback control. This represents a modification of the semi-active guiding systems previously presented, which is quite minor from the technical point of view, but really crucial from the ethical point of view. The surgeon loses final control of the action with many possible implications on system safety. The benefit of this approach is not obvious (in our opinion). Such systems have been proposed by at least two groups in the field of neurosurgery.[9,162]

In more complex cases, the need for a partially automated action is more obvious. In Ref. 44, a robot is described that can make a series of small conical shapes in order to remove a prostate transurethrally (Figure 5.23). This is a complex action that requires a lot of cuts, and thus is quite demanding in terms of accuracy, concentration, and time. Therefore, the use of a constrained active system for that case seems very interesting.

In another example, a specific robot architecture makes it possible to move a tool around a fixed pivot point.[149] This is very important in the case of robot-assisted laparoscopy, in which the robot carries an endoscope or even a tool that must always pass through the entry point in the abdomen[62] (Figure 5.24). See a similar system in Ref. 59 and another architecture that uses a passive joint in Ref. 135.

Prototypes of constrained systems have been also proposed for eye surgery.[74,125]

5.6.3.2 Non-Constrained Active Guiding Systems

Systems that deliver a radiation dose or heat through external beams can be considered active. For safety reasons, the mechanical architecture of standard radiation systems is decoupled into three patient table translations and two beam accelerator rotations. However, many other architectures are possible. A six-axis robot has been used to manipulate an external radiation generator for radiosurgery without requiring patient table motions.[4] In a more recent version, authors of this work have proposed to install the patient on a giant Stewart platform, which is a parallel architecture that provides a lot of stiffness and stability to the robot. External magnetic fields also have been used to control the displacements of a metallic seed inside the brain of a patient.[132] Both systems are still in development.

There are also a few other examples of projects involving active robots. For instance, the miniature system presented in Ref. 80 has been designed to move inside the intestine and to perform some specific tasks. The system presented in Ref. 152 was designed to perform corneal transplantation automatically.

However, to our knowledge, the only non-constrained active robot that has been used successfully on many patients is the Robodoc™ system developed by Taylor et al.[148,150] (Integrated Surgical Systems, Sacramento, CA). In this system, the robot machines a cavity in the femur that fits exactly the shape of the hip implant. The position and orientation of this implant is defined on pre-operative CT images and registered into the robot space through the use of small pins inserted into the patient's bones. A similar work is also underway for total knee arthroplasty, in order to obtain a good prosthesis fitting and position.[55] A compact version of robots for orthopedic surgery has also been proposed by using a parallel architecture.[26]

This category of active systems also includes advanced teleoperation, in which multimodal data can be taken into account. We classify teleoperation devices in active systems because the slave robot is really active, even if the master system is manipulated by the surgeon. Here, the challenge is to make an efficient cooperation between the operator and the robotic system possible, by assigning some subtasks to each one at the three levels of perception, decision, and action, while keeping an acceptable level of safety. Teleoperation is interesting in two main cases. First, teleoperated robots can enhance the dexterity of the surgeon, which is interesting when the dimensions

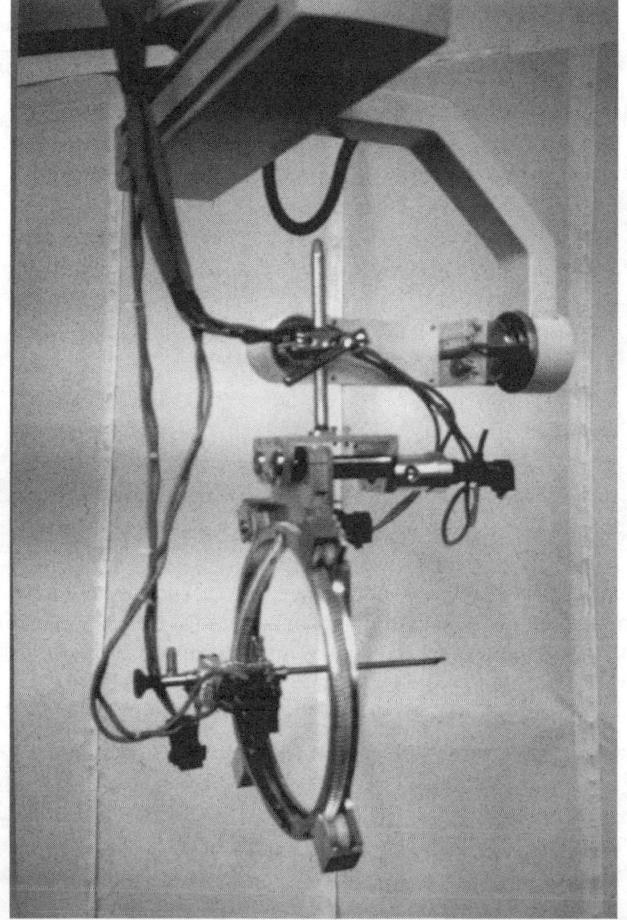

a

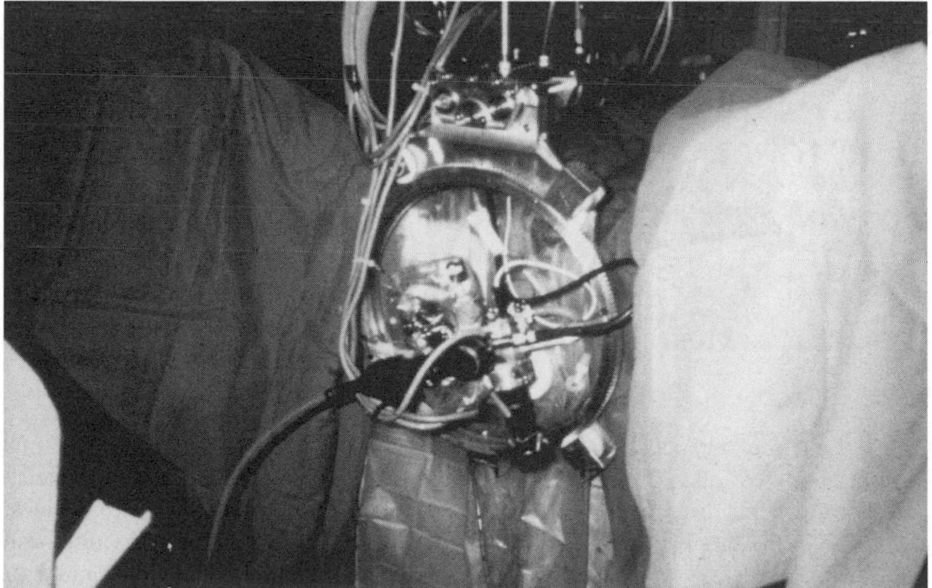

b

FIGURE 5.23 An active robot for prostatectomy. The architecture of the robot is constrained to make small conical shapes. (a) Robot architecture. (b) System in use for prostatectomy. (Courtesy of Brian Davies, Imperial College of London, England.)

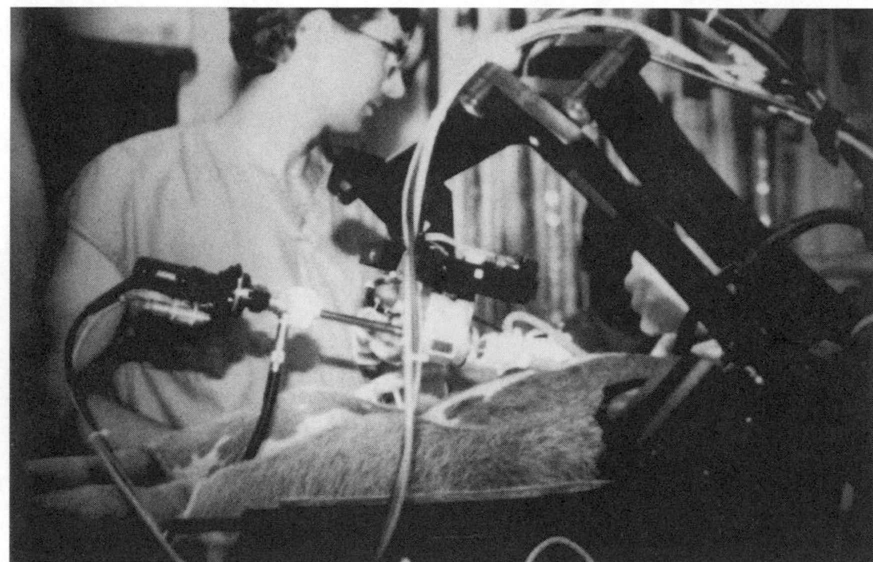

FIGURE 5.24 A constrained active robot used for carrying an endoscope during laparoscopy. At the beginning of an operation, the center of motion of the robot is placed at the entry point of the abdomen. Then the operator manipulates the rotation degrees of freedom by remote control through vocal commands. (Courtesy of Russell H. Taylor, IBM T.J. Watson Research Center, NY.)

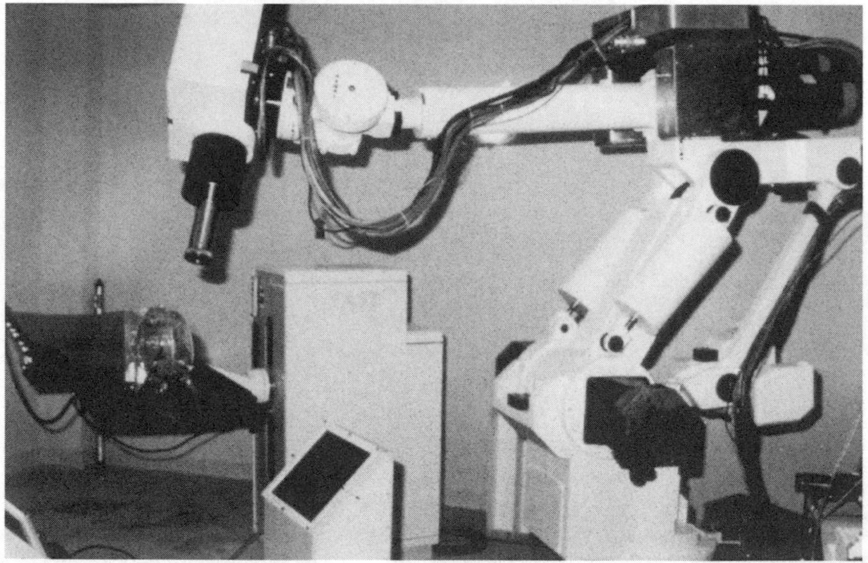

FIGURE 5.25

of the surgical field are very small (i.e., in microsurgery), or when a miniature tool must be introduced in the body by following a non-linear path. Such systems are under development, with the main focus on eye microsurgery.[35,83,114,138] Second, teleoperation can be interesting when the surgeon cannot be in the surgical field. This happens because of possible contamination problems or excessive X-ray dose delivery, but also when the specialized surgeon is far away from the patient (ships, ambulances, battlefields, etc.). Although preliminary work exists in this domain, research is still necessary to provide efficient clinical results.

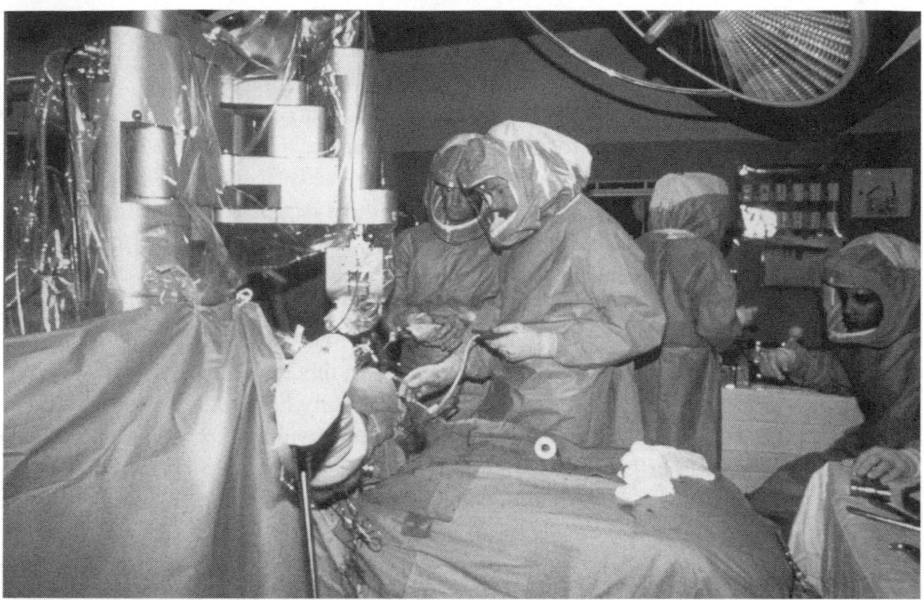

FIGURE 5.26

5.7 CONCLUSIONS

Many medical or surgical interventions can benefit from the use of computers. Through progress of technology and growing consciousness of the possibilities of real clinical improvements through computers, the tools that were in the past the privilege of a very few operations (mostly stereotactic neurosurgery) are now becoming available in many surgical fields. Although several technical issues remain to be solved, there is virtually no limit to the introduction of computers in any surgical field. This tendency can take on many varied forms. At Grenoble Hospital and TIMC laboratory, three golden rules have guided our projects for more than 10 years.

- ***Rule 1:*** *Conceive systems for which the clinical added value is well defined.* This is probably the main issue since real results of a new technique can usually be demonstrated only after a long period of clinical validation. Discussions among several experienced and non-experienced surgeons, scientists, and industrial partners are necessary to avoid developing systems that have no significant medical value. Measuring the clinical added value of CIST technology is a difficult task, especially when trying to answer the crucial question of patient benefits. At the current level of CIST maturity, most of the existing systems make surgery more rational than it was before, by improving the success of operation on a statistical rather than individual basis. The efficiency of a system must be assessed by measuring various factors that correspond to the different clinical objectives of a particular application. Moreover, the introduction of a particular CIST system has clinical implications that surpass its initial objectives, because minor transforms of a particular system can create a new system that solves another clinical problem efficiently. What is happening is really a matter of new technology introduction and not just of a particular system's use.
- ***Rule 2:*** *Develop generic tools that can be applied to many different clinical applications.* This concept enables fast and safe developments, and it also transforms a series of applications into a common scientific problem. Interestingly, not only different techniques but also different medical specialties are gathered in this framework. The methodology

based on the loop perception/decision/action presented in this chapter provides a sound basis for these projects.

- ***Rule 3:*** *Create an efficient collaboration between the surgeon and the system, through simple interfaces.* The purpose of CIST technology must never be to replace the surgeon but rather to provide advanced tools that help him or her do the job better than could be done without the system. It is necessary to keep the surgeon in the loop such that competence is shared between the surgeon and the system. It seems that the surgical strategy must always be defined or at least actively controlled by the surgeon. However, the limit is much less clear in the case of the surgical action. Is it necessary to leave the control of the final action to the surgeon? In our opinion, the answer is definitely yes. The main reason is that an action made by the surgeon and controlled by the system is safer than an action made by the system (a robot in this case) and passively controlled by the surgeon. Moreover, having a look at what is really needed, we think that the main challenge is to help the surgeon to benefit from all the available *information* gathered in the system before and during the operation. In many cases, passive systems are sufficient. When the dexterity of the surgeon must be enhanced, we think that a semi-active system such as the PADYC device presented earlier (Section 5.6.2), or a teleoperation system such as the ones under development (see Section 5.6.3.2) provide efficient solutions.

From the technical point of view, computer-integrated surgery and therapy offers a variety of interesting research problems. At the perception level, intra-operative feedback should be enhanced, through the development of small, inexpensive, and accurate 3D localizers, interventional MR imaging, 3D ultrasound imaging systems, microsensors, and the like. Efforts in fast, accurate, and reliable segmentation methods that are easy to handle are necessary to provide high-level representations of anatomy from raw data. Improving the decision and reasoning step of CIST technology raises a major long-term challenge, which is to build mechanical, morphological, physiological, and functional models of anatomic structures, in order to make possible the definition of complex surgical strategies and to simulate interventions in a perfectly realistic manner. Also, this step requires the development of efficient virtual reality and augmented reality devices such as 6D force-feedback systems or light, fast, and accurate semitransparent displays. Merging all the models, data, and devices necessitates more and more automated anatomy-based registration methods, with special emphasis on real-time elastic registration. At the action level, the development of semi-active guiding systems such as the PADYC and teleoperation systems represent a serious challenge. Designing microsystems for specific tasks constitutes another challenge. Considering the increasing number of researchers, clinicians and companies involved in CIST, most of these challenges have a very good chance of being met during the years to come.

ACKNOWLEDGMENTS

A large part of the results presented in this chapter have been provided by the CAMI team, directed by Jocelyne Troccaz and including 25 researchers of TIMC laboratory, as well as many medical and surgical departments of Grenoble University Hospital. TIMC projects are partially supported by grants from the French Ministeries of Health and Research (PHRC), CNRS, European Community (Telematics in Health Care: IGOS Project, BIOMED: CRIGOS Project), INSERM and CNAMTS (GMCAO Project), Rhône-Alpes Region, IMAG, Université Joseph Fourier, in collaboration with industrial partners (Praxim, Sofamor-Danek, Surgical Navigation Technologies, Aesculap, Northern Digital, Image Guided Technologies, Maquet, Elf, Digital, Mecasserto, Matra, Siemens, Varian, EDF).

REFERENCES

1. Clinical investigation of medical devices for human subjects. European Norm NF EN 540, Oct. 1993.
2. L. Adams, A. Knepper, W. Krybus, D. Meyer-Ebrecht, G. Pfeiffer, R. Ruger, and M. Witte. Orientation aid for head and neck surgeons. *ITBM (Innovation and Technology in Biology and Medicine) — Special Issue on Robotic Surgery,* 13(4):409–424, July 1992.
3. L. Adams, W. Krybus, D. Meyer-Ebrecht, R. Rueger, J.M. Gilsbach, R. Moesges, and G. Schloendorff. Computer assisted surgery. *IEEE Computer Graphics and Applications,* pages 43–51, May 1990.
4. J. Adler, A. Schweikard, R. Tombropoulos, and J.-C. Latombe. Image-guided robotic radiosurgery. In *First Symposium on Medical Robotics and Computer Assisted Surgery (MRCAS'94),* pages 291–297. Pittsburgh, PA 1994.
5. L.K. Arata and A.P. Dhawan. Iterative principal axes registration: a new algorithm for retrospective correlation of MR-PET brain images. In J.P. Morucci, editor, *IEEE Engineering in Medicine Biology Society (EMBS),* pages 2776–2777. Paris, 1992.
6. K.S. Arun, T.S. Huang, and S.D. Blostein. Least-squares fitting of two 3-D point sets. *IEEE Transactions Pattern Analysis and Machine Intelligence,* PAMI-9(5):698–700, 1987.
7. N. Ayache. *Vision Stéréoscopique et Perception Multisensorielle,* InterEditions, Paris, 1989.
8. N. Ayache, P. Cinquin, I. Cohen, L. Cohen, F. Leitner, and O. Monga. Segmentation of complex medical objects: a challenge and a requirement for computer assisted surgery planning and performing. In R. Taylor, S. Lavallee, G. Burdea, and R. Mosges, editors, *Computer Integrated Surgery,* MIT Press, Cambridge, MA, 1996.
9. F. Badano and F. Danel. The NEURO SKILL Robot: a new approach for surgical robot development. In *Second Symposium on Medical Robotics and Computer Assisted Surgery Proceedings (MRCAS'95),* pages 318–323. Wiley, New York, 1996.
10. E. Bainville, P. Chaffanjon, and P. Cinquin. Computer generated visual assistance to a surgical intervention: the retroperitoneoscopy. In *AAAI 94 Applications of Computer Vision in Medical Image Processing, Spring Symposium,* Stanford, CA, 1994.
11. E. Bainville, P. Chaffanjon, and P. Cinquin. Computer generated visual assistance to a surgical operation: the retroperitoneoscopy. *Computers in Biology and Medicine,* 25(2):165–171, May 1995.
12. R. Bajcy and S. Kovacic. Multiresolution elastic matching. *Computer Vision, Graphics, and Image Processing,* 46:1–21, 1989.
13. D.H. Ballard and C.M. Brown. *Computer Vision.* Prentice-Hall, Englewood Cliffs, NJ, 1982.
14. J. Balter, K. Lam, H. Sandler, F. Littles, R. Bree, and T. Ten Haken. Automated localization of the prostate at the time of treatment using implanted radioopaque markers: technical feasibility. *International Journal of Radiation Oncology Biol. Phys.,* 33(5):1281–1286, 1995.
15. C. Barbe, L. Carrat, O. Chavanon, and J. Troccaz. Computer assisted pericardiac surgery. In *Computer Assisted Radiology (CAR'96),* pages 781–786. Springer-Verlag, Berlin, 1996.
16. C. Barbe, J. Troccaz, B. Mazier, and S. Lavallee. Using 2.5D echography in computer assisted spine surgery. In *IEEE Engineering in medicine and Biology Society Proceedings,* pages 160–161, IEEE, 1993.
17. G. Baroni, G. Ferrigno, and A. Pedotti. Optoelectronic techniques for patient repositioning in radiotherapy. In *Technology and Health Care 3,* pages 251–262. Elsevier, 1996.
18. N.H. Barth. An inverse problem in radiation therapy. *International Journal of Radiation Oncology Biol. Phys.,* 18:425–431, 1990.
19. P.J. Besl. The free-form surface matching problem. In H. Freeman, editor, *Structure Transfer Between Sets of Three Dimensional Medical Imaging Data.* Academic, New York, 1990.
20. P.J. Besl and N.D. McKay. A method for registration of 3-D shapes. *IEEE Transactions on Pattern Analysis and Machine Intelligence,* 14(2):239–256, 1992.
21. G. Bettega, V. Dessenne, B. Raphael, and P. Cinquin. Computer assisted mandibular condyle positioning in orthognathic surgery. *Journal of Oral Maxillo Facial Surgery,* (54):553–558, 1996.
22. F. Betting, J. Feldmar, N. Ayache, and F. Devernay. A new framework for fusing stereo images with volumetric medical images. In *Conference of Computer Vision, Virtual Reality, Robotics in Medicine (CVRMed'95), LNCS Series 905,* pages 30–39. Springer, Berlin, 1995.

23. E. Bittar, S. Lavallee, and R. Szeliski. A method for registering overlapping range images of arbitrarily shaped surfaces for 3-D object reconstruction. In *SPIE Vol. 2059, Sensor Fusion VI,* 1993.
24. F.L. Bookstein. Principal warps: Thin-plate splines and the decomposition of deformations. *IEEE Transactions on Pattern Analysis and Machine Intelligence,* 11(6):567–585, 1989.
25. G. Borgefors. Distance transformations in arbitrary dimensions. *Computer Vision, Graphics, and Image Processing,* 27:321–345, 1984.
26. G. Brandt, K. Radermacher, S. Lavallee, H.W. Staudte, and G. Rau. A compact robot for image-guided orthopedic surgery: concept and preliminary results. In Troccaz et al., editors, *CVRMed-MRCAS'97 Proceedings LNCS Series 1205,* pages 767–776. Springer-Verlag, 1997.
27. I. Bricault. *Endoscopie bronchique assist;aaee par ordinateur. R;aaesolution multi-niveaux d'un probl;ageme d'optimisation sc;agene/mod;agele.* Ph.D. thesis, Universit;aae Joseph Fourier, Grenoble, France, 1997.
28. I. Bricault, G. Ferretti, and P. Cinquin. Computer assisted bronchoscopy: aims and research perspectives. In *Second Symposium on Medical Robotics and Computer Assisted Surgery Proceedings (MRCA'95),* pages 124–131. Wiley, New York, 1995.
29. M. Bro-Nielsen and K. Gramkow. Fast fluid registration of medical images. In K.H. Hoehne et al., editors, *Visualization in Biomedical Computing (VBC'96), LNCS Series 1131,* pages 267–276. Springer-Verlag, Berlin, 1996.
30. L.G. Brown. A survey of image registration techniques. *ACM Computing Surveys,* 24(4):326–376, 1992.
31. L. Brunie, S. Lavallee, and Szeliski R. Using force fields derived from 3D distance maps for inferring the attitude of a 3D rigid object. In G. Sandini, editor, *Second European Conference on Computer Vision (ECCV'92), LNCS Series 588,* pages 670–675, Springer-Verlag, 1992.
32. L. Brunie, S. Lavallee, J. Troccaz, P. Cinquin, and M. Bolla. Pre- and intra-irradiation multimodal image registration: principles and first experiments. *Radiotherapy Oncology,* (29):244–252, 1993.
33. U. Cerchiari, G. Del Panno, C. Giorgi, and G. Garibotto. 3-D correlation technique for anatomical volumes in functional stereotactic neurosurgery. In V. Cappellini, editor, *Time-Varying Image Processing and Moving Object Recognition,* pages 147–152. Firenza, Italy, 1986.
34. G. Champleboux, S. Lavallee, P. Sautot, and P. Cinquin. Accurate calibration of cameras and range imaging sensors, the NPBS method. In *IEEE International Conference on Robotics and Automation,* pages 1552–1558. Nice, France, 1992.
35. S. Charles. Dexterity enhancement for surgery. In *First Symposium on Medical Robotics and Computer Assisted Surgery (MRCA'94),* pages 140–160, Pittsburgh, 1994.
36. G.E. Christensen, S.C. Joshi, and M.I. Miller. Individualizing anatomical atlases of the head. In K. Hoehne and R. Kikinis, editors, *Visualization in Biomedical Computing (VBC'96),* pages 343–348. Springer-Verlag, 1996.
37. P. Cinquin. Gestes Medico-Chirurgicaux Assistes par Ordinateur. *Annales de Radiologie* (in French), 36(6):386–406, 1993.
38. P. Cinquin et al. Computer assisted medical interventions at TIMC laboratory: passive and semi-active aids. *IEEE Engineering in Medicine and Biology — Special Issue on Robots in Surgery,* 14(3):254–263, 1995.
39. A. Colchester, J. Zhao, K. Holton-Tainter, C. Henri, N. Maitland, P. Roberts, C. Harris, and R. Evans. Development and preliminary evaluation of VISLAN, a surgical planning and guidance system using intra-operative video imaging. *Medical Image Analysis,* 1(1):73–90, March 1996.
40. A. Collignon, D. Vandermeulen, P. Suetens, and G. Marchal. 3D multi-modality medical image registration using feature space clustering. In *Conference of Computer Vision, Virtual Reality, Robotics in Medicine (CVRMed'95), LNCS Series 905,* pages 195–204. Springer-Verlag, 1995.
41. D.L. Collins, G. Le Goualher, R. Venugopal, A. Caramanos, A.C. Evans, and C. Barillot. Cortical constraints for non-linear cortical registration. In K. Hoehne and R. Kikinis, editors, *Visualization and Biomedical Computing,* pages 307–316. Springer-Verlag, 1996.
42. S. Cotin, H. Delingette, and N. Ayache. Real time volumetric deformable models for surgery simulation. In K. Hoehne and R. Kikinis, editors, *Visualization and Biomedical Computing, VBC'96,* pages 535–540. Springer-Verlag, 1996.

43. C. Cutting, F. Bookstein, and R. Taylor. Applications of simulation, morphometrics, and robotics in cranio-facial surgery. In R. Taylor, S. Lavallee, G. Burdea, and R. Mosges, editors, *Computer-Integrated Surgery: Technology and Clinical Applications,* pages 641–662. MIT Press, Cambridge, MA, 1996.
44. B.L. Davies and R.D. Hibberd. Robotic surgery at Imperial College London. In *International Conference on Advanced Robotics (ICAR'93),* pages 305–310. Tokyo, Japan, 1993.
45. B.L. Davies, S.C. Ho, and R.D. Hibberd. The use of force control in robot assisted knee surgery. In A. DiGioia, R. Taylor, and T. Kanade, editors, *First Symposium on Medical Robotics and Computer Assisted Surgery (MRCAS'94),* pages 258–262. Pittsburgh, PA, 1994.
46. Y. Delnondedieu and J. Troccaz. PADyC: A passive arm with dynamic constraints. A two degrees of freedom prototype. In *Second Symposium on Medical Robotics and Computer Assisted Surgery Proceedings (MRCAS'95),* pages 173–180. Wiley, New York, 1995.
47. V. Dessenne, G. Bettega, S. Lavallee, P. Cinquin, and B. Raphael. Computer-assisted mandibular condyle positioning in orthognathic surgery. In *Second Symposium on Medical Robotics and Computer Assisted Surgery Proceedings (MRCAS;95),* pages 215–221. Wiley, New York, 1995.
48. V. Dessenne, S. Lavallee, R. Julliard, P. Cinquin, and R. Orti. Computer assisted knee anterior cruciate ligament reconstruction: first clinical tests. In *Conference of Computer Vision, Virtual Reality, Robotics in Medicine (CVRMed'95), LNCS Series 905,* pages 476–480. Springer-Verlag, 1995.
49. V. Dessenne, S. Lavallee, R. Orti, R. Julliard, S. Martelli, and P. Cinquin. Computer assisted knee anterior cruciate ligament reconstruction: first clinical tests. *Journal of Image Guided Surgery,* 1(1):59–64, 1995.
50. S. Dunn, G. Burdea, and R. Goratowski. Robotic control of intraoral radiography. In R. Taylor et al., editors, *Computer-Integrated Surgery: Technology and Clinical Applications,* pages 519–528. MIT Press, Cambridge, MA, 1996.
51. P.J. Edwards, D.L.G. Hill, D.J. Hawkes, R. Spink, A.C.F. Colchester, A. Strong, and M. Gleeson. Neurosurgical guidance using the stereo microscope. In *Conference of Computer Vision, Virtual Reality, Robotics in Medicine (CVRMed'95), LNCS Series 905,* pages 555–564. Springer-Verlag, 1995.
52. P.A. van den Elsen, E.J. Pol, and M.A. Viergever. Medical image matching — a review with classification. In *IEEE Engineering Medicine and Biology,* 12(1):26–39, March 1993.
53. A.C. Evans, W. Dai, L. Collins, P. Neelin, and S. Marett. Warping of a computerized 3-D atlas to match brain image volumes for quantitative neuroanatomical and functional analysis. In *SPIE Vol. 1445, Medical Imaging V,* pages 236–247. Philadelphia, 1991.
54. A.C. Evans, D.L. Collins, P. Neelin, and T.S. Marrett. Correlative analysis of three-dimensional brain images. In R. Taylor, S. Lavallee, G. Burdea, and R. Mosges, editors, *Computer-Integrated Surgery: Technology and Clinical Applications,* pages 99–114. MIT Press, Cambridge, MA, 1996.
55. M. Fadda, T. Wang, M. Marcacci, S. Martelli, P. Dario, G. Marcenaro, M. Nanetti, C. Paggetti, A. Visani, and S. Zaffagnini. Computer-assisted knee arthroplasty at Rizzoli Institute. In *First Symposium on Medical Robotics and Computer Assisted Surgery (MRCA'94),* pages 26–31. Pittsburgh, 1994.
56. J. Feldmar and N. Ayache. Locally affine registration of free-form surfaces. In *IEEE Computer Society Conference on Computer Vision and Pattern Recognition (CVRPR'94),* pages 496–501. Seattle, 1994.
57. J. Feldmar, N. Ayache, and F. Betting. 3D-2D projective registration of free-form curves and surfaces. Technical Report 2434, INRIA, France, 1994.
58. P. Finlay. Orthosista: an active surgical localiser for assisting orthopaedic fracture fixation. In *Second Symposium on Medical Robotics and Computer Assisted Surgery Proceedings (MRCAS'95).* Wiley, New York, 1995.
59. P.A. Finlay and M.H. Ornstein. Controlling the movement of a surgical laparoscope. *IEEE EMBS,* 14(3):289–291, 1995.
60. K.T. Foley et al. Spinal stereotactic surgery. In *AANS Proceedings,* April 1995.
61. T. Fortin, J.L. Coudert, G. Champleboux, P. Sautot, and S. Lavallee. Computer-assisted dental implant surgery using computed tomography. *Journal of Image Guided Surgery,* 1(1):53–58, 1995.
62. J. Funda, R. Taylor, S. Gomory, B. Eldridge, K. Gruben, and M. Talamini. An experimental user interface for an interactive surgical robot. In *First Symposium on Medical Robotics and Computer Assisted Surgery (MRCAS'94),* pages 196–203. Pittsburgh, PA, 1994.

63. I. Gastambide. Utilisation des splines pour le calibrage d'images irm (in French). Technical report. TIMB-IMAG, Grenoble, France, 1992.
64. B. Geiger and R. Kikinis. Simulation of endoscopy. In *Conference of Computer Vision, Virtual Reality, Robotics in Medicine (CVRMed'95), LNCS Series 905,* Nice, France, pages 277–281. Springer, 1995.
65. K.G. Gilhuijs, K. Drukker, A. Touw, P. Van de Hen, and M. Van Herk. Interactive three dimensional inspection of patient setup in radiation therapy using digital portal images and computer tomography data. *International Journal of Radiation Oncology Biol. Phys.,* 34(4):873–885, 1996.
66. G.T. Gillies, R.C. Ritter, W.C. Broaddus, M.S. Grady, M.A. Howard III, and R.G. McNeil. Magnetic manipulation instrumentation for medical physics research. *Review Scientific Instrumentation,* 63(3):533–562, 1994.
67. C. Giorgi, U. Cerchiari, G. Broggi, N. Contardi, P. Birk, and A. Struppler. An intra-operative interactive method to monitor stereotactic functional procedures. *Acta Neurochirurgica,* Suppl. 39:10–12, 1987.
68. S.J. Goerss, P.J. Kelly, B.A. Kall, and G.J. Alker. A computed tomographic stereotactic adaptation system. *Neurosurgery,* 3(10):375–379, 1982.
69. W.E.L. Grimson, T. Lozano-Perez, W.M. Wells, G.J. Ettinger, S.J. White, and R. Kikinis. An automatic registration method for frameless stereotaxy, image guided surgery, and enhanced reality visualization. In *IEEE Computer Society Conference on Computer Vision and Pattern Recognition (CVPR'94),* pages 430–436. Seattle, WA, 1994.
70. A.R. Gunkel, W. Freysinger, W.F. Thumfart, and M.J. Truppe. Application of the ARTMA image-guided navigation system to endonasal sinus surgery. In *Computer Assisted Radiography (CAR'95),* pages 1147–1151. Springer-Verlag, Berlin, 1995.
71. A. Hamadeh, P. Cinquin, S. Lavallee, and R. Szeliski. Anatomy-based registration for computer-integrated surgery. In N. Ayache, editor, *Conference of Computer Vision, Virtual Reality, Robotics in Medicine (CVRMed'95), LNCS Series 905,* pages 212–218. Springer-Verlag, 1995.
72. A. Hamadeh, P. Sautot, S. Lavallee, and P. Cinquin. Towards automatic registration between CT and X-ray images: cooperation between 3D/2D registration and 2D edge detection. In *Second Symposium on Medical Robotics and Computer Assisted Surgery Proceedings (MRCAS'95),* pages 39–46. Wiley, New York, 1995.
73. N. Hata, W. Wells, M. Halle, S. Nakajima, P. Viola, R. Kikinis, and F. Jolesz. Image guided microscopic surgery system using mutual information based registration. In K. Hoene and R. Kikinis, editors, *Visualization and Biomedical Computing (VBC'96),* pages 317–325. Springer-Verlag, 1996.
74. S. Hayat, P. Vidal, and J.C. Hache. A prototype of microtelemanipulator for the radical keratotomy. In *International Conference on Advanced Robotics (ICAR'93),* pages 331–336. Tokyo, Japan, November 1993.
75. D. Henry, J. Troccaz, and J.L. Bosson. Virtual echography: simulation of an ultrasonic examination. In H.U. Lemke, editor, *Computer Assisted Radiology (CAR'95),* pages 1055–1060. Springer-Verlag, Berlin, 1995.
76. D. Hill, C. Studholme, and D. Hawkes. Voxel similarity measures for automated image registration. In *Visualization in Biomedical Computing (VBC'94),* pages 205–216. SPIE, Bellingham, WA, 1994.
77. B.K.P. Horn. Closed-form solution of absolute orientation using unit quaternions. *Journal of the Optical Society of America,* 4(4):629–642, 1987.
78. I. Hunter, L. Jones, T. Doukoglou, S. Lafontaine, P. Hunter, and M. Sagar. Ophthalmic microsurgical robot and simulator. In H. Das, editor, *SPIE 2351, Telemanipulator and telepresence technologies,* pages 184–190, 1994.
79. IGOS. *Image Guided Orthopaedic Surgery.* European Project HC 1026 Telematics DGXIII, 1996.
80. K. Ikuta, M. Tsukamoto, and S. Hirose. Shape memory alloy servo actuator system with electric resistance feedback and application to active endoscope. In *IEEE Conference on Robotics and Automation,* pages 427–430. Philadelphia, 1988.
81. H. Iseki and K. Amano. CT-guided stereotactic surgery in combination with intraoperative monitoring by sector type ultrasonography. *Asian Medical Journal,* 28(3):157–167, 1985.
82. J.J. Jacq and C. Roux. Automatic registration of 3D images using a simple genetic algorithm with a stochastic performance function. In *IEEE Engineering in Medicine and Biology Society Proceedings,* pages 126–127. San Diego, CA, October 1993.

83. P.S. Jensen, M.R. Glucksberg, J.E. Colgate, K.W. Grace, and R. Attariwala. Robotic micromanipulator for ophthalmic surgery. In *First International Symposium on Medical Robotics and Computer Assisted Surgery (MRCAS'94),* pages 204–210. September 1994.
84. H. Jiang, R.A. Robb, and K.S. Holton. A new approach to 3-D registration of multimodality medical images by surface matching. In *Visualization in Biomedical Computing (VBC'92), SPIE Vol. 1808,* pages 196–213, 1992.
85. F.A. Jolesz and S.M. Blumenfeld. Interventional use of magnetic resonance imaging. *Magnetic Resonance Quarterly,* (10):85–96. 1994.
86. B.A. Kall. Comprehensive multimodality surgical planning and interactive neurosurgery. In P.J. Kelly and B.A. Kall, editors, *Computers in Stereotactic Neurosurgery,* pages 209–229. Blackwell Scientific Publications, Boston, MA 1992.
87. P.J. Kelly and B.A. Kall. *Computers in Stereotactic Neurosurgery.* Blackwell Scientific Publications, Boston, MA, 1992.
88. T.C. Kienzle III, S.D. Stulberg, M. Peshkin, A. Quaid, J. Lea, A. Goswami, and C.W. Wu. A computer-assisted total knee replacement surgical system. In R. Taylor, S. Lavallee, G. Burdea, and R. Mosges, editors, *Computer-Integrated Surgery.* MIT Press, Cambridge, MA, 1996.
89. U. Kliegis, R. Ascherl, and H. Kaercher. Anatomical models in surgery planning — applications and manufacturing techniques. In H. Lemke, editor, *Computer Assisted Radiology (CAR'95),* pages 885–892. Springer-Verlag, Berlin, 1995.
90. Y. Kosugi, E. Watanabe, and J. Goto. An articulated neurosurgical navigation system using MRI and CT images. *IEEE Transactions on Biomedical Engineering,* 35(2):147–152, 1988.
91. Y.S. Kwoh, J. Hou, E.A. Jonckheere, and S. Hayati. A robot with improved absolute positioning accuracy for CT guided stereotactic brain surgery. *IEEE Transactions on Biomedical Engineering,* 35(2):153–160, 1988.
92. J. Lavallee, S. Troccaz, L. Gaborit, P. Cinquin, A.L. Benabid, and D. Hoffmann. Image guided robot: a clinical application in stereotactic neurosurgery. In *IEEE International Conference on Robotics and Automation,* pages 618–625. Nice, France, 1992.
93. S. Lavallee. *Geste Medico-Chirurgicaux Assistes par Ordinateur: Application a la Neurochirurgie Stereotaxique.* Ph.D. thesis, Grenoble University, France, December 1989.
94. S. Lavallee. A new system for computer assisted neurosurgery. In K. Yongmin, editor, *IEEE Engineering in Medicine and Biology Society (EMBS),* pages 926–927. Seattle, WA, November 1989.
95. S. Lavallee. Registration for computer integrated surgery: methodology, state of the art. In R. Taylor, S. Lavallee, G. Burdea, and R. Mosges, editors, *Computer Integrated Surgery.* MIT Press, Cambridge, MA, 1996.
96. S. Lavallee and P. Cinquin. Computer assisted medical interventions. In K.H. Hohne, editor, *NATO ARW, Vol. F60, 3D Imaging in Medicine,* pages 301–312. Springer-Verlag, Berlin, 1990.
97. S. Lavallee, P. Cinquin, R. Szeliski, O. Peria, A. Hamadeh, G. Champleboux, and J. Troccaz. Building a hybrid patient's model for augmented reality in surgery: a registration problem. *Computers in Biology and Medicine,* 25(2):149–164, 1995.
98. S. Lavallee, P. Sautot, J. Troccaz, P. Cinquin, and P. Merloz. Computer assisted spine surgery: a technique for accurate transpedicular screw fixation using CT data and a 3D optical localizer. In *First Symposium on Medical Robotics and Computer Assisted Surgery (MRCAS'94),* pages 315–322. Pittsburgh, PA, 1994.
99. S. Lavallee, P. Sautot, J. Troccaz, P. Cinquin, and P. Merloz. Computer assisted spine surgery: a technique for accurate transpedicular screw fixation using CT data and a 3D optical localizer. *Journal of Image Guided Surgery,* 1(1):65–73, 1995.
100. S. Lavallee and R. Szeliski. Recovering the position and orientation of free-form objects from image contours using 3-D distance maps. *IEEE PAMI (Pattern Analysis and Machine Intelligence),* 17(4):378–390, 1995.
101. S. Lavallee, R. Szeliski, and L. Brunie. Matching 3-D smooth surfaces with their 2-D projections using 3-D distance maps. In *SPIE Vol. 1570 Geometric Methods in Computer Vision,* pages 322–336. San Diego, CA, July 1991.

102. S. Lavallee, R. Szeliski, and L. Brunie. Anatomy-based registration of 3-D medical images, range images, X-ray projections, 3-D models using octree-splines. In R. Taylor, S. Lavallee, G. Burdea, and R. Mosges, editors, *Computer-Integrated Surgery,* pages 115–143. MIT Press, Cambridge, MA, 1996.
103. S. Lavallee, J. Troccaz, P. Sautot, B. Mazier, P. Cinquin, P. Merloz, and J.P. Chirossel. Computer assisted spine surgery using anatomy-based registration. In R. Taylor, S. Lavallee, G. Burdea, and R. Mosges, editors, *Computer-Integrated Surgery,* chapter 32. MIT Press, Cambridge, MA, 1996.
104. F. Leitner, F. Picard, R. Minfelde, H.J. Schulz, P. Cinquin, and D. Saragaglia. Computer-assisted knee surgical total replacement. In J. Troccaz, E. Grimson, and R. Moesges, editors, *CVRMed-MRCAS Proceedings, LNCS Series 1205,* Springer-Verlag, 1997.
105. L. Lemieux, D.R. Fish, and N.D. Kitchen. A patient-to-computed-tomography image registration method based on digitally reconstructed radiographs. *Medical Physics,* November 1994.
106. D.G. Lowe. Fitting parameterized three-dimensional models to images. *IEEE PAMI (Pattern Analysis and Machine Intelligence),* 13(5):441–450, May, 1991.
107. H. Maitre and Y. Wu. Software tools to standardize and automate the correlation of images with and between diagnostic modalities. *Pattern Recognition,* 20(4):443–462, 1987.
108. G. Malandain and J.M. Rocchisani. Registration of 3D medical images using a mechanical based method. In *IEEE EMBS — 3D Advanced Image Processing in Medicine,* pages 91–95. Rennes, France, November 1992.
109. M. Marcacci, P. Dario, M. Fadda, G. Marcenaro, and S. Martelli. Computer-assisted knee arthroplasty. In R. Taylor et al., editors, *Computer-Integrated Surgery: Technology and Clinical Applications,* pages 417–423. MIT Press, Cambridge, MA, 1996.
110. C.R. Maurer, J.M. Fitzpatrick, M.Y. Wang, and R.J. Maciunas. Correction of geometrical distorsion in MR image registration. In *IEEE Engineering in Medicine and Biology Society Proceedings,* pages 122–123. San Diego, CA, October 1993.
111. Q. Mei, S.J. Harris, F. Arambula-Cosio, M. Nathan, R. Hibberd, J. Wickham, and B. Davies. PROBOT: a computer integrated prostatectomy system. In K. Hoehne and R. Kikinis, editors, *Visualization and Biomedical Computing (VBC'96),* pages 581–590. Springer-Verlag, 1996.
112. Y. Menguy, P. Cinquin, N. Laieb, J. Troccaz, M. Bolla, P. Vassal, A. Dusserre, J.Y. Giraud, and S. Dal Soglio. Optimization in conformal therapy for prostatic cancer. In *Proceedings of the XIth International Conference on Computers in Radiation Therapy,* Manchester, March 1994.
113. P. Meseure, J.F. Rouland, P. Dubois, S. Karpf, and C. Chaillou. SOPHOCLE: a retinal laser photocoagulation simulator overview. In N. Ayache, editor, *Conference of Computer Vision, Virtual Reality, Robotics in Medicine (CVRMed'95), LNCS Series 905,* pages 105–114. Springer-Verlag, 1995.
114. M. Mitsuishi, T. Watanabe, H. Nakanishi, T. Hori, H. Watanabe, and B. Kramer. A tele-micro-surgery system with co-located view and operation point. In *Second Symposium on Medical Robotics and Computer Assisted Surgery Proceedings (MRCAS'95).* Wiley, New York, 1995.
115. A.M. Mohsen et al. The CAOS projects (computer assisted orthopaedic systems). In *First Symposium on Medical Robotics and Computer Assisted Surgery (MRCAS'94),* pages 49–56. Pittsburgh, PA, 1994.
116. O. Monga, S. Benayoun, and O.D. Faugeras. From partial derivatives of 3D density images to ridge lines. In *IEEE Computer Society Conference on Computer Vision and Pattern Recognition (CVPR'92),* pages 354–359. Champaign, IL, June 1992.
117. R. Mosges and S. Lavallee. Multimodal information for computer-integrated surgery. In R. Taylor, S. Lavallee, G. Burdea, and R. Mosges, editors, *Computer-Integrated Surgery: Technology and Clinical Applications,* pages 5–20. MIT Press, Cambridge, MA, 1996.
118. R. Mosges, G. Schlondorff, L. Klimek, D. Meyer-Ebrecht, W. Krybus, and L. Adams. Computer assisted surgery: an innovative surgical technique in clinical routine. In H.U. Lemke, editor, *Computer Assisted Radiology (CAR'89),* pages 413–415. Springer-Verlag, Berlin, 1989.
119. L.P. Nolte, L. Zamorano, Z. Jiang, Q. Wang, F. Langlotz, E. Arm, and H. Visarius. A novel approach to computer assisted spine surgery. In *First Symposium on Medical Robotics and Computer Assisted Surgery (MRCAS'94),* pages 323–328. Pittsburgh, PA, September 1994.
120. R. Orti, S. Lavallee, R. Julliard, P. Cinquin, and E. Carpentier. Computer assisted knee ligament reconstruction. In *IEEE Engineering in Medicine and Biology Society Proceedings,* pages 936–937. San Diego, CA, 1993.

121. C.A. Pelizzari, G.T.Y. Chen, D.R. Spelbring, R.R. Weichselbaum, and C.-T. Chen. Accurate 3-D registration of CT, PET, and/or MR images of the brain. *Journal of Computer Assisted Tomography,* 13(1):20–26, 1989.
122. O. Peria, A. Francois-Joubert, S. Lavallee, G. Champleboux, P. Cinquin, and S. Grand. Accurate registration of SPECT and MR brain images of patients suffering from epilepsy or tumor. In *First Symposium on Medical Robotics and Computer Assisted Surgery (MRCA'94),* pages 58–62. Pittsburgh, PA, 1994.
123. M. Peshkin, J.E. Colgate, and C. Moore. Passive robots and haptic displays based on nonholonomic elements. In *IEEE International Conference on Robotics and Automation,* 1996.
124. B. Peuchot, A. Tanguy, and M. Eude. Virtual reality as an operative tool during scoliosis surgery. In *Conference of Computer Vision, Virtual Reality, Robotics in Medicine (CVRMed'95), LNCS Series 905,* pages 549–554. Springer-Verlag, 1995.
125. C.J. Pournaras, R.D. Shonat, J.L. Munoz, and B.L. Pretig. New ocular micromanipulator for measurements of retinal and vitreous physiologic parameters in the mammalian eye. *Experimental Eye Research,* (53):723–727, 1991.
126. W.H. Press, B.P. Flannery, S.A. Teukolsky, and W.T. Vetterling. *Numerical Recipes in C: The Art of Scientific Computing,* second edition. Cambridge University Press, Cambridge, England, 1992.
127. K. Radermacher, G. Rau, and H. Staudte. Computer-integrated orthopaedic surgery: connection of planning and execution in surgical intervention. In R. Taylor, S. Lavallee, G. Burdea, and R. Mosges, editors, *Computer-Integrated Surgery,* pages 451–464. MIT Press, Cambridge, MA, 1996.
128. K. Radermacher, H.W. Staudte, and G. Rau. Computer assisted orthopaedic surgery by means of individual templates — aspects and analysis of potential applications. In *First Symposium on Medical Robotics and Computer Assisted Surgery (MRCAS'94),* pages 42–48. Pittsburgh, PA, September 1994.
129. S. Ranade and A. Rosenfeld. Point pattern matching by relaxation. *Pattern Recognition,* 12:269–275, 1980.
130. H.F. Reinhardt. Neuronavigation: a ten years review. In R. Taylor, S. Lavallee, G. Burdea, and R. Mosges, editors, *Computer-Integrated Surgery.* MIT Press, Cambridge, MA, 1995.
131. E. Rekow and B. Nappi. CAD/CAM automation and expert systems for design and fabrication of dental restorations. In R. Taylor et al., editors, *Computer-Integrated Surgery: Technology and Clinical Applications,* pages 543–554. MIT Press, Cambridge, MA, 1996.
132. R.C. Ritter, M.S. Grady, M.A. Howard III, and G.T. Gillies. Magnetic stereotaxis: computer-assisted, image-guided remote movement of implants into the brain. *ITBM (Innovation and Technology in Biology and Medicine) — Special Issue on Robotic Surgery,* 13(4):437–449, July 1992.
133. R.A. Robb and D.P. Hanson. The ANALYZE software system for visualization and analysis in surgery simulation. In Taylor et al., editors, *Computer-Integrated Surgery,* chapter 10. MIT Press, Cambridge, MA, 1996.
134. D.W. Roberts, J.W. Strohbein, J.F. Hatch et al. A frameless stereotaxic integration of computerized tomographic imaging and the operating microscope. *Journal of Neurosurgery,* 545–549, 1986.
135. J. Sackier and Y. Wang. Robotically assisted laparoscopic surgery: from concept to development. *Surgical Endoscopy,* (8):63–66, 1994.
136. P. Sautot, P. Cinquin, S. Lavallee, and J. Troccaz. Computer assisted spine surgery: a first step towards clinical application in orthopaedics. In *14th IEEE Engineering in Medicine and Biology Conference,* pages 1071–1072, Paris, November 1992.
137. L.R. Schad, R. Boesecke, W. Schlegel, G.H. Hartmann, V. Sturm, L.G. Strauss, and W.J. Lorenz. Three dimensional image correlation of CT, MR and PET. Studies in radiotherapy treatment planning of brain tumors. *Journal of Computer Assisted Tomography,* 11(6):948–954, 1987.
138. P. Schenker, H. Das, and T. Ohm. A new robot for high dexterity microsurgery. In *CVRMED'95, Computer Vision Virtual Reality and Robotics in Medicine Conference,* pages 115–122. Springer-Verlag, 1995.
139. C. Schiers, U. Tiede, and K.H. Hoehne. Interactive 3D registration of image volumes from different sources. In H.U. Lemke, editor, *Computer Assisted Radiology (CAR 89),* pages 667–669. Springer-Verlag, Berlin, 1989.
140. D.A. Simon, M. Hebert, and T. Kanade. Techniques for fast and accurate intrasurgical registration. *Journal of Image Guided Surgery,* (1):17–29, 1995.

141. K.R. Smith, K.J. Frank, and R.D. Bucholz. The neurostation: a highly accurate minimally invasive solution to frameless stereotactic neurosurgery. *Computerized Medical Imaging and Graphics,* 18(4):247–256, 1994.
142. G.C. Stockman, S. Kopstein, and S. Benett. Matching images to models for registration and object detection via clustering. *IEEE Transactions on Pattern Analysis and Machine Intelligence,* PAMI-4:229–241, 1982.
143. C. Studholme, J. Little, G. Penny, D. Hill, and D. Hawkes. Automated multimodality registration using the full affine transformation: application to MR and CT guided skull base surgery. In K. Hoehne and R. Kikinis, editors, *Visualization and Biomedical Computing (VBC'96),* pages 601–606. Springer-Verlag, 1996.
144. R. Szeliski and S. Lavallee. Matching 3-D anatomical surfaces with non-rigid deformations using octree-splines. In *IEEE Workshop on Biomedical Image Analysis.* IEEE Computer Society, Seattle, WA, 1994.
145. R. Szeliski and S. Lavallee. Matching 3-D anatomical surfaces with non-rigid deformations using octree-splines. *International Journal of Computer Vision (IJVC),* 18(2):171–186, 1996.
146. R.H. Taylor, C.B. Cutting, Y.Y. Kim, A. Kalvin, D. Larose, B. Haddad, D. Khoramabadi, M. Noz, R. Olyha, M. Bruun, and D. Grimm. A model-based optimal planning and execution system with active sensing and passive manipulation for augmentation of human precision in computer-integrated surgery. In *Second International Workshop on Experimental Robotics.* Springer-Verlag, 1991.
147. R.H. Taylor, S. Lavallee, G.C. Burdea, and R.W. Mosges. *Computer-Integrated Surgery: Technology and Clinical Applications.* MIT Press, Cambridge, MA, 1996.
148. R.H. Taylor, B.D. Mittlestadt, H.A. Paul, W. Hanson, P. Kazanzides, J.F. Zuhars, B. Williamson, B. Musits, E. Glassman, and W.L. Bargar. An image-directed robotic system for precise orthopaedic surgery. *IEEE Transactions on Robotics and Automation,* 10(3):261–275, 1994.
149. R.H. Taylor, H.A. Paul, C.B. Cutting, B. Mittelstadt, W. Hanson, P. Kazanzides, B. Musits, Y.Y. Kim, A. Kalvin, B. Haddad, D. Khoramabadi, and D. Larose. Augmentation of human precision in computer-integrated surgery. *ITBM (Innovation and Technology in Biology and Medicine) — Special Issue on Robotic Surgery,* 13(4):450–468, July 1992.
150. R.H. Taylor, H.A. Paul, B.D. Mittelstadt, E. Glassman, B.L. Musits, and W.L. Bargar. A robotic system for cementless total hip replacement surgery in dogs. In *Second Workshop on Medical & Healthcare Robotics,* pages 79–89. D.T.I., Newcastle, UK, 1989.
151. ISG Technologies. Viewing wand operator's guide. Technical report, ISG Technologies Inc., 1993.
152. N. Tejima, H. Funakubo, T. Dohi, I. Sakuma, T. Tanishima, and Y. Nomura. A new microsurgical robot system for corneal transplantation. *Precision Machinery,* 2:1–9, 1988.
153. J.P. Thirion and S. Benayoun. Image surface extremal points, new feature points for image registration. Technical Report 2003, INRIA, France, August 1993.
154. J.P. Thirion, O. Monga, S. Benayoun, A. Gueziec, and N. Ayache. Automatic registration of 3D images using surface curvature. In *IEEE International Symposium on Optical Applied Science and Engineering,* San Diego, CA, July 1992.
155. K.D. Toennies, G.T. Herman, and J.K. Udupa. Surface registration for the segmentation of implanted bone grafts. In H.U. Lemke, editor, *Computer Assisted Radiology (CAR 89),* pages 381–385. Springer-Verlag, Berlin, 1989.
156. J. Troccaz, S. Lavallee, and E. Hellion. PADYC: a passive arm with dynamic constraints. In *ICAR (International Conference on Advanced Robotics),* pages 361–366. JIRA, Tokyo, 1993.
157. J. Troccaz, Y. Menguy, M. Bolla, P. Cinquin, P. Vassal, N. Laieb, L. Desbat, A. Dusserre, and S. Dal Soglio. Conformal external radiotherapy of prostatic carcinoma: requirements and experimental results. *Radiotherapy Oncology,* (29):176–183, 1993.
158. J. Troccaz, Y. Menguy, M. Bolla, P. Cinquin, P. Vassal, N. Laieb, and S.D. Soglio. Patient set-up optimization for external conformal radiotherapy. In A. DiGioia, T. Kanade, and R. Taylor, editors, *First Symposium on Medical Robotics and Computer Assisted Surgery (MRCAS'94),* pages 306–313. Pittsburgh, PA, September 1994.
159. J. Udupa and R. Goncalves. Imaging transforms for volume visualization. In R. Taylor, S. Lavallee, G. Burdea, and R. Mosges, editors, *Computer-Integrated Surgery,* pages 33–57. MIT Press, Cambridge, MA, 1996.

160. M. Van Herk and H.M. Kooy. Automatic three-dimensional correlation of CT-CT, CT-MRI, and CT-SPECT using chamfer matching. *Medicine Phys.*, 21(7):1163–1178, 1994.
161. P. Vassal, J. Troccaz, N. Laieb, P. Cinquin, M. Bolla, and E. Berraud. Introducing computer vision sensors in radiotherapy for accurate dose delivery. In Wiley, editor, *Second Symposium on Medical Robotics and Computer Assisted Surgery Proceedings (MRCAS'95),* pages 16–23. Wiley, New York, 1995.
162. N. Villotte, D. Glauser, P. Flury, and C.W. Burckhardt. Conception of stereotactic instruments for the neurosurgical robot minerva. In *14th IEEE Engineering in Medicine and Biology Conference,* pages 1089–1090. Paris, November 1992.
163. K. Waters. Synthetic muscular contraction on facial tissue derived from computer tomography data. In R. Taylor, S. Lavallee, G. Burdea, and R. Mosges, editors, *Computer-Integrated Surgery,* pages 191–200. MIT Press, Cambridge, MA, 1996.
164. S. Webb. *The Physics of Medical Imaging.* Medical Science Series. IOP Publishing, Bristol, UK, 1988.
165. W.M. Wells, P. Viola, H. Atsumi, S. Nakajima, and R. Kikinis. Multi-modal volume registration by maximization of mutual information. *Medical Image Analysis,* 1(1):35–52, March 1996.
166. J. Zhang, M.F. Levesque, C.L. Wilson, R.M. Harper, J. Engel, R. Lufkin, and E.J. Behnke. Multimodality imaging of brain structures for stereotactic surgery. *Radiology,* 175(2):435–441, 1990.
167. R. Ziegler, W. Mueller, G. Fischer, and M. Goebel. A virtual reality medical training system. In *Conference of Computer Vision, Virtual Reality, Robotics in Medicine (CVRMed'95), LNCS Series 905,* pages 282–286. Springer-Verlag, 1995.

6 3D CT Angiography

Willi A. Kalender and Mathias Prokop

CONTENTS

6.1 INTRODUCTION

Spiral CT angiography (CTA) is a relatively new volumetric or truly three-dimensional approach to vascular imaging, but it also makes use of older and known techniques. The assessment of vascular structures and of vascular supplies to tissues and lesions has been an important CT application for many years. It has always required the administration of an intravascular contrast agent, most commonly an intravenous bolus injection of iodinated contrast medium. Because the human body can tolerate only limited amounts of such materials, the concentration, the injection rate, and the duration of injection have to be limited. Consequently, the desired high intravascular contrast can be maintained only for a short time of typically less than 1 min, and therefore the procedure in most cases has been limited to the evaluation of single sections. Often it has been performed in a dynamic fashion; that is, the same anatomic level was scanned repeatedly to monitor contrast medium flow patterns. This particular CT application, commonly known as "dynamic CT,"

0-8493-3179-X/00/$0.00+$.50

received a lot of attention in the early 1980s and has been advocated since then for differentiating tumorous lesions according to their enhancement behavior. Thus it aimed at determining the type of vascular supply and tissue perfusion, but scarcely at assessing vessels directly. Imaging of complete vascular trees was practically impossible with conventional CT because it took too long to obtain the necessary number of single sections while maintaining adequate contrast during that period of time.

It is worthwhile noting that magnetic resonance imaging (MRI) was applied to examine vascular anatomy much earlier than conventional CT, although total scan times were of the same order of magnitude or even longer. MRI in general does not depend on administration of contrast medium and is thus independent of the time constraints given by the timing, length, and height of a contrast medium bolus. However, the most recent and most promising new techniques in MR angiography (MRA) also involve administration of an intravenous contrast bolus of Gd-DTPA or similar materials. This so-called contrast-enhanced MRA or Gd-MRA is subject to similar constraints and provides similar advantages, such as CT: timing of the contrast bolus becomes critical but acquisition time can be markedly reduced, and spatial resolution is high even in regions such as chest or abdomen which are strongly affected by breathing effects. A detailed comparison of the various techniques which are available for angiography or, in a broader sense, for the assessment of vessels can be found in Ref. 1. This chapter will focus on spiral CT angiography, the 3D technique which is used most frequently these days.

The possibility of scanning complete organs or body sections in adequately short time intervals of 20 to 40 s by X-ray CT was first offered by spiral CT. Vascular imaging under synchronous administration of a contrast medium bolus became one of the most spectacular applications of spiral CT very early. First reports were already published in 1991, with the early work concentrated in Germany;[2–4] the breakthrough was achieved in 1992, with important contributions from Napel, Rubin, and co-workers at Stanford[5,6] and other groups in the United States. Since then a large number of studies have been completed and a vast amount of reports in the literature have appeared. A partial review of this material is given in Section 6.4.

The new application was made popular under the name CT angiography. This name reflected the fact that maximum intensity projection (MIP) images of the scanned volume resemble classical angiograms to a high degree. CT angiograms do not provide the same fine detail as film- or image intensifier-based angiography; hence they are mostly used for imaging larger vessels. But they represent a true 3D examination and allow viewing of the scanned volume from any direction, with the desired projection chosen retrospectively. Also, they carry important additional information on the surrounding organs and tissues. Experienced radiologists first view CTA exams like any other regular CT examination and only continue with 3D displays after they have established their diagnosis. Therefore it is important to consider CT angiography in a broader sense: it is more than generating angiographic views by spiral CT — it is the assessment of the vasculature and the organs supplied by the respective vessels in one CT examination (Figure 6.1). Image processing, rendering, and evaluation play an important and integral part in this examination, which make it a particularly interesting example for this book.

CTA examinations can vary widely in the way they are conducted and with respect to scan, reconstruction, and evaluation parameters chosen. A single spiral scan of a small volume with very thin slices is adequate for imaging the vessels at the base of the skull; 3D displays are of great importance here. Repeated scans of complete organs, such as the liver, with thicker slices are indicated to detect lesions which only show high positive or negative contrast in the arterial, portal, or venous phase; reconstruction of the vascular architecture is of limited interest here. In this chapter, we will present the basic and common features of all CTA techniques, include information on practical aspects such as contrast medium application, discuss image quality aspects in detail, and give an overview of clinical applications.

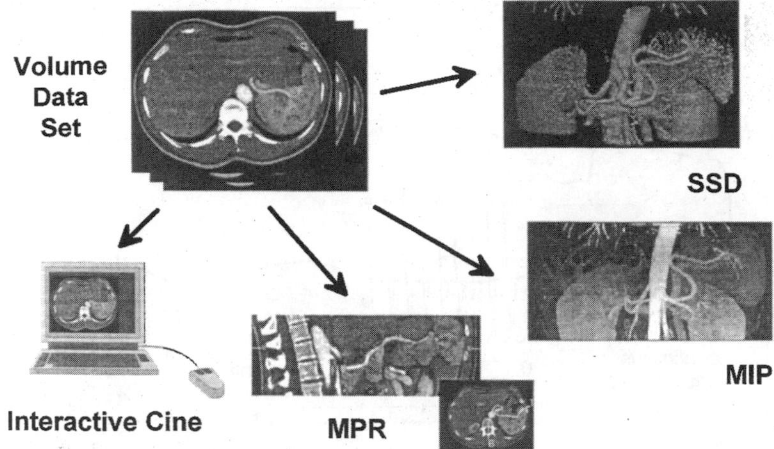

FIGURE 6.1 Spiral CT angiography allows assessment of vascular anatomy in a comprehensive fashion, providing soft-tissue and angiographic information in a single exam. Interactive multiplanar reformation (MPR) cine runs are often considered as the method of choice to establish diagnosis. Maximum intensity projection (MIP) images in arbitrary orientation resemble classical angiograms to a high degree and are a preferred way of viewing and documenting.

6.2 THE CTA EXAMINATION

6.2.1 Spiral CT Scanning

Spiral CT allows continuous volume data acquisition instead of the traditional way of scanning slice by slice successively. It was presented for the first time in 1989[7] and has gained a dominant role since then. Reviews can be found in Refs. 8 and 9.

The basic principle is relatively simple. Contrary to conventional CT, which is limited to scanning a single section over typically 360° in planar geometry, spiral CT is a volume scanning procedure in non-planar geometry with the scan extending over many rotations and the patient being shifted continuously through the gantry. The scanning principle is illustrated schematically in Figure 6.2. While the X-ray tube and detector system rotate around the patient with data being acquired continuously, the patient travels at a speed of typically one to two slice thicknesses per 360° rotation. In practice this means values of typically 1 to 20 mm/s. Relative to the patient, the focus of the X-ray tube describes a spiral or helical path, which led to the two names commonly used for this scanning procedure. Spiral and helical can be considered synonymous in this context: spiral is more descriptive and more widely accepted — consider a spiral staircase as opposed to a helical staircase; helical is unambiguous in a mathematical sense, but not as commonly used. Both terms are accepted in the literature;[10] we will use the original term, spiral.

The technological basis for spiral CT was provided by the introduction of continuously rotating CT measurement systems. Slip rings were used as means for transferring the necessary electrical energy to the rotating gantry part and for transmitting the measured data from the rotating part to the computer system. They replaced the cables connecting the fixed and rotating parts of the gantry, which were traditionally used in CT scanners and which limited scanning to single 360° turns, alternating in clockwise and counterclockwise direction.

The selection of basic scan parameters for spiral CT is the same as in conventional CT (Table 6.1). The parameter values may differ slightly, with limitations possible for spiral scan modes. For example, maximal tube currents have to be lower in spiral CT to avoid excessive heating

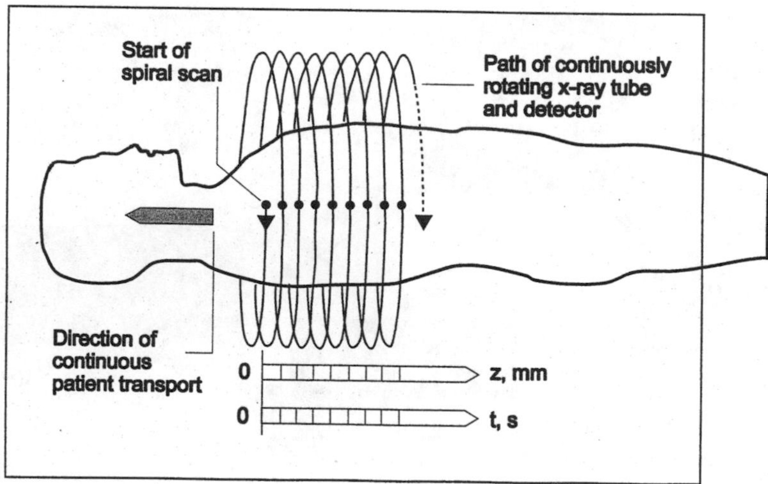

FIGURE 6.2 Spiral CT scan principle. While data are acquired continuously, the patient is transported through the measuring field at constant speed. (Reprinted with permission from Kalender WA, Seissler W, Klotz E, Vock P. *Radiology* 1990;176:181–183.)

of the x-ray tube during the extended scan times. In normal practice, however, total scan times of up to 60 s with up to 300 mA (which are available now in high-end scanners) are sufficient to cover most applications. The additional parameter to be selected in spiral CT is the table feed d in millimeters per 360° rotation. On the scanners used during the first 5 years of spiral CT, which all operated at 1 s for a single 360° scan, the value corresponded directly to the speed d' in millimeters per second. Nowadays there are scanners available with scan speeds per rotation from 0.75 to 2.0 s. The value of d is mostly chosen as less than or equal to 2 larger than one slice thickness. The ratio of table feed d to slice thickness S is commonly termed *pitch*, a dimensionless quantity which is of great interest for image quality, patient dose, and practical considerations, as will be outlined below with reference to practical examples.

Reconstruction of each single image in spiral CT is done the same way as in conventional CT, using the same hardware and the same algorithms and reconstruction kernels. However, an additional step of data processing, the so-called slice, section, or z interpolation, is necessary. Before image reconstruction can be started planar data sets have to be calculated from the acquired volume data set for the desired image positions. This is mostly done by linear interpolation along the z direction, but arbitrary algorithms can be used in principle.[9,11,12] The decisive difference to conventional CT is the inherent advantage that the reconstruction increment (RI), the positions, and spacing of successive images can be chosen freely and retrospectively in spiral CT. Reconstructing overlapping images (i.e., typically two to three images per slice width) provides improvements in 3D image quality and can get us closer to the ideal of isotropic spatial resolution.[13,14] The choice of reconstruction parameters is independent of the scan parameters and can be made retrospectively and without the need for renewed scanning.

6.2.2 Image Quality in Spiral CT

When spiral CT was introduced, there was a lot of concern that image quality might be impaired due to moving the patient and the resulting non-planar scan geometry. As it turned out and has been proven in a number of studies since then, spiral CT offers image quality characteristics quite similar to conventional CT with significant differences only with respect to spatial resolution in the third dimension (i.e., along the longitudinal axis or z direction). Equivalence in image quality characteristics for conventional and spiral CT has to be expected. For example, spatial resolution

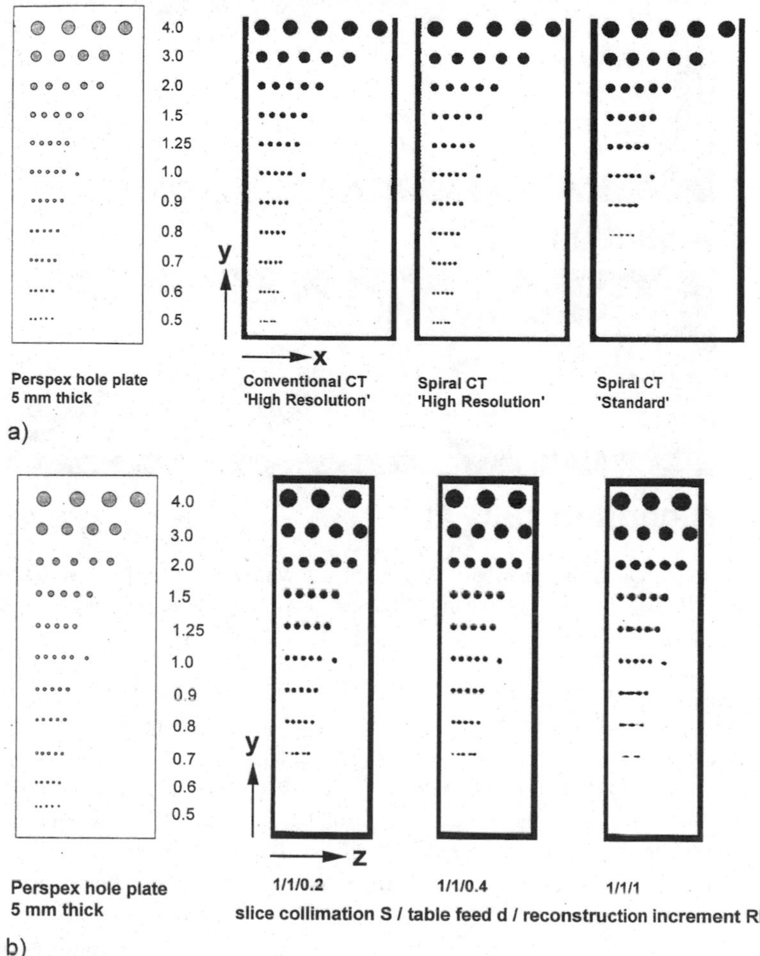

FIGURE 6.3 Spiral CT offers image quality equivalent to conventional CT in most respects. (a) Spatial resolution in the *xy* scan plane is the same for both scan modes, but depends on the reconstruction algorithm. (b) Spatial resolution in the *z* direction, measured in reformatted planes or in 3D, is improved in spiral CT, but requires reconstruction of at least two images per slice width.

has to be the same because we use the same X-ray source, geometry and detection system and the same reconstruction algorithm (Figure 6.3a). The same considerations hold true for most other parameters (e.g., CT numbers, contrast, linearity, and so forth). There are small differences in noise characteristics which will depend on the type and implementation of the *z* interpolation algorithm. These aspects have been reviewed in detail previously.[9]

A decisive difference is the shape of slice sensitivity profiles (SSPs). While SSPs are close to the ideal form of a rectangle in conventional CT, they are smoothed out in spiral CT due to the patient transport. It has been shown that the SSP in spiral CT results as a convolution of the original SSP and a triangular motion function.[15] The base width of the triangle depends on the *z* interpolation algorithm and on the table feed *d* (i.e., the triangle will be wider for higher pitch factors). The resulting SSP shape with extended tails is undesirable and certainly a disadvantage. However, the continuous sampling along the *z* direction, as opposed to discrete image positions in conventional CT at a distance of typically one slice width only, is a clear advantage which should improve spatial resolution in the *z* direction. It has been shown that the latter effect dominates and that 3D spatial resolution in spiral CT is higher than in conventional CT.[13,14] Actually, in spiral CT we come close

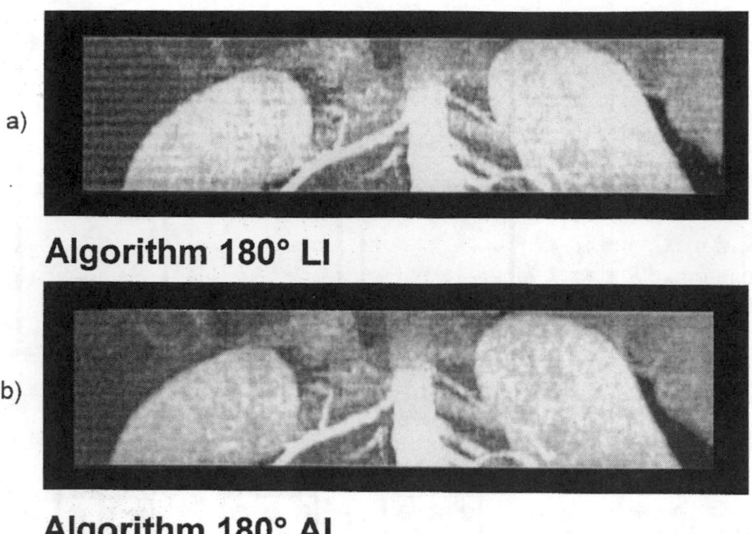

FIGURE 6.4 Inhomogeneous noise distribution in spiral CT which varies with z position may give rise to horizontal stripes in MIP displays (a). These can be reduced or eliminated by specially designed z algorithms (b).[20]

to the ideal of isotropic spatial resolution for the first time. This is an aspect which is of great importance to CT angiography. The desired high 3D spatial resolution can be reached only with thin slice techniques, and these are used in CT angiography in most cases (Figure 6.3b).

With respect to artifacts, there are also only a few differences between conventional CT and spiral CT. Known phenomena like beam hardening due to high contrast medium concentration will affect both scan modes to the same degree. No specific artifacts attributable to spiral CT have been observed in the original transverse images. There is one phenomenon, however, in MIP images which has to be attributed to spiral CT z interpolation. Horizontal stripes are often observed in MIP images in peripheral homogeneous tissue regions. These are due to non-homogeneous noise distributions which change with z position. We were able to demonstrate that these effects can be removed (Figure 6.4); however, such algorithms are not yet widely available.

As a summary of the dicussion on image quality aspects, we can state that there are few differences between conventional and spiral CT and that there are very few detrimental effects. Very clearly, an increase in spatial resolution along the z axis with improved 3D spatial resolution can be claimed for spiral CT. Spiral scan modes are the only possibility to do CT angiography in any case, and they offer the most adequate performance.

6.2.3 Choice of Scan Parameters

A CTA examination is, in most cases, preceded by a standard CT examination without contrast medium application. This prior exam may be indicated for routine diagnostic purposes, but it will definitely serve to determine the range to be examined. Knowing the desired scan range R in millimeters, the following parameters must be selected: the total scan time T in seconds, the slice thickness S in millimeters, and the necessary table speed d' in millimeters per second. Total scan times T cannot be selected arbitrarily. The upper limit for T is given by the contrast medium technique and the patient's tolerance (e.g., renal function); in addition to the limits on contrast medium dose and injection rates, the patient's ability to hold still during the time of the exam has to be taken into consideration. For most patients, the upper limit for the time of suspended respiration is about 30 s. In areas where there is no respiratory motion (e.g., skull base, carotids, legs) or where respiration does not influence the vessels of interest (e.g., pelvic arteries in the lower abdomen), scan time can be increased to 40 s or more. Thus, total scan times T of 30 to 40 s are typically recommended in the literature. It should be noted, however, that quotation of a 30-s scan time, for example, traditionally implied 30 scanner rotations. With new scanner designs operating at scan speeds t of 0.75 to 2.0 s per 360° rotation, this will imply a range of 40 to 15 rotations. Forty or more is desirable since CTA is preferably a thin-slice technique; 15 is insufficient for many examinations. This stresses the need for and advantage of fast scanners. To simplify the discussion, we will assume a maximum scan time of 40 s and a rotation time of 1 s per 360°.

With the scan range R given and a maximal scan time of 40 s or less chosen, the maximal table speed d' in millimeters per second results immediately:

$$d' = R/T. \tag{6.1}$$

Recalling the simple relations on table speed d', slice thickness S, and pitch p (Table 6.1)

$$d' = S \times p/t \tag{6.2}$$

and the limitation of pitch to values between 1 and 2, the range of slice widths available for a given exam is determined. As pointed out above, thinner SSPs and higher spatial resolution in the z direction will result if we select thinner slice collimations and a higher pitch for a given table speed. This is the tendency with CTA because we want to image structures of relatively high contrast and high structural complexity. In CTA 1- to 2-mm slice collimation and pitch values of 1.5 or higher are rather common. For tube voltages, standard values of 120 kVp are generally chosen. The choice of tube currents will depend as usual on the diameter of the body section to be examined and the noise level that can be tolerated. Tube currents and dose values for spiral CTA exams generally need not be increased, as compared to standard spiral exams of the same region. Typical combinations of scan parameters for a few common CTA examinations are assembled in Table 6.2.

6.2.4 Contrast Medium Application and Timing

To keep the desired contrast medium concentration in the vascular territory of interest over the full duration of the scan constant is a decisive and, maybe, the most difficult part of the CTA exam. Intra-individual differences in circulation time pose considerable problems; variations in bolus passage time from the forearm to the abdomen of 10 to 30 s are frequently found. Such uncertainty is relatively large in comparison to the spiral scan, which lasts only 30 to 40 s. Thus, if the scan is started 10 s too soon, one third of the range is scanned without adequate contrast enhancement, which may often mean that the total examination is lost. Determination of the delay between start of injection and start of the spiral scan therefore is critical. Several projects are currently in progress which aim at providing support for timing the start of the scan in individual patients or even triggering it automatically.

In the majority of cases, an intravenous injection is chosen, normally via the antecubital vein. However, if the high contrast medium concentration in the subclavian vein or the vena cava superior may lead to disturbing artifacts in imaging the supra-aortic vessels, an entry point in the lower extremities may be chosen or the scan may be performed in a caudo-cranial direction in order to hit the brachiocephalic veins at a later point in time when the contrast medium is partially washed out by normal blood. Typical volumes of contrast medium vary between 80 and 150 ml. They are preferably injected by a power injector with a flow of 3 to 5 ml/s. All this is considered standard practice; the new challenge with spiral CT examinations — both in standard organ scanning with contrast medium and for vasular exams or CTA — is the high demand for accurate timing of the bolus.

TABLE 6.1
Scan and Reconstruction Parameters in Conventional and Spiral CT (Typical Values)

		General scan parameters
Voltage	V	80 to 140 kVp
Tube current	I	100 to 400 mA
Power	P	10 to 60 kW
Slice collimation	S	1 to 10 mm
Scan time per 360° rotation	t	0.75 to 2.0 s
		Scan parameters specific to conventional CT
Scan increment	SI	Arbitrary, mostly equal to S
Number of 360° scans	n	20 to 60
Scan range	R	$(n - 1) \cdot SI + S$ mm
		Scan and reconstruction parameters specific to spiral CT
Spiral scan time	T	24 to 100 s
Table feed per 360° rotation	d	1.0 to 20.0 mm
Table speed	d'	1.0 to 26.0 mm/s
Pitch	p	1.0 to 2.0 = d/S (dimensionless)
Number of 360° rotations per scan	n	20 to 80
Scan range	R	30 to 1500 mm $= (n - 1) \cdot d + S$ mm
z interpolation algorithm		Mostly 360° or 180° linear interpolation
Reconstruction increment	RI	0.1 to 5 mm
$S/d/RI$		Specifies the scan and reconstruction parameters (e.g., 3/5/1 means a scan with $S = 3$ mm, $d = 5$ mm, $RI = 1$ mm)

TABLE 6.2
Typical Scan Parameters and Dose Values for Some Typical CTA Examinations

Vascular region	Circle of Willis	Carotid arteries	Thoracic aorta	Renal arteries
Scan time (T, s)	40	30	30	30
Scan range (R, mm)	40–60	120–150	150–270	90–150
Table speed (d', mm/s)	1–2	4–5	5–9	3–5
Slice width (S, mm)	1	2–3	3–5	2–3
Reconstruction increment (RI, mm)	0.5–1	1–2	2	1
Tube voltage (kVp)	120	120	120	120
Tube current (mA)	150–200	150–200	150	200
Contrast medium (ml)	120	120	120	150
Injection rate (ml/s)	3–4	3–4	3–4	4–5
Delay[a] (s)	20	20	20	20
Critical organ	Lens	Thyroid	Lung	Liver
Organ dose[b] (mSv)	2.6	9.7	9.0	5.9
Effective dose (mSv)	0.5	0.6	2.3	1.6

[a] Determined by a test bolus or by a bolus triggering method.

[b] Values calculated for 120 kV on a Siemens SOMATOM PLUS for "standard man." For "standard woman," a CTA examination of the thoracic aorta would incur an organ dose to the breast of ~10.2 mSv and an effective dose of ~3.1 mSv.

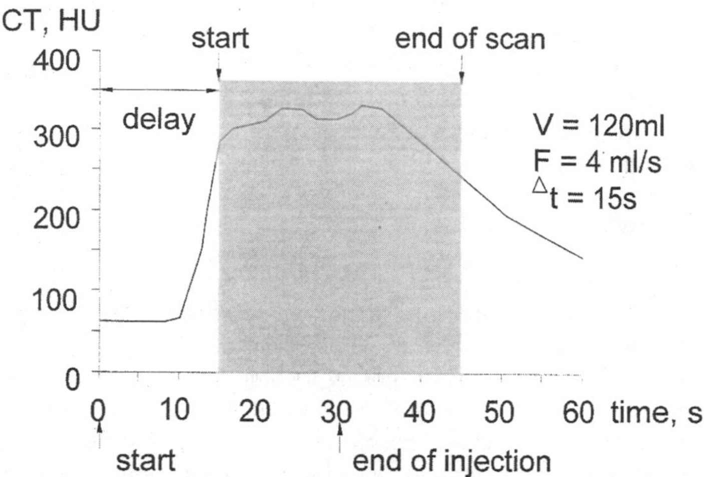

FIGURE 6.5 Sketch of the temporal course of a CTA examination. Determination of the delay between the start of contrast medium injection and the start of the spiral scan is a crucial task.

To provide high contrast in the vascular region to be examined in a reliable fashion, the delay between start of contrast medium injection and start of spiral scan has to be estimated or measured. Currently various methods are in use:

1. Selection of a start delay solely based on experience, taking into account the condition of the individual patient; sometimes empirical formulae based on the pulse rate are used.
2. Injection of a test bolus of typically 10 to 15 ml and successive CT scans in 2- to 5-s intervals to determine the bolus transit time from the injection site to the organ of interest.
3. Monitoring of the contrast medium bolus arrival in the arterial system by CT and starting the spiral scan semi-automatically.[16]
4. Monitoring of the contrast medium bolus arrival in the arterial system by other means and starting the spiral scan semi-automatically or automatically.[17]

Although Method 1 has been used for many years it is considered by many radiologists to be too error prone for CTA applications. Today, Method 2 is the most widely advocated approach because it can be carried out without special technical prerequisites. However, it demands an extra injection of contrast medium and additional exposure to detect the test bolus. In both Methods 1 and 2, a value for the delay Δt results, which allows preprogramming of the total procedure (Figure 6.5).

Approaches 3 and 4 have not been generally established yet. In both these cases technical effort is demanded to detect the arrival of the contrast medium bolus in the arterial system, but it allows us to dispense with the additional short examination required by Method 2. In Method 3, CT scans are taken in the region of interest — which is not necessarily equal to the scan start position — at short time intervals. Images are reconstructed and checked for contrast medium enhancement. If contrast medium is detected (this decision cannot be fully automatic because a number of disturbances might erroneously lead to an increase in signal!), the patient has to be moved to the scan start position, a spiral scan mode has to be loaded, and the scan must be started. While the timing information may be optimal because it can be obtained in the region of interest, a delay between time of arrival and start of the spiral scan has to be accepted. Present technical solutions demand at least 6 s delay. A further disadvantage is the fact that dose is imparted to the patient solely for timing purposes. Therefore, alternatives are considered under Method 4, in which the arrival of the contrast medium bolus is to be detected by external means without CT scanning. Measurements on peripheral body parts such as the earlobe or a finger are considered. The detection mechanism can be absorption of low-energy radiation by the contrast medium itself or absorption of visible light by a dye added to the contrast medium.[17] Inherent advantages of this approach are the possibilities to place the patient in the scan start position and to start the scan instantly. Efforts at validating the different techniques are still in progress, and alternative proposals may arise.

6.2.5 Patient Dose Considerations

Concern about patient dose in X-ray procedures has always been high and is increasing as alternative imaging modalities such as MRI and ultrasound, which do not use ionizing radiation, steadily improve in their performance. The advent of volume scanning by spiral CT met with reservations in some instances. The thought was that exposing a complete volume would lead to higher doses than exposing single slices only. We will try to show that, on the contrary, spiral CT offers the potential to reduce dose. It is assumed and understood that always the same anatomic range is investigated, no matter if by one volume scan or by many contiguous single slices.

There are a number of mostly practical reasons why in spiral CT lower dose will be imparted to the patient than in conventional CT:

1. In spiral CT, tube currents often have to be set to lower values than in conventional CT due to the above-mentioned technical limitations.
2. The need to retake single scans which sometimes results from a lack of patient cooperation is largely reduced in spiral CT.
3. The practice of taking overlapping scans in conventional CT for high-quality 3D displays is replaced by the possibility of calculating arbitrarily many overlapping images from one spiral scan without renewed exposure.
4. The possibility to use pitch values greater than 1 leads to an immediate reduction in dose as compared to contiguous single slice scanning, with the dose reduction equal to the pitch factor.

Pitch values greater than 1 are common practice in CTA, as was discussed above and is reflected in Table 6.2. Nevertheless, there is justified concern whenever a new type of X-ray procedure is introduced. The benefits of CTA are unquestioned in most cases and will be discussed again below. The risk, which is mostly tied to the patient's exposure to ionizing radiation, should be assessed also as closely as feasible. It is useful and even necessary to provide quantitative estimates of organ dose and effective dose values. The results of respective efforts[18] are listed in Table 6.2. It should be noted that organ dose values are mostly around 10 mSv or lower and that effective dose values are in the range of 0.5 to 3.0 mSv. These values can offer only a rough orientation because scan parameters, scan range, geometry, patient thickness, and so forth will influence dose in each individual case considerably. Thus CTA exposures on an average are slightly lower than those in classical projection angiography. The level of natural background radiation of 2.4 mSv per year can also be used as a point of reference.

6.3 VISUALIZATION OF THE 3D DATA SET

Various possibilities and strategies for evaluation, diagnosis, and display of the 2D CT images which represent the 3D scan volume are described in different chapters of this book. The brief summary offered here shall hint to some problems specific to CTA. In this context it is important to stress again that the full diagnostic information is contained in the original axial images. Successive processing into 3D displays is valuable and often the only way to fully grasp the complex situation, but it always means a reduction in information content and it can generate artifacts.

Therefore, interactive viewing of the original CT images in arbitrary multiplanar reformations (MPRs) is considered the method of choice for diagnosing. Reviewing the images in this fashion, mostly by control of a mouse, and selecting the optimal cut by going back and forth is a very convenient and efficient procedure.[13] Such interactive MPR evaluations can also be demonstrated very nicely and convincingly by video recordings. The procedure exploits the tremendous inherent advantage of spiral CT pointed out before: optimum contrast for small details is achieved if we slide the slice (or a slab of arbitrary thickness) through the scan volume instead of being limited to single incremented scans as in conventional CT. This type of assessment has also been extended to the evaluation of thin slabs in MIP representation — the sliding-thin-slab (STS) MIP display as suggested by Napel et al.[19]

3D displays reduce the tremendous amount of data given by a set of typically 100 to 200 images into a single image to enhance and selectively display the finding of interest. Here we mention only shaded surface display (SSD) and MIP images, which are most commonly used in CT angiography (Figure 6.6). In SSDs all CT value information is given up. A surface image is generated with gray values assigned in a way to simulate shading by a fictitious light source assumed in an arbitrary position to give a realistic 3D impression. Surfaces are determined by a threshold criterion in most cases today (Figure 6.6a) (i.e., a global value is chosen for the complete image set to determine bone surfaces or vessel surfaces). This procedure must be limited in performance because CT values of small vessels, for example, will be decreased as compared to thicker vessels because they do not fill the slice completely. Loss of small vessels in SSDs or pseudostenoses can result (Figure 6.6c,e). These effects are well known from skeletal imaging, where "fenestration" effects may occur when a particularly thin part of a bony surface is represented with CT values below the threshold value: a hole in the bony surface will be artificially generated. MIP displays are less susceptible to this type of artifact but they exhibit some weaknesses also (Figure 6.6d,f). The assessment of the degree of stenosis is critical in any case. Again, careful selection of a multiplanar display in several orientations will be the most reliable way of diagnosing. SSDs and MIPs can often be complementary in the information they offer. And for both techniques it can be advantageous to view the images resulting from different projections in an interactive cine mode or movie fashion. Here again, similar to the 2D case, it can be very helpful to select the appropriate projection by going back and forth in position and to compare neighboring views. Perspective volume rendering of CTA data, discussed in the literature as virtual angioscopy, provides fascinating animated views of intravascular anatomy, but clinical value and applications remain to be proven.

6.4 CLINICAL APPLICATIONS

Although the first applications of what is now called CT angiography have been around since 1991, there is still comparatively little quantitative data on the diagnostic accuracy of this method. This may be due to the excellent visualization of many vessels of interest that has resulted in the immediate substitution of arterial angiography, the "gold standard," by CTA.[22–25] The diagnostic performance of CTA is strongly dependent on the appropriate choice of imaging parameters and also on the region of interest. The evaluation and 3D rendering approach will also vary with the clinical questions. All this necessitates an anatomy-oriented discussion.

6.4.1 Circle of Willis

The arteries of the circle of Willis pose the hardest challenges for CTA: they are small, run mostly within the scan plane, and are closely related to the bony structures of the skull base. Given a sufficiently narrow slice width of 1 to 1.5 mm, detection and evaluation of all relevant vessels is possible, however. The main indication for CTA is the detection of cerebrovascular aneurysms in cases of acute subarachnoid hemorrhage: these patients require CT for detection of acute hemorrhage, and CTA may be added to immediately determine the origin of the bleeding. For giant

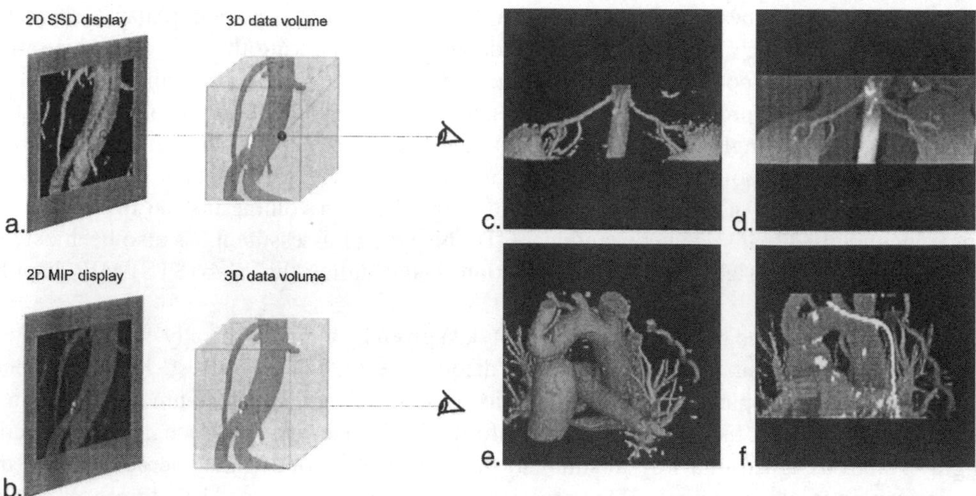

FIGURE 6.6 3D displays of vascular anatomy are essential to demonstrate the diagnostic finding in a single view. Different approaches may exhibit both advantages and disadvantages when compared to each other directly. The original axial CT images should always be referred to for diagnosis and in cases of doubt. (a) Shaded surface display (SSD) images are mostly based on thresholding and display that point in the 3D data volume for which a selected CT value is reached or surpassed for the first time along a ray from an assumed observer position to the image plane. (b) Maximum intensity projection (MIP) images display the maximal CT value along the projection ray from an assumed observer position to the image plane. (c,d) Suspicion of a stenosis of the renal artery. A pseudodefect is seen in the left main renal artery due to inconsistent contrast enhancement in SSD (c), whereas the MIP display (d) correctly shows the uncritical situation in the region of the renal arteries. (e,f) Membrane-like restenosis and poststenotic dilatation after surgery of an isthmus stenosis of the aorta. Diagnosis is easy and clear with SSD (e), whereas MIP images do not yield the relevant information (f).

anuerysms, CTA can be superior to DSA because thrombosed portions are directly visualized. As compared to MRA, fewer flow-related artifacts occur in the aneurysmatic lumen. Aneurysms larger than 5 mm can be securely detected,[26] and some authors even suggest that those as small as 2 mm can be evaluated. This, however, requires careful screening of the primary data set using interactive cine displays or multiplanar reformats. SSDs will be the preferential technique for display of CTA data sets because removal of the bones of the skull base is not mandatory. MIPs are able to display smaller vessels but require time-consuming editing of overlying bones. Semi-automated editing techniques may become available soon, either using morphological information or subtraction techniques.

6.4.2 Carotid Arteries

The carotid arteries run perpendicular through the scan plane and would therefore be perfect for CTA. For full evaluation of the carotid arteries from their origin at the aortic arch to the intracranial portion, a large scan range would be required. In addition, the uppermost portion of the carotid arteries runs through the skull base in the region of the carotid siphon and is hard to separate from the surrounding bony structures. Thus, usually only the extracranial portions are examined by CTA, with most of the current publications concentrating only on the region of the carotid bifurcation. This may limit the clinical usefulness in those cases that require a full diagnostic workup of the whole length of the supra-aortic arteries.

As compared to MRA, calcifications can be visualized. On SSD or MIP, however, these calcifications may obscure stenoses and may obviate the evaluation of the carotid lumen.[27] Therefore it is necessary to interactively evaluate the primary axial data set or use reformats that are adapted to the course of the carotid arteries. Diagnostic accuracy is high and may even be superior to i.a. DSA because the cross-sectional area rather than the projected diameter can be used for quantification of stenoses.[28]

6.4.3 Pulmonary Embolism

Detection of pulmonary embolism with spiral CT was suggested early by Remy-Jardin et al.[29] This imaging task is less dependent on the choice of a narrow slice width. Evaluation of CTA data relies almost exclusively on axial sections with occasional use of multiplanar reformats.[30] MIPs or SSDs are generally of little use since they are not able to demonstrate intraluminal thrombi surrounded by contrast-enhanced blood.

Comparison studies have shown that CTA is as reliable as DSA to diagnose patients with suspected pulmonary emboli but may be superior in determining the number of arterial segments involved.[31] As opposed to DSA or angiography, even mural thrombi are detected that may be missed on the angiographic images if there is no contour irregularity. In contrast to the gold standard of conventional film angiography, CTA and DSA are much less reliable in detecting involvement of peripheral arterial branches (beyond the level of subsegmental arteries). It is not yet clear, however, whether this is of general clinical relevance, especially since conventional film angiography equipment is being substituted by DSA in many institutions. For the detection of pulmonary embolism, CTA becomes a direct competitor to ventilation/perfusion scintigraphy and appears to be superior to this technique because CTA is able to directly visualize thrombi and other causes that may simulate pulmonary embolism on scintigraphic studies.

6.4.4 Thoracic Aortic Aneurysms

The thoracic aorta was examined very early with CTA but there were limits to the general acceptance due to artifacts that commonly arise from highly concentrated contrast medium within the brachiocephalic veins or the superior vena cava. There are four basic ways to reduce these artifacts:

1. Reduction of the concentration of the intravenously applied contrast medium to 100 to 150 mg iodine per milliliter.
2. Caudo-cranial scan direction in order to hit the areas with high venous contrast at the end of the scan, thus increasing the probablity of fewer artifacts due to wash-out effects.
3. A saline chaser bolus administered in order to further enhance the wash out effect.
4. Femoral contrast injection in order to avoid all high-contrast artifacts within the scan range (cranio-caudal scan direction should be chosen because of early enhancement of the jugular veins).

For practical purposes, a combination of Techniques 2 and 3 seems most appropriate, while Technique 4 should be considered when maximum quality images are required for pre-operative planning and 3D reconstructions.

Thoracic aneurysms can be easily evaluated using spiral CT. SSDs are superior to MIPs in all but the simplest of cases: superimposing vessels make it impossible to distinguish foreground from background on MIP images. The diagnostic value is comparable to that of MRI and is superior to DSA in most cases because mural thrombi are directly visualized and arbitrary projection angles are available for 3D displays. The latter are of major importance to surgeons in cases of aneurysms of the aortic arch and the proximal descending aorta: here it is necessary to determine the exact position of the aneurysms relative to the supra-aortic vessels. In younger patients, however, pulsation of the ascending aorta may deteriorate the quality of reformats or SSD.

6.4.5 Abdominal Aortic Aneurysms

For the pre-operative workup of abdominal aortic aneurysms, CTA should include the celiac artery and should extend down to the iliac bifurcations if not the femoral bifurcations. Due to the long scan range, z axis resolution is relatively low. In order to obtain optimum results, a total scan time of 40 to 50 s should be used if available. Slice collimation should not exceed 5 mm and may even be reduced to 3 mm or less.[25] Although widely used, larger collimations suppress fine detail and yield inferior results, especially for the assessment of renal or visceral artery stenoses. Detection of stenoses is the most critical imaging task that requires the smallest effective slice thickness possible. Identification of accessory renal arteries is reliably possible on axial images but requires an overlapping image reconstruction.

Diameter measurements and detection of mural thrombus or calcification pose no problems for CTA. The spatial relationship of the neck of the aneurysm and the renal arteries is best appreciated on SSD images if the renal arteries are large, and on MIP images for smaller arteries. Spiral CTA provides a rapid and thorough examination of the abdominal aorta that eliminates the need for arterial angiography.[32] The only indication left for arterial angiography is the supraselective evaluation of the blood supply of the spinal cord prior to thoraco-abdominal aortic surgery. Gd-MRA has recently been able to produce images of quality similar to CTA,[33] but the high costs of the intravenous contrast agent will probably limit its use.

6.4.6 Aortic Dissection

In aortic dissections, CTA is able to directly visualize the intimal flap and mural thrombi. Thus, CTA is superior to angiography in most cases. The great majority of aortic side branches can be attributed to the true-or-false channel. Transaxial sections are the primary display modality for assessment of vascular diameter, intimal flap, entry and re-entry sites, and perfusion of the true-or-false channel. Multiplanar reformats may be helpful in the aortic arch and in cases of complex dissections. MIPs may demonstrate differential opacification of the channels but only rarely show the intimal flap. SSD images can be advantageous for comprehensive display. A threshold range that includes only the aortic wall and intimal flap[34] may provide additional information in complex dissections. Virtual reality approaches using perspective volume rendering may further improve the pre-operative workup for complex cases.

Due to its higher spatial resolution, and its insensitivity to flow artifacts, CTA is often superior to MRA with respect to small branching arteries and thrombus in the false lumen.[35] Due to the short time the patient has to remain on the table, CTA is becoming the method of choice for evaluating dissections. CTA is ideal for monitoring chronic dissection and for assessment before elective surgery. In acute dissections, CTA represents the fastest non-invasive imaging modality with high diagnostic yield.

6.4.7 Renal Arteries

CTA has been proven to be an excellent screening procedure for renal artery stenosis. Accurate imaging requires thin slice collimation of 2 to 3 mm.[25] Optimal results are obtained if CTA evaluation includes not only MIP or SSD images but also the primary transaxial data set. In a series of 62 arteries, MIP images provided a sensitivity of 93% and a specificity of 83% whereas SSD reduced the sensitivity to 59% with a specificity of 82%.[36] When the primary axial data set and interactive reformatting were used, another series (80 patients, 198 arteries) yielded a sensitivity of 99% for the detection of significant stenoses (<50%) with a specificity of 93%.

CTA is sufficient for pre-operative evaluation of the anatomy of renal donors. For this indication, SSD was superior to axial images in demonstrating perihilar branches.[23] In patients with renal artery aneurysms, CTA is often superior to DSA in demonstrating the spatial relationship of branching arteries relative to the aneurysm.

6.4.8 Visceral Arteries

Pre-operative spiral CT examinations (in the arterial phase) prior to partial liver resection or liver transplantation provided sufficient angiographic information to reliably assess anatomy and variants of hepatic arterial supply and accompanying atherosclerotic changes in the visceral arteries.[24] These examinations may serve as a pre-operative splanchnic vascular mapping that alleviates additional risky, costly, and time-consuming arteriograms.

In patients with abdominal tumors such as pancreatic carcinoma, the pre-operative assessment of vascular involvement is essential for planning further treatment. 3D models of vascular structures may improve diagnosis in a selected patient group.[37] However, even if spiral CT provides optimized intravascular contrast, the differentiation of vascular infiltration versus encasement remains difficult. In our opinion, the primary image data set is the most essential display mode.

Chronic visceral ischemia with involvement of the main arteries can be readily diagnosed, although color duplex sonography may be less costly and invasive. Stenoses of the celiac axis or the superior mesenteric artery are frequent incidental findings in CTA performed for other reasons (aorta or renal arteries).

6.4.9 Pelvic and Peripheral Arteries

Pelvic arteries are usually examined in combination with peripheral arteries, requiring a large scan range. Although there are first reports in the literature,[38,39] this imaging task exceeds the volume that can be currently covered by CTA with reasonable spatial resolution and contrast volume. Hence, indications for CTA are limited to the pre- and post-therapeutic assessment[38] of limited subvolumes. MIP images allow for optimal display of arterial calcifications and may thus alter the choice of an interventional radiologic procedure.

6.5 DISCUSSION

Spiral CT angiography is now an accepted and widely applied technique. It is suitable for the examination of all body regions; a few examples are given in Figure 6.7. A review of the extensive literature and of the clinical applications is beyond the scope of this chapter. It is of interest, however, to discuss the performance characteristics of spiral CTA in a clinical context and to briefly compare it to competing imaging modalities. This shall also cover general and practical aspects. For a detailed comparison to competing angiographic procedures, the reader is referred to the recent review article by Mistretta.[1] The results of the discussion below are compiled in a simple qualitative form in Table 6.3. It is understood that this can give only a rough overview and that it will be subject to change with time. Nevertheless, it may be helpful for general orientation.

CTA is a relatively non-invasive technique which can be applied to the evaluation of all vascular regions in the human body. Vessels as small as 3 mm in diameter can be diagnosed reliably. Its invasiveness is limited to puncturing a vein and applying contrast medium. Placing a catheter and injecting arterially is done only in very few special procedures such as CT arterial portography (CTAP), for which the catheter is placed during a preceding fluoroscopic exam. Demands on the experience of the investigator are therefore only moderate. The most critical part in conducting the exam with respect to the experience required is the timing of the contrast medium bolus. The total time required for conducting the exam is comparatively low. If the CTA exam is combined with a CT procedure it typically demands only an additional 10 min. The time on the scanner will be further reduced because independent workstations with the possibility of image reconstruction and evaluation will become available.

The selectivity of a CTA exam with respect to evaluating the venous and the arterial vasculature separately is very limited due to the long duration of injection and scan which results in opacification of all vessels. Differentiation between a high-grade arterial stenosis or an occlusion may therefore be difficult: as opposed to conventional angiographic techniques, no information is provided on

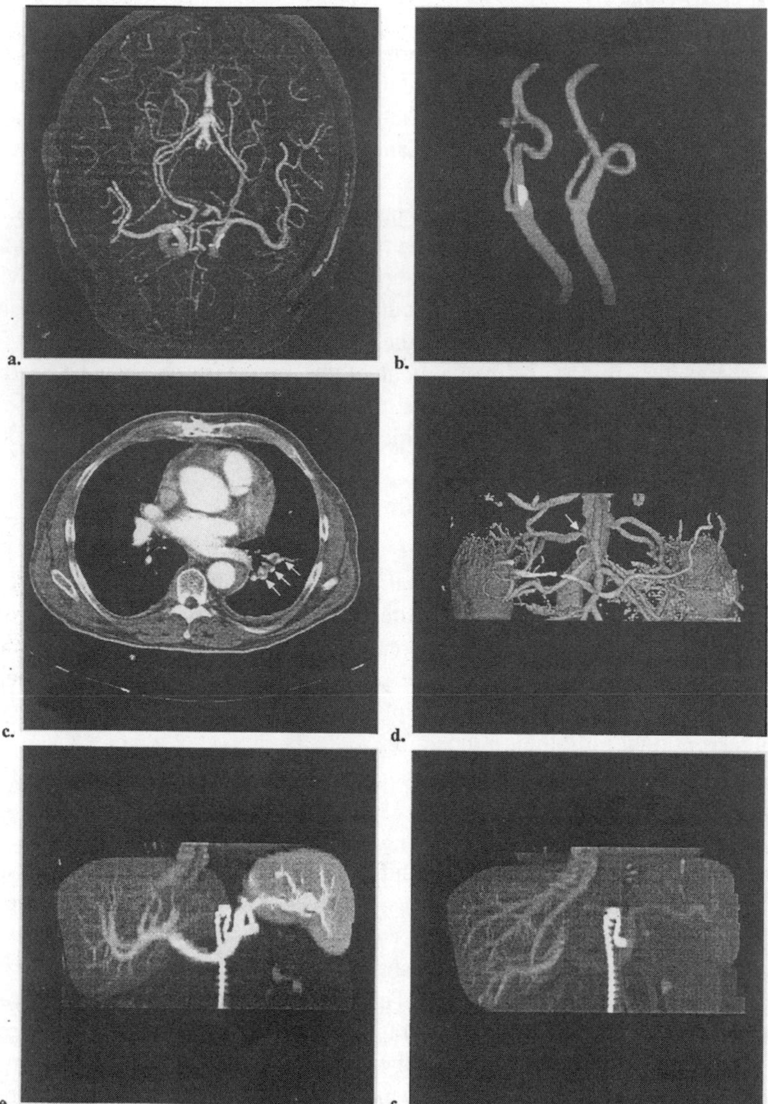

FIGURE 6.7 CT angiography can be applied for the examination of larger vessels of all body regions. (a) MIP display of the circle of Willis. (b) MIP display of the calcified plaque of the right carotid artery. No stenosis. (c) Axial image display of multiple lung emboli in segmental lung arteries. (d) SSD showing a high-grade stenosis of the right renal artery. (e,f) Pre-operative CT arterial portography in dual phase technique. Selective display of the portal (e) and the venous (f) system.

whether the vessel is opacified in an antegrade fashion (stenosis) or via collaterals (occlusion). In addition, early venous enhancement, such as of the renal or jugular veins, may lead to superimposition of arterial and venous structures. CTA does not provide any information about flow, but it does not suffer from flow-induced artifacts either. Its particular strength in comparison to classical angiography and ultrasound is given by the fact that full information about extraluminal tissues and organs is provided in a single exam.

Image quality in CTA is limited in several respects, when compared to classical radiography. Spatial resolution is much lower; experienced investigators claim diagnosis of vascular structures as small as 2 to 3 mm in diameter. Temporal resolution is very limited also; the frame rates of

TABLE 6.3
Comparison of Angiographic Procedures

	DSA	US	CTA	MRA
General aspects				
Anatomic region	+	–	+	+
Invasiveness	–	+	–	+
Experience of investigator	0	–	0	–
Time	0	0	+	0
Cost	–	+	0	–
Selectivity	+	0	0	0
Flow information	0	+	0	+
Extraluminal information	–	+	+	0
Image quality				
Spatial resolution	+	0	0	0
Temporal resolution	+	+	–	0
Free choice of projection	–	0	+	+
Background suppression	+	0	–	+
Artifacts	+	0	+	–

Note: Compared to the other modalities, – = disadvantage, 0 = no significant difference, and + = advantage.

DSA are orders of magnitude higher. Resolution of the arterial and venous phases is only partially possible with CTA. The only application with temporal resolution is CTAP, where separate displays of the portal and venous circulation are obtained with arterial injection (Figure 6.7e,f).

A definite advantage of CTA is that a complete 3D image set is available which can be viewed with arbitrary techniques and, above all, in arbitrary projection. Thereby it is possible to view vascular trees in a direction where superimposed structures do not obscure the view. To do so it is often necessary to edit the data set. This is still time consuming but the respective hardware and software tools are improving dramatically. Thereby a background suppression, which is inherent in DSA and MRA but not in CTA, can be provided retrospectively. CTA is not free of artifacts, but they are very subtle and do not disturb the diagnosis, as might be the case in MRA.

CTA has developed into a relatively mature technique within a very short time. Nevertheless we can expect further technical advances and improvements of contrast media and contrast medium bolus techniques, which will make CTA more easy to perform and hopefully will further increase its diagnostic value. 3D image processing, rendering, and evaluation is a rapidly developing field which will certainly contribute also. For example, vessel tracking in general, quantitative determination of the degree of a stenosis, virtual angioscopy, and similar efforts may provide valuable tools to the radiologist in the near future.

REFERENCES

1. Mistretta CA. Relative properties of MR angiography and competing vascular modalities. *JMRI* 1993;3:685–698.
2. Gmeinwieser J, Wunderlich A, Gerhardt P, Strotzer M. Dreidimensonale Rekonstruktion von atemverschieblichen Organen und Gefäβstrukturen aus Spiral-CT-Datensätzen. *Röntgenpraxis* 1991;44:2–8.
3. Bautz W, Strotzer M, Lenz M, Dittler H, Kalender WA. Preoperative evaluation of the vessels of the upper abdomen with spiral CT: Comparison with conventional CT and arterial DSA. *Radiology* 1991;181(P):261.

4. Prokop M, Schaefer C, Doehring W, Laas J, Nischelsky J, Galanski M. Spiral CT for three-dimensional imaging of complex vascular anatomy. *Radiology* 1991;181:293.
5. Napel SA, Marks MA, Rubin GD, et. al. CT angiography with spiral CT and maximum intensity projection. *Radiology* 1992;185:607–610.
6. Rubin G, Napel S, Dake M, Walker P, McDonnell C, Marks M, Jeffrey RB. Spiral CT creates 3-D neuro, body angiograms. *Diagn Imaging* 1992;August.
7. Kalender WA, Seissler W, Klotz E, Vock P. Spiral volumetric CT with single-breath-hold technique, continuous transport, and continuous scanner rotation. *Radiology* 1990;176:181–183.
8. Kalender WA. Technical foundations of spiral CT. *Semin Ultrasound CT MRI* 1994;15:81–89.
9. Kalender WA. Principles and performance of spiral CT. In: Goldman LW, Fowlkes JB, eds. *Medical CT and Ultrasound: Current Technology and Applications*. Advanced Medical Publishing, Madison, WI, 1995, 379–410.
10. Kalender WA. Spiral or helical CT: Right or wrong? *Radiology* 1994;193:583.
11. Polacin A, Kalender WA, Marchal G. Evaluation of section sensitivity profiles and image noise in spiral CT. *Radiology* 1992;185:29–35.
12. Crawford C, King K. Computed tomography scanning with simultaneous patient translation. *Med Phys* 1990;17:967–982.
13. Kalender WA, Polacin A, Suess C. A comparison of conventional and spiral CT: An experimental study on the detection of spherical lesions. *J Comp Assisted Tomogr* 1994;18:167–176.
14. Kalender WA. Three-dimensional spiral CT: Is isotropic imaging possible? *Radiology* 1995;197:578–580.
15. Kalender WA, Polacin A. Physical performance characteristics of spiral CT scanning. *Med Phys* 1991;18:910–915.
16. Kopka L, Funke M, Fischer U, Vosshenrich R, Oestmann JW, Grabbe E. Parenchymal liver enhancement with bolus-triggered helical CT: Preliminary clinical results. *Radiology* 1995;195:282–284.
17. Kalender WA, Suess C. Different approaches to trigger contrast-enhanced CT scans. *Radiology* 1996 (in press).
18. Kalender WA, Svatos M, Niendorf E. Calculation of effective dose in CT. *Radiology* 1993;189(P):347.
19. Napel S, Rubin GD, Jeffrey RB. STS-MIP: A new reconstruction technique for CT of the chest. *J Comp Assisted Tomogr* 1993;17:832–838.
20. Polacin A, Kalender WA. Evaluation of spatial resolution and noise in spiral CT. *Radiology* 1994;193(P):170.
21. Prokop M, Schaefer C, Leppert AGA, Galanski M. Spiral CT angiography of thoracic aorta: Femoral or antecubital injection site for intravenous administration of contrast material? *Radiology* 1993;189(P):111.
22. Bluemke DA, Chambers TP. Spiral CT angiography: An alternative to conventional angiography (editorial; comment). *Radiology* 1995;195(2):317–319.
23. Rubin GD, Alfrey EJ, Dake MD, Semba CP, Sommer FG, Kuo PC, Dafoe DC, Waskerwitz JA, Bloch DA, Jeffrey RB. Assessment of living renal donors with spiral CT. *Radiology.* 1995;195(2):457–462.
24. Winter TC III, Freeny PC, Nghiem HV, et al. Hepatic arterial anatomy in transplantation candidates: Evaluation with three-dimensional CT arteriograms. *Radiology* 1995;195:363–370.
25. Galanski M, Prokop M, Chavan A, Schaefer CM, Jandeleit K, Nischelsky JE. Renal arterial stenoses: Spiral CT angiography. *Radiology* 1993;189(1):185–192.
26. Wilms G, Gryspeerdt S, Bosmans H, Boulanger T, van Hoe L, Marchal G, Baert AL. Spiral CT of cerebral aneurysms. *J Belge Radiol* 1995;78(2):75–78.
27. Cumming MJ, Morrow IM. Carotid artery stenosis: A prospective comparison of CT angiography and conventional angiography. *AJR* 1994;163(3):517–523.
28. Marks MP, Napel S, Jordan JE, Enzmann DR. Diagnosis of carotid artery disease: Preliminary experience with maximum-intensity-projection spiral CT angiography. *AJR* 1993;160:1267–1271.
29. Remy-Jardin M, Remy J, Wattinne L, Giraud F. Central pulmonary thromboembolism with spiral volumetric CT with the single-breath-hold technique — comparison with pulmonary angiography. *Radiology* 1992;185:381–387.
30. Remy-Jardin M, Remy J, Cauvain O, Petyt L, Wannebroucq J, Beregi JP. Diagnosis of central pulmonary embolism with helical CT: Role of two-dimensional multiplanar reformations. *AJR* 1995;165:1131–1138.

31. Steiner P, Phillips F, Wesner D, et al. Primärdiagnostik iund Verlaufskontrolle der akuten Lungenembolie: Vergleich zwischen digitaler Subtraktionsangiographie und Spiral CT. *RÖFO* 1994;161:285–291.
32. Rubin G, Dake M, Napel S, McDonnell CH, Jeffrey R. Abdominal spiral CT angiography: A minimally invasive three-dimensional alternative to angiography. *Radiographics* 1994;14:5–9.
33. Prince MR, Narasimham DL, Stanley JC, Chenevert TL, Williams DM, Marx MV, Cho KJ. Breath-hold gadolinium-enhanced MR angiography of the abdominal aorta and its major branches. *Radiology* 1995;197:785–792.
34. Adachi H, Ino T, Mizuhara A, Yamaguchi A, Kobayashi Y, Nagai J. Assessment of aortic disease using three-dimensional CT angiography. *J Cardiac Surg* 1994;9(6):673–678.
35. Sommer T, Fehske W, Holzknecht N, et al. Aortic dissection: A comparative study of diagnosis with spiral CT, multiplanar transesophageal echocardiography, and MR imaging. *Radiology* 1996;199:347–352.
36. Rubin GD, Dake MD, Napel S, Jeffrey RB Jr, McDonnell CH, Sommer FG, Wexler L, Williams DM. Spiral CT of renal artery stenosis: Comparison of three-dimensional rendering techniques. *Radiology.* 1994;190(1):181–189.
37. Zeman RK, Davros WJ, Bermann P, et al. Three-dimensional models for abdominal vasculature based on helical CT: Usefulness in patients with pancreatic neoplasms. *AJR* 1994;162:1425–1429.
38. Lawrence JA, Kim D, Kent KC, Stehling MK, Rosen MP, Raptopoulos V. Lower extremity spiral CT angiography versus catheter angiography. *Radiology* 1995;194(3):903–908.
39. Richter CS, Biamino G, Ragg C, Felix R. CT angiography of the pelvic arteries. *Eur J Radiol.* 1994;19(1):25–31.

7 Volume Visualization in Radiation Treatment Planning

Charles A. Pelizzari and George T.Y. Chen

CONTENTS

ABSTRACT

Radiation treatment planning (RTP), historically an image-intensive discipline and one of the first areas in which 3D information from imaging was clinically applied, has become even more critically dependent on accurate 3D definition of target and non-target structures in recent years with the advent of conformal radiation therapy. In addition to the interactive display of wireframe or shaded surface models of anatomic objects, proposed radiation beams, beam modifying devices, and calculated dose distributions, recently significant use has been made of direct visualization of relevant anatomy from image data. Dedicated systems are commercially available for the purpose of geometrically optimizing beam placement, implementing in virtual reality the functionality of standard radiation therapy simulators. Such "CT simulation" systems rely heavily on 3D visualization and on reprojection of image data to produce simulated radiographs for comparison with either diagnostic-quality radiographs made on a simulator or megavoltage images made using the therapeutic beams themselves. Although calculation and analysis of dose distributions is an important component of radiation treatment design, geometric targeting with optimization based on 3D anatomic information is frequently performed as a separate step independent of dose calculations.

7.1 INTRODUCTION

Identification of target volumes to be irradiated and normal structures to be spared irradiation is critical to the planning of radiation treatment. This statement is true for all forms of radiotherapy: teletherapy, in which beams of photons or energetic particles are aimed at the target from outside the patient; brachytherapy, in which radioactive sources are implanted directly into the tumor or placed in nearby body cavities; and radioimmunotherapy, in which labeled biologically active agents are injected and carry radioisotopes to tumors. In this chapter we discuss only teletherapy, for which image-based treatment planning is most highly developed.

0-8493-3179-X/00/$0.00+$.50

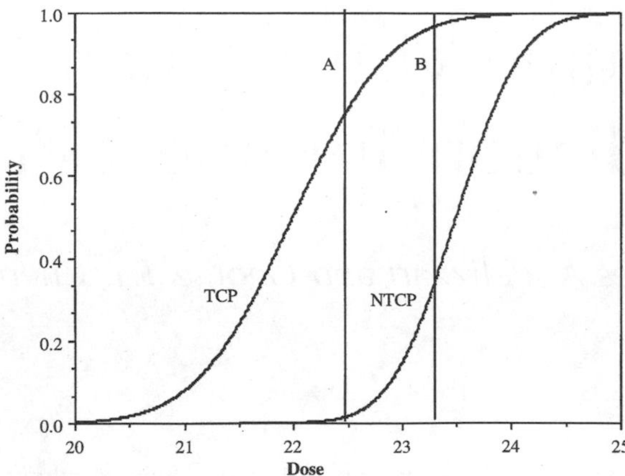

FIGURE 7.1 Schematic variation of tumor control probability (TCP) and normal tissue complication probability (NTCP) with dose.

The need for accurate identification of target and critical normal structures arises from the fact that for many tumor sites, the ability of radiotherapy to achieve local tumor control is limited by the dose that can be delivered to the tumor while maintaining safe levels of irradiation of normal tissues. The tumor control probability (TCP) increases with increasing dose, so to maximize this probability the dose delivered to the target should be high. Unfortunately, for organs adjacent to the target, some of which may unavoidably receive a dose close to the full tumor dose, the normal tissue complication probability (NTCP) for a particular complication endpoint will also increase with increasing dose, as shown schematically in Figure 7.1. If the NTCP curve lies to the right of the TCP curve, as shown, then a dose level can be chosen which corresponds to a large TCP and a small NTCP. The greater the horizontal separation between the two curves, the more favorable the situation; unfortunately in practice the separation may not be large, and for some complications the NTCP curve may lie to the left of the TCP curve. Dose to these normal tissues must be limited to values significantly lower than the prescribed tumor dose. Increasing the dose to the tumor unavoidably increases dose to some normal tissues, since teletherapy beams must enter through the patient's body. In the case of photon and neutron beams, which do not exhibit a finite range as do charged particles, the beams also exit through normal tissues. Thus as the dose is increased from level A to level B in Figure 7.1, TCP increases but so does NTCP.

The difficulty and the importance of avoiding irradiation of normal tissues varies from site to site. Some normal tissues inevitably are located adjacent to the target and, in some situations, present dose limiting constraints. For example, the prostate is in contact with the bladder on its anterior-superior margin and with the rectum on its posterior margin. This can be seen in Figure 7.2, which shows a volume-rendered 3D view from a treatment planning CT scan with a rectangular right lateral viewport exposing the prostate, bladder, and rectum. To the extent that the high dose volume cannot be made to conform to the prostate exactly, some portions of these organs will receive high doses, ranging up to the full prescribed dose. There are several effects which lead to the necessity of incorporating margins in the definition of each radiation field, thus extending the high dose volume beyond the nominal tumor boundary. This increases the volume of adjacent normal tissues, such as bladder and rectum in the case of prostate irradiation, exposed to high dose. Depending on the severity of the complications that may result from such irradiation, the ability to increase dose to the tumor is thus constrained by the potential increase in NTCP. The thrust of 3D conformal radiotherapy[1] is to reduce unnecessary irradiation of normal tissue by precise definition of tumor and normal anatomic structures from 3D imaging data; by design of irradiation geometries which minimize the inclusion of normal tissues in high dose regions, while fully irradiating the tumor; by accurate control and/or measurement of patient position during irradiation;

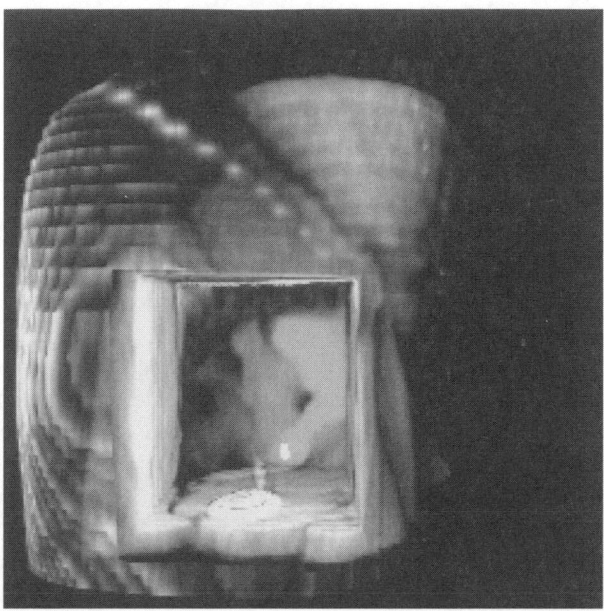

FIGURE 7.2 Right lateral volume-rendered view from a pelvic CT scan. A transparent viewport representing a rectangular radiation field has been inserted into the patient's right side, revealing the prostate, bladder, and rectum at the midsagittal plane.

and by accurate transfer of patient positioning information between image-based planning, simulation, and treatment. As we will see, several of these steps rely heavily on 3D image-derived information.

7.2 BACKGROUND — THE PROCESS OF RADIATION THERAPY

To understand the process of planning and delivery of radiation therapy, it is important to recognize as pointed out by Fuks et al. that "radiation therapy, like surgery, is a local-regional mode of treatment, capable of curing human cancers only when the primary tumors are still confined to their original local or local-regional anatomic sites."[1] The aim of radiotherapy is thus to achieve local tumor control and to prevent or limit the spreading of disease from the primary tumor site to other parts of the body, by delivering a high dose to a specified target volume. It is also significant that the radiobiology of tumor and normal tissues leads to a necessity for delivery of a tumoricidal radiation dose in multiple small fractions, rather than in a single large irradiation. As a result, a prescribed dose of 70 Gray may be delivered in 200 cGy fractions in 35 daily treatments. For each fraction, the radiation beams must be aligned with the patient with sufficient accuracy to ensure that the target is within the beams and that normal tissues are not unnecessarily irradiated. As more and more precise treatment techniques are devised in order to shrink target volumes and spare normal tissues, the importance of reliable patient alignment becomes ever greater. This translates directly into a need to maintain precise control over the coordinate transformation relating the virtual patient model in image space to the physical patient in the treatment room.

The planning and delivery of radiation therapy divide naturally into several phases. Initially, the volume within the patient to be treated is identified. This involves not only the identification of the palpable or visible tumor but also estimation, on the basis of clinical information, image data, and knowledge of the particular disease in question, of areas beyond the identifiable tumor which must be treated to achieve local control and to limit spreading of the cancer. A standard nomenclature has been proposed[2] for the description of these regions. The gross tumor volume

(GTV) is defined as the gross palpable or visible extent of the tumor. The clinical target volume (CTV) is the volume which contains microscopic or subclinical disease. Various subcategories of CTV are defined, such as areas of gross nodal disease and areas of subclinical disease surrounding the gross tumor. The planning target volume (PTV) is derived from the CTV by incorporation of uncertainties in CTV location due to patient motion, organ motion due to physiologic processes (e.g., breathing or bladder filling and emptying), and inaccuracies in treatment delivery resulting from limitations of precision in treatment machine alignment, potential errors in repeated daily patient positioning, etc. The PTV is defined as that volume within the static patient that if treated to the full prescribed dose, given all identified sources of uncertainty in organ and patient position, ensures the CTV will receive full dose. It is typically defined via the expansion of CTV by margins determined by the various uncertainties being accommodated. The object of radiation treatment design is then to arrive at a plan which delivers the prescribed dose throughout the PTV with acceptable doses to critical normal tissues, and with acceptable homogeneity of dose within the PTV. Definition of these volumes involves manual or automated segmentation from 3D image data sets such as CT and MRI either alone or used in combination,[3–6] together with estimates of subclinical spread, regional involvement, and position uncertainties. Synthesis of CT or MRI with information from nuclear medicine images such as PET, lymphoscintigraphy, or SPECT[6–8] has also been found helpful in defining areas of viable tumor, which may sometimes be difficult to assess from MRI alone.[9] Since anatomic scans used for RTP frequently contain 50 or more slices, and several structures of interest must be defined, a large amount of time is inevitably devoted to image segmentation in planning each case.[10] Development of image segmentation tools for RTP has thus been a topic of continuing interest over the years. In recognition of the importance of improving efficiency in this area, a multi-institution NCI contract to develop portable software tools had an image segmentation tool as one of its endpoints.[11,12]

Geometric optimization of radiation beam configurations, for a virtual patient model composed of the segmented target and non-target structures of interest, may be done manually or with the aid of computer optimization methods. For each beam orientation, an appropriate aperture shape is readily defined by viewing the target from the point of view of the radiation source and surrounding the target with a suitably chosen margin, as illustrated in Figure 7.3. Not only can the aperture be conformed to the target, but critical normal structures can also be avoided by this means. Candidate beam orientations may be chosen based on analysis of the volumes of normal structures irradiated by beams from all directions.[13,14] Such “beam's-eye view” targeting was recognized early on as one of the most valuable benefits of incorporation of 3D information into the RTP process.

Targeting of beams on the virtual patient cannot be carried out in isolation without consideration of the actual patient and treatment equipment, however. Some beam orientations are physically impossible to achieve — an inferior field irradiating the lung for example, or an orientation which causes a collision between the gantry and the couch of the therapy machine or the gantry and the patient. Furthermore, treatment of the entire target volume for many disease sites involves combinations of fields which do not share a common iso-center, and ensuring the accurate matching of borders of such fields within the actual patient is a difficult problem. Figure 7.4 illustrates a lateral neck field whose inferior border is matched to an anterior supraclavicular field. This matching requires precise 3D control of the patient orientation as well as correct values for the orientation and size of the fields (note that the divergence of each beam depends on its size, since the distance to the source is fixed). It is essential that when these fields are delivered during treatment, the borders match as well as they do in the computer model, otherwise hot or cold spots will occur on the match plane, possibly leading to failure to control the tumor (cold spot in the target) or a complication (hot spot in a critical normal structure). *Simulation* is the name given to the process of immobilizing and marking the patient so that each field can be repeatedly set up and delivered correctly. Traditionally, this has been done using a therapy simulator, which is an X-ray machine reproducing the geometry and motions of the actual therapy unit, but which produces a diagnostic quality rather than a megavoltage X-ray beam. The patient is immobilized on the couch of the

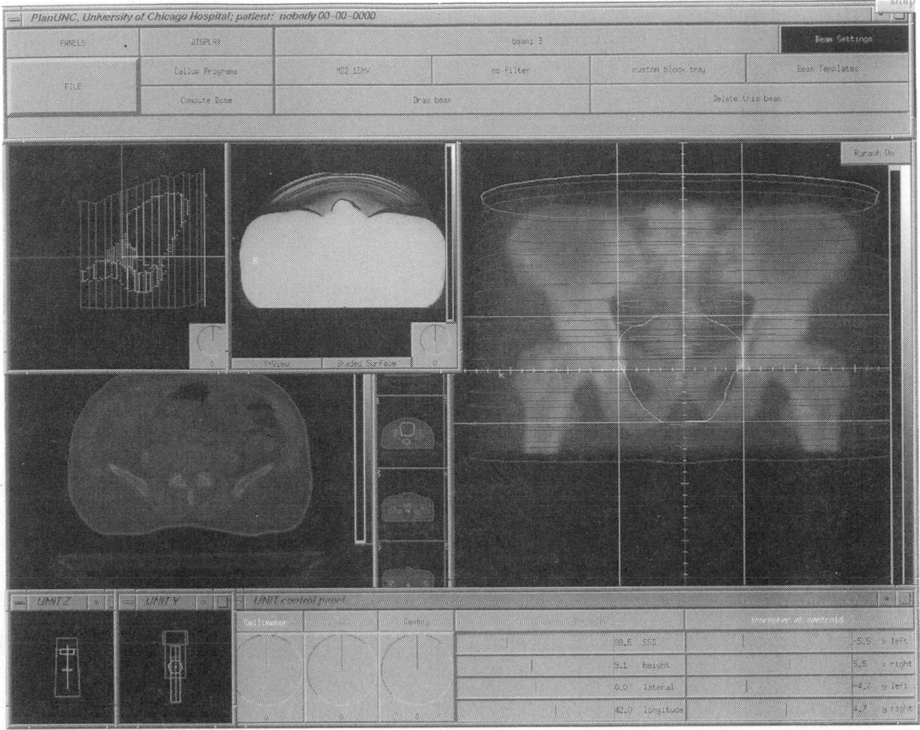

FIGURE 7.3 Main screen of the University of North Carolina radiation treatment planning system, PlanUNC. This is the control panel for the original virtual simulator. On the right, a beam aperture has been drawn by enclosing the prostate and seminal vesicle contours from each CT slice with a user-specified margin, as seen from the point of view of an anterior field. A digitally reconstructed radiograph is also included as a backdrop to the beam's-eye view.

simulator exactly as he or she will be on the therapy machine, and each radiation field is set up. Marks are placed on the patient or on the immobilization device to facilitate repeated setup using a coordinate reference frame defined with wall-mounted lasers and/or light fields projected from the source position through the beam apertures. Finally, radiographs are made to verify that the desired anatomy is actually in the beam. Since bony structures dominate these films, it is highly desirable to have predicted radiographs calculated from the image data set for each planned beam for comparison. Overlay of projections of segmented structures on computed radiographs, and comparison with actual radiographs from the simulator, allows assessment of how well an actual beam irradiates the tumor and avoids normal structures.

Dosimetric optimization, details of which are beyond the scope of this chapter, may be used to choose between a number of apparently favorable geometric beam arrangements and to optimize the weighting of doses from a number of beams in a given arrangement. With appropriately weighted integrations of calculated doses over the volume of tumor and normal structures segmented from image data, estimates of TCP and NTCP can be made. Although sufficient clinical data to accurately define the parameters of NTCP models, in particular, are not available, relative ranking of candidate plans based on such calculations is still possible. Clearly the ability to make such calculations hinges on accurate definition of the 3D regions of integration. Note that for this purpose, simply visualizing the structures of interest and their relationships is not sufficient — the position of the region of interest must be known in the same coordinate system in which the dose calculation has been done. A geometric definition of the regions of interest, derived for example from slice-by-slice image segmentation or explicit voxel classification, is essential. Thus a direct

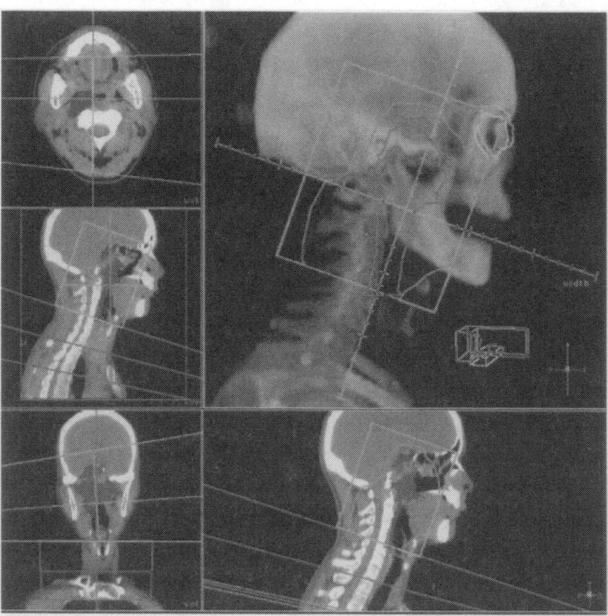

FIGURE 7.4 Example of non-coplanar field matching in the Picker AcQSim CT simulator. In the lower right window, a lateral field is shown to have its lower border matching the superior plane of an anterior supraclavicular field. (upper right) Computed radiograph from the lateral beam's perspective. (other panels) Multiplanar reformations of the 3D CT data.

volume visualization method such as opacity-weighted voxel compositing[15] alone is not adequate for this purpose unless special care is taken to recover the coordinates of objects visible in the rendered scene.[16]

Delivery of a radiation treatment involves fabrication of beam apertures matching those in the computer-generated plan, repeated immobilization of the patient on the therapy machine, and setup of the individual radiation fields for each fractional irradiation. Accurate transfer of coordinates from the image space and the virtual patient model, to the radiotherapy simulator, to the treatment machine is essential for successful delivery of a computer-planned treatment. In this sense, the problem of image-based radiation therapy planning and delivery is very similar to other image-guided procedures such as frameless stereotactic neurosurgery[17] and numerous robotic procedures in which correct registration of machine to patient coordinates must be maintained. As we shall see, one of the essential functions of modern CT simulators is to assist in defining and maintaining these coordinate transformations.

7.3 3D VISUALIZATION IN TREATMENT PLANNING — HISTORICAL PERSPECTIVE

Radiation therapy planning was one of the earliest areas in which use of 3D patient information from CT was applied to clinical problems. In the mid-1970s, the group at Rhode Island Hospital developed CT-based treatment planning systems utilizing patient surface and internal structure contours on multiple slices which were digitized from CT films and, at first, plotted on a monochrome video monitor or on paper as viewed from the perspective of candidate beam directions.[18] Hard-copy perspective plots from each beam's point of view were used for design of field apertures and blocks. Subsequently, use of an interactive color graphics system replaced monochrome plots, and coupled with a calculation of dose on multiple planes, allowed interactive display of dose on arbitrarily oriented sections through the patient.[19] Since no CT information in digital form was used, only contours from films, the 3D display was limited to wireframe models. It is interesting to note that the feature of these early systems which seemed most compelling was the ability to visualize anatomic relationships from the perspective of the radiation source for any beam orientation. As we shall see, this is also the defining capability of what have recently come to be known as CT simulation systems. Beam orientation could also be controlled via knobs interfaced to the graphics system, presaging the use a decade later of physical or on-screen knobs to control a virtual simulator (see below).

Accurate consideration of 3D patient geometry is essential in treatment planning for heavy charged particle radiotherapy, which also was an area of intense development in the late 1970s and into the 1980s. Goitein et al.[20,21] described a 3D treatment planning system, used for both proton and megavoltage X-ray plans, that incorporated a number of capabilities that have since become accepted as standards. Delineation of structures directly from CT image data using interactive graphic displays was supported, with sagittal and coronal reformatted images displayed along with the transverse slices to assist in the appreciation of anatomy. Calculation of simulated radiographs from the CT, for a particular beam quality and orientation, for comparison with actual radiographs was introduced as a method of verification that actual treatment beams matched those that had been planned. The use of such digitally reconstructed radiographs (DRRs) has also become a standard capability of CT simulation systems. The display of structures or DRRs from the perspective of the radiation source was given the name beam's-eye view and once again its utility was stressed:

> The source of radiation is a very natural viewpoint from which to gauge anatomic relationships. If the user's eye is hypothetically placed at that point and directed along the central axis of a hypothetical radiation beam, the relative disposition of structures is readily apparent and judgments as to what would and would not be included in the beam can readily be made. If the user is able interactively to move his eye around to all locations accessible to a radiation source, he can explore which directions provide the greatest separation between, say, the target volume and critical normal structures. Beam-shaping apertures can be designed from these vantage points. These advantages have, of course, been appreciated by others.[21]

Departure from an all-inclusive monolithic 3D treatment planning program and repackaging of beam's-eye view targeting, field aperture design, and generation of DRRs into a virtual simulator as a stand-alone application was pursued at the University of North Carolina during the mid- to late 1980s.[22,23] Taking advantage of the rapid increase in computational and graphic capabilities of mid-range workstations, the virtual simulator effectively implemented in virtual reality the process of radiotherapy simulation described earlier, combining the advantages of visualization of internal structures from 3D image data with visualization of projected fields on the external surface of the patient, as one would see in an actual simulation. Simulated radiographs from any beam could be produced, although for high image quality these became somewhat time consuming to calculate. Control of the geometric parameters of the virtual beams was through a control panel adjusting parameters characteristic of an actual simulator (see Figure 7.3). Although the capabilities of the virtual simulator were largely those previously described by McShan, Goitein, and others, the conceptualization of this collection of tasks as an enhanced virtual analog to conventional simulation was highly appropriate, and set the stage for the generation of CT simulators to come.

7.3.1 Volume Visualization in Beam Targeting

A number of investigators have applied general-purpose volume visualization software to the problem of RTP.[24,25] The visualizations produced by Gehring are particularly elegant, allowing inclusion of geometrically defined objects such as radiation beams and models of segmented structures, along with calculated dose distributions, together with anatomic views directly rendered from voxel data. An example from the stereotactic radiosurgery planning system developed by

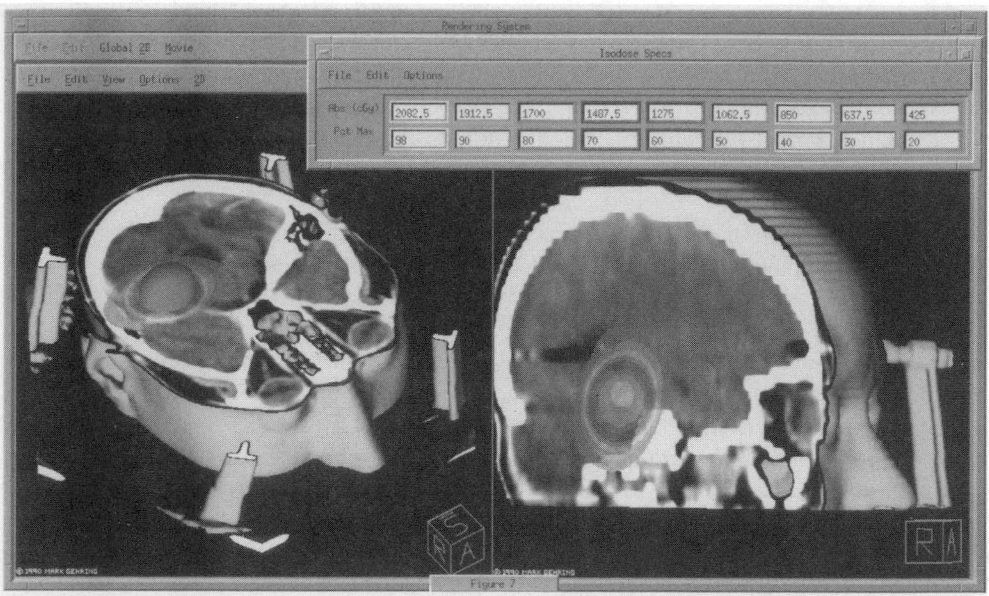

FIGURE 7.5 Visualization of idealized high dose region, calculated dose distribution, CT data, and patient surface from the University of Wisconsin stereotactic radiosurgery planning program of Gehring and colleagues.

Gehring and co-workers at the University of Wisconsin is shown in Figure 7.5. Examples from the Pinnacle^3 radiation treatment planning system sold by ADAC, based on Gehring's software, are shown in Figures 7.6 and 7.7. These figures illustrate one style of visualization for planning stereotactic radiosurgery, an external beam irradiation technique where a high dose of radiation, typically in the range of 15 to 20 Gy, is delivered in a single fraction. Such treatments are frequently applied in cases of arteriovenous malformations (AVMs) in the brain, acoustic neuromas, and other well-localized non-malignant lesions, as well as some metastases in the brain. Precise localization is essential to minimize the unnecessary irradiation of normal brain or of critical structures such as optic nerves, chiasm, or brainstem which may be adjacent to regions receiving such high doses. The patient is usually immobilized with a stereotactic frame rigidly fixed to the skull, to ensure that uncertainties due to patient motion are held below 1 mm. In the most frequently used technique, many beams of circular cross-section along multiple non-coplanar arcs focused on the target are delivered. This results in a nearly spherical high dose region, as seen in Figure 7.7.

Due to the great importance of critical structure avoidance, the confined nature of target volumes, and the predictable size and shape of the dose distribution for multiple confocal arc beams, targeting using beam's-eye view displays is relied upon even more heavily in the planning of stereotactic radiosurgery than in other forms of external beam therapy. Since the high dose region can be well approximated by a sphere of known diameter, a geometric representation of the structures of interest along with an idealized spherical high dose region is nearly as informative as a calculated dose distribution. The XKnife radiosurgery treatment planning system developed at Harvard by Kooy and colleagues and sold by RSA utilizes this type of visualization in a system optimized for interactivity, as shown in Figures 7.8 and 7.9. All regions of interest, both target and critical normal structures, are segmented and geometric models of them are generated. These models can then be manipulated rapidly in a high-quality shaded surface display to aid in identification of beam directions that are particularly favorable or unfavorable. Interactivity is maximized by limiting the complexity of the display, and the beam's-eye view targeting phase proceeds rapidly to generate beam configurations fully irradiating the target while avoiding normal structures. More elaborate

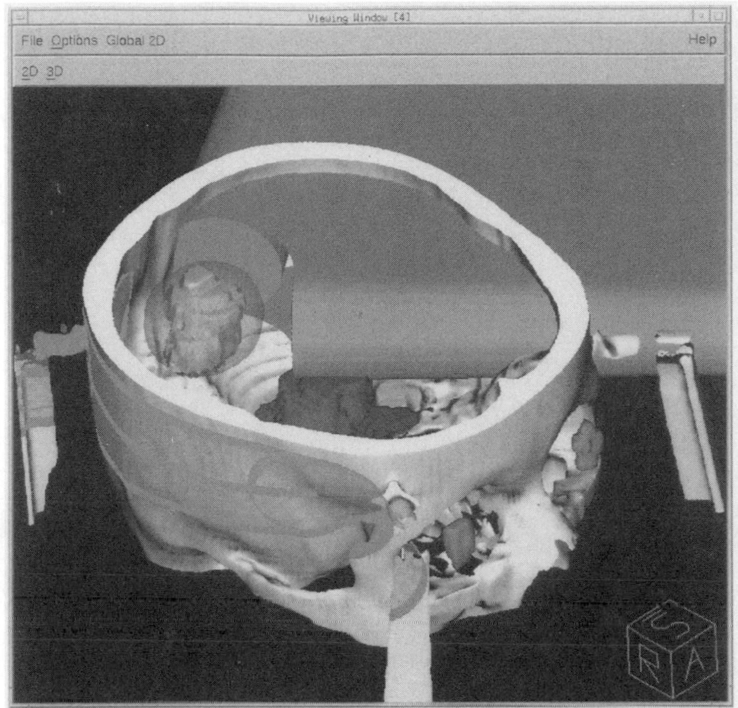

FIGURE 7.6 Example of visualization of several radiosurgery fields from the ADAC Pinnacle[3] treatment planning program (see text).

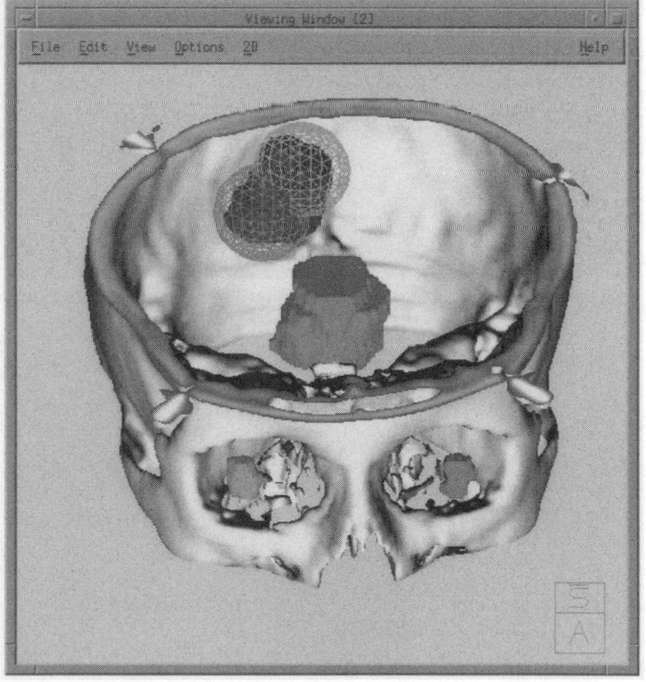

FIGURE 7.7 Visualization from Pinnacle[3] for a radiosurgery case incorporating both geometrically and volumetrically rendered components.

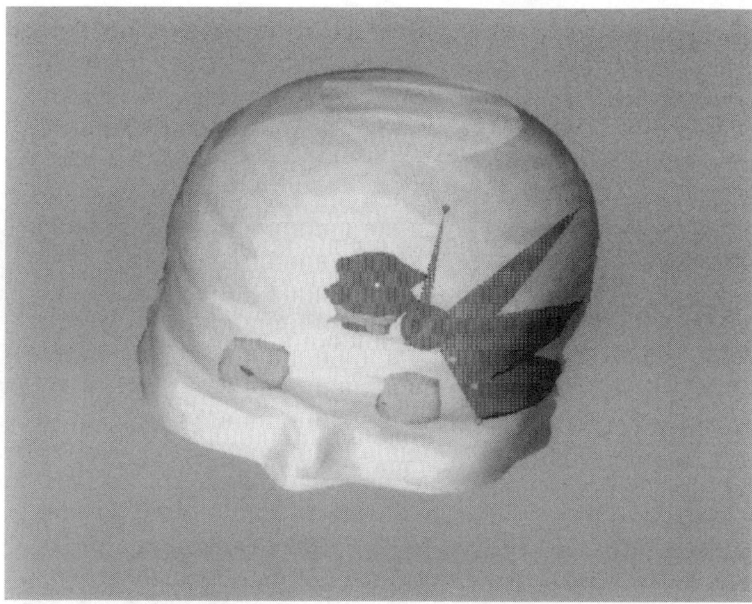

FIGURE 7.8 Display from the RSA's XKnife radiosurgery planning program. Simple geometric models of only the essential objects are used to maximize interactivity.

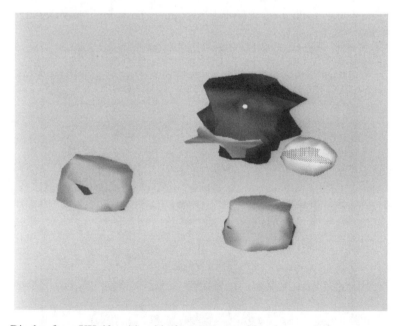

FIGURE 7.9 Display from XKnife with critical structures and iso-dose surfaces.

displays including reformatted CT data and calculated doses may be viewed outside the interactive beam's-eye view targeting procedure. In Figure 7.8 normal structure regions of interest are shown together with a sphere representing the idealized high dose region. In Figure 7.9 an iso-dose surface from a calculated dose distribution is included as a separate transparent surface.

Several groups have investigated the use of direct volume visualization in the virtual radiotherapy simulation process. Until quite recently, the computational demands for interactive visualization from extensive data sets such as those used in RTP have restricted the applicability of these techniques. Early studies using the Pixar with its ChapVolumes volume rendering library[15] were rather successful in diagnostic applications.[26–28] The Pixar's architecture was well optimized for volume rendering, and a high-quality rendered view could be produced from a full-resolution 3D data set in about a minute — not interactive by any means, but still in a tolerable range. Unfortunately, the system was best suited for production of orthographic rather than perspective projections, while perspective is essential for beam's-eye view targeting. Thus attempts to use the Pixar ChapVolumes system for RTP were not particularly successful. A very ambitious demonstration project at the University of North Carolina involved a high-speed network link among a virtual simulation workstation, a dedicated graphics supercomputer for volume rendering, and a supercomputer for dose computation.[29] Subsecond rendering times could be achieved with acceptable image quality, although widespread availability of such facilities seems unlikely. Texture mapping hardware capable of performing this type of rendering is readily available today from vendors such as Silicon Graphics, but not in inexpensive mass-market computers. Software-based volume rendering is more widely applicable, although it is far less interactive due to the considerable computational demands.[16] Considerable progress has been made in recent years in reducing the computation time for voxel-based rendering, and near-interactive performance (~1 s per view) is in fact possible at the current state of the art.[30,31] However, a composited volume rendering method that does not require an explicit segmentation step to define structures or classify voxels produces a rendered view which is itself only a 2D picture of a 3D scene rather than a picture of geometrically identified objects. Although 3D objects may be perceived in the scene, their coordinates in the 3D image space are neither required in order to produce the rendering nor directly available from it. Since accurate coordinate information is required for both radiation therapy planning (e.g., for calculation of dose-volume histograms) and delivery (for registration of virtual to physical space), this would appear to seriously limit the utility of direct 3D visualization in the RTP process. In fact, these methods do rely on assignment of visual attributes (color, opacity) to voxels based on their membership in interesting classes, and thus on an implied segmentation, albeit a probabilistic or fuzzy one. Udupa and Odhner[30] have taken advantage of this implied fuzzy segmentation to allow recovery of coordinates of points in the 3D image space most likely to represent structure boundaries. Grzeszczuk and Pelizzari[32,33] have recovered object coordinates through a z-buffer, which records for each pixel in a rendered view, the length from the viewpoint to the point at which the opacity integral along that ray exceeds a threshold. Combined with the known viewing transformations, this gives a reasonable approximation to the 3D voxel coordinate on the visible surface. Knowing these coordinates, it is possible to merge other information such as calculated dose with the rendered image, as in Figure 7.10. Furthermore, partial visible surfaces of a given object from several views may be combined to build a segmented model of the object; the volume-rendered images thus become a segmentation aid. An example of this is shown in Figure 7.11, where a contrast-infused spiral CT scan of a patient with a cerebral AVM has been used to produce several rendered views. On three of these views the visible surface of the AVM has been extracted and the three partial surfaces combined to aid in definition of the target volume.

As mentioned earlier, Sherouse, Chaney, and colleagues at North Carolina introduced the notion of virtual simulation, a logically separate 3D visualization step for the beam targeting phase of RTP, which replicates in software the functions traditionally performed with a radiotherapy simulator machine. In the virtual simulation process, beam's-eye view targeting is used to position radiation beams relative to a virtual patient model created from 3D CT and/or MRI image data. Target volumes and normal structures of interest are identified from the 3D image data, are used in beam's-eye view beam placement, and may be superimposed on calculated radiographs replicating those which would be made on the actual simulator. This ability to mix 3D information from image data with radiographs is one of several desirable features of virtual, as contrasted to conventional, simulation. A conventional simulation film depicts the anatomy irradiated by a given field with some certainty, but does not allow accurate assessment of how well structures seen in a

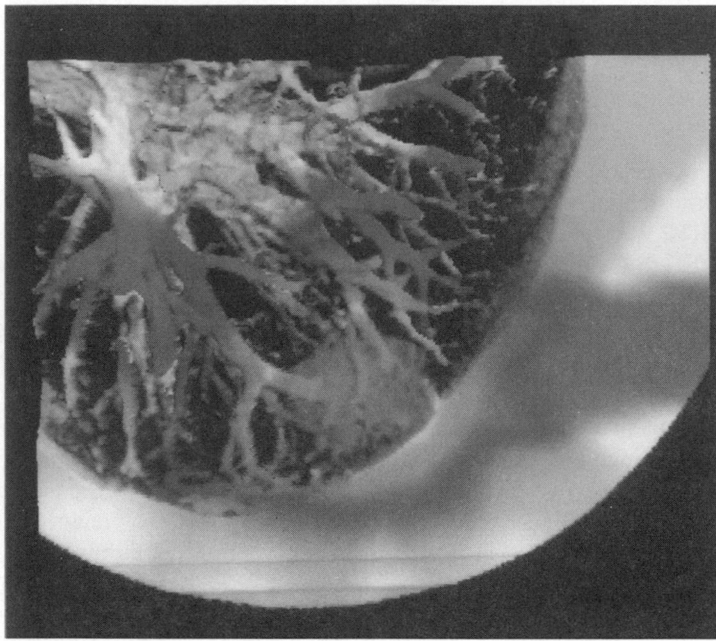

FIGURE 7.10 Volume-rendered view of a lung tumor from an inferior viewpoint. Using a z-buffer to retain 3D coordinates, color has been mapped onto each pixel according to calculated radiation dose for a five-field plan, from high (red) to low (blue).

3D image data set relate to the beam. Since the 3D image data is the source of the most accurate identification of both target and normal structures, it is of great interest to see the position of these structures within radiographs generated from each individual radiation beam. The UNC virtual simulator (Figure 7.3) provides this functionality, as do several RTP programs and other CT simulator programs, both commercial and non-commercial. One interesting feature of the Picker AcQSim CT simulator, illustrated in Figure 7.12, is the ability to compute not only beam's-eye view radiographs but also beam's-eye view volume renderings, using an opacity-weighted compositing algorithm quite similar to that used by Drebin, Grzeszczuk, and others. In the case of AcQSim, this compositing is performed in near real time using proprietary voxel processing hardware.[34]

7.4 DISCUSSION

Although use of beam's-eye view radiographs calculated from the CT data in principle allows more complete assessment of the involvement of tumor and normal structures in a beam, traditional radiographic simulation retains an important practical advantage. With conventional simulation, there is no question that the patient is actually irradiated as the radiograph demonstrates. With a calculated radiograph made from image data, there is no guarantee that when the patient is set up on a simulator or the treatment machine, the physical beam will intersect the patient exactly as the virtual one appears to do. In order to ensure that a calculated radiograph, or any beam's-eye view for that matter, accurately reflects beam delivery it is critical to control, or at a minimum to know, the transformation between the *image* coordinate system in which the virtual patient model exists and from which the beam's-eye view or calculated radiograph is made, and the *physical* coordinate system of the therapy machine. It is of course the relative position of the patient in these two coordinate systems that is important. The widespread use of CT simulators has resulted in a renewed recognition of the necessity to measure and/or control the patient position at each step of the

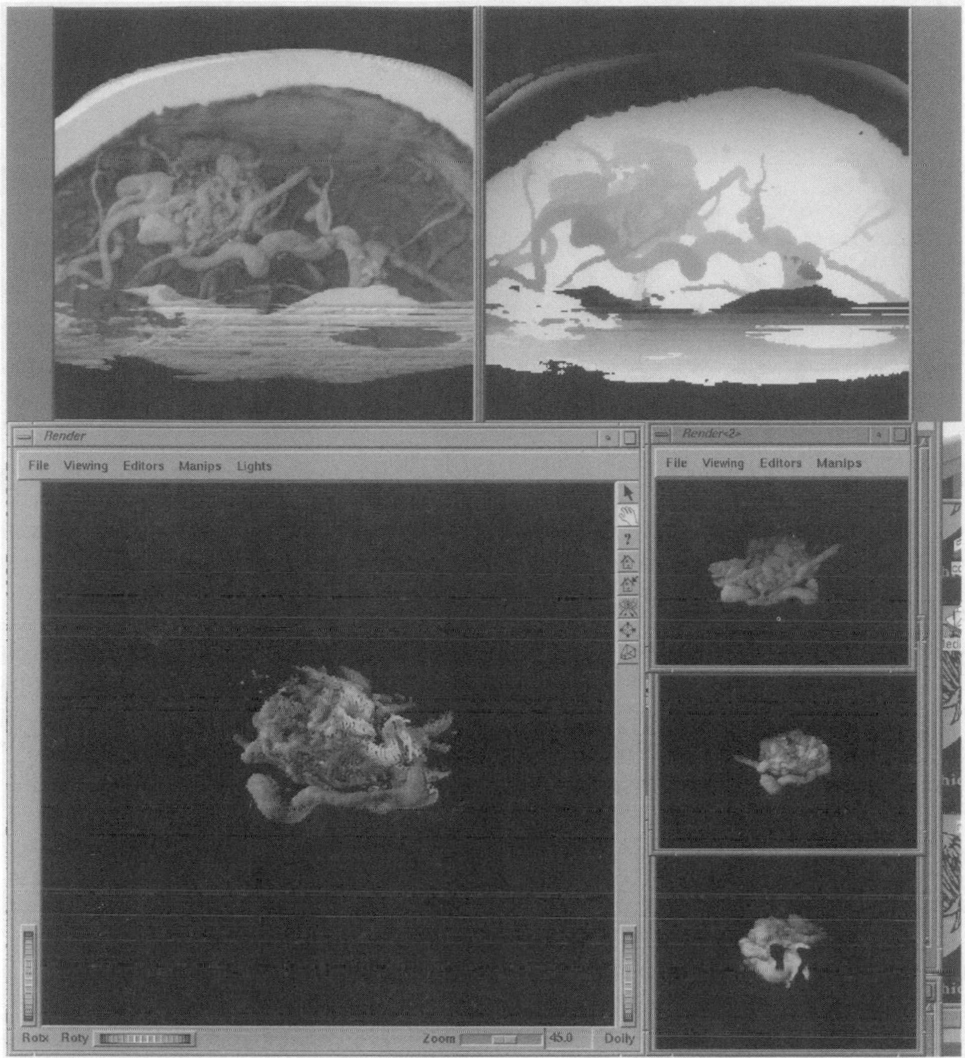

FIGURE 7.11 Example of 3D aided segmentation for a cerebral AVM. Rendered view (upper left) and corresponding z-buffer (upper right, darker = closer to viewpoint). Partial surfaces of the AVM (lower right) from the top view and two others have been combined into a single 3D target volume (lower left).

treatment planning and delivery procedure. There are two separate issues to be dealt with: localization and immobilization. By localization we mean that the patient is in the *correct position* relative to the treatment machine; that the physical beam is oriented relative to the physical patient just as the virtual beam was to the virtual patient. By immobilization we mean that once the patient is positioned on the treatment couch, he or she will remain in the *same position* throughout the treatment. Both of these conditions need to be met in order to maximize the irradiation of the target volume and minimize irradiation of non-target tissues. Historically, a single device such as a body cast or a stereotactic head frame has been used for both localization and immobilization. When the patient is tightly immobilized in the holding device, and the device is aligned with the treatment machine, one assumes that the patient is correctly positioned. Some investigators, notably the University of Florida radiosurgery group,[35] have advocated separating the immobilization and localization functions by arranging to measure the patient position after immobilization, and to make corrections if it is not within a specified tolerance of the correct position. A number of

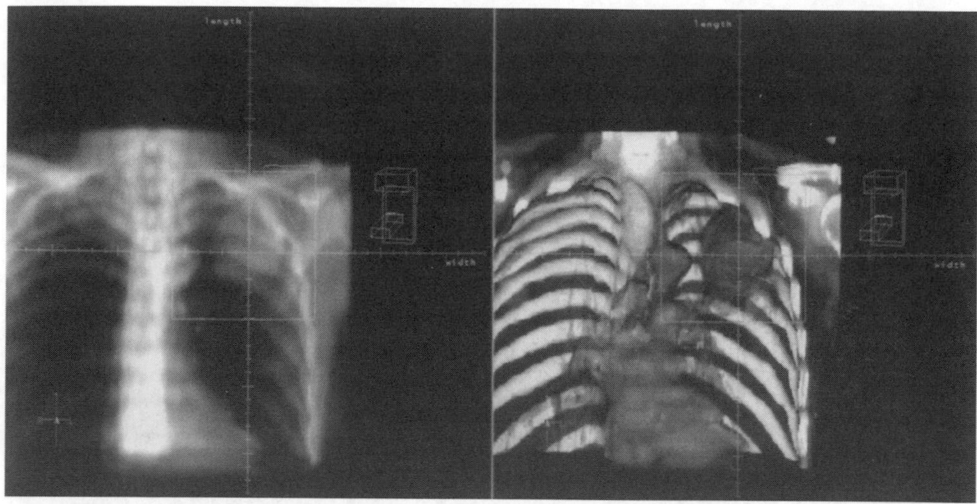

FIGURE 7.12 Example from AcQSim of digitally reconstructed radiograph (left) and volume rendering (right) of a lung tumor, from the same beam's-eye view.

possibilities exist for measuring the patient position in such a scheme; the Florida group has used a bite block instrumented with trackable LEDs to measure the position of fractionated radiosurgery patients, allowing adjustment of patient position well within 1 mm. Reliable measurement of patient position is more difficult in other areas of the body, but the recognition that immobilization and localization are separate and sometimes even conflicting requirements is an important one. As more precise targeting of beams is attempted in the continuing development of conformal radiotherapy, improvements in both areas will be required.

7.5 CONCLUSION

Presentation of patient anatomy in 3D views derived from image data is an important part of radiation therapy planning. For some purposes, segmented models of tumor and normal anatomic structures are needed; for example, in the calculation of tumor control and normal tissue complication probabilities by functional integration of dose distributions throughout the relevant volumes. Thus, significant time is spent in the treatment planning process in segmentation of tumor and normal structures from 3D image data sets. For other purposes, such as choosing beam entrance angles and aperture shapes to minimize irradiation of critical normal structures while fully irradiating target volumes, direct volume visualization without segmentation can be useful. Geometric optimization of beams and matching of multiple beam borders can be readily carried out using virtual simulation. Reliable registration of image-defined virtual space with the physical space of the simulator and treatment machine, which must be achieved within a few millimeters for each of thirty to forty fractions in a multi-week treatment, remains a challenging problem.

ACKNOWLEDGMENTS

We are grateful to Mark Gehring (Geometrix, Inc.), Colin Sims and Barry Werner (Picker International), and Michael Williams (Radionics) for images generated by their respective software systems, and to Frank Bova (University of Florida) for supplying the contrast-infused AVM brain CT. Thanks also to Ed Chaney and Tim Cullip (University of North Carolina) for providing the PlanUNC software and for valuable consultations on its installation and use.

REFERENCES

1. Fuks, Z., et al., Three-dimensional conformal treatment: a new frontier in radiation therapy, in *Important Advances in Oncology,* V.T. DeVita, S. Hellman, and S.A. Rosenberg, Editors. 1991: J.B. Lippincott, Philadelphia. p. 151–172.
2. ICRU, New ICRU dose specification for external radiotherapy. 50 : International Committee for Radiation Units and Measurements, 1993.
3. Kessler, M.L., et al., Integration of multimodality imaging data for radiotherapy treatment planning. *Int J Radiat Oncol Biol Phys,* 1991. 21: p. 1653–1667.
4. Thornton, A.F., et al., The clinical utility of magnetic resonance imaging in 3-dimensional treatment planning of brain neoplasms. *Int J Radiat Oncol Biol Phys,* 1992. 24: p. 767–775.
5. Phillips, M.H., et al., Image correlation of MRI and CT in treatment planning for radiosurgery of intracranial vascular malformations. *Int J Radiat Oncol Biol Phys,* 1991. 20: p. 881–889.
6. Schad, L.R., et al., Three dimensional image correlation of CT, MR, and PET studies in radiotherapy treatment planning of brain tumors. *J Comp Assisted Tomogr,* 1987. 11(6): p. 948–954.
7. Kramer, E.L. and M.E. Noz, CT-SPECT fusion for analysis of radiolabeled antibodies: applications in gastrointestinal and lung carcinoma. *Nucl Med Biol,* 1991. 18(1): p. 27–42.
8. Scott, A.M., et al., Clinical validation of SPECT and CT/MRI image registration in radiolabeled monoclonal antibody studies of colorectal carcinoma. *J Nucl Med,* 1994. 35: p. 1976–1983.
9. Holman, B.L., et al., Computer-assisted superimposition of magnetic resonance and high resolution Tc-99m HMPAO and TL-201 SPECT images of the brain. *J Nucl Med,* 1991. 32: p. 1478–1484.
10. Li, C., D.R. Spelbring, and G.T.Y. Chen, An analysis of image segmentation times for beam's eye view planning. *Med Dosim,* 1991. 8: p. 119–124.
11. Kalet, I., et al., Radiotherapy treatment planning tools first year progress report. Technical Report 90–91, 1990.
12. Tracton, G.S., et al. Medical anatomy segmentation kit: combining 2D and 3D segmentation methods to enhance functionality, in *Mathematical Methods in Medical Imaging.* 1994: SPIE, Bellingham, WA.
13. Myrianthopoulos, L.C., et al., Beam's eye view volumetrics: an aid in rapid treatment plan optimization. *Int J Radiat Oncol Biol Phys,* 1992. 23: p. 367–375.
14. Chen, G.T.Y., et al., The use of BEV volumetrics in the selection of non-coplanar portals. *Int J Radiat Oncol Biol Phys,* 1992. 23: p. 153–163.
15. Drebin, R.A., L. Carpenter, and P. Hanrahan, Volume rendering. *Comp Graphics,* 1988. 22: p. 65–74.
16. Pelizzari, C.A., et al., Volumetric visualization of anatomy for treatment planning. *Int J Radiat Oncol Biol Phys,* 1996. 34(1): p. 205–211.
17. Maciunas, R.L., ed. *Interactive Image-Guided Neurosurgery.* 1993: American Association of Neurological Surgeons, Park Ridge, IL.
18. Reinstein, L.E., et al., A computer-assisted three-dimensional treatment planning system. *Radiology,* 1978. 1217: p. 259–264.
19. McShan, D.L., et al., A computerized three-dimensional treatment planning system utilizing interactive colour graphics. *Br J Radiol,* 1979. 52: p. 478–481.
20. Goitein, M. and M. Abrams, Multidimensional treatment planning: I. Delineation of anatomy. *Int J Radiat Oncol Biol Phys,* 1983. 9: p. 777–787.
21. Goitein, M., et al., Multidimensional treatment planning: II. Beam's eye view, back projection, and projection through CT sections. *Int J Radiat Oncol Biol Phys,* 1983. 9: p. 789–797.
22. Sherouse, G.W., et al. Virtual simulation: concept and implementation, in *The Use of Computers in Radiation Therapy.* Bruinvis, I.A.D., van der Giessen, D.H., van Kleffens, H.J., and Whitkamper, F.W., Eds., 1987: North Holland, Amsterdam, p. 429–432.
23. Sherouse, G.W. and E.L. Chaney, The portable virtual simulator. *Int J Radiat Oncol Biol Phys,* 1991. 21: p. 475–482.
24. Gehring, M.A., et al., A three-dimensional volume visualization package applied to stereotactic radiosurgery treatment planning. *Int J Radiat Oncol Biol Phys,* 1991. 21: p. 491–500.
25. Bourland, J.D., J.J. Camp, and R.A. Robb. Volume rendering: application to static field conformal radiosurgery, in *Visualization in Biomedical Computing.* 1992: SPIE, Chapel Hill, NC.
26. Fishman, E.K., et al., Volumetric rendering techniques: applications for three-dimensional imaging of the hip. *Radiology,* 1987. 163: p. 737–738.

27. Levin, D.N., et al., The brain: integrated three-dimensional display of MR and PET images. *Radiology,* 1989. 172: p. 783–789.
28. Levin, D.N., X. Hu, K.K. Tan, et al., Surface of the brain: 3D MR images created with volume-rendering. *Radiology,* 1989. 171: p. 277–280.
29. Rosenman, J.G., et al., VISTAnet: interactive real-time calculation and display of 3D radiation dose: an application of gigabit networking. *Int J Radiat Oncol Biol Phys,* 1992. 25: p. 123–129.
30. Udupa, J.K. and D. Odhner, Shell rendering, *IEEE Computer Graphics and Applications*, 1993. 13: p. 58–67.
31. Lacroute, P. and M. Levoy. Fast volume rendering using a shear-warp factorization of the viewing transformation, in *SIGGRAPH '94*. 1994: ACM SIGGRAPH, Orlando, FL.
32. Pelizzari, C.A., et al., Interaction with 3D image data through volume rendered views. *Med Phys,* 1995. 22: p. 922 (abstract).
33. Grzeszczuk, R.P. and C.A. Pelizzari. Real-time merging of visible surfaces for display and segmentation, in *Visualization in Biomedical Computing*. 1996: Springer-Verlag, Berlin, p. 93–98.
34. Goldwasser, S.M., et al., Techniques for the rapid display and manipulation of 3-D biomedical data. *Comp Med Imaging Graph,* 1988. 12: p. 1–24.
35. Wichman, B., et al., Frameless stereotactic repeat fixation system. *Med Phys,* 1996. 23: p. 1167 (abstract).

8 3D Imaging: Musculoskeletal Applications

Elliot K. Fishman and Brian Kuszyk

CONTENTS

8.1 INTRODUCTION

The role of three-dimensional imaging has evolved over the past two decades. Three-dimensional imaging was initially hailed as a visualization technique to allow the surgeon to better understand complex anatomy in a more intuitive form than through a series of transaxial slices.[1–3] Although our clinical colleagues in orthopedics, plastic surgery, neurosurgery, and other subspecialties found the images to be of value, most radiologists felt the images were of little benefit and routinely did not provide three-dimensional imaging services in their hospital. Today our clinical colleagues more than ever are requesting three-dimensional imaging displays but still meet with resistance (or disinterest) at many sites. Yet changes are slowly occurring despite tradition, and 3D imaging is becoming a more widely available tool.

The ability to affect patient care and clinical decision making is the key to the successful integration of three-dimensional imaging into the radiology mainstream. However, changes are now occurring and are being driven by such diverse (yet in some ways similar) forces as computer networking, PACS systems, and the World Wide Web. The continuing decrease in systems hardware

0-8493-3179-X/00/$0.00+$.50

costs also suggests that more opportunity for diffusion of 3D workstations into the clinical environment including the operating room will occur.

The specific clinical applications where three-dimensional imaging is used will vary from institution to institution depending on the clinical workload and local expertise. Space does not allow us to address all of the applications but the more classic ones will be addressed. However, before we discuss applications let us review some of the principles of 3D imaging and what techniques are currently available.

8.2 CT SCANNING PROTOCOLS: THE ROLE OF SPIRAL CT

In the past, one of the most limiting features of three-dimensional imaging was the inability to obtain satisfactory data sets for rendering. This limitation was based on the compromise between the speed of data acquisition (8 to 10 single scans per minute), the length of the area to be scanned, and the ability of the patient to remain motionless during the examination. Although the latter issue was less of a problem in areas less prone to motion such as the knee and ankle, it posed significant problems in areas such as the shoulder, sternoclavicular joints, and pelvis where inadvertent motion or even uneven respiratory efforts could create artifact that limited the study quality or created potential artifacts that could lead to false positives or false negatives. These problems were compounded by the facts that in many cases these were trauma patients whose pain and discomfort made them less than ideal candidates to remain motionless during a 5- to 15-min period. In order to complete the examination as quickly as possible and still acquire a quality study, some compromise in terms of slice thickness and interscan spacing had to be made.

With the introduction of spiral CT many of these problems have been overcome.[4–6] Spiral CT provides second or subsecond slice acquisition, which in turn allows acquisition of the entire volume of data over a 24- to 50-s period, depending on the specific scanner make and model. Therefore, a study can use narrower collimation and still complete the examination in the period of a single patient breath hold. Additionally, since spiral CT is a true volume acquisition the postprocessing of the data set can be done at any interval down to 1 mm. The combination of narrow slice collimation (2 to 3 mm), close interscan reconstruction interval (1 to 3 mm), and lack of patient interscan or intrascan motion should be ideal for a three-dimensional imaging study (Table 8.1). An additional benefit of the spiral CT scan is the ability to image the vascular system in either the arterial or venous phase (or both) by carefully timing the contrast injection and data acquisition. This technique, referred to as CT angiography, can create angiographic-like images and in many applications replace the need for conventional angiography.

TABLE 8.1
Scanning Protocols for Musculoskeletal Imaging

Scan Parameters	Trauma: Large Part Scanning (i.e., acetabulum, pelvis)	Trauma: Small Part Scanning (i.e., wrist, ankle)	Soft-Tissue Mass	Infection
Time (sec)	.75–1.0	.75–1.0	.75–1.0	.75–1.0
mAs	250–300	250–300	250–300	250–300
kVp	120	120	120	120
Collimation (mm)	3	1.5–2	3–5	3–5
Pitch	1–1.6	1–1.5	1–2	1–2
Reconstruction interval	3	1	2–5	3–5
Algorithm	Standard or high resolution	High resolution	Standard	Standard
IV contrast	Yes/no	No	Yes	Yes

One of the initial limitations of spiral CT was the low mAs values (110 to 145 mAs), which were especially problematic in musculoskeletal imaging. However, advances in both tube technology and generator design have overcome these limitations and current mAs values for spiral and non-spiral studies are essentially equal. Typically, mAs settings for spiral CT are in the 250 to 320 range.

8.3 REAL-TIME INTERACTIVE THREE-DIMENSIONAL IMAGING

Interactive rendering has been possible for some time now, even on PCs, using software packages such as 3DVIEWNIX[7] via shell rendering techniques.[8] Interactive manipulation including peeling, cutting, separating, and mirroring has also been possible on such systems.[9,10] The introduction of the latest generation of workstations with specialized graphics engines has carried interaction between the user and the CT data set to an even higher level.[11] Previous 3D imaging systems required significant user time in steps ranging from data editing (e.g., disarticulation of the hip from the acetabulum) to creating the actual three-dimensional views. We previously did our three-dimensional imaging on a Pixar Image Computer (Pixar Inc., Richmond, CA) and a Sun Microsystems workstation (Sun Microsystems, Mountain View, CA).[12] Both of these were state-of-the-art imaging systems in the late 1980s and early 1990s. Our standard technique was to create video loops of 64 frames along a preselected axis, usually parallel or perpendicular to the patient. The creation of a single study would take between 20 and 45 min, depending on the number of scans in the study. Once a study was generated the user could view the images but had little ability to change the image parameters. However, the system's use of motion as well as the realistic (as well as accurate) nature of the images made it a valuable clinical tool.

During the subsequent years further developments in hardware led to capabilities that were possible to take advantage of in software. Computer systems with increasing capabilities were introduced by such leading hardware vendors as Silicon Graphics (Mountain View, CA), Hewlett Packard (Palo Alto, CA), and Sun Microsystems (Mountain View, CA). Besides decreasing the price from prior systems, the newer systems had increased capabilities. These newer systems, for example, could be programmed to provide a range of image reconstruction algorithms including shaded surface display, maximum intensity projection, and volume rendering.

We are currently using a Silicon Graphics workstation for all of our three-dimensional image reconstructions. The Onyx and Infinite Reality workstations provide a wide range of capabilities including real-time rendering, interactive volume rendering, and stereo display.[11] Running a custom-designed software package which was built upon the Silicon Graphics libraries and our prior work (Advanced Medical Imaging Laboratory, Department of Radiology, Johns Hopkins Hospital), we have found that we can interactively use sliding cut planes for image editing and that the complex and time-consuming editing tools of the past are no longer needed. Interactive three-dimensional rendering with the ability to interactively change the opacity and data look-up tables provides the radiologist with a variety of capabilities. The coupling of these newer technologic advances in computers with the better data sets of spiral CT have made a significant impact in making three-dimensional imaging a key part of a radiology department.

8.4 IMAGE RENDERING METHODS

Although a detailed discussion of the advantages and disadvantages of the various reconstruction algorithms is beyond the scope of this chapter, it is important to briefly comment on some of the basic concepts that must be considered in daily clinical practice. The three main image rendering methods that are classically used in imaging are shaded surface display, maximum intensity projection, and volume rendering. There has been much discussion in the literature as to the advantages and disadvantages of binary classification schemes and the relative advantages of volume rendering.[13–15] Nevertheless, most available workstations today provide only shaded surface display for the user and so this is probably the most common technique used. There are many segmentation approaches available in the literature (see Chapter 1) that provide a binary description of the objects in the image data. When a shaded surface display is employed to render these object descriptions, no matter how sophisticated the segmentation and surface display methods are, they cannot account for object graduations that are inherent in the original objects and that are captured in the acquired images. Maximum intensity projection is typically reserved for vascular imaging, where its results have been fairly successful. Our tendency is to use maximum intensity projection as a supplement to volume rendering in vascular imaging.

We currently exclusively use volume rendering for all of our orthopedic applications. Volume rendering, which is a percentage classification technique, provides an accurate display of data so that we can individually image soft tissue, muscle, and bone. The technique as implemented on newer workstations is interactive, which gets around many of the problems of the past for which the technique was relatively slow due to its complexity. We have found that volume rendering is very accurate and can detect fractures even when they are non-displaced. The potential for artifacts or false information is more easily avoided in the volume rendering technique. We feel that the flexible opacity gradients are particularly advantageous in orthopedic imaging, where bones of varying density are seen in a single scene. For example, in imaging the shoulder the humerus, clavicle, and scapula all are of different density. With volume rendering we can clearly show each bone in detail. With techniques such as thresholding and shaded surface display, attempts to make the humerus look good will make the scapula look too thin and have pseudoforamen within it. Several different thresholds may be needed to minimize this problem. Similarly, in order to show the scapula well the humerus and joint space may be inaccurately illustrated. The images that make up the clinical cases in this chapter are all done with volume rendering.

Even within volume rendering there are numerous techniques for its implementation. We have stayed fairly true to the technique as described by Drebin, Carpenter, and Hanrahan in their classic paper.[13] Multiple institutions are developing their own forms of volume rendering and the future will undoubtedly bring new and exciting algorithms that will increase the quality of our images.

The importance of imaging algorithms can never be overemphasized. It is important to remember that the radiologist and referring physician are looking at the final 3D images. If the 3D images are not of the quality expected based on the CT data set, then 3D imaging will never become a mainstream application. It is important therefore that the techniques used optimize the accuracy of the data set and present images with high fidelity.

8.5 STEREOSCOPIC VIEWING OF THREE-DIMENSIONAL CT DATA

Although the initial display for 3D CT data was select images on standard x-ray film, the value of viewing the 3D images interactively with motion has become the accepted mode of display for 3D data sets. In some systems the display may have had motion capabilities, but only minimal user interaction may have been provided because the motion was in a preselected “flight plan” in a set axis like the x or z axis. Current workstations provide absolute freedom for selection of 3D image plane or perspective, which allows one to more quickly and efficiently select a specific tissue plane or orientation. Newer workstations also provide stereo-ready monitors which can be used to enhance data display. One solution we have found helpful is to use stereo-ready monitors and a sequential electrostereoscopic system like CrystalEyes (StereoGraphics Corporation, San Rafael, CA). This system uses an infrared emitter to sequence the left and right eye image at around 120 frames per second. The technique is simple — so, for example, when the left stereo pair image is displayed the left lens is open and the right lens is closed. The technique also allows for multiple users to simultaneously view the data, which is valuable in the true clinical setting. Developments in display technology, including holography and virtual reality displays, may play a major role in the future of medical imaging.

8.6 CLINICAL APPLICATIONS

8.6.1 Pelvic Ring and Acetabulum: Trauma

Pelvic trauma is most commonly a result of a high-speed motor vehicle accident. The rapid evaluation of the pelvis is critical for patient triage and management. A full examination of the pelvis must also include evaluation of potential bladder and/or vascular injuries. Successful hemodynamic, neurologic, and orthopedic stabilization requires prompt, accurate, and non-invasive assessment. In the most severe cases, such as would be seen in a shock trauma center, the "golden hour" immediately following major trauma is the window of time in which medical intervention is most effective. This golden hour concept underscores the improved outcomes which can result from rapid diagnosis and treatment.

Previously, it has been demonstrated that three-dimensional imaging with motion display provided a comprehensive examination of the pelvic ring.[16–22] The combination of two-dimensional imaging including multiplanar reconstruction in the coronal and sagittal planes plus three-dimensional imaging provides a highly accurate examination regardless of the extent of pelvic injury. The more complicated injuries, including fracture with dislocation, combined femur and pelvic fracture, as well as concomitant injury to the lower spine, sacrum, and pelvis, will benefit most from a 3D study. In these studies the entire pelvis is examined interactively through a full range of views that would be impossible without the computer's assistance. The views that are routinely most helpful are the views from directly above and below the pelvis as well as split views of both hemipelvis from at least two projections laterally. Interactive editing is very helpful in these situations. Clinical studies have shown that the use of three-dimensional imaging can affect management in up to nearly 30% of cases of pelvic trauma, resulting in a change of the chosen management plan[16] (Figures 8.1 to 8.3).

Although most cases of bony trauma were previously evaluated without intravenous enhancement with iodinated contrast (i.e., Omnipaque-350 Nycomed Inc., Princeton, NJ) the use of spiral CT allows a true angiographic study of the pelvic vessels while the bony pelvis is being examined. If the CT scan shows active bleeding then the decision can be made quickly and accurately as to whether surgery or angiographic embolization is preferable.[23]

The combination of ever faster CT scanners and the trend to placing CT scanners in the emergency rooms of hospitals is a strong impetus for the use of CT imaging in the evaluation of skeletal trauma. The pure convenience of a nearby available scanner (i.e., no 15 to 60 min wait for an available scanner which might be located on the other side of the hospital) increases the use of CT for the evaluation of skeletal trauma. The use of a spiral CT scanner results in a motion-free study with data sets that are excellent for 3D imaging in less time then it normally takes to obtain a set of pelvic films and develop them. That even assumes that the plain films are of adequate quality and require no repeat images. With 3D systems being part of the scanners' software or workstations being an arm of the scanner, this area of imaging is likely to prosper and grow.

8.6.2 Non-Traumatic Pelvic Pathology

There are a number of non-traumatic uses for spiral three-dimensional imaging of the pelvis where information can be provided that is critical for patient management.[24–26] In the pediatric patient there are a number of specific applications for 3D imaging. These include the pre- and/or post-operative evaluation of the patient with congenital hip dislocation. In these cases, a short spiral CT scan at a low mAs value (decreased radiation dose) can define the success of surgical reduction. We also use three-dimensional imaging in patients with slipped capital femoral epiphysis to look at either the extent of original involvement or the post-operative result.

In the oncologic patient three-dimensional imaging has several potential roles (Figure 8.4). In the patient with a suspected metastasis, three-dimensional imaging can supplement the transaxial and multiplanar images to better define the true extent of disease prior to therapeutic intervention.

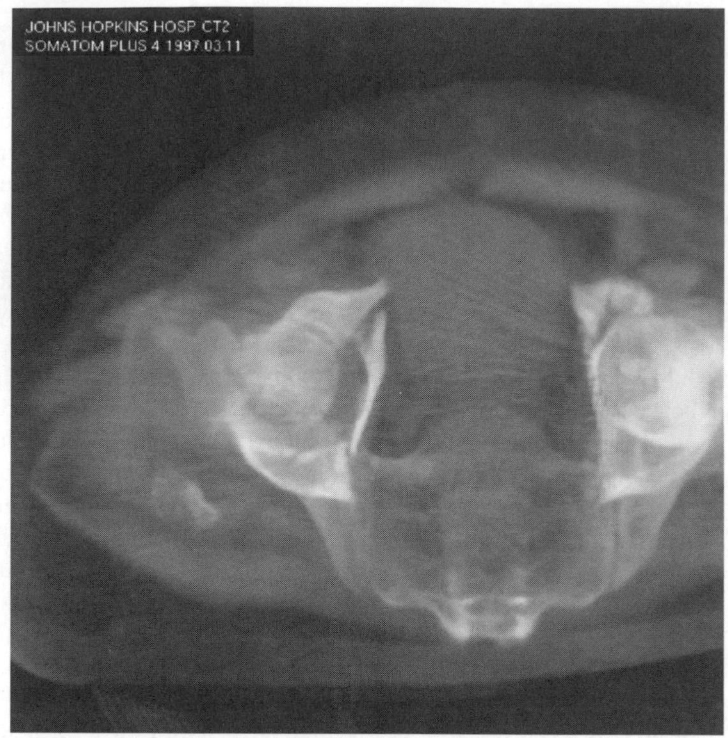

FIGURE 8.1A

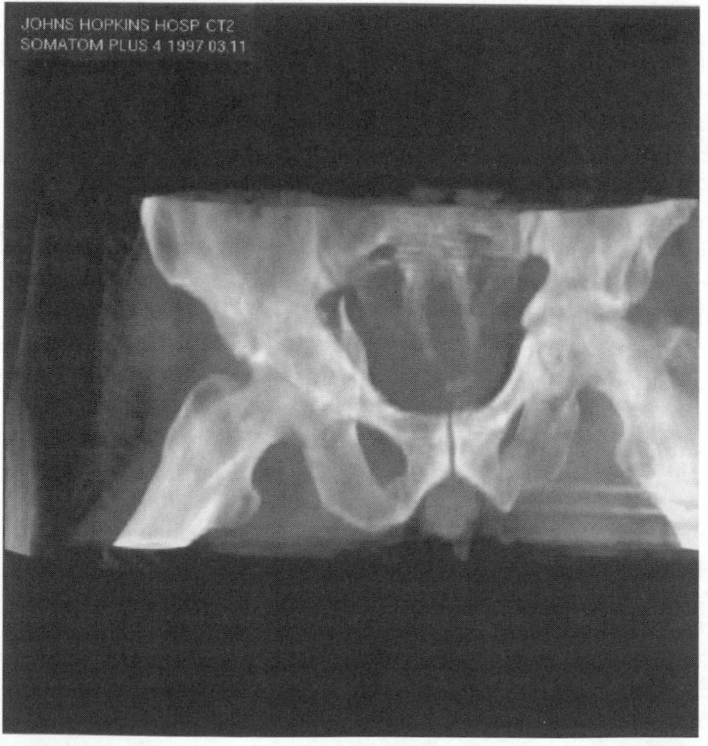

FIGURE 8.1B

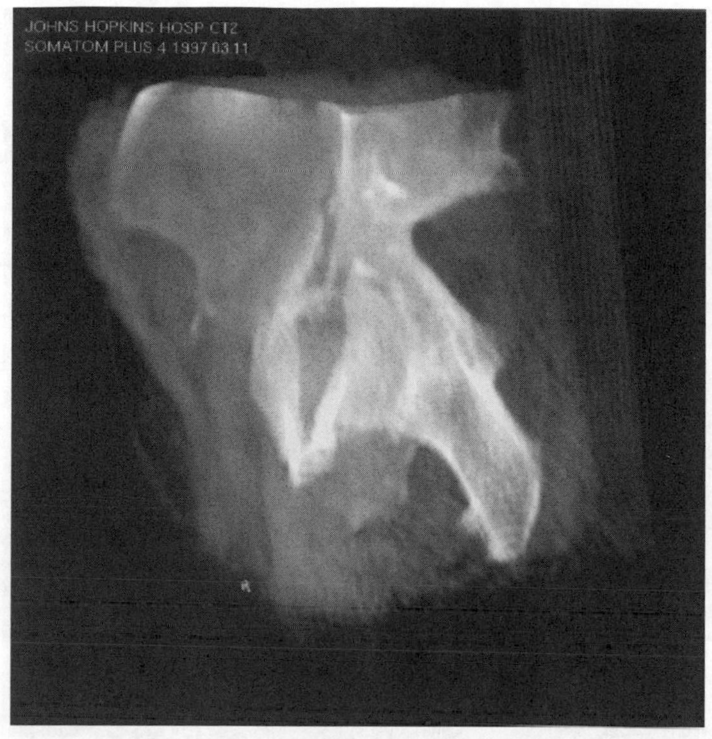

C

FIGURE 8.1 Three-dimensional views of acetabular fractures. The patient has evidence of acetabular fractures bilaterally. The study was done to identify the extent of the right fracture, and the images are focused on that area. A series of views from varying obliquities including inferior oblique (A), anterior-posterior (B), and cutaway lateral (C) pelvic view. They demonstrate that the right medial acetabular wall has been displaced superiorly and medially with multiple small fragments. The right femoral head has been impacted superiorly and medially. The left acetabular fracture with involvement of the medial wall is also noted but displacement on that side is minimal. This patient subsequently underwent open reduction with repair of the right acetabular joint space.

Volume rendering with a more transparent setting is especially valuable. Similarly, in patients with primary skeletal tumors, three-dimensional imaging may provide important information about extent of disease, including whether an attempt at surgical cure is even possible. We have found that the 3D volume images can give excellent representation of both the bony and muscle components of disease.

In patients with malignant tumors 3D imaging may be helpful in designing radiation therapy protocols. Many of the newer radiation therapy simulations include 3D capabilities for more accurate target planning. This may be especially helpful in areas where a toned-down therapy port is critical.

8.6.3 The Knee and Knee Joint

The knee joint is another anatomic zone where multiplanar reconstruction and three-dimensional imaging have been of clinical value in both diagnosing the extent of injury as well as deciding on therapeutic intervention.[27] Most of the pathology that we examine in the region of the knee is related to trauma. Occasionally we evaluate tumors for pre-operative planning, but the majority of cases revolve around trauma, most commonly to the tibial plateau or femoral condyles. In these cases the CT examination is done with narrow collimation to detect the presence of joint fragments

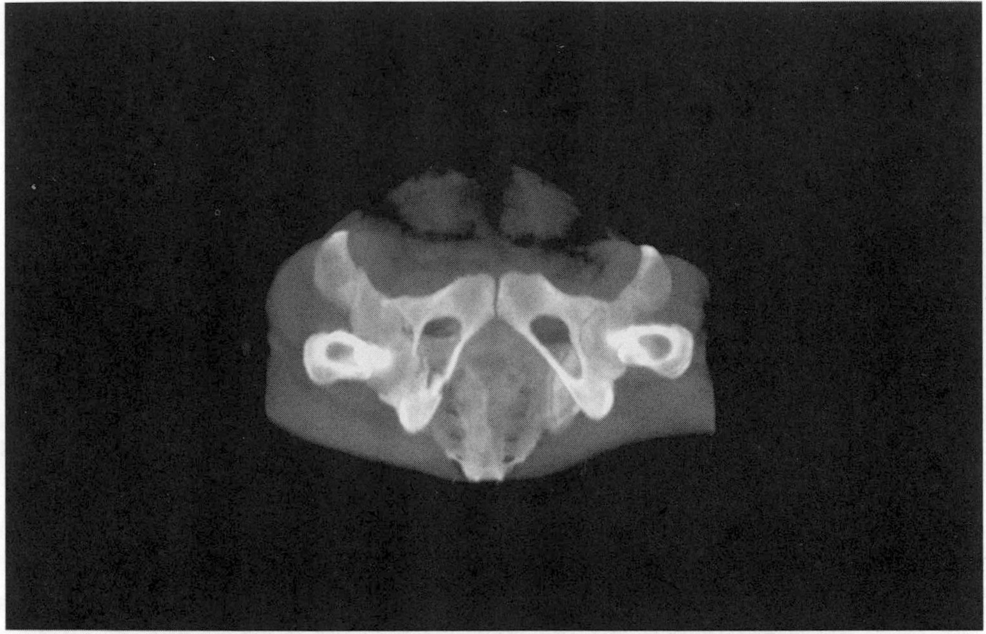

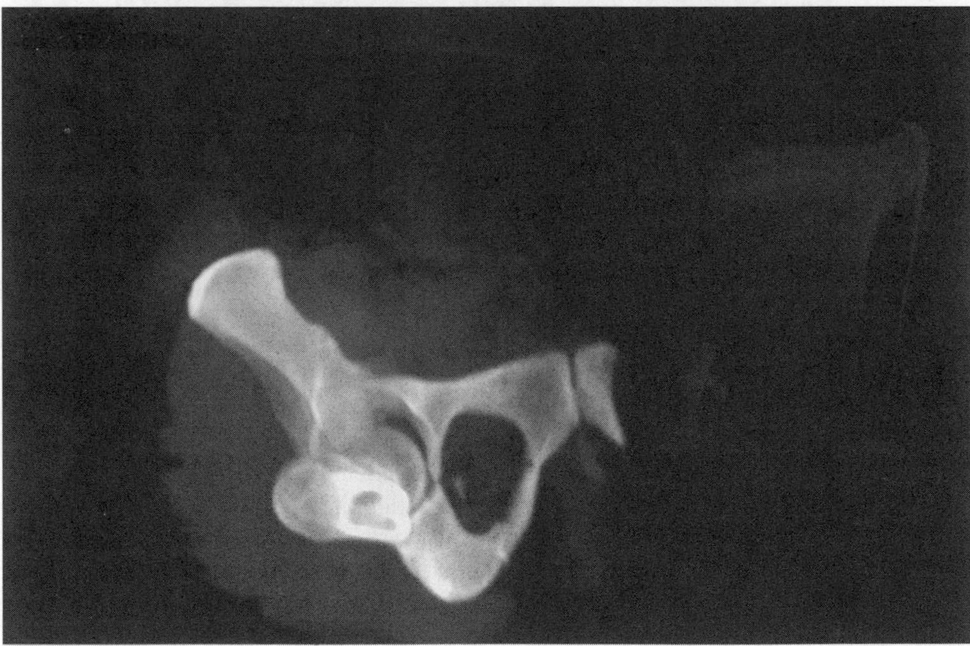

FIGURE 8.2 Fracture and dislocation of right hip and acetabulum. Three-dimensional images in select planes with the use of editing to define the orientation of a fracture of the posterior column of the right acetabulum with dislocation of the femur.

and extension of injury with involvement of the joint space. The lateral or sagittal views are especially important for determining the degree of downward displacement of bone in tibial plateau fractures (Figure 8.5). If the plateau is displaced more than 4 or 5 mm most orthopedic surgeons will feel that surgical intervention is necessary to repair the fracture to maintain joint function. Although plain radiography can often define the extent of injury, the multiplanar and 3D images tend to be best for defining the true displacement and orientation of fracture fragments that arise

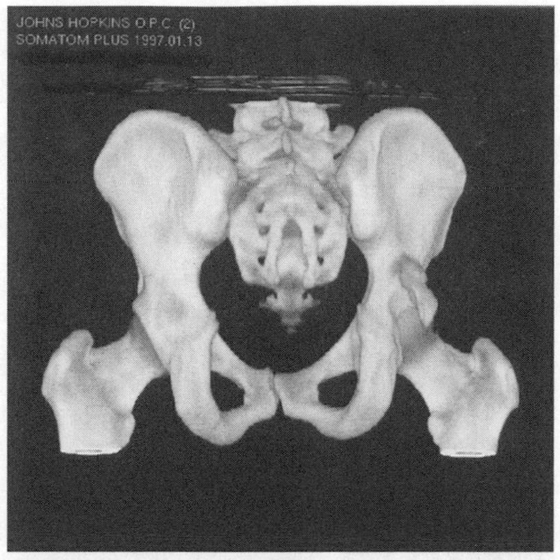

A

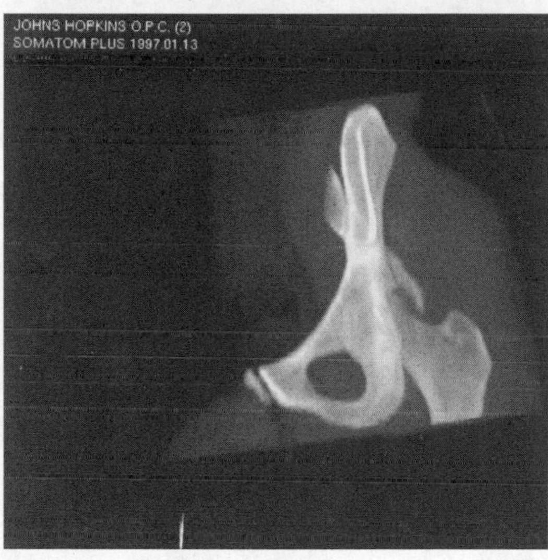

B

FIGURE 8.3 Missed posterior lip fracture with resultant repeated dislocations of the hip. The patient had several episodes of spontaneous dislocation of the hip several months after trauma. At the time of initial injury no evidence of acetabular fracture was seen. 3D reconstructions from posterior (A) and edited oblique (B) view demonstrate the posterior lip fracture. The major portion of the posterior acetabular wall has been displaced superior-laterally which would make the patient prone to posterior dislocations with only a minimal positional change. The ability to obtain varying opacities of bone with volume rendering is defined on this study. Undoubtedly a CT scan with 3D reconstructions earlier would have disclosed the initial fracture which was overlooked.

off the plateau.[27] Recent studies have suggested that MR is also very valuable in this area. Although this is undoubtedly true, one of the key advantages of multidimensional CT imaging is the speed with which a study can be performed. In our experience, the entire CT scan and reconstructive process will take less than 5 min, making it a very flexible examination, especially if the CT scanner is located in or in close proximity to the emergency room.

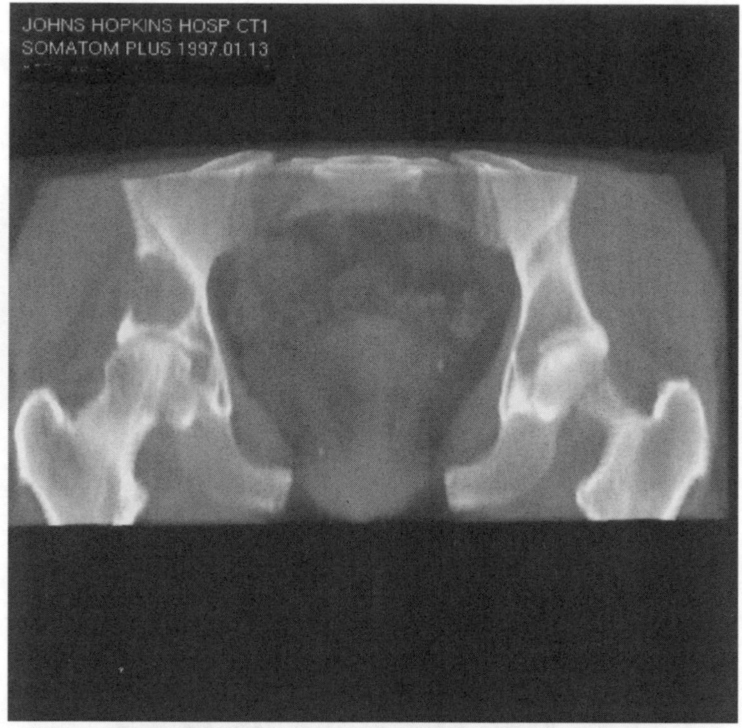

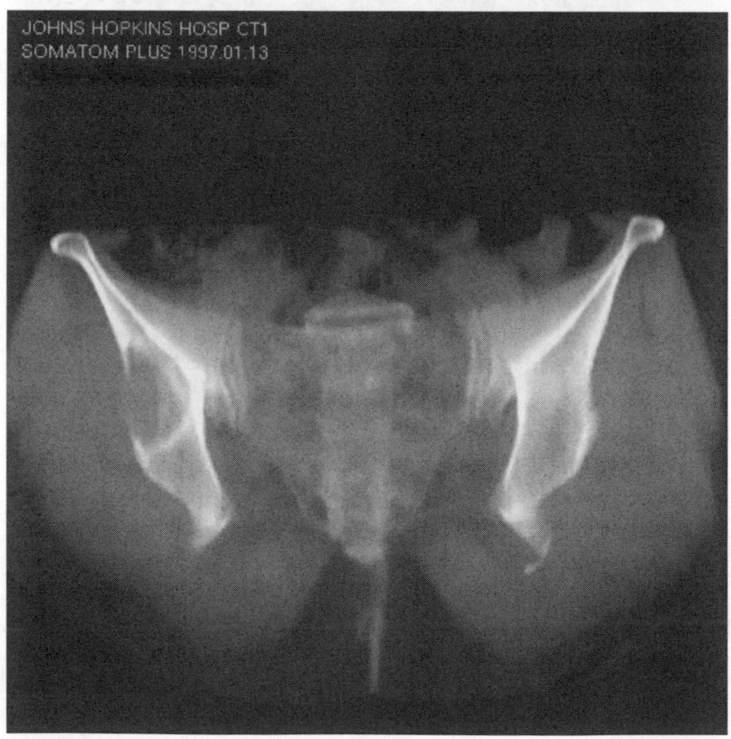

FIGURE 8.4 Metastasis to right iliac bone. The patient has a history of breast cancer and had hip pain. 3D reconstructions were done which demonstrated a large lytic lesion at the level of the right acetabulum extending to the joint surface. The full extent of the lesion and its relationship to the weight-bearing surface of the acetabulum is defined on these studies.

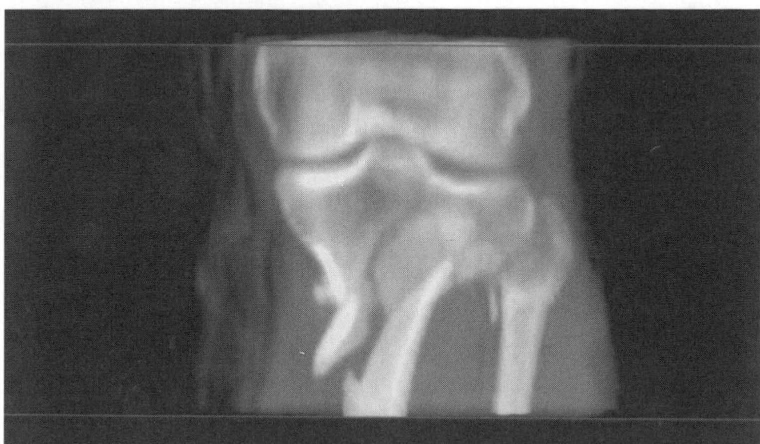

FIGURE 8.5 Tibial plateau fracture. 3D reconstructions demonstrate a spiral fracture of the tibial plateau. The fractural line extends up to the joint surface. Although the joint surface was not displaced downward, the spiral nature of the fracture is demonstrated with several small bony fragments seen. An incidental fibular fracture is also defined.

8.6.4 Ankle Fractures

The ankle, or the talocrural joint, is often involved in trauma.[28] Most fractures are produced by combinations of rotation with supination or pronation, with a minority produced by axial forces. Complete imaging assessment of the traumatized ankle must include evaluation of bony integrity, soft tissue and ligamentous structures, and the preservation or loss of normal spatial relationships between component parts. Even small tibio-talar shifts or alterations can significantly reduce the normal articular contact surface (Figure 8.6).

In evaluating pre- and post-reduction plain films of the ankle, one seeks clues to ligamentous integrity in the configuration of the mortise and the extent of displacement at fracture sites.

Transaxial CT has proven its superiority over plain film in demonstrating bone and soft-tissue trauma. CT, removing the element of superimposition-limiting plain films, often shows fractures either missed or underestimated by plain film and more precisely maps fragment displacement and rotation. Although CT cannot separate ligaments from adjacent soft tissue to the extent possible with MRI, it surpasses plain films at defining joint effusion, soft-tissue swelling, and tissue plane effacement, which may suggest the extent of trauma. It is also more sensitive to cortical disruptions or avulsions resulting from ligamentous or tendinous forces.

In the ankle, as in the tibial plateau or the vertebral disc and end plate, some of the primary structures of interest — the tibial plafond, the central portion of the mortise, and the talar dome — are horizontally oriented and therefore parallel the conventional plane of scanning. Therefore, although transaxial CT gives better bone and tissue detail than plain film, the addition of multiplanar reformatting (sagittal and coronal images) allows more precise demarcation of the anatomy in question.

Current scanners and workstations provide integration of all images — transaxial, coronal, and sagittal — on one screen, which, with the traveling cross-haired reference axes, allows precise localization and confirmation of findings from three perspectives.

In comparing CT to existing plain film parameters commonly used to assess fractures, we find that the plain film criteria do not necessarily translate directly to CT. We believe that the CT images give a more precise impression of displacement and rotation. The degree of apparent plain film displacement and distraction at a distal fibular fracture, for instance, is thought to be a good indicator of more distal tibio-fibular and fibular-talar disruption. Our CT experience has not supported this; we find the more distal joints often to be more stable than would be expected given the degree of more proximal loss of alignment.

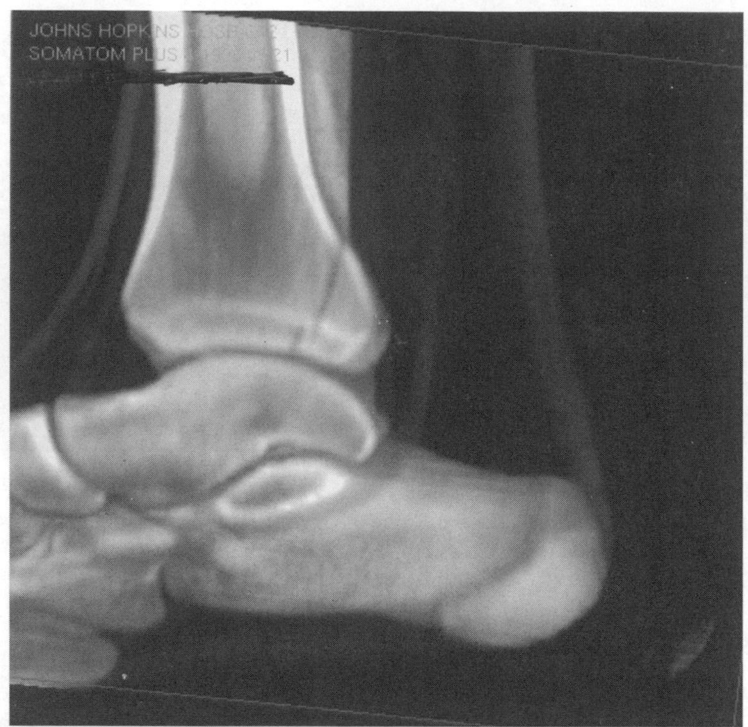

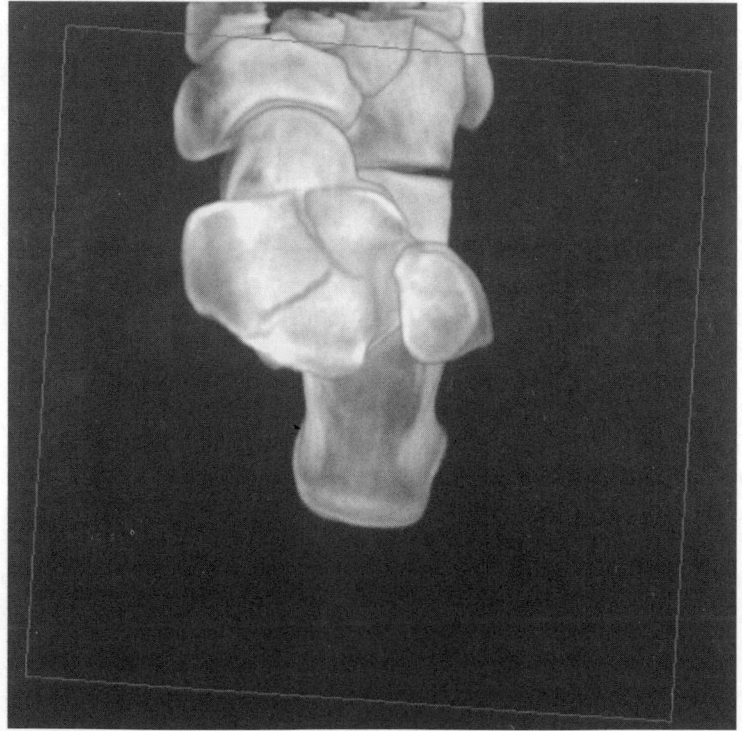

FIGURE 8.6 3D reconstructions demonstrate fracture of the tibia with the fracture line extending through the epiphyseal plate and to the joint surface. 3D reconstructions from cutaway views clearly define the full extent of the injury. This study demonstrates that the detail of fracture definition with even a minimally displaced portion of the fracture or non-displaced portion can be well defined.

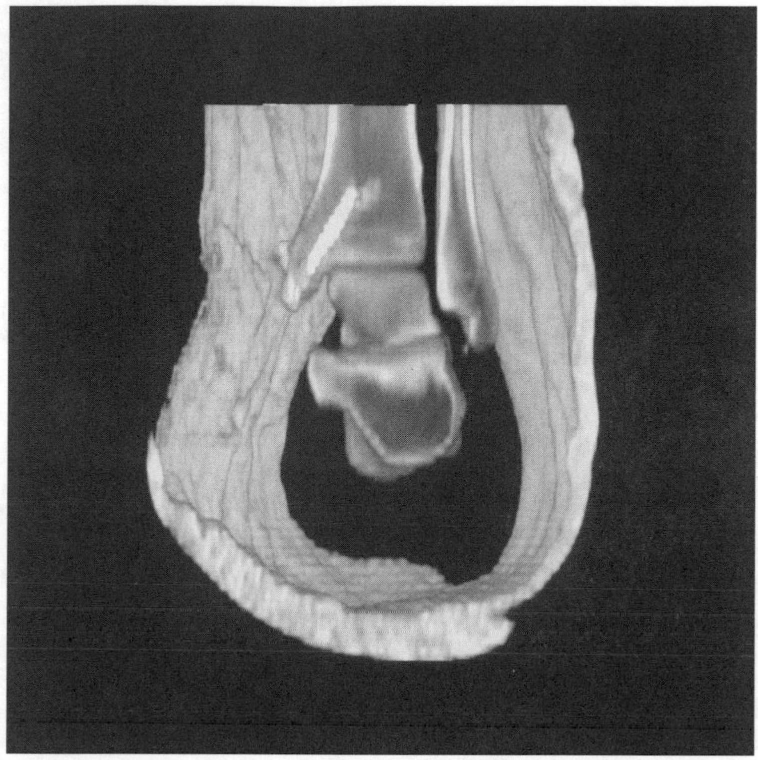

FIGURE 8.7 Tibial fracture with repair. 3D reconstructions demonstrate a screw through the medial malleolus of the tibia. This study was done in cast to determine if there was satisfactory joint space alignment. There is, and it is clearly defined on the study.

Preserving both sides for comparison allows us to evaluate the differences in several key measurements and angles which are commonly measured in and around the ankle joint. In our experience, differences in these indices between the injured and normal sides may be more useful than absolute values, which may not be useful in a given individual.[28]

The fractured posterior tibial lip must also be assessed for percent involvement of the articular surface, best done by reviewing sagittal and transaxial series together, and for determining the degree to which fracture distraction or displacement has created a gap or step-off in the articular surface.

Review of the coronal and sagittal series best identifies osteochondral defects or fractures involving the talar dome; we can also pinpoint any intra-articular fragments prior to surgery or arthroscopy. The true 3D images are useful in defining more globally the true extent of injury. They are especially valuable in cases of more complex injury including fracture with dislocation of the ankle mortise. Interactive 3D plane selection allows the visualization of the extent of injury without the need for cast removal. Cast removal had often been a serious time-consuming effort on some imaging systems, but with interactive editing it is a transparent process (Figure 8.7). Three-dimensional imaging is also valuable in the evaluation of calcaneal fractures, especially when surgical management is contemplated (Figure 8.8).

8.6.5 The Shoulder and Shoulder Joint

Routine radiographic evaluation of the shoulder and shoulder girdle is often limited by a number of technical factors, including poor patient positioning, improperly exposed radiographs, or overlapping shadows on the standard radiographic views. Routine transaxial CT scanning overcomes

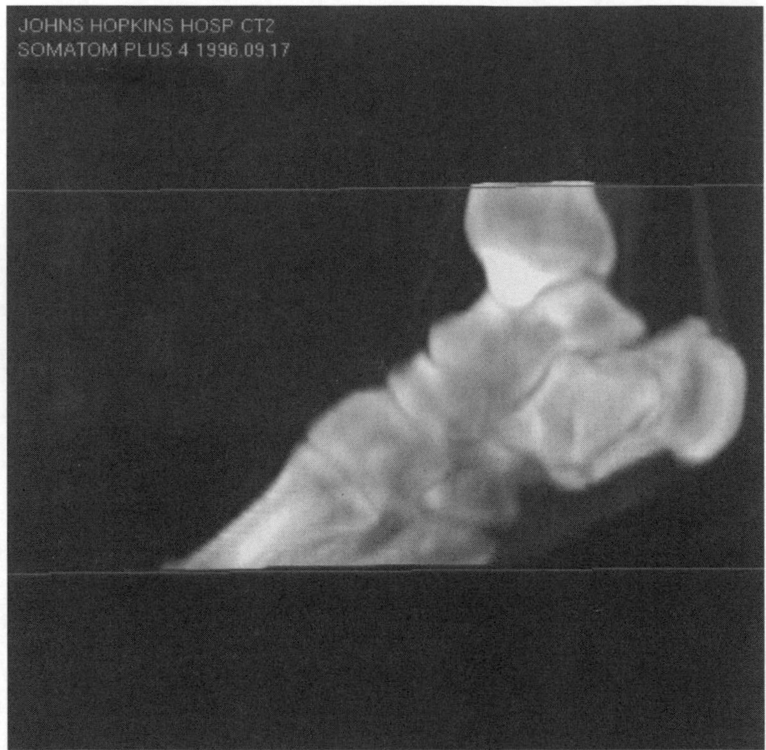

FIGURE 8.8 Calcaneal fracture. 3D reconstructions demonstrate a comminuted fracture of the calcaneus. The lateral oblique view demonstrates a loss of height in the calcaneal surface as well as the multiple fracture lines, particularly in the anterior and midportions of the calcaneus.

many of these limitations by requiring less patient cooperation, providing a more optimal view without overlapping radiographic lines, and the ability to visualize soft tissue and bone. 3D CT provides an even more comprehensive visualization of this area.[29,30]

The clinical problems for which 3D CT of the shoulder have proven valuable include acute trauma, acute or chronic dislocations, suspected scapular injuries, and evaluation of axillary masses. In all cases, the spiral CT imaging technique is used. This helps eliminate problems with respiratory motion. Sections 3 mm thick are usually satisfactory in these cases. We prefer to reconstruct the data at 2-mm intervals.

The ability to disarticulate the scapula, sternum, or humerus in 3D CT images helps to optimize the information generated in any individual case. We have found it particularly valuable to edit the scapula off the chest wall and visualize it directly. Scapular fractures are easily missed on routine radiographs, because of overlapping structures, which can be eliminated from view with edited 3D views. The value of volume rendering is particularly well demonstrated in imaging the scapula. The body of the scapula is often paper-thin, yet the acromion and glenoid are of thicker bone. The 3D images generated are able to simultaneously show features of both of these areas.

The major clinical use of 3D of the shoulder has been in trauma. The presence and extent of a fracture, as well as the presence or absence of an associated dislocation, are best demonstrated on 3D images. Associated injuries to the sternum and clavicle or sternoclavicular joint can be imaged at the same time. Sternoclavicular injuries are well demonstrated on z axis rotations. This display projects the sternum/clavicle relationship from directly above and below, optimizing the detection of even the most subtle dislocation. Edited x axis views are obtained to define the extent of humeral injury. Usually the humeral head need not be disarticulated from the glenoid cavity for an adequate evaluation. However, when joint fragments are suspected from the transaxial images

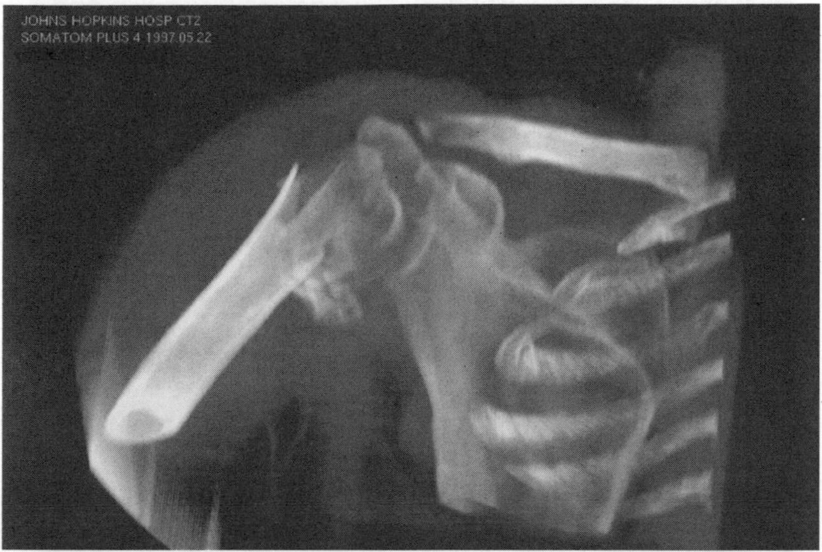

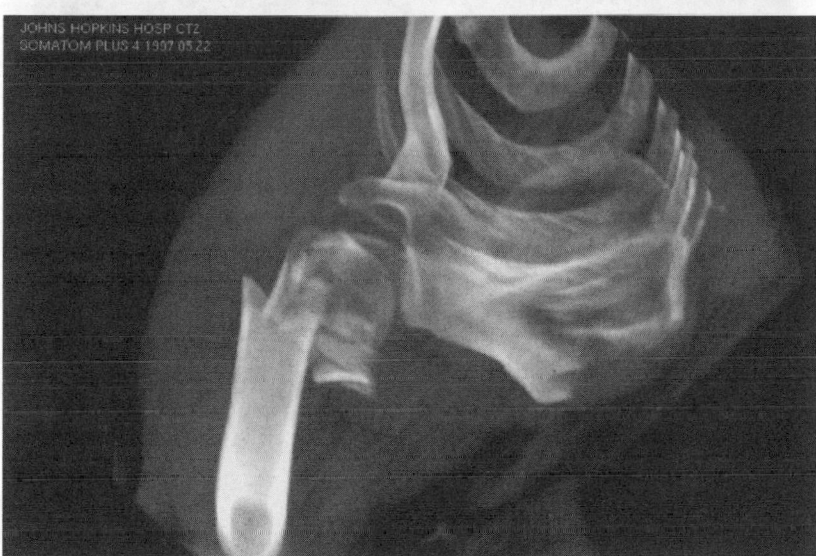

FIGURE 8.9 Comminuted humeral head fracture. The selected 3D views demonstrate the true extent of the fracture as well as the integrity of the joint space. The angulation and orientation of the fracture fragments are well defined.

or the fracture appears to extend medially, then disarticulation is advised. 3D reconstructions with a high degree of transparency is particularly helpful in these cases. The presence or absence of a dislocation is best seen on the z axis views (Figure 8.9).

Although most trauma cases require bone reconstructions only, 3D reconstructions of the soft tissue and muscle are helpful in other cases. Patients with a clinically palpable mass or with symptoms related to a suspected mass in the region of the neurovascular bundle are ideal candidates for 3D imaging. The presence and extent of a mass can be well documented for further therapeutic intervention. As 3D images of the soft tissues and internal organs improve, evaluation of the axilla and brachial plexus may become an important clinical indication for study (Figure 8.10).

Similarly, in cases of musculoskeletal infection 3D imaging may be of value in determining muscle, soft-tissue, and skeletal involvement.[31] We have found this especially valuable in

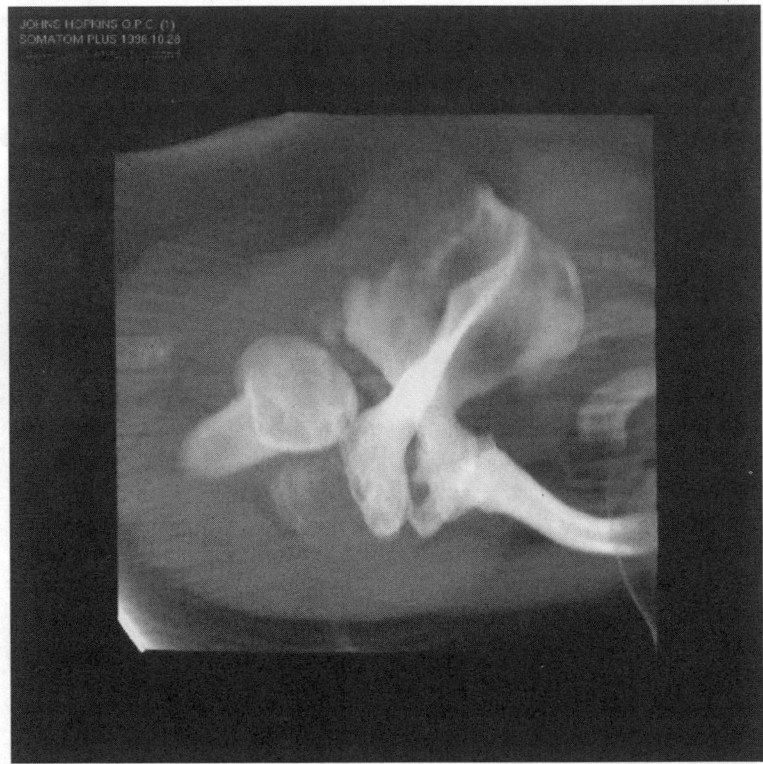

FIGURE 8.10 Charcot's joint. 3D reconstructions demonstrate a markedly deformed humeral head and a lack of clearly defined glenoid process. Multiple small bony fragments are seen in the region of the joint space. This was due to a Charcot's joint.

diagnosing IV drug abusers with infection near the sternoclavicular joint. The involvement of the sternoclavicular joint as well as the bony sternum or clavicle is especially useful in pre-operative planning.

8.6.6 Spine

3D reconstruction has found a number of successful applications in the evaluation of the spinal column.[32–35] The major areas of use include trauma, oncology, infectious etiologies, and degenerative disease. MRI is especially useful in determining cord compression or involvement and may be an adjunct to the 3D CT exam.

In the traumatized patient the presence and extent of the fracture is important. Although in most cases the routine transaxial views are sufficient for the detection of a fracture, its true extent is best documented on a 2D or 3D display. The 2D display is especially helpful in the detection and definition of small bone fragments which may extend into the spinal canal. Associated hematomas either in an extradural location or in the paraspinal zones are best seen on the transaxial CT slices or on reformatted coronal/sagittal planes. An interactive 2D display is especially useful in the sacrum, where an oblique reconstruction along the major plane of the sacrum presents the foramen in an end-on appearance. This allows one to evaluate foraminal involvement in trauma or neoplastic involvement. Three-dimensional images can also be helpful in defining these planes.

The 3D images can be useful in the spine by providing visualization of overlapping structures to the orthopedic surgeon, neurologist, or neurosurgeon. The clinical applications include the following.

8.6.6.1 Trauma

Although most instances of spinal trauma are vividly displayed on transaxial CT, the use of multiplanar and 3D imaging can help with the more difficult cases. Unusual lines created by congenital variations, poor patient positioning, or unusual fractures are often best explained on the reformatted views. These views are also of special value in patients with prior surgery with pins or plates in place and the resultant artifacts.

The 3D presentation is especially helpful in evaluating encroachment on the spinal canal, neural foramina, or adjacent joint spaces. To optimize these findings the use of edited 3D views is encouraged. The neural foramina are particularly well seen when the spine is cut in half along a sagittal plane. This view also allows for a full evaluation of the texture of the vertebral bodies if 3D reconstruction is done with volume rendering. Several authors have suggested that 3D reconstruction can determine whether there is proper union following spinal fusion or detect unsuspected fractures where plain CT is negative.[36] However, these ideas should be viewed with some skepticism on several grounds. There has been no proof that thresholded images can accurately detect subtle fractures or define fusion. In fact, information to the contrary exists. Drebin et al. have shown that thresholded images cannot accurately detect small fractures or define cranial sutures.[22] Observer bias with subsequent choices of threshold level can produce the wrong results. Several papers have suggested that 3D images created with percentage classification and volume rendering can be correct in these areas. Our experience with phantoms bears out our conclusions.[22] Although classification parameters and opacity values undoubtedly affect the accuracy of fracture detection with the percentage classification technique and volume rendering, no studies have been done to define optimal values of these parameters.

8.6.6.2 Tumors

A combination of 2D and 3D images is helpful in determining the extent of primary and malignant tumors. Transaxial CTs are often obtained to help in difficult cases where clinical exam, plain X-rays, or bone scan are equivocal or contradictory. Detection of the extent of a destructive lesion as well as the presence or absence of an associated mass can be made with the routine scans. The 3D image adds a better understanding of the extent of a lesion, especially when two or more vertebrae segments are involved. The full 3D display can also prove useful in the construction of radiation therapy portals. We have found the 3D reconstructions especially valuable in cases where sacral involvement is present (Figures 8.11 to 8.13).

8.6.6.3 Infection

Infection of the spine or disc space by hematogenous or direct means is an uncommon phenomenon. Tuberculous involvement of the spine (Pott's disease) is now a rare presentation. However, in those cases with osteomyelitis 3D display can help define the extent of involvement and be used for pre-operative planning. The rise in the immunosuppressed population as well as drug abuse have led to an increase in spinal infection in our clinical practice. In these cases CT scanning must be done to try to define real or potential cord involvement.

8.6.7 Craniofacial

One of the first areas analyzed in detail with 3D imaging was the craniofacial region and skull.[2,37,38] Some of the more common uses include evaluation of craniofacial trauma as well as pre-operative evaluation of craniofacial anomalies, orbital tumors, and tumors and inflammatory disease of the sinuses.

The images are a valuable adjunct to the surgeon by allowing him or her to precisely visualize the abnormality to be corrected at operation. The surgeon could use the images created as a template

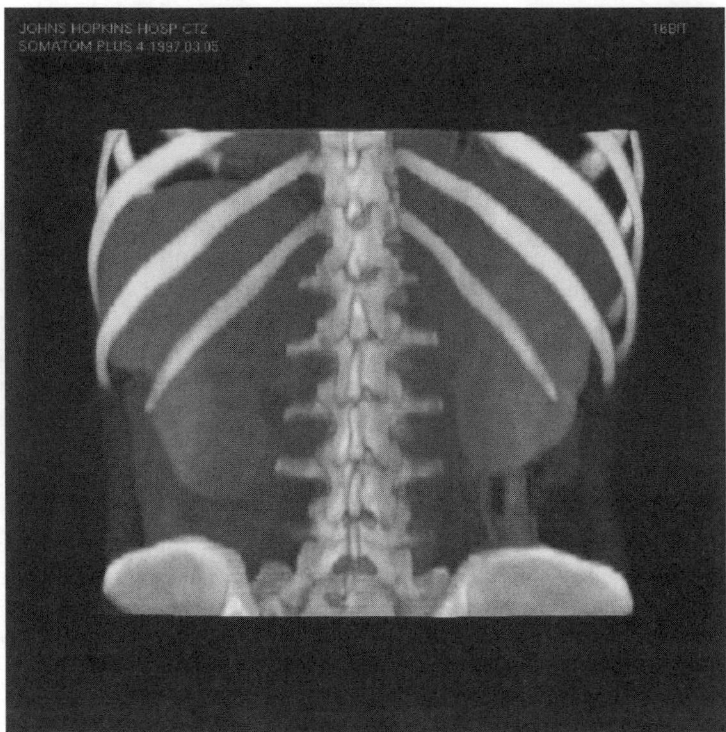

FIGURE 8.11 Normal lumbar spine. 3D reconstructions were done for evaluation of possible trauma to the lumbar spine. Notice the excellent detail of the posterior elements and spinous processes seen on these 3D reconstructions.

for surgical planning and rehearsal. 3D CT has been most helpful in complex congenital anomalies such as Apert's syndrome and Crouzon's syndrome.

Images of the skull can be generated with either opaque or transparent bone, depending on the clinical problem being evaluated. We have found transparent bone most valuable in visualizing pathology of the sinuses, mastoids, and orbits. An opaque bone reconstruction is most helpful around the zygomatic arches and the mandible. The use of intravenous contrast is helpful in defining vascular anatomy, which may eliminate the need for conventional angiography in select cases (Figures 8.14 and 8.15).

8.6.8 Muscle and Soft Tissue

Although most of the work on 3D orthopedic imaging has been on reconstruction of bony structures, advances in computer software now allow for high-quality displays of soft-tissue structures.[39,40] This ability opens up a wide range of new potential applications of 3D imaging in such varied areas as evaluation of soft-tissue tumors, plastic surgery, radiation therapy planning, surgical simulation, and correlative imaging (simultaneous data display of CT and/or MRI and/or PET data).

The detection, definition, and display of a soft-tissue or muscular mass is important in determining the optimal management of the individual patient (Figure 8.16). The extent of a tumor, its relationship to adjacent bone or muscle, as well as its vascularity are all important pieces of information. We have used 3D imaging, combined with a review of the transaxial and 2D data, for defining the extent of a planned surgery.

Evaluation of the chest wall and axilla is especially important in the patient with a history of breast cancer. Tumor recurrence is common in the axilla, occurring most commonly around the

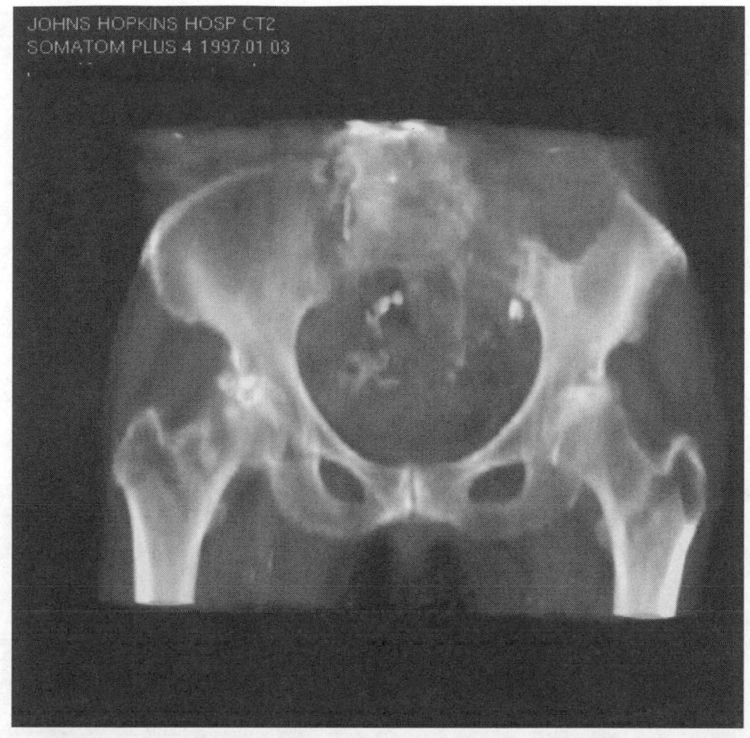

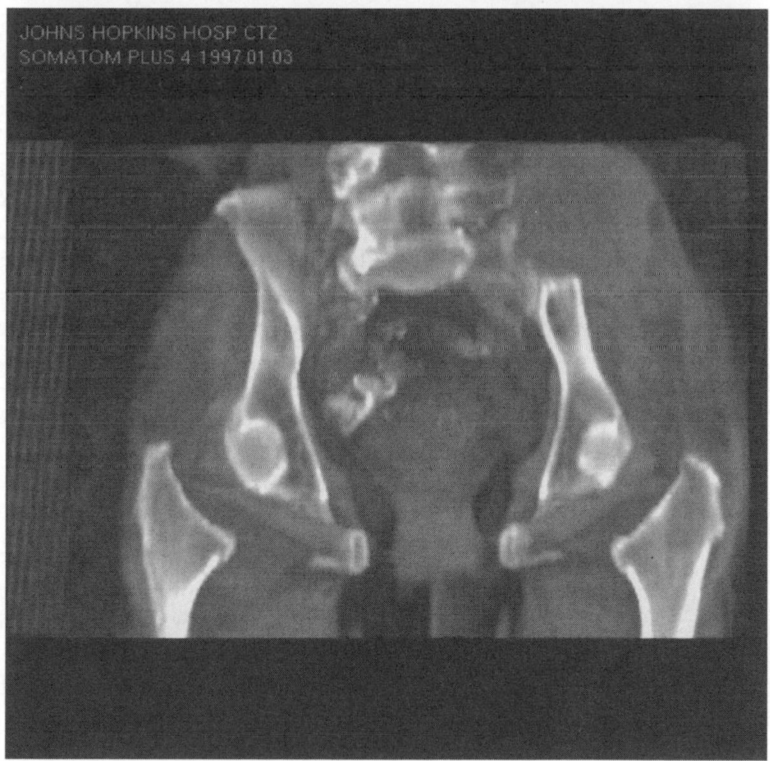

FIGURE 8.12 Three-dimensional reconstruction of a lytic lesion with soft-tissue mass arising off the left iliac crest. This lesion was a plasmacytoma. Extension to and involvement of the sacrum was also seen on this study.

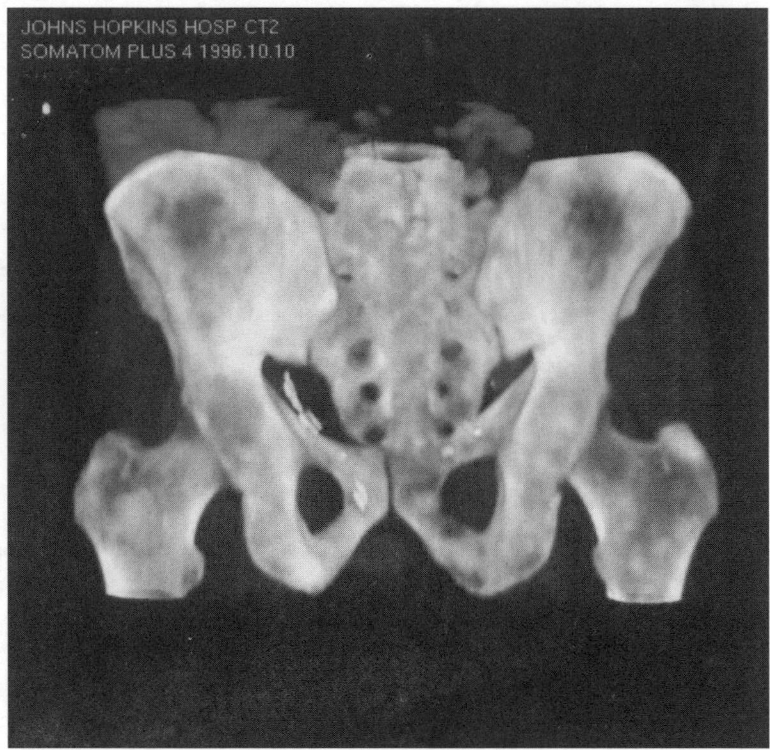

FIGURE 8.13 Prostate cancer and blastic bone metastasis. 3D reconstructions demonstrate multiple blastic lesions throughout the bony pelvis including the ileac wings, sacrum, and bilateral femurs. Note that in volume rendering the clear definition of sclerotic lesions can be seen due to the correct use of opacity.

region of the axillary and vein (near neuromuscular bundle). Other common areas of recurrence are in the chest wall, the internal mammary nodal region, and the supraclavicular nodes.

The detection of recurrence may be difficult to distinguish from postsurgical scarring or fibrosis, particularly when viewing only transaxial images. A multidimensional display with 2D and 3D images can better define the normal anatomy and extent of disease. These images can then be used as a basis for surgical resection or radiation therapy planning. Three-dimensional imaging may also prove useful in the evaluation of soft-tissue infection, mainly in helping to plan therapy. The extent of involvement can help determine whether percutaneous drainage or open drainage will need to be done. Once again, the use of CT angiography can be helpful in these cases.

8.7 CONCLUSION

This chapter has attempted to review some of the more common clinical applications of 3D musculoskeletal imaging (Figures 8.17 and 8.18). With increased user sophistication, improvements in computer hardware and software, as well as a close collaboration with our clinical colleagues, new and more sophisticated applications continue to develop. The use of 3D CT as both a diagnostic and therapeutic imaging study will undoubtedly prosper in the years to come.

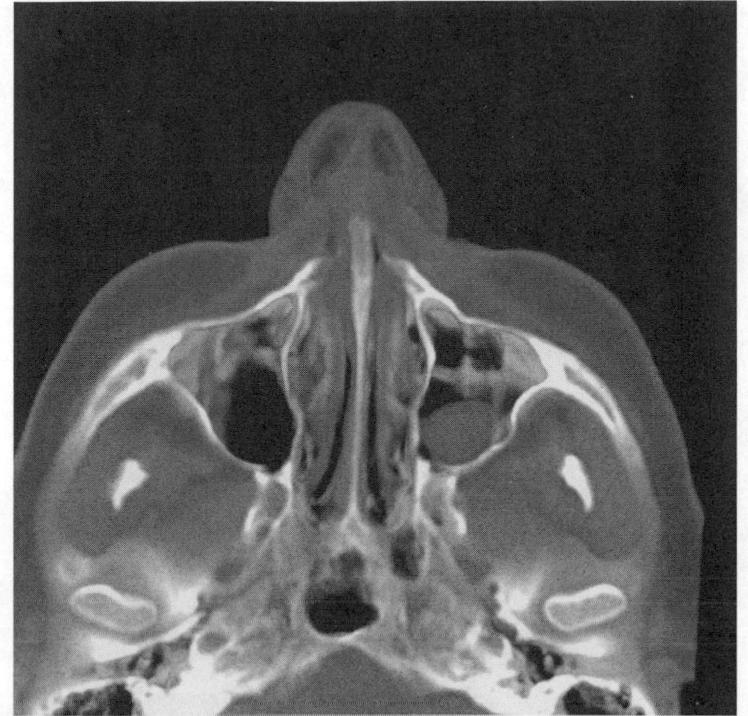

A

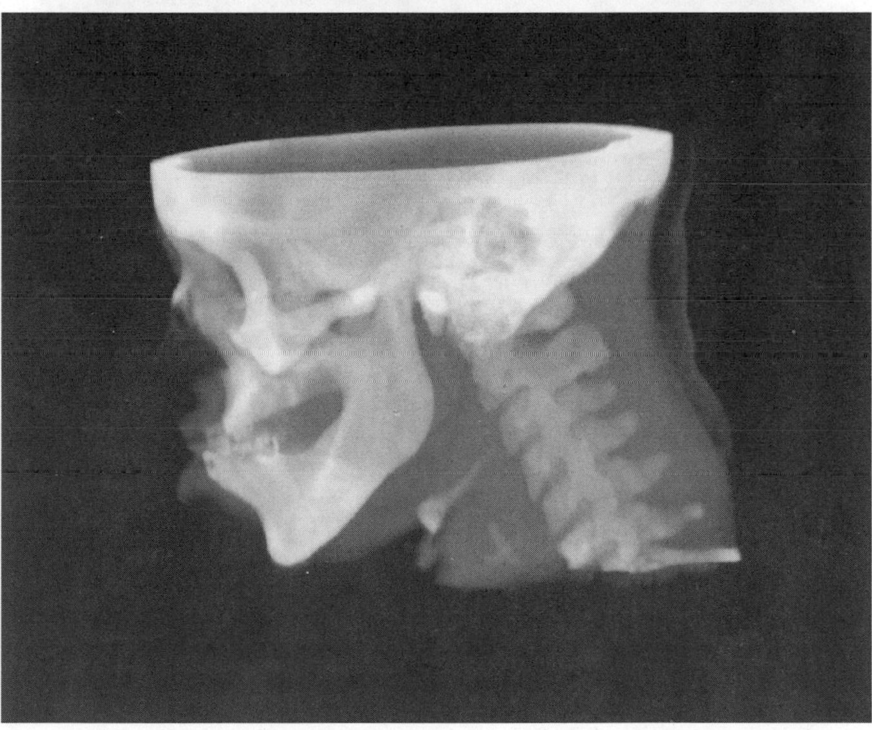

B

FIGURE 8.14 (A) Polypoid lesion in the left maxillary sinus. 3D reconstructions were done for evaluation of possible bony tumor in the left maxillary sinus. A small polypoid mass was seen, although there was no evidence of bony destruction noted. Note the fine detail of the bony structures of the sinuses and base of skull seen on this volume-rendered view. (B) More transparent reconstruction of facial bones.

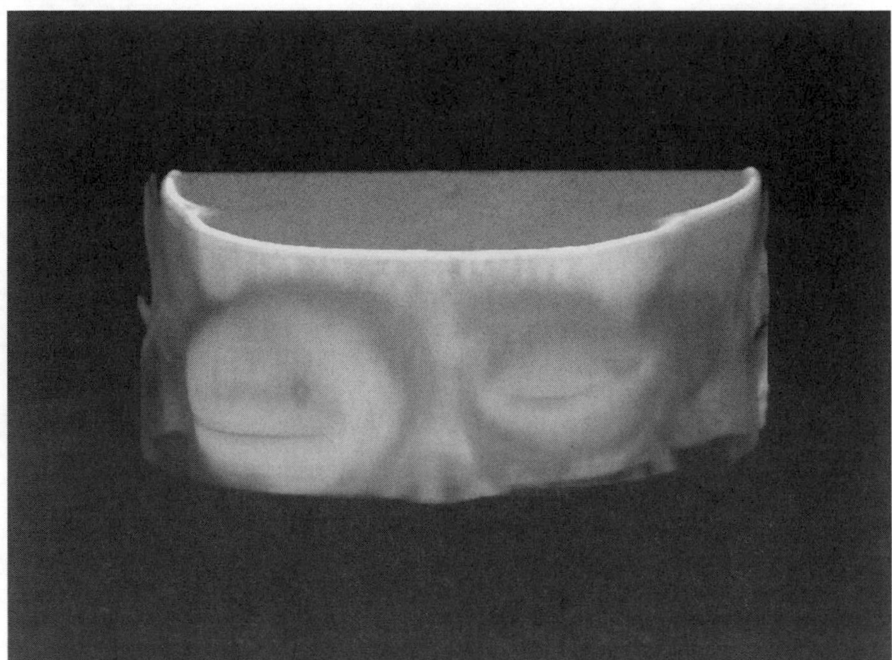

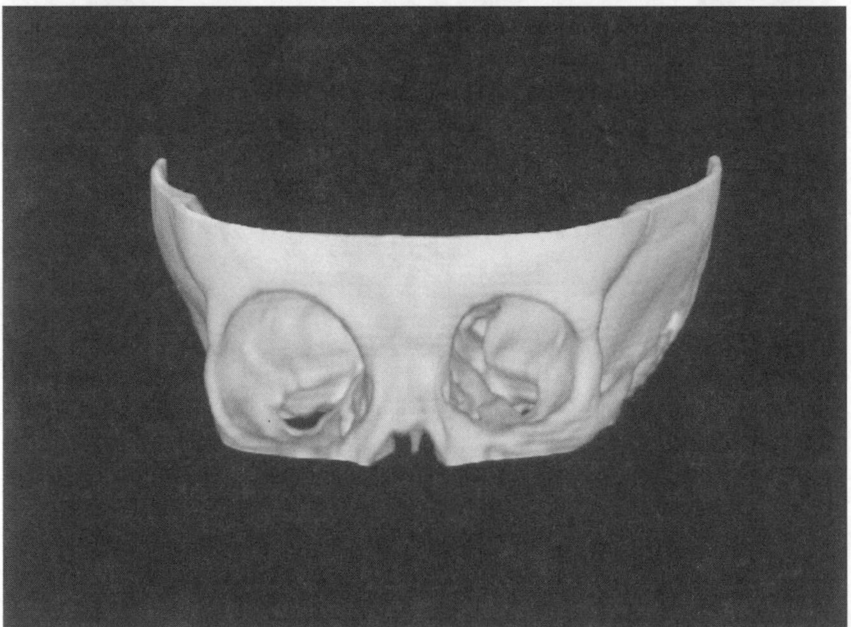

FIGURE 8.15 Orbital expansion due to tumor. Three-dimensional reconstructions demonstrate expansion and remodeling of the right orbit due to orbital tumor. The fine bony detail possible with spiral CT and 3D volume rendering are well illustrated in this case.

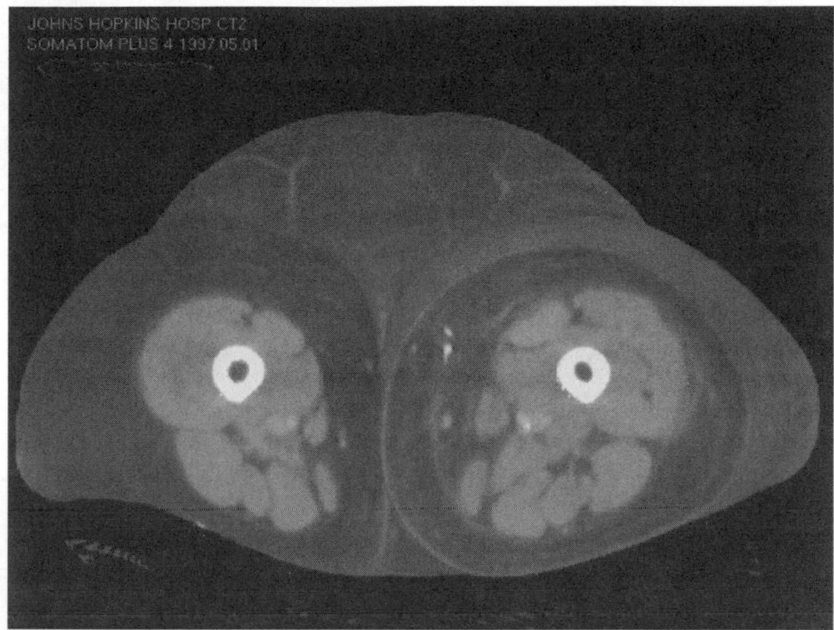

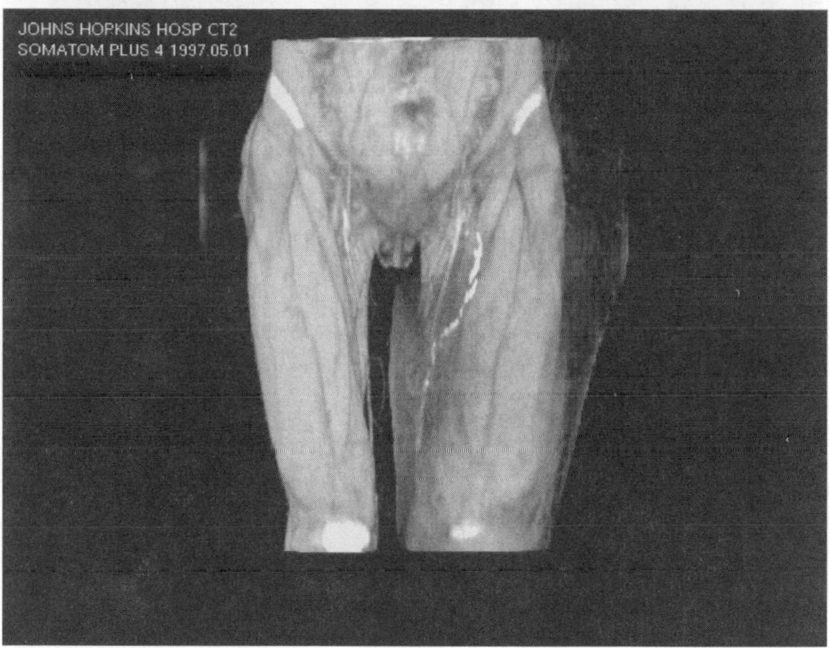

FIGURE 8.16 Soft-tissue inflammation. The 3D reconstructions were done for evaluation of possible mass in the left thigh. They demonstrate that the total muscle mass appears to be slightly enlarged on the left side, but the key finding is the increased extent and density of the subcutaneous tissues. This was caused by a mild cellulitis. No underlying tumor as suspected clinically was seen. The cellulitis was due to mild inflammation.

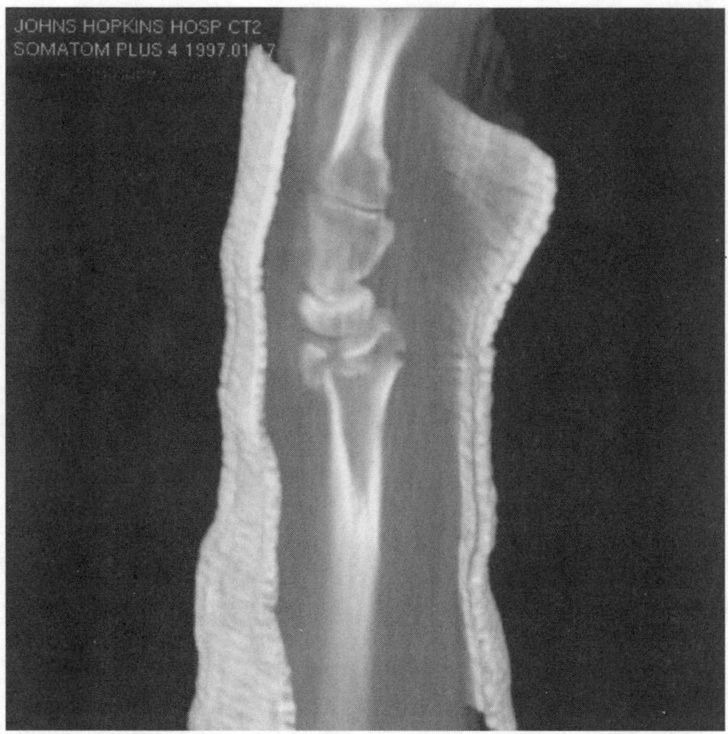

FIGURE 8.17 Radial fracture. 3D reconstructions demonstrate fracture of distal radius which was scanned in the cast. The multiple fracture lines involved in the epiphyseal place are seen with the impaction of the fracture noted on this view.

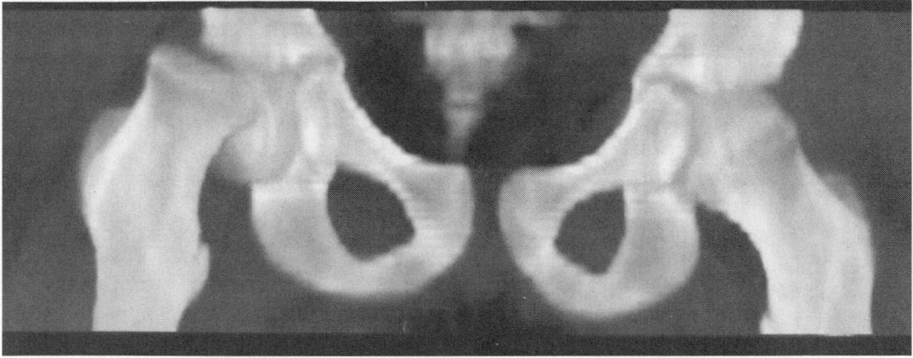

A

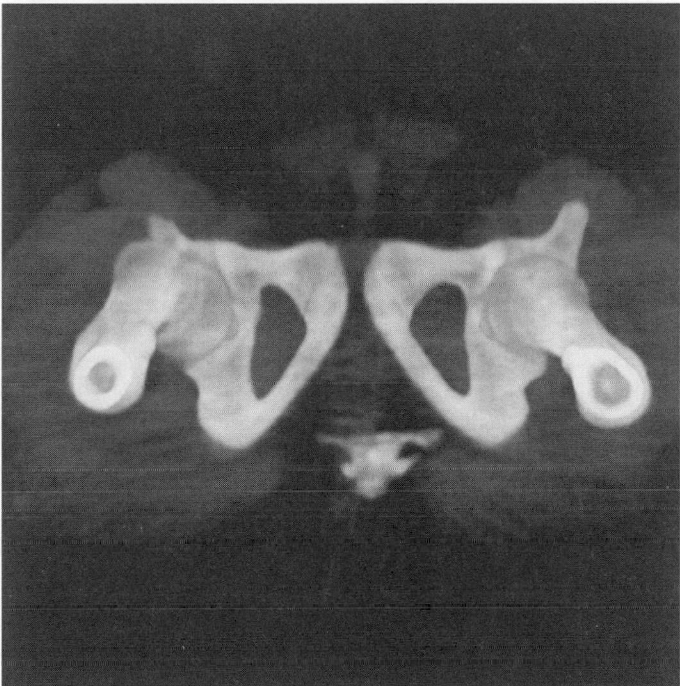

B

FIGURE 8.18 Right slipped capital femoral epiphysis. 3D reconstructions demonstrate the slipped capital femoral epiphysis with the femoral head rotating medially and posteriorly relative to the shaft of the femur. The anterior-posterior (A) and pelvic inlet (B) views clearly define the position of the femoral head and its relationship to the proximal femur.

REFERENCES

1. Totty WG, Vannier MW. Complex musculoskeletal anatomy: analysis using three-dimensional surface reconstruction. *Radiology* 1984; 150:173–177.
2. Vannier MW, Totty WG, Steven GW et al. Musculoskeletal applications of three-dimensional surface reconstruction. *Orthop Clin NA* 1985; 16(3):543–555.
3. Pate D, Resnick D, Andre M et al. Perspective: three-dimensional imaging of the musculoskeletal system. *AJR* 1986; 147(3):545–551.
4. Ney DR, Fishman EK, Kawashima A, Robertson Jr DD, Scott Jr WW. Comparison of helical and serial CT with regard to three-dimensional imaging of musculoskeletal anatomy. *Radiology* 1992; 185:865–869.
5. Kasales CJ, Mauger DT, Sefczek RJ et al. Multiplanar image reconstruction and 3D imaging using a musculoskeletal phantom: conventional versus helical CT. *J Comp Assisted Tomogr* 1997; 21(1):162–169.
6. Fishman EK, Wyatt SH, Bluemke DA, Urban BA. Spiral CT of musculoskeletal pathology: preliminary observations. *Skeletal Radiol* 1993; 22:253–256.
7. Udupa JK, Odhner D, Samarasekera S, Goncalves R, Iyer K, Venugopal K, Furuie S. 3DVIEWNIX: an open, transportable, multidimensional, multimodality, multiparametric imaging software system. *SPIE Proc* 1994; 2164:58–73.
8. Udupa JK, Odhner D. Shell rendering. *IEEE Comp Graphics Appl* 1993; 13(6):58–67.
9. Udupa JK, Odhner D. Fast visualization, manipulatioin, and analysis of binary volumetric objects. *IEEE Comp Graphics Appl* 1991; 11(6):53–62.
10. Odhner D, Udupa JK. Shell manipulation: interactive alteration of multi-material fuzzy structures. *SPIE Proc* 1995; 2431:35–42.
11. Cabral B, Cam N, Foran J. Accelerated volume rendering and tomographic reconstruction using texture mapping hardware. In: *ACM/IEEE Symposium on Volume Visualization.* 1994. Washington, DC.
12. Ney DR, Fishman EK, Magid D, Kuhlman JE. Interactive real-time multiplanar CT imaging. *Radiology* 1989; 170:275–276.
13. Drebin RA, Carpenter L, Hanrahan P. Volume rendering. *Comp Graph* 1988; 22(4):65–74.
14. Lorensen WE, Cline HE. Marching cubes: a high resolution 3D surface reconstruction algorithm. *Comp Graph* 1987; 21(4)163–169.
15. Ney DR, Drebin RA, Fishman EK, Magid D. Volumetric rendering computed tomography data: principles and techniques. *Comp Graph Appl* 1990; 10(2):24–32.
16. Scott Jr WW, Fishman EK, Magid D. Acetabular fractures: optimal imaging. *Radiology* 1987; 165:537–539.
17. Magid D, Fishman EK, Brooker Jr AF, Riley Jr LH. Volumetric three-dimensional image processing: an introduction to orthopaedic applications. *Contemp Orthop* 1988; 16(2):29–34.
18. Burk Jr DL, Mears DC, Kennedy WH, Cooperstein LA, Herbert DL. Three-dimensional computed tomography of acetabular fractures. *Radiology* 1985; 155:183–186.
19. Fishman EK, Magid D, Drebin RA, Brooker Jr AF, Scott Jr WW, Riley Jr LH. Advanced three-dimensional evaluation of acetabular trauma: volumetric image processing. *J Trauma* 1989; 29(2):214–218.
20. Fishman EK, Drebin RA, Magid D, Scott Jr WW, Ney DR, Brooker Jr AF, Riley Jr LH, St. Ville JA, Zerhouni EA, Siegelman SS. Volumetric rendering techniques: applications for three-dimensional imaging of the hip. *Radiology* 1987; 16(7):56–61.
21. Marsh JL, Vannier MW. Surface imaging from computerized tomographic scans. *Surgery* 1983; 94(2):159–165.
22. Drebin RA, Magid D, Robertson DD, Fishman EK. Sensitivity of three-dimensional imaging for detecting fracture gaps. *J Comp Assisted Tomogr* 1989; 13(3):487–489.
23. Cerva DS, Mirvis SE, Shanmuganathan K, Kelly IM, Pais SO. Detection of bleeding in patients with major pelvic fractures: value of contrast-enhanced CT. *AJR* 1996; 166:131–135.
24. Fishman EK, Magid D, Mandelbaum BR et al. Multiplanar (MPR) imaging of the hip. *RadioGraph* 1986; 6:7–54.
25. Magid D, Fishman EK, Scott Jr WW et al. Femoral head avascular necrosis: CT assessment with multiplanar reconstruction. *Radiology* 1985; 157:751–756.

26. Fishman EK, Magid D, Robertson DD, Brooker Jr AF, Weiss PJ, Siegelman SS. Metallic hip implants: CT with multiplanar reconstruction. *Radiology* 1986; 160:675–681.
27. McEnery KW, Wilson AJ, Pilgram TK, Murphy Jr WA, Marushack MM. Fractures of the tibial plateau: value of spiral CT coronal plane reconstructions for detecting displacement in vitro. *AJR* 1994; 163:1177–1181.
28. Magid D, Fishman EK, Ney DR, Kuhlman JE. Two- and three-dimensional CT analysis of ankle fractures. *Radiology* 1988; 169(P):265.
29. Lucet L, Le Loet X, Menard JF et al. Computed tomography of the normal sternoclavicular joint. *Skeletal Radiol* 1996; 25:237–241.
30. Kuhlman JE, Fishman EK, Ney DR, Magid D. Complex shoulder trauma: three-dimensional CT imaging. *Orthopedics* 1988; 11(2):1561–1563.
31. Tecce PM, Fishman EK. Spiral CT with multiplanar reconstruction in the diagnosis of sternoclavicular osteomyelitis. *Skeletal Radiol* 1995; 24:275–281.
32. Petersilge CA, Emery SE. Thoracolumbar burst fracture: evaluating stability. *Semin Ultra CT MRI* 1996; 17(2):105–113.
33. Tehranzadeh J, Palmer S. Imaging of cervical spine trauma. *Semin Ultra CT MRI* 1996; 17(2):93–104.
34. Wojcik WG, Edeiken-Monroe BS, Harris Jr JH. Three-dimensional computed tomography in acute cervical spine trauma: a preliminary report. *Skeletal Radiol* 1987; 16(4):261–269.
35. Kilocyne RF, Mack LA. Computed tomography of spinal fractures. *Appl Radiol* 1987; 16(7):40–54.
36. Wojcik WG, Edeiken-Monroe BS, Harris JH. Three-dimensional computed tomography in acute cervical spine trauma: a preliminary report. *Skeletal Radiol* 1987; 16:261–269.
37. Hemmy DC, David DJ, Herman GT. Three-dimensional reconstruction of craniofacial deformity using computed tomography. *Neurosurgery* 1983; 13(5):534–541.
38. Vannier MW, Marsh JL, Warren JO. Three-dimensional CT reconstruction images for craniofacial surgical planning and evaluation. *Radiology* 1984; 150:173–177.
39. Fishman EK, Drebin RA, Hruban RH, Ney DR, Magid D. Three-dimensional reconstruction of the human body. *AJR* 1988; 18(1):53–59.
40. Fishman EK, Ney DR, Magid D, Kuhlman JE. Three-dimensional imaging of the vascular tree. *Dyn Cardio Imaging* 1989; 2(1):55–60.

9 Tarsal Joint Kinematics Via 3D Imaging

Bruce Elliot Hirsch, Jayaram K. Udupa, and Eric Stindel

CONTENTS

9.1 INTRODUCTION

The study of joint biomechanics is made difficult by the inaccessibility of most of the joints in the body. Although there are methods for studying the nature of the motion which occurs at any articulation, they are usually indirect and do not permit measurement of the motion of the actual bones. Those methods that do measure the actual bony motion are invasive, and not practical for routine use. There is a need, therefore, for a technique which quantifies and displays the motion

0-8493-3179-X/00/$0.00+$.50

of the bones of individual patients, without putting them at any risk. In this chapter we describe such a technique, which is based upon the quantitative analysis of three-dimensional (3D) reconstructions of bones from magnetic resonance (MR) images.

Certain animations described in this chapter can be seen at the MIPG Web site. The URL for that Web site is http://www.mipg.upenn.edu.

9.2 BIOMECHANICS

Most movement of vertebrates is accomplished through the movement of bones. Whatever the cause of that movement — muscle action, external forces, or other factors — the bones move and carry with them the soft tissues.

Such motions occur at the joints, which are places where separate bones meet. A great deal of the control of the motion is to be found in the shape and nature of the articulating bone surfaces, and in the type, properties, and location of the associated soft tissues. At one extreme, the resulting joints may be specialized to prevent movement, as are the sutures of the skull, and at the other they may permit essentially unrestricted motion over a wide angular range, as in the human shoulder.

The morphology of the articular structures thus sets the limits of what motions can occur at any individual joint. Within these limits the movements which take place at any given time are controlled by other factors: gravity makes our hands drop; muscles move our jaws in chewing; momentum helps propel us in walking. The interaction of these factors, especially the selection of muscles active at a particular moment, determines the exact nature of the displacement between apposing bones.

We describe here a method, based upon the 3D reconstruction and interpretation of sectional image data, which is proving beneficial in the elucidation of joint function. After determining that 3D reconstructions from sectional image data were reliable representations of small bones[1] we realized that this could lead to the development of a valuable tool for measuring and demonstrating small movements among the bones of a joint.[2,3] For reasons described below, we felt it necessary to use magnetic resonance imaging (MRI) data for our studies rather than computed tomography (CT), which is the modality generally used for the 3D reconstruction of bone; once the bones were rendered as objects, principal component analysis and rigid body mechanics were used to describe their motions.[2] A brief summary of our work has been published before,[4] as has a more technical explanation.[5]

This technique has been used to study the foot function of people with normal feet, as well as of patients with various abnormalities. It is the purpose of these studies to learn more about the normal and abnormal motions which occur at some of the joints among the foot bones. It is hoped that they will lead to a better understanding of the morphological changes in various pathologies, and of the functional deficiencies which accompany them.[6]

9.2.1 KINEMATICS

Our interest in the study of the biomechanics of the foot is derived from both practical and intellectual considerations. In distinction from the anatomically more generalized hand, the human foot is an organ which has become highly modified for only one purpose: locomotion.[7,8] This puts significant strain on its components, especially when one considers the wide variety of activities in which humans take part. In addition, social factors enter into the scene. As the population ages, as many as 95% or more of the geriatric population will have at least one foot complaint, and often many more.[9,10] As other examples, athletic fadism and high-heeled shoes can lead to significant injury. Considering these contributing factors, it is important to understand, evaluate, and have the information at hand to properly treat normal and abnormal foot biomechanics. It is probably fair to say that practically every podiatric or orthopedic complaint in the foot is the result of, or causes, some biomechanical abnormality.

A full understanding of the biomechanics of skeletal joints requires considerable information. A partial catalog of such knowledge includes position and orientation of the bones and associated soft tissues; changes in those factors as the joint moves; shape, location, orientation, and cartilage properties of the articular surfaces; areas of contact between bones and the forces across them; the effects of muscular action, gravity, momentum, and other forces on the joint; relationships among the bones; proportions of the bones and their effect on other structures; the joint space and how it changes… The list goes on. Certain of these biomechanical descriptors can be observed only during actual joint function, but others can be studied when the joint is passive, or even in cadavers.

The study of joint biomechanics can be broken down into two interrelated parts. The first is *kinematics*, which is that aspect of joint biomechanics that depends upon articular geometry and upon the passive effects of joint structures. The second aspect is *kinetics*, which is considered when the effects of forces external to a joint, such as muscle action or gravity, are involved. The technique described in this chapter provides only kinematic data. Because the collection of image data requires several minutes, we must hold our subjects' feet still for that length of time. Therefore, we cannot take into account the effect of forces which cause motion, and we limit our analysis to a kinematic description of a joint's function.

As two bones move relative to each other, the changes in their relative positions may involve rotations or linear displacements (translations). In fact, all biological joint motions combine both rotations and translations in varying proportions.

Since joints are all within the body and cannot be observed directly, it is often difficult to determine just how the bones move in any given action. Various approaches have been developed to get around this difficulty. Our field of interest is the mechanical function of the foot, which proves to be an area where the previous methods for studying joints are hard to apply, although many have been tried. They give some insight into the function of the foot joints, but leave many questions unanswered.

A variety of methods have been designed over the years in an effort to understand how joints function, and some of them are described in the following paragraphs. Some have been applied in living subjects and others were used in cadaver studies. Although work in live subjects can clearly be more useful, at least in concept, it is not always possible. Some of the methods have been of limited use because they were designed for specific situations, such as an instrumented prosthesis.[11] Others involve the surgical insertion of pins, and are thus too invasive for regular use.[12–16]

External linkage devices have been designed which attach, for example, to the leg and foot[17,18] or wrist.[19] They allow movements around axes which are set to coincide, as much as possible, with an average joint axis. Such devices often include goniometers, which can help measure the extent of motion that occurs, but they give little information about the nature of the motion within a joint in a given activity.

One approach to studying joint biomechanics in cadavers is to dissect the bones of a joint, move them in a way which mimics actual movements, and observe what happens at the articular surfaces. Various methods are used in the effort to replace the bones in their original positions and move them in their actual paths,[20,21] and the value of these methods obviously depends upon the precision with which the bones can be positioned and the accuracy with which a biological motion can be duplicated. The destruction of soft tissues, absence of muscle action, and individual variability ensure that these methods can only approximate the actual joint actions. Other cadaver experiments are designed to measure motions among bones which are left connected in more-or-less dissected specimens.[22,23]

Another approach is to use X-rays of a joint in two or more positions to provide information about the biomechanics of a joint. However, radiographs are inherently two dimensional, whereas all motions are three dimensional (even though most motion might be in one plane). To get around this, van Langelaan[24] developed a technique for three-dimensional X-ray stereophotogrammetry, in which he determined the position of small metal balls inserted into the foot bones of a cadaver. The cadaver foot was moved and the 3D locations of the balls were calculated at various foot positions. The technique was later utilized in a small number of living subjects, both normal[25–27] and with foot abnormalities.[28] The dose of X-rays required, plus the invasiveness of surgically inserting the metal balls, renders this technique impractical.

Only one technique, the analysis of the positions of surface markers, has really been widely adopted for the *in vivo* study of joints. It involves measuring the motion of markers placed on the skin around a joint. The positions of these markers, which are usually photoreflective, are recorded by two or more video cameras as they move within a calibrated space. The locations on the skin selected for the markers are chosen because they are thought to accurately represent what happens to the bones within the skin. As much as possible the markers are placed in locations where the bones are close to the surface and where the skin is tightly bound to the underlying periosteum, because in such locations skin (and therefore marker) movement is thought to represent most accurately what the bones are doing. Since there are methods to accurately describe the location of the markers in a defined 3D coordinate space, the accuracy of the method depends upon how truly the markers reproduce the motion of the bones. If the skin and other tissues between a marker and a bone are loose or moveable, there may not be any direct correlation between them. Although it may be possible to place the markers in acceptable positions near some joints, at least for some motions,[29,30] it is practically impossible to find good positions near some other joints.

The foot bones are a good example of bones that cannot be well represented by surface markers. (The anatomy of the foot is described below.) They are small and close together, and where they are close to the skin, the skin is loose and moveable. In other areas they are separated from the skin by tendons, a relatively thick layer of fat, or other soft tissues. Skin motion artifact in the posterior part of the foot may be over 4 mm relative to the underlying bones, a considerable distance when such small bones are being studied.[31] Additionally, the movements in each of the individual tarsal joints is small, so that the degree of motion to be detected may exceed the limits of accuracy of the systems used. A similar limitation applies to the ankle joint, because it is impossible to locate a reliable external indicator of the talus. It is easier to find reasonable (though probably not foolproof) skin locations over the calcaneus. Most studies of *in vivo* ankle motion which have been published therefore do not measure motion at the ankle joint alone, but incorporate motion at the subtalar joint as well.[25–27,32]

The ability to see internal parts of a joint with slice-based imaging, such as CT or MRI, has stimulated an interest in applying it to the examination of joint biomechanics. Two-dimensional CT slices have been utilized in examining the changes in talar tilt in a cadaver foot when the lateral supporting ligaments were cut.[33] Several studies on the knee have used magnetic resonance images to determine the relative position of the patella.[34–37] Such evaluations are becoming more common in clinical practice, since the manufacturers of MR scanners now include in their systems the ability to image a single slice plane at high speed and play the successive images as a movie. All of these studies and patient evaluations, unfortunately, are two dimensional, and are unable to illustrate the 3D nature of motion. Neuman et al.[38] utilized 2D slices in their study of arytenoid cartilage movement, but they used multiple slices and therefore were able to calculate a 3D axis of rotation. Since they did not create 3D renditions of the cartilages, the motion they describe can be difficult to visualize.

The unsolved difficulty in all of these techniques is that it is impossible to measure directly and exactly how specific, individual bones move in a living person. To get around this, we have developed a method for studying the biomechanics of skeletal joints in such a way that the changing positions of the actual bones are quantified, described, and displayed. It is based on computerized 3D reconstructions of MR images of bones from body segments in various positions, the computation of the position and orientation of the bones relative to the MR scanner coordinate system, and the changes in those parameters as the bones move.[1,2,4,5,39–44] Because this method allows the determination of kinematic parameters of joints within intact bodies, we refer to it as *internal kinematics*. This chapter describes the application of internal kinematics to some of the important joints of the foot. There have been reports of other biomechanical analyses of various joints from

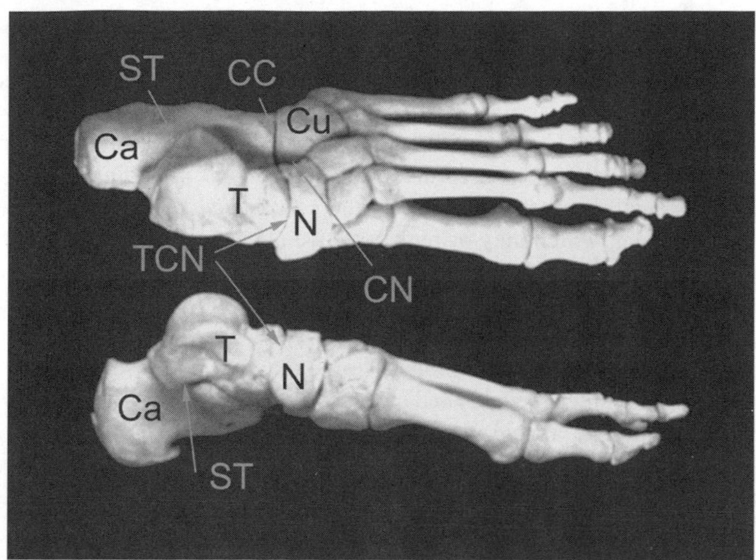

FIGURE 9.1 The bones of the foot and ankle, shown in a dorsal view at the top and a medial view at the bottom. The bones discussed in this chapter are labeled Ca = calcaneus; Cu = cuboid; N = navicular; T = talus. The joints involved in the kinematics described here are ST = subtalar joint; TCN = talocalcaneonavicular joint; CC = calcaneocuboid joint; CN = cuboideonavicular joint.

3D images, including the temporomandibular,[45,46] carpal,[47–49] finger,[50,51] knee,[52] cricoarytenoid,[38,53] and spinal joints,[54] but they have generally been restricted in scope. There has also been a report in which a method similar to ours was applied to the evaluation of one subject's foot and ankle.[55] These studies generally used CT as the image data source, which renders them impractical for extensive *in vivo* studies because of the radiation doses involved.

Internal kinematics provides a means of obtaining much of the data necessary for an understanding of a given joint's biomechanics. Such information includes the three-dimensional geometry of the bones involved, their relationships, and how these relationships change with motion. These data can be presented not only in numerical format, but as graphics and animations, which improve the ability to understand what is happening. Further development will lead to data on the soft tissues and joint spaces.

9.3 ANATOMY OF THE FOOT

The skeleton of the foot can be divided into several regions made up of several types of bones. The posterior half, approximately, is the *tarsal* region, formed of a number of small chunky bones. They are involved in energy storage and release, in controlling the distribution of forces within the foot, and as they take different positions in different parts of the gait cycle, they control the flexibility of the foot as a whole. The metatarsal bones, located more anteriorly between the tarsal bones and the toes, are relatively long in proportion to the foot as a whole, and serve to lengthen the lever arm during propulsion. The phalanges or toe bones are used to provide balance and fine control to foot movement.

The four most posterior tarsal bones are the talus, calcaneus, cuboid, and navicular (Figure 9.1). The talus is the bone that actually articulates with the leg bones, and thus forms a key structure in control of foot activity. It is in the intrinsic foot joints surrounding the talus — the *peritalar joints* — where the oblique motions of the foot which define normal function occur. These motions are *pronation* and *supination*, which control the foot's adaptation to the ground and, very importantly, regulate the shift which takes place in each step as it switches between its flexible and rigid states.

There are a number of joints connecting these four bones (Figure 9.1):

- The relatively large articulation between the posterior parts of the talus and the calcaneus is called the *subtalar joint.*
- The head of the talus articulates with one or two small facets on the anterior part of the calcaneus and with the navicular in the *talocalcaneonavicular joint.*
- The calcaneus and the cuboid articulate at the *calcaneocuboid joint.*
- There is also a joint, which may or may not have a synovial cavity, between the cuboid and the navicular. It is called the *cuboideonavicular joint.*

Because of the close, interlinked nature of these joints, action at one causes motion at the others. For example, movement of the subtalar joint requires corresponding movement at the talocalcaneonavicular joint, since the talus and calcaneus are involved in both. This kind of situation is reflected in the description of a *transverse tarsal* (also known as *midtarsal*) *joint*, which is really the talonavicular part of the talocalcaneonavicular joint and the calcaneocuboid joint considered as one complex entity. It is generally thought that the motion of the foot is controlled by the types of movements that can occur at the subtalar and transverse tarsal joints.[12,21,56–58]

Open chain kinetics refers to a situation when the foot is non-weight-bearing and free to move without external constraints, as during the swing phase of a step. In this situation *pronation* is defined as a motion in which the distal part of the foot everts (the outer edge lifts up), abducts (the toes point away from the midline of the body), and dorsiflexes (bends upward). *Supination* is the opposite motion. Although these motions seem complicated, they are determined by the shape of the articular surfaces and can be roughly described as rotations around an axis oblique to the cardinal (anatomical) reference planes of the foot. Such an overall twisting of the foot obviously involves many of its joints, but most of this movement occurs at the subtalar and transverse tarsal joints. (Part of this motion also occurs at the ankle joint, which was not included in this study.[26,59]) In certain situations the foot is more-or-less fixed in place, as when it is supporting the body and bearing weight. Motion in this situation involves *closed chain kinetics*, where movement of one or more of the bones is restricted. Therefore, in order for a given relative motion among the bones to remain the same, a different bone or bones will have to alter its movement.

9.4 INTERNAL KINEMATICS

Three-dimensional reconstruction of sectional image data has proven both feasible and useful in evaluating the structure and relationship among small bones, such as those of the foot[1,60] and hand.[47] There are various situations (e.g., difficult fractures,[61–63] tarsal coalitions,[62] production of custom implants,[64] and surgical planning[6]) where the descriptive aspects of 3D imaging have the potential to greatly affect treatment.

However, the 3D images contain more than just visual information. The practical difficulties in determining the true 3D *in vivo* motions of the foot joints motivated us to develop the method of studying kinematics we call *internal kinematics*. This method allows us to identify each bone of interest and determine how it moves as the foot goes from one position to another. It relies upon the identification of each bone in magnetic resonance image data of the foot in each position, computerized three-dimensional reconstruction of the bones, and the use of this derived data to determine the rotations and translations which occur. Since several minutes are required to gather the MR image data in each position, this method does not allow us to study the kinetics of the joints.

We have applied the method to the study of the joints distal to the talus (the subtalar and transverse tarsal joints, collectively referred to as the *peritalar joints*), but it is applicable to the analysis of any skeletal joint that can be appropriately imaged.[65] This non-invasive image-based method seems to be the only approach, except for that of Lundberg,[25] involving the surgical insertion of metal balls, which provides direct three-dimensional data on the movement of bones in living subjects.

TABLE 9.1
Subjects Studied

	Male	Female
Clinically normal	8	4
Calcaneonavicular coalition, pre-operatively	5	
Calcaneonavicular coalition, post-operatively	1	
Pes planus, pre-operatively	2	3
Pes planus, post-operatively	1	
Other	3	1

In the following sections, we describe our subjects and the imaging methods used to collect image data from them, explain the methods used to analyze those data, and discuss the validation studies done to ensure that the methods are reliable. This is followed by a description of bone morphology, an account of normal and abnormal movements as revealed by internal kinematics, a discussion of some of the difficulties which had to be overcome during the development of the technique, and an explanation of the use of this technique in understanding normal and abnormal foot function.

9.5 MATERIALS AND METHODS

9.5.1 Subjects

We have collected image data on 12 clinically normal volunteers. In addition, we have studied several subjects who, although functioning adequately, had abnormal feet. We also evaluated other patients, some of whom underwent corrective surgery because of a congenital calcaneonavicular coalition or flat feet. The postsurgical patients have been re-examined post-operatively (or will be, when healing is complete). The 28 subjects imaged and analyzed are described in Table 9.1.

9.5.2 Magnetic Resonance Imaging

Our first images from cadavers demonstrated that it is possible to get high-resolution 3D images of the small bones of the foot from CT slices.[1] Although it would have been easier for us to continue using CT as an image data source because it would have been so much simpler to segment the bones, radiation exposure was a prohibiting factor. The radiation exposure in CT imaging is low enough that it is acceptable for clinical usage, but since our research subjects are imaged as many as eight times in a session, with their feet in as many positions, the cumulative dose would be prohibitive. Therefore, we decided to use MR image data, even though it meant that we had to develop new segmentation tools.

All subjects were imaged in a General Electric Signa 1.5 T magnetic resonance scanner, using a particular protocol commonly abbreviated as GRASS. The images included the posterior part of the foot, including the talus, calcaneus, navicular, and cuboid, and the distal ends of the tibia and fibula. Sixty contiguous sagittal slices 1.5 to 1.7 mm thick (depending on the size of the foot, so

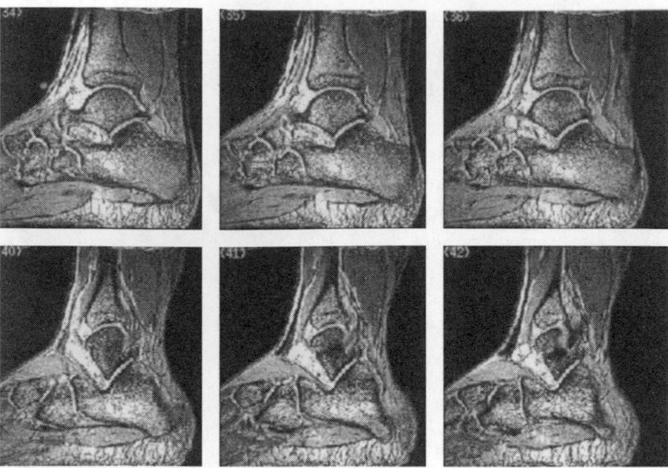

FIGURE 9.2 Six representative sagittal slices in an MR data set from a normal subject.

that its entire width was included) were imaged at each time instance, with a 14- to 16-cm field of view, 256 × 256 matrix, and .75 NEX. The pixels in the slice plane were about 0.6 mm across. At various positions from extreme pronation to extreme supination, the foot was held immobile long enough to collect an image data set. Several representative slices from one data set are shown in Figure 9.2.

9.5.3 Control of Foot Movement

Our early subjects were asked to move their feet in increments from one position to another, holding still at each position for imaging. However, we quickly realized that even motivated subjects were unable to keep their feet still for the time required without support. In addition, they were not able to break their total motion into uniform stages, which would be required for the production of smooth, realistic movies.

A plastic jig was therefore developed to hold the foot and ensure that it moves in a defined, controlled manner. The jig is designed to pronate and supinate the foot around an axis which is considered a typical axis for subtalar motion, one that deviates 23° antero-medially in a transverse plane and 42° antero-superiorly in a sagittal plane.[20] We hold the foot in place with adhesive and Velcro™ tapes, and the leg is mechanically fixed to the scanner table with straps. In most cases we begin with the foot in 20° of pronation, and it is moved in 10° increments to 50° of supination, for a total of eight positions unless a limited range of motion or subject discomfort prevents this. At each position, which we refer to as a "time instance," we obtain an MR image data set of the posterior part of the foot. Figure 9.3 shows the jig holding a subject's foot in extreme pronation and in extreme supination.

9.5.4 Software

Further processing is done using 3DVIEWNIX, a software system for 3D reconstruction, visualization, and analysis, which was developed by the Medical Image Processing Group at the University of Pennsylvania, and which we have been using in a variety of imaging problems in a number of anatomic regions.[66,67] First, each bone of interest is segmented in each slice of each time instance, using a semi-automatic method (described below) which minimizes the time required for an operator to complete this part of the procedure.[68] Second, the surface of each bone is computed, as are its centroid and principal axes. Third, starting with the second time instance, each bone is registered with its position in the previous time instance; the change in position required for registration

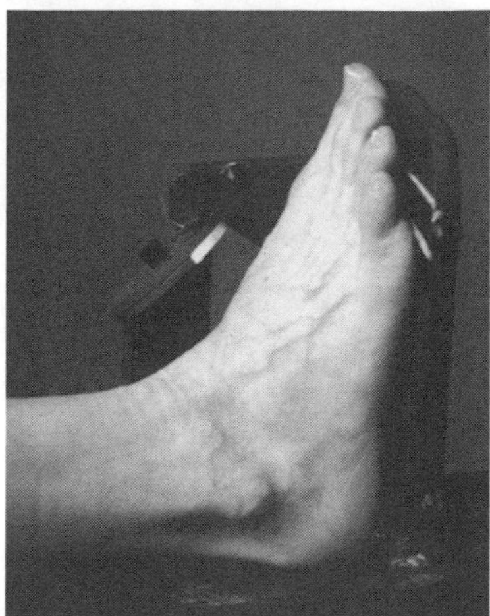
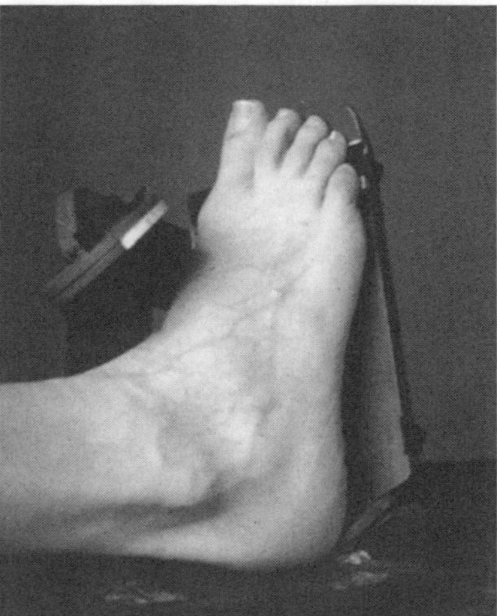

FIGURE 9.3 A foot is in place in the jig used to hold and control subjects' feet during imaging. At the left, the foot is in 20° of pronation, and at the right it is in 50° of supination. These positions are near the extremes of a normal subject's range of motion.

provides a description of the sequential motions of the bone. Finally, the images are displayed and the data are analyzed. Each step is further described below.

9.5.5 Segmentation

Of the two approaches to displaying three-dimensional images, volume and surface rendering, the latter is more suitable to our needs. It permits the precise definition of the boundary surface of each bone, so that the volume and shape parameters of the bones can be calculated. Surface rendering necessitates the identification of the bones' surfaces, a process called "segmentation." In our study of the peritalar joints we segment the talus, calcaneus, cuboid, and navicular bones.

The difficulty in the segmentation of bone from MR images arises because it, like other dense connective tissues, gives a very weak MR signal. Its apparent similarity to other connective tissues, particularly the tendons and ligaments which lie near or attach to it, often makes it difficult to determine the precise bone boundary in a particular region. For this reason, automatic segmentation is not always able to separate bone from connective tissue and the process requires the interaction of a knowledgeable operator to deal with the confusion generated by this resemblance. However, manual segmentation is extremely time consuming and is not always consistent or repeatable. Therefore, we developed two variations on a semi-automatic theme, called "live wire" and "live lane," which compute the optimal boundary under user guidance.[68] Both methods operate in a slice-by-slice fashion. In our tests, and in tests done on a similar program in another laboratory, the use of live wire segmentation is not only 1.5 to 3 times faster than manual segmentation, but it is also much more accurate and repeatable.[68,69]

In live wire, the user denotes one point on the boundary with a mouse click then moves the cursor to another point on the object border (Figure 9.4). The optimum boundary, based upon the characteristics of features established for that type of image and boundary, is computed in real time. If it is satisfactory, the operator clicks the mouse to fix the second point and uses it as the starting location for the next boundary segment. If the segment is not satisfactory, the operator can move the cursor to a spot closer to the starting point and, as the boundary re-adjusts, can decide when to accept this segment. This process is repeated until the whole boundary of the object is outlined. In some situations, the complete boundary of a bone in one slice can be computed with as few as two or three clicks.

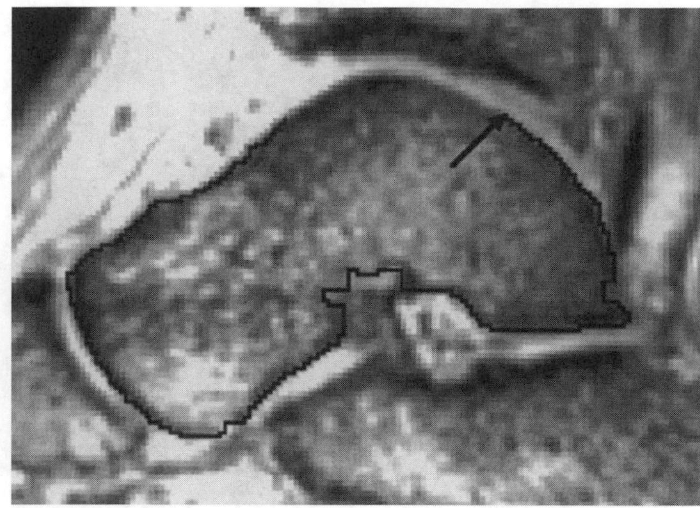

FIGURE 9.4 The live wire method is used to determine the boundary of a bone. The black line is an example of a boundary determined in this way. The arrow indicates the current position of the cursor.

Live lane is similar, with one exception. In live wire, the program examines the whole image to determine the optimum line segment. With the live lane method, as the mouse is moved, a band between 10 and 90 pixels wide across the cursor position is identified. Only the area within this band is considered in determining the boundary, so the operator can exhibit close control on the location of the boundary line. Both methods give similar results.[68]

9.5.6 Computation of Object Surfaces

The result of segmentation is a set of files, each containing slice-by-slice binary images of a bone. Since the reconstruction of 3D images in 3DVIEWNIX requires cubic voxels, a shape-based interpolation algorithm is used to reduce the thickness of the original slices and interpolate additional ones.[70] The dimensions of each voxel in these new slices are equal to the dimensions of the original voxels in the plane of sectioning; in our data this is about 0.55 to 0.60 mm. The slices are filtered with a Gaussian smoothing filter[71] and rendered with algorithms described by Udupa et al.[72]

9.5.7 Measurement of Motion

Although it is possible to use other methods such as registration of surface landmarks to align bones,[2,3,50,51] we have found that the use of the centroid and principal axes is easier.[73–76] It was very difficult to identify the small features necessary for accurate registration, and we were also concerned that digitization artifacts and partial volume effects could lead to unpredictable shifts in the positions of the landmarks. The bone axes system defined by the centroid and the principal axes of the bones (see Section 9.7.1) appears to be robust and provides some vital parameters to study the morphology, architecture, and kinematics of the joints, as will be described later. The registration process assumes that we are dealing with rigid body motion. It involves translating the centroid of a bone in one time instance until it coincides with the centroid of that same bone in the previous instance, relative to the coordinate system of the MR scanner, and then rotating the bone about one axis until the principal axes coincide.[5] The direction and amount of translation, the position and orientation of the axis of rotation, and the amount of rotation provide a description of the motion that occurred as the bone moved during supination of the foot. These data are available for each bone contributing to a joint. Given these data, we also compute the motion of any bone relative to

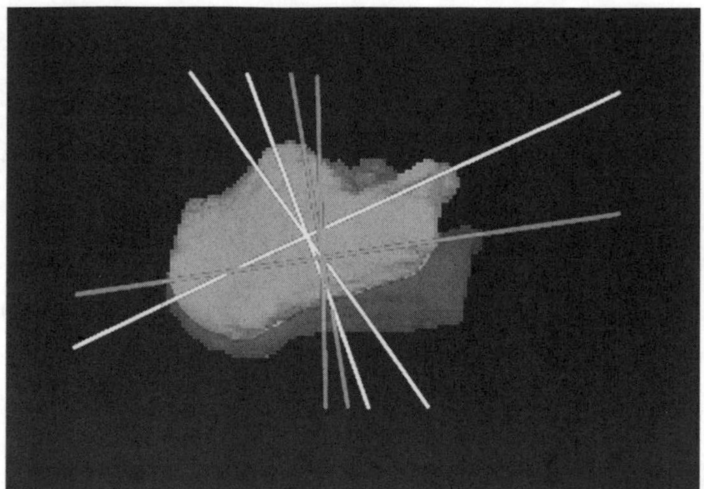

FIGURE 9.5 A calcaneus is shown in two positions: pronated (lighter gray) and supinated. The principal axes of the bone in each position are also shown; in the pronated position they are green, and in the supinated position they are red.

any other given bone and express this data in two components: translation and rotation. Figure 9.5 shows a bone in two positions and its principal axes.

Rigid body motion requires that the principal axes system of each object remains constant with respect to the object from one time instance to another. This is true for the small bones we segment because the entire object contributes to the 3D reconstruction. However, only parts of the tibia and fibula, the long bones of the leg, appear in the field of view. Therefore, the principal axes system will remain constant from time instance to time instance only if the exact same part of each bone appears in each data set. This is not the case, however, because the motion of the foot in the jig also changes the position of the leg. Recognizing this problem, we have not attempted to measure ankle motion up to now. Recently we have developed a method called "iso-shaping" to cut off an identical part of each long bone in each time instance, creating a set of objects with the same parts included in the surface model and, therefore, resulting in the same principal axes systems.[65] With iso-shaping, it will be possible to include the ankle joint in our future studies.

9.5.8 Animations

These motion data are used to create various animations, or movies, of the moving bones, and can also be utilized to derive other information about the nature of the joint motion. An animation is prepared by creating a 3D image (surface rendition) of the bone or bones of interest, in each sequential position of the foot, and then displaying them one after the other. However, because there are no more than eight frames in such a movie it gives a jerky presentation. To get around this, intermediate positions are interpolated from the original frames, increasing the number of frames in the movie to about 40.[66,70] This provides a smooth presentation.

The features of the bone set in the movie can be adjusted to show whatever might be of interest. The display of one or more bones can be turned off, the bones can be colored, the angle of view is adjustable, and various lighting effects can be created. Also, the movements can be displayed as they occurred (absolute motion) or adjusted so that the motion is displayed relative to one selected bone, which then appears not to move at all (relative motion).

By combining bones from different individuals in one display, comparisons which would otherwise be difficult to visualize become much easier to comprehend. For example, a normally moving bone can be included in the movie of an abnormal foot, by registering the two feet, to

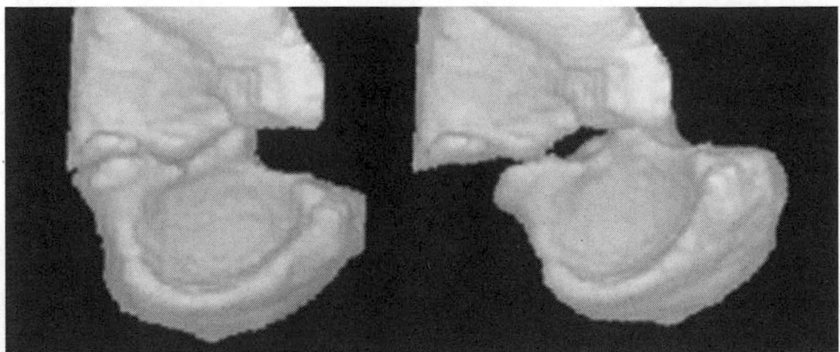

FIGURE 9.6 This illustration demonstrates the effect of applying normal motion to a foot with a calcaneonavicular coalition. On the left, the calcaneus and navicular are shown in pronation. The supination movement of the navicular of a normal subject was then applied to this abnormal bone. The two bones no longer remain in contact in some areas, and in others they intersect. This can serve as a guide to a surgeon, indicating the amount of bone that must be resected to allow normal motion. (Reprinted from Udupa, J. K., Hirsch, B. E., Hillstrom, H. J., Bauer, G. R., and Kneeland, J. B., *IEEE Trans. Biomed. Eng.*, 45, 1387, 1998.)

show how the abnormality affects motion. As another example, a navicular from a patient with a calcaneonavicular coalition, where the presence of an abnormal joint restricts motion, was made to move like a normal bone. In this way the enlarged navicular appeared to enter into the calcaneus, and the amount of overlap indicated to the surgeon how much of the abnormally shaped navicular had to be resected (Figure 9.6).

For all the subjects studied, animations were prepared showing the bones as the feet were moved from pronation to supination. It was found that the motions are easier to study if they are expressed relative to one bone, say the calcaneus or talus. This provides a common reference and eliminates the effect of extraneous movement such as a motion of the foot as a whole. Moreover, choosing the appropriate reference bone makes it easier to describe a motion in terms of conventionally used relationships. For example, open chain (non-weight-bearing) subtalar pronation-supination is often described according to the way the calcaneus moves relative to the talus. A variety of such animations can be prepared, showing any combination of the bones from any point of view. These animations have been studied to describe the motions of each of the bones.

9.5.9 Kinematic Analysis

An important issue is the means of presenting the results of these analyses in terms that are practically useful to clinicians and others who might use the data. For example, clinicians tend to think of joint motions as rotations around *an* axis related to the cardinal body planes, but such descriptions are subjective and not anchored in any descriptions that can be precisely transposed to the coordinate system of the scanner. Moreover, clinical examinations are not capable of picking up very small movements, such as most intertarsal motion or the small translations that generally accompany rotations. The difficulty is that our data, which include mathematical descriptions of the rotations and translations, are not easily understood in clinical terms. Therefore, we have begun to look for other ways of describing the motions which will be useful for determining in a clinical sense whether a joint functions normally.

One example of the approach we are taking is to find expressions of the data that are clear by themselves and do not require any mathematical background or applied biomechanical experience. The included angle determined by two lines which connect the centroids of any three tarsal bones changes in a consistent way as the foot goes through its range of motion. In abnormal joints these angles undergo different sorts of changes, but may be brought back toward the normal range by surgery. This is further discussed in Section 9.7.3.2.

9.6 VALIDATION

There are several steps in the process of determining the motions occurring at a joint which required testing and validation. These processes include segmentation and the computation of motion.

9.6.1 SEGMENTATION

Because the measurements of motion depend upon the accurate determination of each bone's surface, it is important that the segmentation is reliable and repeatable. The manual step-by-step and bit-by-bit delineation of the boundary of an object in a single slice by an expert is often considered to be the "gold standard" by which other procedures are judged. However, such manual segmentation is, in fact, not always reliable or consistent.[68,69] We have come to realize that even where the edges are visually clear, it is just about impossible for different human operators to trace a boundary exactly at the same location in the image. In our experience there are two circumstances where this is particularly true. The first is in areas where different structures of similar gray levels are in contact. In these cases — for instance, where a ligament or tendon attaches to a bone — it can be very difficult to make a decision about the precise location of the bone edge. The second situation is where the edge of a bone is approximately parallel to the plane of sectioning, and volume sharing occurs over a large area. The boundary is vague in this example, and in all likelihood there is no line that truly represents it. Consistency in deciding where to draw the line, from slice to slice and data set to data set, is very important, and probably more important than trying to decide upon a true edge.

We have tested the automatic segmentation techniques of live wire and live lane in representative data from our subjects.[68] The purpose of these experiments was to compare the repeatability and speed of these methods to manual segmentation. Various slices including the talus and calcaneus were presented to each of three experimenters, to be segmented manually or by one of the live methods. The slice order and the method used for each slice were randomized. We found that the live methods were significantly more repeatable than manual segmentation. In addition, they were always faster for two of the three experimenters who took part in the comparisons, and sometimes they were faster for the third experimenter as well. Overall, the live methods were 1.5 to 3 times faster (with statistical significance) than manual tracing.[68,69]

9.6.2 MOTION

It is important that the amount of motion computed for each joint at each time instance be correct. We have undertaken a number of experiments to determine the accuracy of our calculated rotations and translations. These experiments involved test objects, isolated bones, and comparisons between our method and another method of measuring motion.

In the first experiment, an acrylic frame was constructed of three orthogonal panels, and small plastic boxes of identical size were placed on them in precisely known positions and orientations.[41] One box was placed at the corner where the three planes met. Each box was filled with Magnevist™ MR contrast medium. Three reflective markers were placed on each of the boxes. Therefore, the same objects could be used for internal kinematics and for stereometric analysis by video recording of the positions of the reflective markers. In motions combining translation and rotation, the internal kinematic measurements were within 0.8° and 2.6 mm of the actual values. The values as determined by stereometry were within 2.1° and 1.6 mm.

Another experiment designed to compare the two methods involved placing markers on the heel of a cadaver foot, as well as on rods inserted into the talus, navicular, and cuboid.[40] The results were similar with the two techniques, and the slight differences could be explained by possible movement of the skin markers as well as handling of the specimen between the two study locations.

In a third experiment, a cleaned, dried talus was suspended in a plastic box filled with Magnevist contrast medium.[5] The box and its contents were placed on a prepared support and imaged in three

TABLE 9.2
Average Correlation Coefficients for Operator-Dependent Segmentation Parameters

	Intra-Operator Correlation Coefficients	Inter-Operator Correlation Coefficients
Orientation of the first two principal axes	0.983	0.978
Centroid location	0.984	0.996
Lengths of the principal axes, as limited by the surfaces	0.955	0.944
Bone volume	0.997	0.983

different positions and orientations, with an accuracy estimated to be better than 0.5° and 0.5 mm. Errors in our computation of rotation and translation were in the range of 0.9 to 1.3° and 0.3 to 2.2 mm. A study of the glenohumeral joint, in which the bones were translated known distances by means of plastic plates with calibrated holes, gave similar results: the translations were accurate to about 0.61 mm, which was approximately one pixel.[65,77]

Because the live methods we use are under the control of the person who does the segmenting there is a possibility that different people may choose different surfaces, or even that one operator may not be consistent, and that the objects created from these segmented boundaries are therefore too inconsistent for reliable use. To see if that was the case we performed an experiment in which two people each segmented the talus, calcaneus, cuboid, and navicular in the MR image data sets of 10 subjects.[42] Each operator segmented each data set twice. For each bone the following parameters were computed: volume, centroid location, length of each principal axis segment within the bone, and orientation of the first two principal axes. Intra- and inter-operator correlation coefficients were calculated for each segmentation parameter. As shown in Table 9.2, these values were very reliable. The most stable parameters were the locations of the centroids and the volumes of the bones. The lengths of the principal axes within the bones were the least stable — although still quite consistent — because they are subject to local variations in the determination of the surface.

Another variable in the process arises because, as the foot moves, the orientation of each bone in the scanner changes. Does this change, reflected in different ways of digitizing the bones, affect their segmentation and thus their principal axes? To test this, 10 data sets of normal subjects were used, each containing one foot scanned in eight different positions.[42] For each subject, one person did all of the segmentation. Our results indicated that the principal axes varied little as a result of differences in orientation. For example, the principal axis segments (defined as the length of each principal axis between its intersections with the bone surface; see further explanation in Section 9.7.1) were quite consistent. The standard deviations of the principal axis segments ranged from 0.3 to 1.4 mm, with an average of 0.8 mm. Therefore, we may conclude that the orientation of a given bone in the scanner does not affect the reliability of the segmentation or of the principal axes system.

9.7 RESULTS

The 3D reconstructions produced in our work hold a considerable amount of data. Some of it concerns the bones as individual isolated entities, primarily matters of shape, size, and proportion. Some data deal with the relationships among bones, such as relative positions and orientations. Other data concern the changes among those relationships as the foot moves, which are kinematic factors.

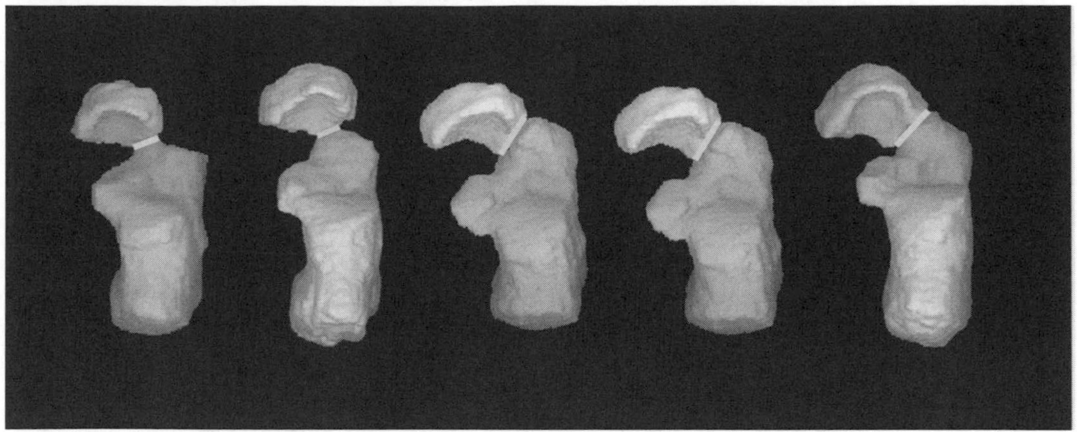

FIGURE 9.7 The calcanei and naviculars of five subjects with calcaneonavicular coalitions. The joints between the bones are indicated by the white lines. The size of this abnormal joint is quite variable, as is the amount of motion it permits.

We break down our results into three categories, representing the three general types of data just described. We call the first category *morphology*, the second *architecture*, and the third *kinematics*.

9.7.1 Morphology

There is much that can be seen and learned simply by looking at visual displays of the reconstructed bones. With careful imaging it is possible to see bony details with a high level of resolution.[1] Although radiographs, sectional images, and (for anatomic purposes) dried bones, reveal a great deal, there are some things that just cannot be seen. These have to do with objects obscured in 2D projection radiographs, particulars of shape and surface form, matters of orientation in space, and details of relationships among bones. In addition, the measurements underlying the images hold information concerning the size, shape and proportion, relationships, and possible abnormalities of the bones, all measured in three dimensions.

As one example, calcaneonavicular coalitions, described in more detail in Section 9.7.3.1, involve an abnormal joint between two bones. One factor in deciding a course of therapy is the extent of the joint. 3D reconstructions can provide this information in a clear manner (Figure 9.7).

Stereo pairs (Figure 9.8) can be useful when the illusion of depth helps clarify relationships.[52] Rotating a reconstruction approximately 5° around a vertical axis, and displaying the two images side by side to create such pairs is easily done via 3DVIEWNIX.

The tarsal bones are, in their details, complicated shapes. However, in order to characterize their morphology and movements we have found it useful to define a coordinate system for each bone, which serves as a reference system for the bones. These "bone axes systems" are defined by the geometric centroid of each bone, plus its three principal axes. Analyses similar to some of ours, derived from CT data, have been used to describe certain architectural features of the carpus.[49,78]

In this system the three axes are orthogonal to each other, and all pass through the centroid (Figure 9.9). The location and orientation of a bone axes system are indicators of the location and orientation of the bone. In addition, three axis segments can be defined, representing the section of each axis between its intersections with the surface. The lengths of these segments, AL_1, AL_2, and AL_3, help describe the size and proportion of each bone.[42] They are measured in millimeters, giving an indication of the bones' actual sizes and shapes. For the four bones we studied, we consistently found that $AL_1 > AL_2 > AL_3$.

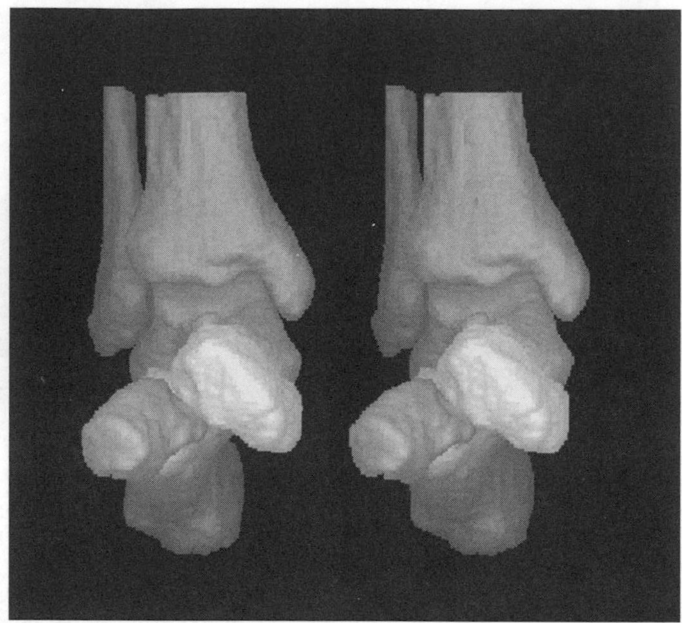

FIGURE 9.8 A stereo pair of the four posterior foot bones and the lower ends of the leg bones in an anterior view.

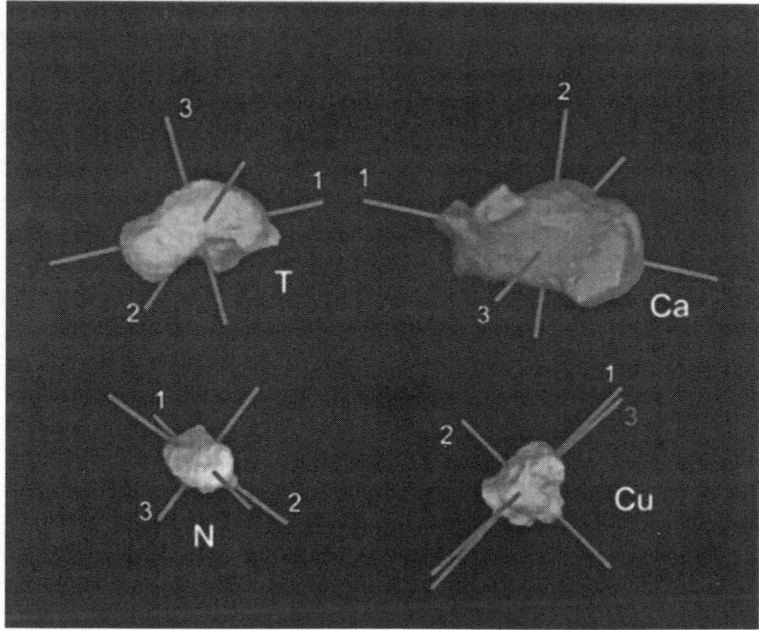

FIGURE 9.9 Medial views of the talus (T), calcaneus (Ca), navicular (N), and cuboid (Cu), with the principal axes of each bone shown. All bones are shown in the same orientation (anterior is on the left) and magnification.

For the calcaneus, cuboid, and talus the first principal axis is oriented in a roughly anterior-posterior direction, but for the navicular it is oriented from side to side. The second principal axes of the calcaneus and cuboid are approximately vertical in their orientation, in the talus it is from side to side, and in the navicular it is anterior-posterior (Figure 9.9).[42]

TABLE 9.3
Length and Volume Parameters of the Tarsal Bones and Relative Sizes

	Linear		Volumetric	
	AL_1 (mm) ± SD	Length Relative to Calcaneus	Volume (cm^3) ± SD	Volume Relative to Calcaneus
Calcaneus	80.37 ± 6.56	1.00	66.72 ± 14.90	1.00
Talus	56.43 ± 3.05	.70	36.38 ± 6.66	.55
Cuboid	34.02 ± 2.04	.42	12.21 ± 2.10	.18
Navicular	39.09 ± 3.04	.49	10.79 ± 2.54	.16

Table 9.3 lists some of the average values for measurements of the four tarsal bones we study and their relation to the calcaneus, in our normal sample. The axis segment length for AL_1 of the calcaneus is 80.37 mm, making it the longest of the bones. The talus averages 70% of the length of the calcaneus. The other two bones are, on average, less than half as long as the calcaneus. The calcaneus is also the largest of the bones on the basis of bulk, with an average volume of 66.72 cm^3. It is almost twice as large as the talus, which has an average volume of 36.38 cm^3, more than five times as large as the cuboid at 12.21 cm^3, and over six times as large as the navicular, whose volume averages 10.79 cm^3.

The proportions of each bone can be characterized by the ratios of the axis segments. We define the following ratios:

$$R_1 = \frac{AL_2}{AL_1} \qquad R_2 = \frac{AL_3}{AL_1} \qquad R_3 = \frac{AL_3}{AL_2}$$

In a sample of 10 subjects the ratios were quite constant for each type of bone, and independent of size. For the talus the mean ratios were 0.7, 0.4, and 0.6; for the calcaneus they were 0.5, 0.3, and 0.7; for the navicular they were 0.7, 0.4, and 0.5; and for the cuboid they were 0.8, 0.6, and 0.8. These ratios describe the overall shape of each of the bones. The cuboid, as its name indicates, is the most block-like of the four bones, and the calcaneus is the most elongated. The talus and navicular have similar proportions, but their long axes are oriented differently. A 3D cluster plot of R_1, R_2, and R_3 showed that each bone type formed a cluster distinct from the others.[42] It is likely that deviations from these proportions will be of value in classifying certain pathologies.

We have begun to apply such quantitative morphological methods to the study of the evolution of human bipedalism, because differences in foot bone proportion and interrelationships are likely to be related to mechanisms of gait. There are, for example, questions about the nature of Neanderthal locomotion that could bear on their lifestyles, and one of the factors that could have affected the way they walked is the proportions of their bones. A sample of six Neanderthal talus casts was imaged and analyzed to compare their proportions to those of modern human bones. We found that the third principal axis segment, which in tali is vertically oriented, is proportionately longer in the fossil group.[42] Trinkhaus[79] made a similar observation by measuring specimens with calipers and calculating length/height and length/breadth measurements. He observed that tali that are relatively foreshortened and taller place more bone mass under the tibia, and tali that are in line with the body weight and calf muscle induce joint reaction forces.[79]

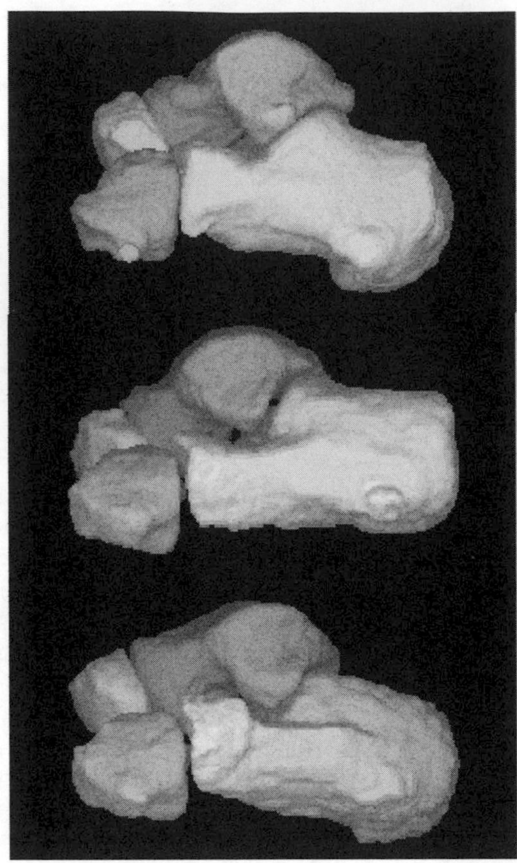

FIGURE 9.10 Comparison of a normal foot to the foot of a patient with congenital pes planus (flat foot): Normal foot (top); abnormal foot (middle); abnormal foot after surgical correction (bottom). All are shown in lateral view.

9.7.2 Architecture

3D reconstructions give a clear view of the relationships among the bones of the feet. This may be of use to surgeons in their assessment of abnormal feet and the effects of reconstructive operations. Figure 9.10 shows a subject with a severe flat foot, before and after corrective surgery, and a normal foot for comparison. The pre-operative organization of the foot (middle panel in Figure 9.10) is clearly abnormal. The calcaneus, instead of appearing tilted upward at its anterior end looks almost flat; the talus has slid forward and down relative to the calcaneus; the cuboid is everted or tilted toward the outer side of the foot. The surgery largely corrected these problems.[39]

Given the wide variety of measurements available to categorize the bones and their relationships, it is reasonable to wonder whether any of them can be used to form a description of normal feet. Alternatively, can changes in any of these parameters be used as a basis for categorizing various types of abnormal feet?

A number of measurements related to the relationships among bones can be derived from the 3D data. So far we have selected three types of measurements as including potentially useful parameters for defining the interosseous relationships.[43] In all cases the parameters are defined for the foot's neutral position. They are, first, the distances between centroids which, when normalized for variation in foot size, give an indication of the proportions of different parts of the foot. They are also likely to change if bones alter their orientation for one reason or another, such as ligament

TABLE 9.4
Architectural Parameters of Normal Feet

	Mean	SD	%CV
dCaCu	64.57	1.61	2.49
dCaNa	69.95	1.99	2.84
dCaTa	46.03	1.20	2.61
dCuNa	38.74	2.24	5.78
dCuTa	60.63	3.29	5.42
dTaNa	44.35	1.80	4.06
aCaCuNa	81.31	2.68	3.29
aCaNaCu	65.68	2.61	3.98
aNaCaCu	33.01	2.12	6.41
aCaCuTa	42.81	1.62	3.78
aCaTaCu	73.68	4.07	5.52
aTaCaCu	63.50	4.59	7.23
aCaNaTa	39.68	1.90	4.78
aCaTaNa	102.77	3.93	3.83
aTaCaNa	39.04	1.95	5.00
aTaNaCu	92.70	3.30	3.56
aNaTaCu	39.49	1.69	4.27
aTaCuNa	47.28	2.38	5.02
ACaCu	122.45	5.51	4.50
ACaNa	65.35	2.40	3.67
ACaTa	144.48	2.53	1.75
ACuNa	65.84	6.85	10.40
ACuTa	129.41	5.79	4.47
ANaTa	86.20	4.33	5.02

Note: The prefix d represents the intercentroid distance between any two bones; a is the angle subtended by three centroids, with the middle bone in the list being at the apex of the angle; and A denotes the magnitude of the angle formed between the major principal axes of any two bones. Ca = calcaneus; Cu = cuboid; Na = navicular; Ta = talus.

Source: From Stindel, E., Udupa, J. K., Hirsch, B.E., and Odhner D., *IEEE Trans. Biomed. Eng.*, in press, 1999. With permission.

damage. Second, the subtended angle formed by two lines connecting any three centroids is an indicator of the arrangement of the bones. Potentially, changes in bone proportions or orientation can affect the "spread" of the bones. The third indicator, the angle between the major principal axes of any two bones, reflects their orientation and possible variations in shape.

There are 24 such architectural parameters for the four bones we studied, and for each we have calculated the mean and variation in our normal population of 10 subjects. Table 9.4 gives the means for each of these parameters in our sample of 10 normal feet, along with the standard deviation and percent coefficient of variation for each parameter.[42]

Given this wealth of data describing the interrelationships among the bones we have studied, it is reasonable to wonder whether it can be of any help in diagnosing or categorizing feet according to abnormalities. We have developed a method for selecting parameters that vary from the normal in certain pathological conditions which may serve this purpose.[43] This method consists of creating a profile of architectural parameters that deviate from the normal population, for each abnormal group. A suspect foot is then classified on the basis of a number of parameters that have been linked to these groups. We believe this is more likely to prove valid than trying to identify only one or two key diagnostic features. Although data from only a small sample of patients has been used in devising this method, we think that it has promise for determining when a patient's foot can be considered functionally abnormal, and the nature and extent of its abnormality. The profiles described in Ref. 43 will be refined as more patients are included in our study.

9.7.3 Kinematics

In this section, we will discuss both the qualitative aspects of kinematics observed from animations and the quantitative aspects derived from mathematical motion descriptions.

9.7.3.1 Qualitative

The motion data computed by rigid body analysis are used to create various animations of the moving bones and can also be utilized to derive other information about the nature of the joint motion. However, just as there is much that can be learned by looking at still images of the bones, a lot can be learned by observing the movies. These animated displays allow, for the first time, the observation of whole bones moving in their natural way *in situ*.

For all the subjects studied, animations were prepared showing the bones as the feet were moved from pronation to supination. It was found that the motions are easier to study if they are expressed relative to one bone, say, the calcaneus or talus. This provides a common visual reference and eliminates the effect of extraneous movement such as a motion of the foot as a whole. Moreover, choosing the appropriate reference bone makes it easier to describe a motion in terms of conventionally used relationships. For example, open chain (non-weight-bearing) subtalar pronation-supination is often described according to the way the calcaneus moves relative to the talus. As another example, movies of the navicular and cuboid relative to the calcaneus were used to study the motions at the transverse tarsal joint. A variety of such animations can be prepared, showing any combination of the bones from any point of view.

Many observations were made during our studies, such as the following examples. In all normal feet, the calcaneus moves as expected at the subtalar joint. It inverts, adducts, and flexes relative to the talus during supination (Figure 9.11). The navicular is also seen to adduct and invert (Figure 9.12). Motion of the cuboid relative to the calcaneus was similar. We noticed that some motion also took place at the cuboideonavicular joint. This articulation is often assumed to have little[80] or no[81] motion; our data disagreed with those authors but agreed with other authors who have measured some motion at the joint.[24,25] However, in walking, the actual range of joint motion is much smaller than the maximum possible,[58] and it is therefore feasible that the cuboideonavicular joint is essentially immobile in normal gait.

No special criteria were used in the selection of the normal subjects, other than clinically normal ankle and foot function. The subjects, therefore, included people with a variety of foot types ranging from feet that were almost flat to feet with high arches. Yet, if any selection of movies is displayed side by side on the computer monitor they can be seen to move in approximate synchrony, like dancers in a chorus line.

Watching the bones in action makes some aspects of the joint functions much more obvious, and therefore leads to a better understanding of foot function. As an example, the foot undergoes a motion called pronation-supination in which it is twisted from side to side (see the explanation in Section 9.3). This motion is known to occur primarily within the foot at two joint complexes: the subtalar and transverse tarsal joints. However, the relative contribution of each of these joint complexes is not known. Root et al.[58] imply that most of it occurs in the subtalar joint, but van Langelaan[24] (in cadavers) and Lundberg et al.[25,26] (in living subjects) found that talonavicular pronation-supination is greater than talocalcaneal. It is apparent from observing our reconstructions

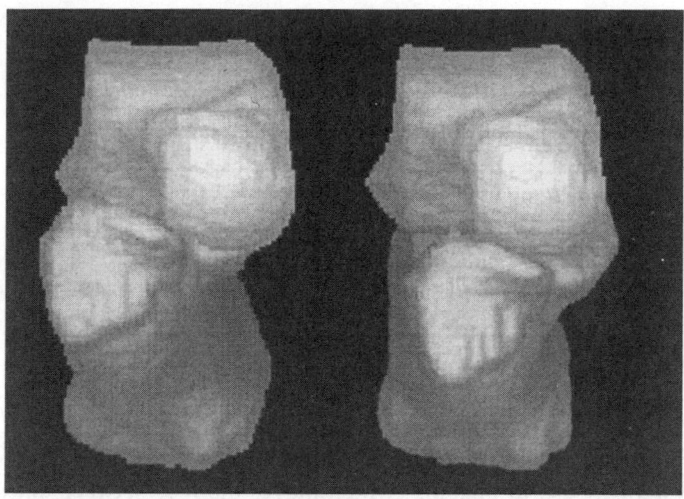

FIGURE 9.11 Anterior views of the talus and calcaneus, with calcaneal motion shown relative to a fixed talus: extreme pronation (left) and extreme supination (right). As the foot supinates the position of the calcaneus changes: it pivots towards the right (adduction), rotates counterclockwise (inversion), and tilts downward (flexion). These motions occur at the subtalar joint.

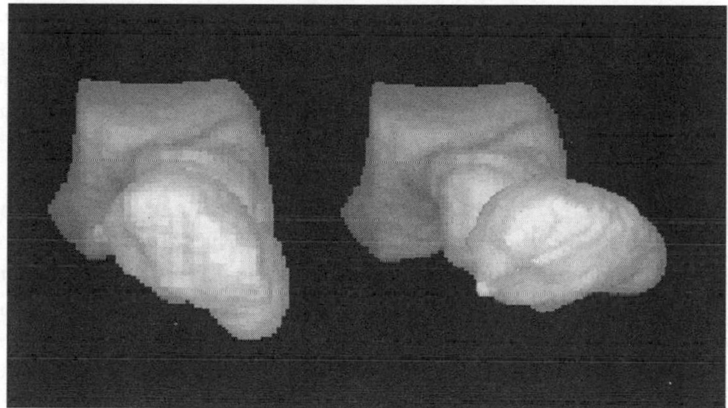

FIGURE 9.12 Anterior views of the talus and navicular of the same foot as in Figure 9.11, with navicular motion shown relative to a fixed talus: extreme pronation (left) and extreme supination (right). The navicular undergoes the same types of motion as the calcaneus does, but the amount of motion is greater. Talonavicular motion takes place at the transverse tarsal joint.

(such as Figures 9.11 and 9.12, although it is more apparent in animations) that more motion occurs in the transverse tarsal than the subtalar joint, at least in our conditions of foot pronation and supination. This puts us in agreement with van Langelaan and Lundberg. The observation is supported by our measurements of joint ranges of motion: the talonavicular joint undergoes 49.2 ± 5.9° of rotation from extreme pronation to extreme supination, whereas the talocalcaneal joint undergoes only 22.3 ± 5.8° of rotation in the same movement (Table 9.5).

9.7.3.2 Quantitative

As indicated in the last paragraph, numerical data underlie the display of motion seen in animation of the kinematics. Examples of these kinds of data follow.

TABLE 9.5
Average Maximum Range of Motion ± SD at Each Joint

Talocalcaneal	Talocuboideal	Talonavicular	Calcaneonavicular	Calcaneocuboid	Cuboideonavicular
		Normal Subjects			
27.2 ± 6.3°	51.8 ± 13.1°	49.2 ± 5.9°	27.2 ± 6.3°	26.8 ± 7.5°	13.5 ± 4.8°
		Calcaneonavicular Coalition Patients			
10.5 ± 8.4°	27.1 ± 15.4°	24.2 ± 12.5°	10.5 ± 8.4°	15.1 ± 9.3°	8.5 ± 4.5°
		Pes Planus Patients			
16.4 ± 6.9°	38.3 ± 4.8°	37.9 ± 8.1°	22.3 ± 5.9°	27.2 ± 3.4°	18.3 ± 5.7°

Most joints are capable of a much greater range of motion than is typically required in normal activities.[58] The system we use in imaging, which moves the foot between extremes of pronation and supination, exceeds the limited range of ordinary use and may approach the actual limits. For each of the joints we studied, we calculated the total rotation it underwent. This information is shown in Table 9.5.

Because articular surfaces are not truly cylindrical or spherical, the position of an axis of rotation must necessarily change, depending on where the joint is in its range of motion.[82] The axes system of a bone will therefore change its orientation — reflecting rotation of the bone — as well as its location, which reflects translation. Early studies tended to acknowledge that axes of rotation change, but their techniques were not sensitive enough to pick up the translations accurately.[21,57] The development of more precise methods permitted van Langelaan to measure the small translations accompanying rotation in cadaver specimens,[24] but he elected to describe his results in terms of a helical axis model. We can also measure translations, but since we do not transform the data to fit any model, our values are not comparable to his.

In our description of the bony architecture of the foot, we defined 24 parameters which specify the relationships of the bones, as described in Section 9.7.2.[43] The values of these parameters change as the foot moves, so that they also provide a means of quantifying various kinematic aspects of foot function. Moreover, just as we found profiles of the architectural parameters that could be used to categorize normal and abnormal feet, it is likely that kinematic abnormalities will be reflected in patterns of change in these characteristics. Some of the changes in pattern that we have observed are described below.

The articular facets that control a bone's motion are on the surface, away from the centroid. As movement takes place at a joint, the centroids of two articulating bones will either approach each other or move farther apart. We have calculated these changes in distance, but they are very small when the joint motions are small. Nevertheless, we have seen patterns of change. For example, in normal feet the distance between the centroids of the talus and calcaneus come about 1.5 mm closer together as the foot goes from extreme pronation to extreme supination, whereas the talus and navicular, on the other hand, separate by about 2.5 mm.[5]

Connecting the centroids of any three bones with two lines creates an angle with the vertex at the centroid of one of the bones, as described in Section 9.7.2 (Figure 9.13). As the centroids move, the size of this included angle will change. We have observed that the angle formed by each trio of bones changes in a consistent way from one extreme of the range of motion to the other. For example, the cuboid-talus-calcaneus angle gradually decreases from roughly 77 to 70° as the foot moves from pronation to supination. At the same time, the talus-navicular-cuboid angle increases from about 91 to 100°.[5,39]

It is generally believed that change in the amount and position of cartilage-to-cartilage contact at a joint is one of the most important factors leading to the development of cartilage degeneration

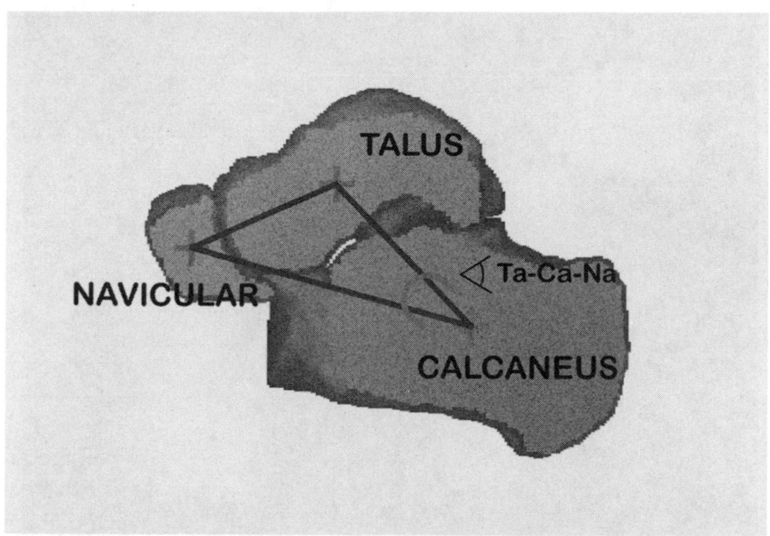

FIGURE 9.13 A diagrammatic illustration of the included angles. The crosses represent the centroids of the bones.

and arthrosis.[83] When the area of contact — which is the area of load transmission — is reduced, the load per unit area can increase beyond the cartilage's physiological capacity to bear it. Similar results can follow when abnormal positioning of bones moves the contact area to a region of the joint surface that is unable to properly bear the load. There has been no technique for measuring or locating the contact area in a living joint. Most studies rely on the insertion of pressure-sensitive film into cadaver joints[84] or other destructive methods. We have developed a method for measuring the distance between two adjacent bones and defining the areas in which the bones are separated by some small distance. As this distance reaches the thickness of the cartilage layers, it approximates the area of contact between those bones.[85]

Early efforts to display the distance between the two bones of the temporomandibular joint[86] have been further developed and animated in the context of the tarsal joints (Figure 9.14).[85] Preliminary experiments (unpublished) were carried out in which sheets of Fuji Prescale Film™, a pressure-sensitive system, were inserted into the ankle of a cadaver while it was in a device that put a load across the joint. This device was made of plastic, so that we were able to collect an MR image data set while the film was in place. These results indicated that the areas of minimum distance displayed through 3D imaging were similar to the areas of pressure transmission as demonstrated with the use of the pressure-sensitive film.

We have begun to apply these methods of analysis to certain pathological conditions. Among the most common of the variant tarsal joints and coalitions is some sort of a union between the calcaneus and the navicular. This can range from a very small joint which appears to have no effect on foot function, to a large joint which effectively locks that part of the foot (Figure 9.7), or even to a bony coalition.[87] Patients with such coalitions typically become symptomatic in their teenage years, as the replacement of flexible cartilage with rigid bone causes strain in other joints, which can no longer compensate adequately. Some such patients require surgery to resect the area of the joint, freeing up the region. However, many patients adjust over time and become pain free. We have imaged four such symptomatic young men, one of whom was imaged again after a surgical resection.

All four of the patients had restriction of motion between the calcaneus and the navicular. Two had practically no mobility, one was quite restricted, and one — who had the smallest area of bony contact — was at the lower limit of the normal population. The patient who required surgical intervention (and was later imaged a second time) had a range of motion at the calcaneonavicular

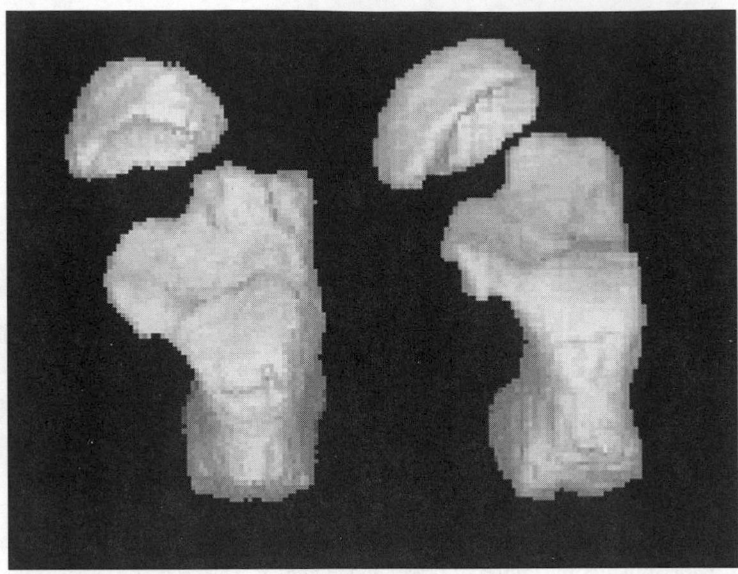

FIGURE 9.14 This dorsal view of the calcaneus and navicular in pronation (left) and supination (right) illustrates the areas where the talus was close to those bones. In this example, the areas where the talus was 4.0 mm or less from the other bones is colored pink and can be considered indicative of joint contact areas. In this example, the joint was not loaded, so the contact areas do not necessarily represent the areas of weight transmission.

TABLE 9.6
Joint Range of Motion Before and After Osteotomy for Calcaneonavicular Coalition

	Talocalcaneal	Talocuboideal	Talonavicular	Calcaneo-navicular	Calcaneocuboid	Cuboideo-navicular
Pre-operative	13.7°	22.2°	16.7°	3.5°	10.9°	8.1°
Post-operative	14.3°	29.2°	25.8°	13.2°	17.0°	20.3°

joint of only 3.5°, compared to an average range in our normal subjects of 27.2° (Table 9.6). Interestingly, the patient whose movement seemed most normal required surgery to control the pain (he will be imaged post-operatively in the future), while the remaining two, apparently worse, did not. Clearly, there are factors other than the extent of coalition affecting the clinical course. These could include the properties and fibrous or cartilaginous nature of the material between the bones, the shape and ligamentous properties of other joints in the foot, and compensatory changes and remodeling in other joints.

Because the calcaneonavicular joint is part of the transverse tarsal joint, which controls pronation and supination, the restriction in these patients limits the maximum range of motion their feet can undergo. In Table 9.5 it can be seen that the amount of angular excursion is reduced at all of the joints of the four patients we studied, generally by about half. Although these patients came for treatment because of pain, they were still able to get about, which indicates that there had been some compensatory adjustment within the foot to allow ambulation. The patient who underwent surgery illustrates this. Pre-operatively he was able to move his foot from extreme pronation to only slight supination — about half the normal range of motion. Considering that the presence of the calcaneonavicular joint caused his transverse tarsal joint to be practically locked, which dramatically reduces pronation-supination there, he had to compensate elsewhere or walking would be extremely difficult. Pre- and post-operative movies of the surgical patient gave some indication of the compensatory motion he was using. The talar motion was seen to be abnormal, in some positions of the foot moving in directions almost opposite to what was expected. This could be related to the adaptive change in the ankle joint, from a hinge to a ball-and-socket joint, which sometimes develops in such patients over time. After resection of the abnormal joint, his talar motion was practically normal. Moreover, the range of motion increased at all the intertarsal joints of this patient (Table 9.6).

Various special animations were created to clarify the biomechanical effects of the restrictions.[53] Examples include the application of motion from a normal foot to the navicular of a calcaneonavicular coalition. In reality the navicular could not move in anything like a normal manner because the outgrowths of the two bones block such motion. However, in the movie it seems as if the navicular moves right into and out of the calcaneus, the amount of such intersection being an indication of the amount of bone that needs to be resected. Figure 9.6 illustrates this form of display.

The included angle of this patient's joints were measured as his foot was moved, both pre- and post-operatively. During that time his cuboid-talus-calcaneus angle *increased* from 69 to 71°, which is opposite to the situation in our normal subjects. After surgery the direction of motion was reversed and was brought within the normal range. A similar reversal of direction and shift into the normal range was observed at the talus-navicular-cuboid angle.[5]

Another common pathological condition is pes planus, frequently known as flat foot. In this situation the arch of the foot is low, which puts strain on the ligaments of the foot joints, reduces the ability of the foot to absorb shocks, reduces its energy storage capabilities, and often leads to pain. In X-rays it can be seen that the calcaneal inclination, which measures the obliquity of the bone, is low. This is also seen in 3D reconstructions of the posterior tarsal bones (Figure 9.15). Pes planus can be congenital, the result of trauma, or degenerative. One form is common in middle-aged women if their tibialis posterior tendon undergoes degeneration and ruptures; that muscle helps support the arches of the foot under stress, and when it is non-functional the arch eventually falls. Various surgical procedures are employed to correct the deformity. We have imaged five pes planus patients and are evaluating the data.[88]

All the patients were able to move their feet into 20° of pronation, like normal feet. However, none were able to supinate as far as the normal population. Perhaps this was because the abnormal starting relationships among the bones meant that the joint contact areas reached the edges of their cartilage sooner than they would in normal feet, that somewhere there was abnormal bone-to-bone contact, or that the ligaments became taut. This limited supination is probably related to the reduced range of motion measured in most of the intertarsal joints (Table 9.5).

9.8 FUTURE DIRECTIONS

The most difficult problem we have faced is the development of an efficient, accurate, and reliable method of segmenting bone in MR images. Most 3D studies involving bones have used CT as the data source, because segmentation can generally be carried out with little difficulty.[45–49,54,55,89] However, because we would be working with living subjects and imaging them a number of times, it was ethically not possible to use CT with its relatively high radiation dose. We were, therefore, forced to use MR images for our data, which made segmentation a difficult process. Bone gives little signal in MR, so that the denser the bone the darker the image. This often makes the bone–soft tissue boundary rather distinct and can sometimes be an advantage; but the tendons and ligaments that attach to bone have similarly low signals, so the exact bone boundary in those regions can be quite obscure.

At the other extreme, the trabecular spaces in the ankle are filled with yellow marrow, which gets its name from its high fat content. Where the cortex is thin and images poorly, the bone may appear to blend indistinguishably with nearby tissues. The most extreme situation among the four

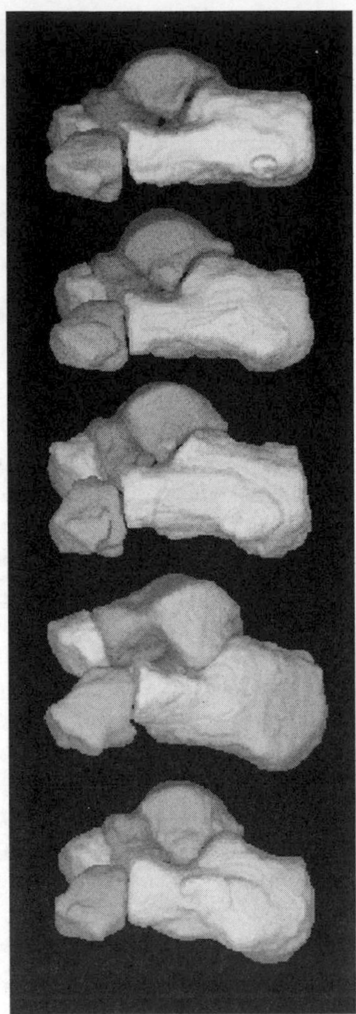

FIGURE 9.15 Lateral views of five pes planus patients, with varying degrees of flattening of the arch.

bones of this study is the area of the cuboid around the attachment of the plantar calcaneocuboid ligament. No cortex can be distinguished, and the mixed trabecular bone–yellow marrow of the cuboid appears virtually the same as the loosely fascicular ligament. Therefore, the cuboid is the most difficult of the four bones to segment, and it is sometimes hard to be sure of the true boundary of the bone.

In our early animations, the motion of the cuboid proved to be difficult to evaluate. It seemed to move more irregularly than was expected from previous understanding of midtarsal joint function, which may be a result of the difficulty in segmenting it. Any errors in such approximations are liable to affect the motions calculated because not only is the bone relatively small, but its secondary and tertiary principal axes are very similar in length. It seems that fairly small errors in segmentation of the cuboid can lead to unrealistic movements. More recent segmentations, however, have led to much smoother animations, which indicates that the bone axes system of the cuboid has become more reliable with the improved segmentation methods.

Although development of the live wire and live lane techniques has greatly improved our ability to segment bones,[68] we hope to further improve the reliability and speed of the process. We intend to develop 3D and 4D extensions of the live methods.[90]

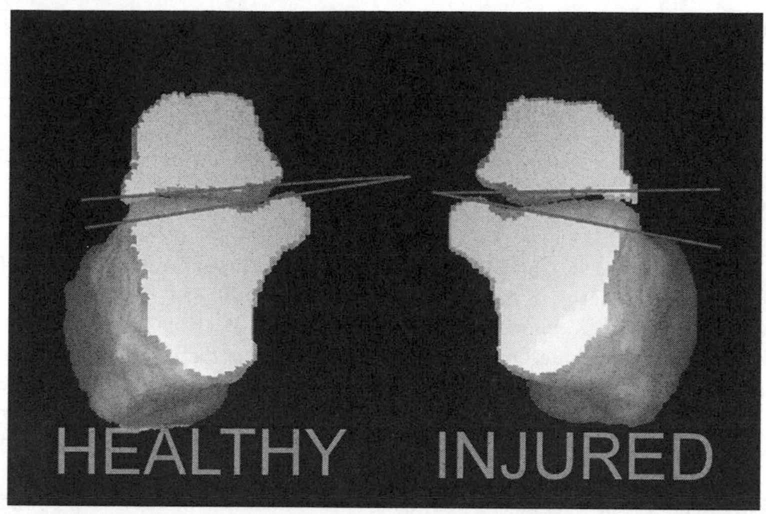

FIGURE 9.16 Frontal sections through the tali and calcanei of a patient with chronic ankle instability, resulting from injury to ligaments on the lateral side of the ankle and subtalar joints. There is an increase in the angle between the bones of the injured foot, indicating that the injury has affected the ligaments that stabilize the subtalar joint.

Internal kinematic analysis will lead to new information about normal and abnormal foot function and can lead to improved diagnosis and treatment of various abnormal conditions. It can be used to visualize and measure relationships in regions that are not visible in plane radiographs and whose 3D configuration cannot be seen in CT or MR. We have, for example, begun to use quantitative 3D analysis of the subtalar joint to evaluate the extent of ligamentous damage at that joint in ankle sprains involving the lateral ligaments (Figure 9.16). In this project we use a non-metallic version of the ankle flexibility tester developed by Siegler et al.[91] to put a defined load on the ankle and subtalar joints.

In addition to the static and subjective diagnostic techniques now used to diagnose and evaluate patients, it will be possible to assess their foot function. Ultimately, we hope to be able to develop a means to visualize and quantify the effects of surgical or non-surgical treatments, and to use that capability to aid in surgical planning.

There are some limits to the use of internal kinematics. MR imaging is more costly than many other diagnostic methodologies, so its use will be justifiable only when simpler methods do not work, or when serious or complicated treatments call for a precise evaluation of the patient. Also, the time required to acquire a data set means that joint motion cannot be measured as the joint functions in real time. However, it may be possible to combine or correlate the data derived from internal kinematics with the data from a real-time gait analysis system, so that one can determine the changes occurring within the joints as the body segments change. It may also be possible to determine which aspects of internal kinematics data are relevant (and to what extent) to the real-time motion observed in gait.

ACKNOWLEDGMENTS

This work has been done in collaboration with a number of investigators, including Drs. Howard Hillstrom and Michelle Butterworth. The study of the calcaneonavicular coalitions is being done in cooperation with Drs. Gary R. Bauer and Enyi Okereke. The pes planus study is being done with Dr. Kieran T. Mahan. Drs. Okereke, Sorin Siegler, and Lee Techner are involved in the work on lateral ankle ligament injuries. Adam L. Michaels carried out the studies comparing our method of determining joint contact area and the use of pressure-sensitive film. Dr. Christine Couture performed the anthropological investigations.

Much of this research was supported by grants from the National Institutes of Health (NIH NS 37172) and the Department of the Army (DAMD 179717271).

REFERENCES

1. Hirsch, B. E., Udupa, J. K., and Roberts, D., Three-dimensional reconstruction of the foot from computed tomography scans, *J. Am. Podiatric Med. Assoc.*, 79, 384, 1989.
2. Hirsch, B. E., Udupa, J. K., Goncalves, R. J., and Roberts, D., Kinematics of joints of the foot via three-dimensional magnetic resonance images, *Proceedings of the First Conference on Visualization in Biomedical Computing*, IEEE Computer Society Press, Washington, D.C.,1990, 232.
3. Hirsch, B. E., Udupa, J. K., and Roberts, D., Joint kinematics can be determined by computerized three dimensional imaging of MRI data, *Anat. Rec.*, 226, 45A, 1990.
4. Hirsch, B. E., Udupa, J. K., and Samarasekera, S., New method of studying joint kinematics from three-dimensional reconstructions of MRI data, *J. Am. Podiatric Med. Assoc.*, 86, 4, 1996.
5. Udupa, J. K., Hirsch, B. E., Hillstrom, H. J., Bauer, G. R., and Kneeland, J. B., Analysis of *in vivo* 3-D internal kinematics of the joints of the foot, *IEEE Trans. Biomed. Eng.*, 45, 1387, 1998.
6. Bauer, G. R., Hillstrom, H. J., Udupa, J. K., and Hirsch, B. E., Clinical applications of three-dimensional magnetic resonance image analysis, *J. Am. Podiatric Med. Assoc.*, 86, 33, 1996.
7. Hirsch, B. E., Structural biomechanics of the foot bones, *J. Am. Podiatric Med. Assoc.*, 81, 338, 1991.
8. Wood Jones, F., *Structure and Function as Seen in the Foot*, 2nd ed., Ballière, Tindall and Cox, London, 1949, 1.
9. Helfand, A. E., Keep them walking, *J. Am. Podiatric Assoc.*, 58, 117, 1968.
10. Helfand, A. E., Gerontology — geriatrics education, *Clin. Podiatric Med. Surg.*, 10, 297, 1993.
11. Hodge, W. A., Fijan, R. S., Carlson, K. L., Burgess, R. G., Harris, W. H., and Mann, R. W., Contact pressures in the human hip joint measured *in vivo*, *Proc. Natl. Acad. Sci. U.S.A.*, 83, 2879, 1986.
12. Close, J. R., Inman, V. T., Poor, P. M., and Todd, F. N., The function of the subtalar joint, *Clin. Orthoped. & Relat. Res.*, 5, 159, 1967.
13. Kaigle, A. M., Pope, M. H., Fleming, B. C., and Hansson, T., A method for the intravital measurement of interspinous kinematics, *J. Biomech.*, 25, 451, 1992.
14. Koh, T. J., Grabiner, M. D., and De Swart, R. J., *In vivo* tracking of the human patella, *J. Biomech.*, 25, 637, 1992.
15. Lafortune, M. A., Cavanagh, P. R., Sommer, H. J., III, and Kalenak, A., Three-dimensional kinematics of the human knee during walking, *J. Biomech.*, 25, 347, 1992.
16. Levens, A. S., Inman, V. T., and Blosser, J. A., Transverse rotation of the segments of the lower extremity in locomotion, *J. Bone Jt. Surg.*, 30-A, 859, 1948.
17. Knutzen, K. M. and Price, A., Lower extremity static and dynamic relationships with rear foot motion in gait, *J. Am. Podiatric Med. Assoc.*, 84, 171, 1994.
18. Wright, D. G., Desai, S. M., and Henderson, W. H., Action of the subtalar and ankle-joint complex during the stance phase of walking, *J. Bone Jt. Surg.*, 46-A, 361, 1964.
19. Palmer, A. K., Werner, F. W., Murphy, D., and Glisson, R., Functional wrist motion: A biomechanical study, *J. Hand Surg.*, 10A, 39, 1985.
20. Inman, V. T., *The Joints of the Ankle*, Williams & Wilkins, Baltimore, 1976, Appendix A.
21. Manter, J. T., Movements of the subtalar and transverse tarsal joints, *Anat. Rec.*, 80, 397, 1941.
22. Hefzy, M. S. and Yang, H., A three-dimensional anatomical model of the human patello-femoral joint, for the determination of patello-femoral motions and contact characteristics, *J. Biomed. Eng.*, 15, 289, 1993.
23. Stähelin, T., Nigg, B. M., Stefanyshyn, D. J., van den Bogert, A. J., and Kim, S.-J., A method to determine bone movement in the ankle joint complex *in vitro*, *J. Biomech.*, 30, 513, 1997.
24. van Langelaan, E. J., A kinematical analysis of the tarsal joints, *Acta Orthoped. Scand.*, 54 (Suppl. 204), 1, 1983.

25. Lundberg, A., Kinematics of the ankle and foot. In vitro roentgen stereophotogrammetry, *Acta Orthoped. Scand.*, 60 (Suppl. 233), 1, 1989.
26. Lundberg, A., Svensson, O. K., Bylund, C., Goldie, I., and Selvik, G., Kinematics of the ankle/foot complex — Part 2: Pronation and supination, *Foot & Ankle*, 9, 248, 1989.
27. Lundberg, A., Goldie, I., Kalin, B., and Selvik, G., Kinematics of the ankle/foot complex: Plantarflexion and dorsiflexion, *Foot & Ankle*, 9, 194, 1989.
28. Löfvenberg, R., Kärrholm, J., and Lundberg, A., Subtalar instability in chronic lateral instability of the ankle, *The Foot*, 2, 39, 1992.
29. Cappozzo, A., Catani, F., Leardini, A., Benedetti, M. G., and Della Croce, U. E., Position and orientation in space of bones during movement: Experimental artefacts, *Clin. Biomech.*, 11, 90, 1996.
30. Reinschmidt, C., van den Bogert, A. J., Nigg, B. M., Lundberg, A., and Murphy, N., Effect of skin movement on the analysis of skeletal knee joint motion during running, *J. Biomech.*, 30, 729, 1997.
31. Tranberg, R. and Karlsson, D., The relative skin movement of the foot: A 2-D roentgen photogrammetry study, *Clin. Biomech.*, 13, 71, 1998.
32. Kepple, T. M., Stanhope, S. J., Lohmann, K. N., and Roman, N. L., A video based technique for measuring ankle-subtalar joint motion during stance, *J. Biomed. Eng.*, 12, 273, 1990.
33. Cass, J. R. and Settles, H., Ankle instability: In vitro kinematics in response to ankle load, *Foot & Ankle*, 15, 134, 1994.
34. Brossmann, J., Muhle, C., Schröder, C., Melchert, U. H., Büll, C. C., Spielmann, R. P., and Heller, M., Patellar tracking patterns during active and passive knee extension: Evaluation with motion-triggered cine MR imaging, *Radiology*, 187, 205, 1993.
35. Niitsu, M., Akisada, M., Anno, I., and Miyakawa, S., Moving knee joint: Technique for kinematic MRI imaging, *Radiology*, 174, 569, 1990.
36. Schutzer, S. F., Ramsby, G. R., and Fulkerson, J. P., Computed tomographic classification of patellofemoral pain patients, *Orthoped. Clin. North Am.*, 17, 235, 1986.
37. Shellock, F. G., Foo, T. K. F., Deutsch, A. L., and Mink, A. L., Patellofemoral joint: Evaluation during active flexion with ultrafast spoiled GRASS imaging, *Radiology*, 180, 581, 1991.
38. Neuman, T. R., Hengesteg, A., Lepage, R. P., Kaufman, K. R., and Woodson, G. E., Three-dimensional motion of the arytenoid adduction procedure in cadaver larynges, *Ann. Otol. Rhinol. Laryngol.*, 103, 265, 1994.
39. Hirsch, B. E., Udupa, J. K., Mahan, K. T., Bauer, G. R., Hillstrom, H. J., and Kneeland, J. B., A new method for the kinematic analysis of joints, *Medical Imaging 1997: Physiology and Function from Multidimensional Images*, vol. 3033, Hoffman, E. A., Ed., SPIE, Bellingham, WA, 1997, 361.
40. Parks, N. L., Hillstrom, H. J., Hirsch, B. E., and Udapa [sic], J. K., Stereometry and 3-D MRI reconstruction for kinematics of the rearfoot: A cadaver study, *Proceedings of the 16th International Conference of the IEEE Engineering in Biology and Medicine Society*, 1994, 562.
41. Smith, N. L., Hillstrom, H. J., Hirsch, B. E., and Udupa, J. K., Comparison of kinematic measurement: Stereometry and 3-D MRI reconstruction, *Proceedings of the 15th Annual International Conference of the IEEE Engineering in Medicine and Biology Society*, Szeto, A. Y. J. and Rangayyan, R. M., Eds., IEEE, San Diego, CA, 1993, 1069.
42. Stindel, E., Udupa, J. K., Hirsch, B. E., Odhner, D., and Couture, C., 3D MR analysis of the morphology of the rearfoot. Application to classification of bones, *Comp. Med. Imaging Graph.*, 23, 75, 1999.
43. Stindel, E., Udupa, J. K., Hirsch, B. E., and Odhner, D., A characterization of the geometric architecture of the peritalar joint complex via MRI: An aid to the classification of foot type, *IEEE Trans. Biomed. Eng.*, in press, 1999.
44. Udupa, J. K., Hirsch, B. E., Samarasekera, S., Goncalves, R. J., Kneeland, B., Barrett, J. P., Butterworth, M., and Tames, P., Analysis of kinematics of joints via three-dimensional imaging, *Medical Imaging 1993: Image Capture, Formatting, and Display*, vol. 1897, Kim, Y., Ed., SPIE, Bellingham, WA, 1993, 152.
45. Chu, S. A., Skultety, K. J., Suvinen, T. I., Clement, J. G., and Price, C., Computerized three-dimensional magnetic resonance imaging reconstructions of temporomandibular joints for both a model and patients with temporomandibular pain dysfunction, *Oral Pathol. Oral Radiol. Endod.*, 80, 604, 1995.

46. Price, C., Connell, D. G., MacKay, A., and Tobias, D. L., Three-dimensional reconstruction of magnetic resonance images of the temporomandibular joint by I-DEAS, *Dentomaxillofac. Radiol.*, 21, 148, 1992.
47. Bresina, S. J., Vannier, M. W., Logan, S. E., and Weeks, P. M., Three-dimensional wrist imaging: Evaluation of functional and pathologic anatomy by computer, *Clin. Plast. Surg.*, 13, 389, 1986.
48. Patterson, R. M., Elder, K. W., Viegas, S. F., and Buford, W. L., Carpal bone anatomy measured by computer analysis of three-dimensional reconstructions of computed tomography images, *J. Hand Surg.*, 20A, 923, 1995.
49. Tagare, H. D., Elder, K. W., Stoner, D. M., Patterson, R. M., Nicodemus, C. L., Viegas, S. F., and Hillman, G. R., Location and geometric description of carpal bones in CT images, *Ann. Biomed. Eng.*, 21, 715, 1993.
50. Van Sint Jan, S. L., Clapworth, G. J., and Rooze, M., Visualization of combined motions in human joints, *IEEE Comp. Graph. Appl.*, 18(6), 10, 1998.
51. Van Sint Jan, S., Giurintano, D. J., Thompson, D. E., and Rooze, M., Joint kinematics simulation from medical imaging data, *IEEE Trans. Biomed. Eng.*, 44, 1175, 1997.
52. Thompson, W. O., Thaete, F. L., Fu, F. H., and Dye, S. F., Tibial meniscal dynamics using three-dimensional reconstruction of magnetic resonance images, *Am. J. Sports Med.*, 19, 210, 1991.
53. Selbie, W. S., Zhang, L., Levine, W. S., and Ludlow, C. L., Using joint geometry to determine the motion of the cricoarytenoid joint, *J. Acoust. Soc. Am.*, 103, 1115, 1998.
54. Lim, T.-H., Eck, J. C., An, H. S., McGrady, L. M., Harris, G. F., and Haughton, V. M., A noninvasive, three-dimensional spinal motion analysis method, *Spine,* 22, 1996, 1997.
55. Metz-Schimmerl, S. M., Bhatia, G., and Vannier, M., Visualization and quantitative analysis of talocrural joint kinematics, *Comp. Med. Imaging Graph.*, 18, 443, 1994.
56. Harris, G. F., Analysis of ankle and subtalar motion during human locomotion, *Inman's Joints of the Ankle*, 2nd ed., Stiehl, J. B., Ed., Williams & Wilkins, Baltimore, 1991, 75.
57. Hicks, J. H., The mechanics of the foot. I. The joints, *J. Anat.*, 87, 345, 1953.
58. Root, M. L., Orien, W. P., and Weed, J. H., *Normal and Abnormal Function of the Foot*, Clinical Biomechanics Corporation, Los Angeles, 1977, 30.
59. Siegler, S., Chen, J., and Schneck, C. D., The three-dimensional kinematics and flexibility characteristics of the human ankle and subtalar joints, *J. Biomech. Eng.*, 110, 364, 1988.
60. McDonald, J. F., Pruzansky, J. D., and Meltzer, R. M., Evaluation of recurrent macrodactyly with three-dimensional imaging, *J. Am. Podiatric Med. Assoc.*, 81, 84, 1991.
61. Allon, S. M. and Mears, D. C., Three dimensional analysis of calcaneal fractures, *Foot & Ankle*, 11, 254, 1991.
62. Morrison, R., McCarty, J., and Cushing, F. R., Three-dimensional computerized tomography: A quantum leap in diagnostic imaging?, *J. Foot Ankle Surg.*, 33, 72, 1994.
63. Gautsch, T. L., Johnson, E. E., and Seeger, L. L., True three dimensional stereographic display of 3D reconstructed CT scans of the pelvis and acetabulum, *Clin. Orthoped. Relat. Res.*, 305, 138, 1994.
64. Bechtold, J. E. and Powless, S. H., The application of computer graphics in foot and ankle surgical planning and reconstruction, *Clin. Podiatr. Med. Surg.*, 10, 551, 1993.
65. Rhoad, R. C., Klimkiewicz, J. J., Williams, G. R., Kesmodel, S. B., Udupa, J. K., Kneeland, J. B., and Iannotti, J. P., A new in vivo technique for three-dimensional shoulder kinematics analysis, *Skeletal Radiol.*, 27, 92, 1998.
66. Udupa, J., Odhner, D., Samarasekera, S., Goncalves, R., Iyer, K., Venugopal, K., and Furuie, S., 3DVIEWNIX: An open, transportable, multidimensional, multimodality, multiparametric imaging software system, *SPIE Proc.*, 2164, 58, 1994.
67. Udupa, J. K., Samarasekera, S., Odhner, D., Iyer, K., Falcão, A. X., Wei, L., Hirsch, B. E., Tian, J., Palagyi, K., Grossman, R., Miki, Y., van Buchem, M., Philips, M., Holland, G., Axel, L., Kneeland, J. B., and Hemmy, D. C., Clinical 3D imaging and analysis with 3DVIEWNIX, *Radiology,* 197(P), 448, 1995.
68. Falcão, A. X., Udupa, J. K., Samarasekera, S., Sharma, S., Hirsch, B. E., and Lotufo, R. de A., User-steered image segmentation paradigms: Live wire and live lane, *Graph. Models Image Proc.*, 60, 233, 1998.
69. Mortensen, E. A. and Barrett, W. A., Interactive segmentation with intelligent scissors, *Graph. Models Image Proc.*, 60, 349, 1998.

70. Raya, S. P. and Udupa, J. K., Shape-based interpolation of multidimensional objects, *IEEE Trans. Med. Imaging*, 9, 32, 1990.
71. Udupa, J. K. and Goncalves, R. J., Imaging transforms for visualizing surfaces and volumes, *J. Digital Imaging*, 6, 213, 1993.
72. Udupa, J. K., Hung, H. M., and Chuang, K. S., Surface and volume rendering in 3D imaging: A comparison, *J. Digital Imaging,* 4, 159, 1991.
73. Udupa, J. K., Hirsch, B. E., Samarasekera, S., Goncalves, R. J., Kneeland, B., Barrett, J. P., Butterworth, M., and Tames, P., Analysis of kinematics of joints via three-dimensional imaging, *Medical Imaging 1993*, vol. 1897, Kim, Y., Ed., SPIE Bellingham, WA, 1993, 152.
74. Hirsch, B. E., Udupa, J. K., and Samarasekera, S., Kinematics of the tarsal joints via 3D MR imaging, *Visualization in Biomedical Computing 1994*, vol. 2359, Robb, R. A., Ed., SPIE, Bellingham, WA, 1994, 672.
75. Spoor C. W. and Veldpaus, F. E., Rigid body motion calculated from spatial co-ordinates of markers, *J. Biomech.*, 13, 391, 1980.
76. Toennies, K. D., Udupa, J. K., Herman, G. T., Wornom, I. L., and Buchman, S. R., Registration of three-dimensional objects and surfaces, *IEEE Comp. Graph. Appl.*, 10, 52, 1990.
77. Rhoad, R. C., Williams, G. R., Kneeland, J. B., Samarasekera, S., Udupa, J. K., and Iannotti, J. P., MRI & 3DVIEWNIX: A non-invasive method for studying shoulder kinematics, *Orthoped. Trans.,* 20, 199, 1996–7.
78. Belsole, R. J., Hilbelink, D. R., Llewellyn, J. A., Dale, M., and Ogden, J. A., Carpal orientation from computed reference axes, *J. Hand Surg.*, 16A, 82, 1991.
79. Trinkhaus, E., *A Functional Analysis of the Neanderthal Foot*. Ph.D dissertation, Univcrsity of Pennsylvania, 1975.
80. Williams, P. L., Ed., *Gray's Anatomy*, 38th ed., Churchill Livingstone, New York, 1995, 725.
81. Elftman, H., The transverse tarsal joint and its control, *Clin. Orthoped.*, 16, 41, 1960.
82. MacConnaill, M. A. and Basmajian, J. V., *Muscles and Movements*, 2nd ed., Robert E. Krieger, Huntington, NY, 1977, chapter 3.
83. Swanson, S. A. V., Articular cartilage, *The Mechanical Properties of Biological Materials*, Vincent, J. V. F. and Currey, J. D., Eds., Society for Experimental Biology Symposium XXXIV, 1980, 377.
84. Driscoll, H. L., Christensen, J. C., and Tencer, A. F., Contact characteristics of the ankle joint. Part 1. The normal joint, *J. Am. Podiatric Med. Assoc.*, 84, 491, 1994.
85. Udupa, J. K., Hirsch, B. E., Samarasekera, S., and Goncalves, R. J., Joint kinematics via three-dimensional MR imaging, *Visualization in Biomedical Computing 1992*, vol. 1808, Robb, R. A., Ed., SPIE, Bellingham, WA, 1992, 664.
86. Udupa, J. K., Roberts, D., and Christiansen, E., Quantified three-dimensional imaging techniques for biomechanical analysis of skeletal joints, *Proceedings of the Eighth Annual Conference of the IEEE/Engineering in Medicine and Biology Society*, 1986, 1079.
87. Downey, M. S., Tarsal coalitions, *Comprehensive Textbook of Foot Surgery*, 2nd ed., vol. 1, McGlamry, E. D., Banks, A. S., and Downey, M. S., Eds., Williams & Wilkins, Baltimore, 1992, 898.
88. Stindel, E., Udupa, J. K., Hirsch, B. E., and Odhner, D., An in vivo analysis of the kinematics of the peritalar joint complex based on MR imaging, MIPG Technical Report No. 251, 1999.
89. Kobayashi, M., Berger, R. A., Nagy, L., Linscheid, R. L., Uchiyama, S., Ritt, M., and An, K.-N., Normal kinematics of carpal bones: A three-dimensional analysis of carpal bone motion relative to the radius, *J. Biomech*, 30, 787, 1997.
90. Falcão, A. X. and Udupa, J. K., Segmentation of 3D objects using live wire, *SPIE Proc.,* 3034, 228, 1997.
91. Siegler, S., Lapointe, S., Nobilini, R., and Berman, A. T., A six-degrees-of-freedom instrumented linkage for measuring the flexibility characteristics of the ankle joint complex, *J. Biomech.*, 29, 943, 1996.

Index

0-8493-3179-X/00/$0.00+$.50